Juvenile Idiopathic Arthritis: Diagnosis and Treatment

Juvenile Idiopathic Arthritis: Diagnosis and Treatment

Editor: Nicholas Greyson

AMERICAN
MEDICAL PUBLISHERS
www.americanmedicalpublishers.com

AMERICAN
MEDICAL PUBLISHERS
www.americanmedicalpublishers.com

Cataloging-in-Publication Data

Juvenile idiopathic arthritis : diagnosis and treatment / edited by Nicholas Greyson.
p. cm.
Includes bibliographical references and index.
ISBN 978-1-63927-396-6
1. Rheumatoid arthritis in children. 2. Rheumatism in children. 3. Arthritis--Age factors. I. Greyson, Nicholas.
RJ482.A77 J88 2022
618.722 7--dc23

American Medical Publishers,
41 Flatbush Avenue,
1st Floor, New York,
NY 11217, USA

ISBN 978-1-63927-396-6 (Hardback)

Contents

Preface

In my initial years as a student, I used to run to the library at every possible instance to grab a book and learn something new. Books were my primary source of knowledge and I would not have come such a long way without all that I learnt from them. Thus, when I was approached to edit this book; I became understandably nostalgic. It was an absolute honor to be considered worthy of guiding the current generation as well as those to come. I put all my knowledge and hard work into making this book most beneficial for its readers.

Juvenile idiopathic arthritis (JIA) is a form of arthritis which occurs in children and adolescents. It is a noninfective, autoimmune, inflammatory disease of the joints, commonly occurring in children between the ages of 1 and 6. JIA often presents nonspecific symptoms initially such as reduced physical activity, lethargy and poor appetite. Its first noticeable manifestation may be limping. Children may become quite ill with flu-like symptoms. Persistent swelling around the knee, wrist, ankle and the joints of the hands and feet is a clinical manifestation of the condition. The diagnosis of JIA is difficult to establish as the symptoms can indicate other causes. Therefore, often times, a combination of blood tests, X-rays, analysis of the fluid from the joint and clinical presentation are done for making a correct diagnosis. The goal of therapy in JIA is to enable the child to regain a normal level of physical and social activity. This is done with physical therapy, social support and pain management strategies. Children may also be treated with intra-articular corticosteroid injections and nonsteroidal anti-inflammatory drugs. This book elucidates the causes, symptoms and pathophysiology of juvenile idiopathic arthritis in a comprehensive manner. It strives to provide a fair idea about the modern practices in the management of JIA. A number of latest researches have been included to keep the readers up-to-date with the global concepts in this medical condition.

I wish to thank my publisher for supporting me at every step. I would also like to thank all the authors who have contributed their researches in this book. I hope this book will be a valuable contribution to the progress of the field.

Editor

1

Synovial membrane protein expression differs between juvenile idiopathic arthritis subtypes in early disease

Sorcha Finnegan[1], Joanne Robson[2], Caitriona Scaife[3], Catherine McAllister[4], Stephen R Pennington[3], David S Gibson[1,5*] and Madeleine E Rooney[1,4]

Abstract

Introduction: Juvenile idiopathic arthritis (JIA) is the most common rheumatological disease of childhood with a prevalence of around 1 in 1,000. Without appropriate treatment it can have devastating consequences including permanent disability from joint destruction and growth deformities. Disease aetiology remains unknown. Investigation of disease pathology at the level of the synovial membrane is required if we want to begin to understand the disease at the molecular and biochemical level. The synovial membrane proteome from early disease-stage, treatment naive JIA patients was compared between polyarticular and oligoarticular subgroups.

Methods: Protein was extracted from 15 newly diagnosed, treatment naive JIA synovial membrane biopsies and separated by two dimensional fluorescent difference in-gel electrophoresis. Proteins displaying a two-fold or greater change in expression levels between the two subgroups were identified by matrix assisted laser desorption ionization-time of flight mass spectrometry with expression further verified by Western blotting and immunohistochemistry.

Results: Analysis of variance analysis ($P \leq 0.05$) revealed 25 protein spots with a two-fold or greater difference in expression levels between polyarticular and oligoarticular patients. Hierarchical cluster analysis with Pearson ranked correlation revealed two distinctive clusters of proteins. Some of the proteins that were differentially expressed included: integrin alpha 2b ($P = 0.04$); fibrinogen D fragment ($P = 0.005$); collagen type VI ($P = 0.03$); fibrinogen gamma chain ($P = 0.05$) and peroxiredoxin 2 ($P = 0.02$). The identified proteins are involved in a number of different processes including platelet activation and the coagulation system.

Conclusions: The data indicate distinct synovial membrane proteome profiles between JIA subgroups at an early stage in the disease process. The identified proteins also provide insight into differentially perturbed pathways which could influence pathological events at the joint level.

Introduction

Juvenile idiopathic arthritis (JIA) consists of a heterogeneous group of diseases which persist for more than six weeks and commence before the age of 16. It is the most common rheumatological disease of childhood, with a prevalence of approximately 1/1,000 [1]. The cause of JIA remains unknown; however, environmental and genetic factors play a role in its pathogenesis and the heterogeneity of the disease would suggest multiple factors are responsible [2]. Adverse outcomes include chronic pain and stiffness, and joint damage and disability as a result of chronic joint inflammation. Despite improved prognoses for JIA patients in recent years, around half of patients will continue to have active joint disease into adulthood [3].

The International League of Associations for Rheumatology (ILAR) classification system divides JIA into seven clinical subgroups [4,5]. The largest subgroup - oligoarticular JIA - accounts for approximately 65% of all cases and refers to children with four or fewer joints involved within six months of diagnosis. Oligoarticular disease is further defined as persistent when it remains confined to

* Correspondence: d.gibson@ulster.ac.uk
[1]Arthritis Research Group, Queen's University Belfast, Centre for Infection and Immunity, Health Sciences Building, 97 Lisburn Road, Belfast BT9 7BL, UK
[5]Northern Ireland Centre for Stratified Medicine, C-TRIC Building, Altnagelvin Hospital campus, Glenshane Road, Londonderry BT47 6SB, UK
Full list of author information is available at the end of the article

four or fewer joints throughout the course of the disease. Oligoarticular JIA is more prevalent in females, with a peak age of onset of one to three years [6]. Polyarticular JIA is defined by the involvement of more than four joints within six months of diagnosis, it accounts for around 10 to 15% of all JIA cases [7].

Very few studies examine the synovial membrane from JIA patients and, of those available, most involved patients with established disease and on disease modifying treatment [8-11]. Our previous immunohistochemical study demonstrated significant differences in the inflammatory infiltrates and levels of vascularisation in the different JIA subgroups. It is still unclear, however, why these changes take place in JIA and why they differ between subgroups. Proteomics offers an unsupervised means to investigate the disease process within the affected tissue.

This study was designed to investigate how the predominant protein expression profile within synovial membrane varies between persistent oligoarticular and polyarticular JIA across a group of newly diagnosed, treatment-naïve patients. We hypothesize that subtype-specific protein expression patterns exist in the early stages of disease. Comparison of the synovial proteome between polyarticular and oligoarticular JIA patients could provide a much needed insight into the pathology underlying these two distinct subtypes.

Materials and methods

Patients

Children with newly diagnosed JIA of less than two years duration were consecutively recruited following informed consent. Medical Ethics Committee approval was obtained for this study at Green Park Healthcare Trust and patient assent and parent informed consent was given (ORECNI 408/03). Recruitment criteria included: involvement of one knee joint that required intra-articular steroid injection, and the patient being steroid and disease-modifying antirheumatic drug (DMARD) naive. Children were classified according to the ILAR criteria at the time of recruitment. Children were then reclassified after two years of follow-up. Detailed clinical examination, biochemical and immunological data, and imaging assessments were obtained. Subgroups were compared with each other as it was not ethically possible to obtain synovial membrane biopsies from healthy paediatric controls.

Tissue collection

Synovial membrane samples were obtained by blind needle biopsy using ultrasound guidance as described previously [12]. Biopsies were obtained prior to the instillation of steroids. Tissue was wrapped in saline soaked gauze, immersed in saline and placed in sterile containers on ice. Biopsies were snap frozen in liquid nitrogen and stored at −80°C.

Sample preparation

Protein was extracted from synovial membrane biopsies in lysis buffer (8.4 M urea, 2.4 M thiourea, 4% 3-[(3-cholamidopropyl)dimethylammonio]-1-propanesulfonate, 2 mM dithiothreitol (DTT), 1% ampholytes). Samples were centrifuged at 12,000 rpm for 15 minutes and the supernatant collected. Protein was precipitated in ice cold acetone at −20°C overnight, pelleted by centrifugation and the pellet air dried to remove residual acetone. The protein pellet was resuspended in difference in-gel electrophoresis (DIGE) lysis buffer (30 mM Tris-Cl, 7 M urea, 2 M thiourea, 4% CHAPS, pH 8.5) and protein concentration was determined using a modified Bradford assay.

Difference in-gel electrophoresis (DIGE)

DIGE was performed as previously described [13] with the exception that isoelectric focusing (IEF) and 2D PAGE were performed on 11 cm Immobiline DryStrip pH 4 to 7 linear. Each gel contained one synovium sample from a polyarticular patient and one synovium sample from an oligoarticular patient (each labelled with either Cy3 or Cy5 dyes). Cy3 and Cy5 dyes were swapped randomly between samples to prevent dye bias. Each gel also contained the internal standard which is a pooled mixture of every patient sample (labelled with Cy2). Voltage and times were adjusted accordingly. Two preparative gels loaded with 300 μg of protein were Coomassie stained and spots excised for identification by mass spectrometry.

Image analysis

DIGE gels were scanned using a Typhoon 9410 imager (GE Healthcare, Bucks, UK). Gel images were analysed using Progenesis Samespots software version 2.0 build 2644.18003 (Nonlinear Dynamics Ltd., Newcastle upon Tyne, UK) as previously described [14]. PermutMatrix [15] was subsequently used to cluster and visualise the spot data as previously described [14].

Tryptic digestion of protein spots and MALDI target spotting

Tryptic digestion of protein bands was performed using a ProGest robot (Genomic Solutions, Holliston, MA, USA) programmed with the long trypsin digestion method. A sterile pipette tip, cut to increase the bore width (approximately 2.0 mm), was used for spot excision. Gel plugs were then transferred to a 96-well plate. This plate is designed with microscopic holes at the bottom of the wells which allows for positive displacement of liquids during reagent changes on the robot. Gel pieces were first equilibrated in 50 μl of 50 mM ammonium bicarbonate and proteins were reductively alkylated with 10 mM DTT and

100 mM iodacetamide followed by de-staining of the protein bands and desiccation of the gel plugs with acetonitrile. Gel plugs were rehydrated with 50 mM ammonium bicarbonate containing 5% trypsin and the proteins were digested for 12 hours at 37°C. Resulting peptides were extracted from the gel plugs with 2 × 25 µl washes of 50% acetonitrile, 0.1% TFA. Peptide extracts were freeze dried and then re-suspended in 10 µl of 0.1% formic acid. A saturated solution of α-cyano-4-hydroxycinnamic acid was prepared in 50% acetonitrile, 0.1%TFA, 10 mM ammonium acetate. For each sample, 1 µl of matrix solution was spotted on the matrix assisted laser desorption ionisation (MALDI) target immediately followed by 1 µl of sample into the matrix spot and the sample/matrix droplet allowed to slowly air dry.

MALDI TOF-TOF analyses, database searching and protein identification

Matrix assisted laser desorption ionisation-tandem time of flight (MALDI TOF-TOF) analyses was performed on a 4800 mass spectrometer (AB Sciex UK Limited, Cheshire, UK) using the following protocol: TOF-MS analyses was first performed on all of the dried target spots using automated data acquisition and processing under the control of Applied Biosystems 4000 series Explorer software (version 3.5) using reflector mode, a mass range of 700 to 4,000 m/z, 1,000 total laser shots per spectrum and a laser intensity of 3,300 V. Following acquisition the TOF-MS spectra were noise corrected, peak de-isotoped and internally calibrated using the trypsin autolysis peaks 842.500 and 2,211.100 m/z. The eight most abundant precursor ions from each spectra were then selected by the software for fragmentation and MS-MS analyses using a 1 kV collision ion dissociation (CID) fragmentation method collecting 4,000 laser shots per spectra with a laser intensity of 3,800 over the mass range.

Peak lists of ion masses were generated by GPS Explorer software version 3.6 (Applied Biosystems) from the calibrated and de-isotoped MS and MS-MS spectra for each sample. Combined lists of MS and MS-MS data were used for database searching with MASCOT version 2.2 (Matrix Science), against all entries in the National Center for Biotechnology Information (NCBI) database. Database search parameters used were the following: digestion enzyme trypsin, single missed cleavage allowed, variable modifications of carboxymethyl cysteine and oxidised methionine, precursor mass tolerance of 50 ppm and fragment ion tolerance of 0.2 Da. HTML pages of MASCOT output were generated for each sample.

The Mowse scoring algorithm was used to determine the significance of the identity. Additional criteria were used to ensure correct protein identifications. These included ensuring the matched peptides were the most abundant peaks in the mass spectrum, the theoretical isoelectric point and molecular weight of the identified protein correlated with the spot's position on the 2D gel, and sequence coverage was high.

Immunohistochemistry

Biopsies were snap frozen in liquid nitrogen for sectioning and stored at −80°C. A total of 7 µm thick frozen sections were cut using a Leica CM 1900 cryostat (Leica Microsystems Nussloch GmbH, Germany) and allowed to air-dry at room temperature for 30 minutes. Primary antibodies used were monoclonal anti-integrin alpha 2b antibody (ITA2B) (Abcam, Cambridge, UK), monoclonal anti-peroxiredoxin 2 (PRDX2) (Sigma, Dorset, UK) and polyclonal anti-myosin regulatory light chain 2 (MYL2) (Sigma, Dorset, UK). Immunostaining was performed using a standard protocol and staining was visualized using the diaminobenzidine (DAB) method [16]. Sections were counterstained with haematoxylin.

Western blotting

Western immunoblot analysis was performed using a standard protocol using the above antibodies against ITA2B, PRDX2 and MYL2.

Results

Patient demographics and clinical features

There were 12 females and 3 males included in the study. The clinical and laboratory data of patients are shown in Table 1.

General laboratory characteristics of JIA patients

There was no significant difference in the age at disease onset between the two groups. VAS pain scores (parent) were significantly higher in the polyarticular as were ESR and CRP levels (Table 1).

2D DIGE analysis

We compared the synovial membrane proteome from seven persistent oligoarticular JIA patients with eight polyarticular JIA patients using 2D DIGE. 2D DIGE analysis revealed an average of 460 spots per pH 4 to 7, 11 cm gel which were matched across all gels (Figure 1). ANOVA revealed 26 spots that were differentially expressed (two-fold or more change in expression levels) between polyarticular and oligoarticular patients ($P \leq 0.05$).

Hierarchical cluster analysis (HCA)

HCA was used to examine the expression patterns of the 26 differentially expressed proteins across the study cohort with results depicted in heat map form (Figure 2). Depicted on the horizontal axis is the patient number and on the vertical axis is the spot number/

Table 1 Demographic and clinical characteristics at the time of biopsy

ILAR subtype	JIA patient study ID	M/F	Disease duration (months)	No. of swollen joints	VAS* pain (parent)	VAS* global physician	WCC*	Hb*	ESR*	CRP* (mg/l)	PC*	ANA*	RF (+/–)
Oligoarticular (n = 7)	1	F	4	1	5	1.9	7.5	11	8	0	407	0	-
	2	M	4	1	0	0.8	12	11	11	0	415	0	-
	3	F	6	3	3.6	2.9	12.1	11	10	5.7	453	0	-
	4	F	10	2	0.3	1.9	6.9	10.7	4	4	315	0	-
	5	F	5	3	7.5	3	12.8	10.6	37	26	407	80	-
	6	M	20	1	1.4	1.9	5.6	14.1	5	0	249	0	-
	7	F	4	3	4.3	1.8	9.1	8.9	62	66.5	460	0	-
	Mean values		**7.6**	**2**	**3.2**	**2**	**9.4**	**11**	**19.6**	**14.6**	**386.6**	**11.4**	
Polyarticular (n = 8)	8	F	2	24	8.7	7.5	12.9	8.3	38	27.5	570	160	-
	9	F	2	9	8.3	3.3	13.9	10.4	22	36.1	232	0	-
	10	F	2	24	4.7	5.7	12.2	10.5	30	67.3	601	0	-
	11	F	2	6	9	4.8	9.9	11.1	26	32.1	446	80	-
	12	F	1	2	7.1	1.5	11.2	10.4	96	47.4	522	ND	-
	13	F	4	15	9.8	3.6	11.8	7.2	110	72	578	0	-
	14	M	10	4	3.3	5.3	10.27	11	20	5.4	314	40	+
	15	F	5	25	6.5	7.4	9.3	8.4	138	181	401	80	+
	Mean values		**3.5**	**13.6**	**7.2**	**4.9**	**11.4**	**9.7**	**60**	**58.6**	**458**	**51.4**	
	t-test p value		**ns**	**ns**	**0.004**	**0.002**	**0.056**	**0.049**	**0.029**	**0.03**	**0.12**	**-**	**-**

ANA, anti-nuclear antibodies; CRP, C-reactive protein; ESR, erythrocyte sedimentation rate; Hb, haemoglobin; ns, not statistically significant at $P \geq 0.05$; PC, platelet count;; RF, rheumatoid factor; *VAS, visual analogue scale; WCC, white cell count.

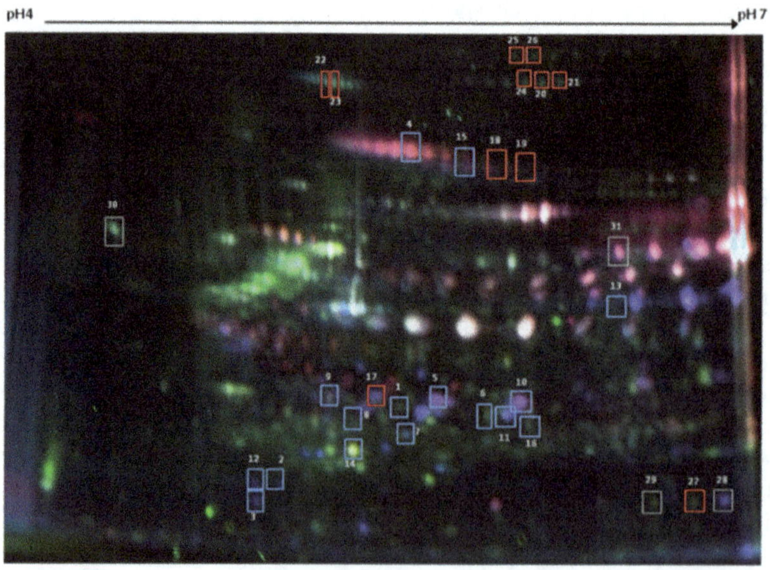

Figure 1 A representative 2D DIGE gel image of JIA synovial membrane proteins. Proteins labeled using fluorescent dyes Cy3 (green) and Cy5 (red). Protein samples were separated on an 11 cm pH4 to 7 IPG strip and on a 12.5% homogenous SDS-PAGE gel. Protein spots analysed by mass spectrometry are highlighted by spot outlines. Spot numbers correspond with those listed in Table 2, Additional file 1: Table S1 and Figure 2. Proteins overexpressed in oligoarticular patients are indicated by red spot outlines; proteins overexpressed in polyarticular are indicated by blue spot outlines. DIGE, difference in-gel electrophoresis; JIA, juvenile idiopathic arthritis.

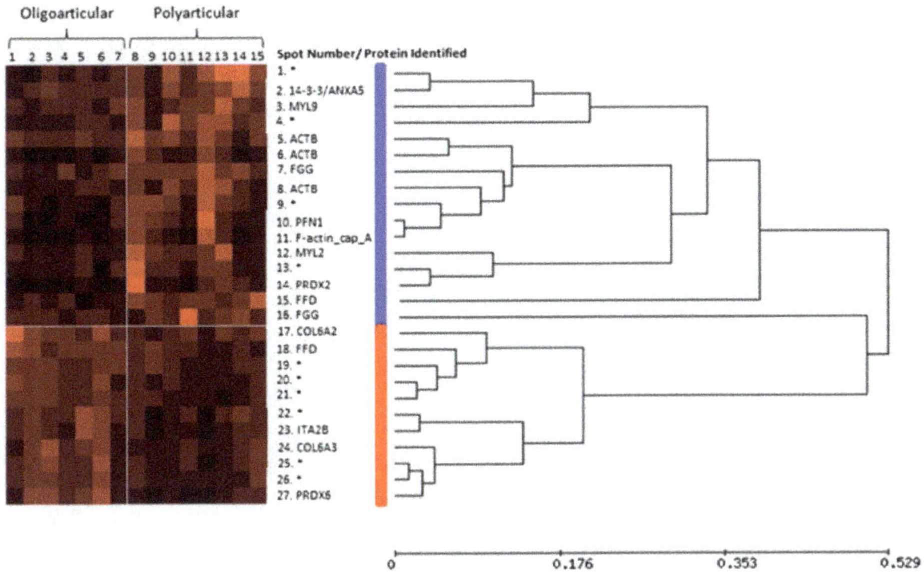

Figure 2 Hierarchical cluster analysis of proteins expressed with statistically significant differences between patient subgroups. The inter-individual and inter-group variation in 19 selected proteins is represented in the form of a heatmap. The protein expression data were reordered by hierarchical cluster analysis (HCA) using Pearson centred correlation (unweighted pair group method with arithmetic mean (UPGMA)), which revealed specific expression patterns. Two main clusters of proteins are highlighted by the coloured bars (blue, red). Each patient sample is represented by a single numbered column (oligarticular 1 to 7 and polyarticular 9 to 15). Spot numbers and protein identifications (UniProt code) are labelled on the vertical axis; unidentified protein spots are indicated by an asterix (*). The relative amount of a protein is denoted by colour intensity within a spectrum of black to red, red being the highest amount.

protein ID. Pearson ranked correlation revealed two distinct clusters of proteins. Cluster 1 contains proteins that were overexpressed in the polyarticular patients, whereas proteins in cluster 2 are overexpressed in the oligoarticular subgroup. It seemed conceivable that these two distinct clusters could be used in combination to differentiate these two disease subgroups.

MALDI-TOF MS protein identification

Differentially expressed proteins were identified by MALDI MS (Table 2). Peptide ion validation data is available as an additional file (Additional file 1: Table S1). Proteins that were overexpressed in the polyarticular group included: chain A of profilin-beta-actin ($P = 0.04$); alpha-1 subunit of F-actin capping protein ($P = 0.03$); beta actin, ($P = 0.04$); beta actin ($P = 0.02$); myosin regulatory light chain 2 (MYL2) isoform B ($P = 0.02$); myosin regulatory light chain 9 (MYL9), isoform a ($P = 0.04$); beta actin variant ($P = 0.005$); peroxiredoxin 2 (PRDX2), isoform a ($P = 0.02$); mixture of protein kinase C inhibitor protein 1 (KCIP-1) and annexin A5 ($P = 0.003$); fibrinogen gamma chain ($P = 0.004$ and $P = 0.05$).

Proteins overexpressed in the oligoarticular group included: collagen type VI, alpha 2 ($P = 0.03$); integrin alpha 2b (ITA2B) ($P = 0.04$); chain C of fibrinogen fragment D ($P = 0.005$); Chain C, crystal structure of fibrinogen fragment D ($P = 0.0002$). Figure 3 shows representative differentially expressed proteins along with a 3D image of the relative quantities of proteins generated using Samespots software (Nonlinear Dynamics Ltd., Newcastle upon Tyne, UK).

The levels of proteins 27 to 31 (listed in Table 2) did not differ between oligoarticular and polyarticular patient groups. There were a number of proteins that could not be identified due to their low abundance in the gel.

Confirmation of protein localisation and expression

Figure 4 shows representative images of MYL2, PRDX2 and ITA2B immunostaining in polyarticular and oligoarticular synovial membrane: (A) MYL2 staining is limited to a small number of discrete cells within the sublining layer in the oligoarticular tissue (arrows), its expression in the polyarticular tissue (B) is more intense. PRDX2 staining is sparse in the oligoarticular tissue (arrows) (C) with more intense staining in the polyarticular tissue (D). ITA2B staining is localised to blood vessels in oligoarticular tissue (E), some ITA2B staining was also observed in the polyarticular tissue (F) around blood vessels (arrows). Figure 5 depicts the synovial membrane expression levels for the aforementioned proteins across a representative subset of the study patients.

Discussion

This is the first study to identify synovial membrane protein expression patterns that discriminate clinical subgroups in early treatment of naive JIA. By understanding the early pathological changes taking place at the disease

Table 2 Mass spectrometry and DIGE quantification data of synovial membrane proteins

Spot number	Protein	Gene symbol	Accession #	Mowse score	% Sequence coverage	Calculatedpl value	Nominal mass (Mr)	Number matched peptides	Normalised volume (Oligo)	Normalised volume (Poly)	ANOVA *P*-value
1	No ID	-	-	-	-	-	-	-	0.73	3.02	0.001
2	Protein kinase C inhibitor protein 1	*KCIP-1*	gi|114629705	88	40	4.78	24,166	14	1.07	2.1	0.03
	Annexin	*A5 ANXA5*	gi|149698420	79	33	4.98	35,977	10	-	-	-
3	Myosin regulatory l ight chain 9	*MYL9*	gi|29568111	52	29	4.8	19,814	8	0.92	2.02	0.04
4	No ID	-	-	-	-	-	-	-	0.79	2.35	0.006
5	Beta Actin	*ACTB*	gi|15277503	76	21	5.55	40,194	9	1.14	2.28	0.04
6	Beta Actin	*ACTB*	gi|15277503	176	37	5.55	40,194	17	0.35	1.24	0.02
7	Fibrinogen gamma chain	*FGG*	gi|930064	94	50	6.49	24,109	11	0.88	2.23	0.004
8	Beta actin variant	*ACTB*	gi|62897625	451	53	5.37	41,738	23	0.56	1.94	0.005
9	No ID	-	-	-	-	-	-	-	0.64	2.04	0.02
10	Chain A, profi l in-beta-actin	*PFN1*	gi|157111829	106/130	44	5.29	41,616	21	0.39	1.76	0.04
11	F-actin capping protein alpha-1	*CAPZA1*	gi|5453597	196	55	5.45	32,902	17	0.3	1.38	0.03
12	Myosin regulatory l ight chain 2	*MYL2*	gi|222144328	86	55	4.26	17,745	10	0.66	2.03	0.02
13	No ID	-	-	-	-	-	-	-	0.62	1.72	0.05
14	Peroxiredoxin	*2 PRDX2*	gi|4758638	348	57	6	25,019	18	0.3	1.73	0.02
15	Chain C, fibrinogen fragment D	*FFD*	gi|2781209	89	42	5.87	36,157	12	2.08	0.58	0.0002
16	Fibrinogen gamma chain	*FGG*	gi|930064	71	44	6.49	24,109	7	0.9	2.14	0.05
17	Collagen, type VI, alpha 2	*COL6A2*	gi|41350923	81	18	5.85	182,860	18	2.77	1.09	0.03
18	Chain C, fibrinogen fragment	*D FFD*	gi|24987625	102	44	5.86	35,155	14	2.1	0.96	0.005
19	No ID	-	-	-	-	-	-	-	1.6	0.9	0.008
20	No ID	-	-	-	-	-	-	-	1.6	0.8	0.02
21	No ID	-	-	-	-	-	-	-	1.4	0.7	0.006
22	No ID	-	-	-	-	-	-	-			
23	Integrin, alpha 2b	*ITGA2B*	gi|119571979	95	15	5.41	103,127	16	1.87	0.64	0.04
24	Alpha 3 type VI collagen	*COL6A3*	gi|62088852	119	17	8.73	182,860	27	1.78	0.78	0.05
25	No ID	-	-	-	-	-	-	-	1.72	0.74	0.04
26	No ID	-	-	-	-	-	-	-	1.56	0.72	0.02
27	Peroxiredoxin 6	*PRDX6*	gi|4758638	348	57	6	25,019	18	-	-	-

Table 2 Mass spectrometry and DIGE quantification data of synovial membrane proteins *(Continued)*

28	Triosephosphate isomerase 1	*TPI1*	gi|17389815	111	53	6.45	26,625	15	-	-	-
29	Albumin, isoform CRA_j	*ALB*	gi|119626073	59	23	6.4	26,233	7	-	-	-
30	Calreticul in precursor variant	*CRT*	gi|62897681	236	29	4.3	46,890	19	-	-	-
31	Fibrinogen, beta chain	*FGB*	gi|70906435	93	34	8.54	55,892	21	-	-	-

Spot trypsin digests were identified using matrix assisted laser desorption ionization (MALDI-TOF/TOF), correlated to compiled peptide data (Matrix Science). *P*-values highlight inter-subgroup comparisons which reached statistical significance ($P < 0.05$) by ANOVA. Full mass spectra peak lists for each identified protein are provided in Additional file 1: Table S1.

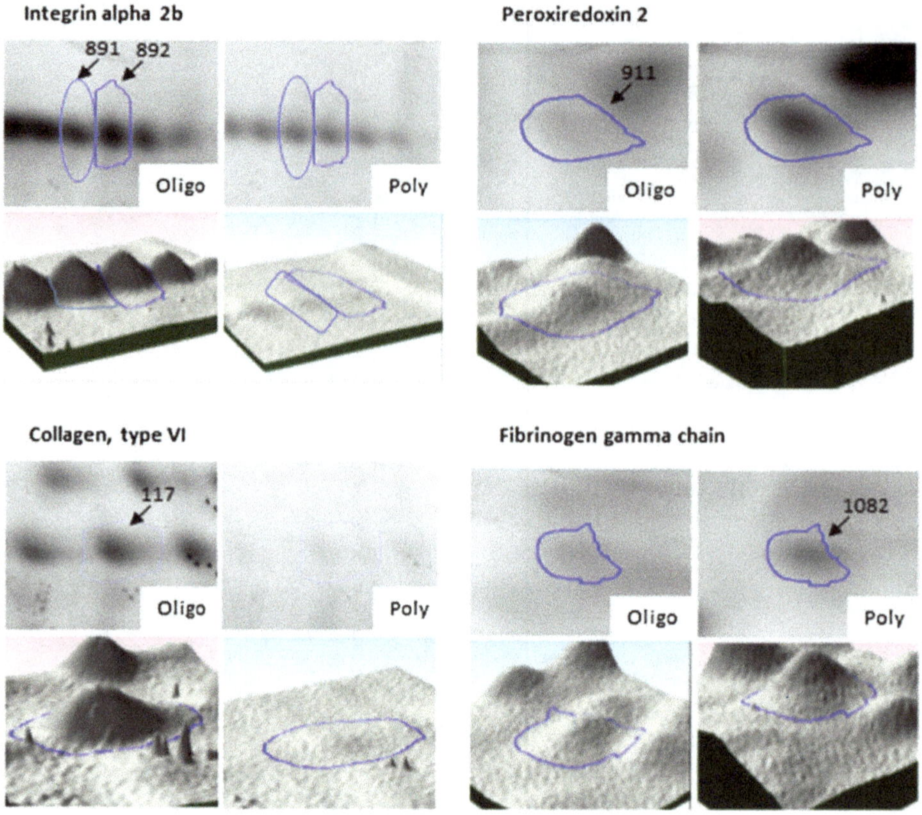

Figure 3 DIGE image analysis of differentially expressed synovial membrane proteins. Spots 22, 23 (integrin alpha 2b) and 24 (collagen) were overexpressed in the oligoarticular group. Spots 14 (peroxiredoxin 2) and 16 (fibrinogen gamma chain) were overexpressed in the polyarticular group. JIA, juvenile idiopathic arthritis.

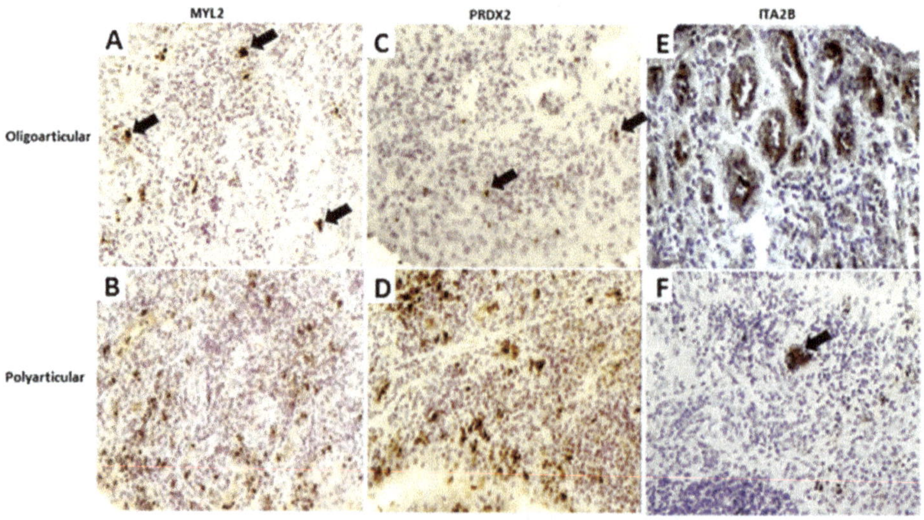

Figure 4 Immunohistochemical staining of differentially expressed synovial membrane proteins. A and **B** Distribution of myosin regulatory light chain 2 (MYL2), **C** and **D** peroxiredoxin 2 (PRDX2), **E** and **F** integrin alpha 2b (ITA2B) in oligoarticular and polyarticular synovial membrane. Sections were counterstained with haematoxylin. Arrows indicate areas of positive staining.

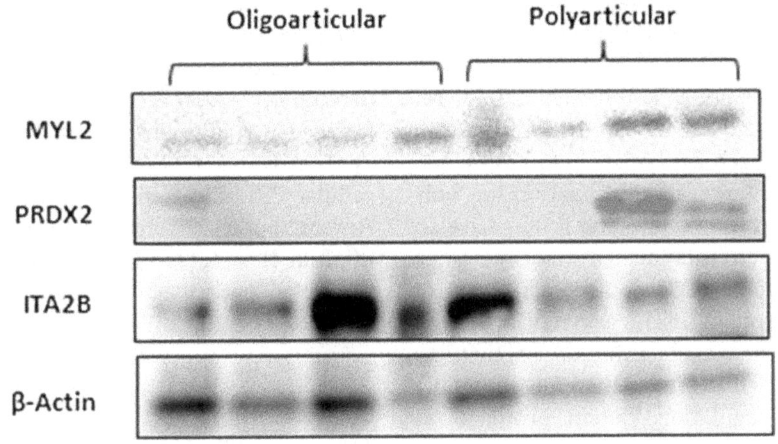

Figure 5 Validation of protein expression changes by Western immunoblot probing for MYL2, PRDX2 and ITA2B. Each lane represents an individual patient synovial membrane protein sample. β-actin was used as a loading control. ITA2B, integrin alpha 2b; MYL2, myosin regulatory light chain 2; PRDX2, peroxiredoxin 2.

site we can begin to elucidate the disease process. There have been a number of proteomic investigations of synovial tissue in adult inflammatory disease [17-19] but not in children. To date, proteomic studies of JIA have focused on synovial fluid and plasma [13,14,20-22], due to the fact that synovial membrane is extremely difficult to acquire. The synovial membrane has an advantage over synovial fluid in that it is the actual site of pathology in JIA. It is also important to note that all synovial membranes used in this study were from treatment-naive early disease-stage patients (average disease duration at time of biopsy was 5.4 months). For the purpose of this study the differences in two JIA subgroups were noted. Although control tissue from healthy subjects would have been useful, such tissue is not obtainable for ethical reasons.

A number of proteins identified in this study were part of a 'charge train' on the 2D gels, indicating post translational modification (PTM). A recently published study by our group indicates that protein modification acts as a surrogate marker of inflammation spread in JIA [23]. Glycosylation of VDBP- Vitamin D-binding protein, which confers macrophage activation activity, was decreased in patients at risk of disease spread. Subtype-specific protein isoforms uncovered within the current study should also be carefully investigated for post translational modifications. In early disease discrete protein isoforms may play a role in the different pathologies observed between oligoarticular and polyarticular synovium. In an earlier study we reported histological features which distinguish these JIA subgroups, including levels of vascularisation and white blood cell infiltration [16]. The likely pathological impact of synovial protein isoforms identified in the current study are subsequently discussed, along with their potential as therapeutic targets.

ITA2B was overexpressed in the oligoarticular group as part of a 'charge train' of spots (Figure 3), strongly suggesting a process of serial post translational modifications. ITA2B contains five N-linked glycosylation points [24]. Furthermore, intense ITA2B immunostaining was observed around blood vessels in the oligoarticular group, relative to polyarticular tissue. ITA2B is a major integrin found on platelet plasma membranes, assisting platelet activation and adhesion and thrombus formation at sites of vascular injury [25]. A previous study reported similar ITA2B expression patterns in rheumatoid arthritis (RA) synovial membrane, restricted to vascular endothelial cells [26]. ITA2B could act as a key target in controlling inflammation, as platelets can elicit cytokine responses from synovial fibroblasts via interleukin-1 in RA patients. The apparent increase in ITA2B observed in oligoarticular patients may result from leaky and tortuous vessels observed in the development of synovitis.

Fibrinogen fragment D was also expressed at higher levels in the oligoarticular group as part of a 'charge train'. The D-dimer of fibrin is a degradation product (FDP) found in the blood following fibrinolysis of a blood clot [27]. Under various inflammatory conditions, including RA, fibrin degradation product levels are increased [28,29], suggesting an imbalance in the coagulation/fibrinolysis system. D-dimers have also been shown to trigger release of IL-1β, IL-6 in peripheral blood monocytes [30]. Fibrinogen is one of several protein targets for citrullination in RA [31] and citrullinated fibrinogen D fragments have been detected in synovial exosomes from patients with RA and osteoarthritis (OA).

In contrast, fibrinogen beta and gamma chains were overexpressed in the polyarticular group. Fibrinogen gamma chains are involved in fibrin polymerization and cross-linking, interacting with platelets and mediating thrombin binding to fibrin [32]. Rosenkranz *et al.* also observed that fibrinogen gamma chain levels were increased in systemic JIA synovial fluid relative to oligoarticular patients [21]. Fibrinogen beta chain is also increased in patients with recurrent joint inflammation [22]. A recent study also demonstrated strong reactivity of JIA sera to anti-citrullinated fibrinogen antibodies [33]. Fibrinogen has been shown to be the target of citrullination not only in JIA but also in adult RA [34], suggesting it may have an important role to play in autoimmunity.

During a normal inflammatory response, activation of coagulation and deposition of fibrin are crucial events that help regulate and contain inflammatory activity to the site of injury or infection. It is, therefore, possible that altered levels of coagulation system proteins reported in polyarticular tissue may indirectly assist in the spread of inflammation to multiple joints, a key characteristic of these patients. It would be intriguing to target these fragments in an animal model of arthritis to determine their function in the synovium.

The collagens are a superfamily of extracellular matrix proteins that play a crucial role in maintaining tissue integrity. Type VI collagen is a prominent constituent of the synovial extracellular matrix [35]. A study by Alexopoulos *et al.* suggests that type VI collagen has an important role in the regulation of normal synovial joint physiology and pericellular matrix displayed significantly reduced mechanical properties in mice lacking type IV collagen. Thus, as the mice aged, accelerated development of joint degeneration, as well as a number of other musculoskeletal abnormalities, was noted [36]. Collagen type VI was found at higher levels in the oligoarticular subgroup. Disease pathology is much less severe in this group, and it is possible that this is due to increased tissue integrity and a more stable extracellular and pericellular matrix in the synovial membrane.

A number of actin family proteins were overexpressed in the polyarticular group. Citrullinated F-actin capping protein alpha-1 subunit autoantigens have been identified in RA synovium [19]. It is thought that one of the pathogenic mechanisms taking place in RA is the promotion of actin polymerization and rearrangement of the actin cytoskeleton. Indeed, a previous study found a number of deregulated genes in synovial fibroblasts known to be involved in actin filament and cytoskeleton organisation [37]. Reorganisation of the actin cytoskeleton and the associated deregulation of ECM adhesion are known to be an intrinsic property of arthritic synovial fibroblasts. The presence of higher levels of these cytoskeletal proteins in the polyarticular group could reflect the severe disease pathology in this group and is consistent with much higher levels of synovial hyperplasia and cytoskeletal reorganisation.

PRDX2 was found at higher levels in the polyarticular group. Peroxiredoxin is involved in redox regulation. Peroxiredoxins constitute a ubiquitous family of antioxidant enzymes that are involved in the control of cytokine-induced peroxide levels [38]. Lymphocytes from RA patients have been shown to have increased levels of intracellular PRDX2 when compared to healthy controls [39]. Autoantibodies against peroxiredoxin have also been identified in RA [40]. Increased levels of PRDX2 in the polyarticular patients may indicate a dysregulated redox response system similar to that observed in adult RA.

Conclusions

There are still substantial gaps in our understanding of JIA disease pathogenesis. As a result, JIA specific treatments have lagged behind the management of other adult arthritides. Identifying pathology specific proteins with functions in key cellular processes may provide help to prioritize putative therapeutic targets. We hypothesize that an imbalance in clotting factors, which primarily control plasma cell activation and thrombus formation, is associated with the involvement of multiple synovial joints in early stage JIA. In the case of polyarticular patients, diminished levels of specific clotting factors may prevent the repair of leaky neovasculature and increase the chances that multiple joints will be affected. Further targeted investigations of the circulating levels of the aforementioned factors in a suitably powered independent study cohort are required to robustly test this theory. Murine knockout models of arthritis which can sequentially test the function of the identified members of clotting pathways could also be used to verify this hypothesis.

Alternately, if the integrin alpha 2b is expressed exclusively on pathogenic vasculature, this property could be exploited to specifically target poorly formed vessels with integrin recognition (RGD) peptides. Integrin homing-RGD peptides have been shown to preferentially target inflamed synovium vessels without damaging other synovial tissues [41]. These small proteins could be linked to therapeutic agents, or clotting agents to clog the vessels which fuel the ensuing synovitis.

In summary, proteomic analysis of synovial tissue from early disease-stage JIA patients has revealed novel pathological protein expression patterns. With further work, molecular pathways which discriminate JIA subtypes could be exploited to develop new treatment strategies which suppress disease and reduce the risk of long term joint damage.

Abbreviations

2D DIGE: Two dimensional fluorescent difference in-gel electrophoresis; 2D PAGE: Two dimensional polyacrylamide gel electrophoresis; ANOVA: Analysis of variance analysis; CHAPS: 3-((3-Cholamidopropyl) dimethylammonio)-1-propanesulfonate; CID: Collision induced dissociation; CRP: C-reactive protein; Da: Dalton; DAB: 3,3'-Diaminobenzidine; DMARD: Disease modifying anti-rheumatic drug; DTT: Dithiothreitol; ECM: Extracellular matrix; ESR: Erythrocyte sedimentation rate; FDP: Fibrin degradation product; HCA: Hierarchical cluster analysis; HTML: Hypertext markup language; IEF: Isoelectric focusing; IL-1β/6: Interleukin 1 beta or 6; ILAR: International league of associations for rheumatology; ITA2B: Integrin alpha 2b; JIA: Juvenile Idiopathic Arthritis; KCIP-1: Protein kinase C inhibitor protein 1; kV: Kilovolt; m/z: Ion mass over charge; MALDI-TOF: Matrix assisted laser desorption ionization-time of flight; MS-MS: Tandem mass spectrometry; MYL2/9: Myosin regulatory light chain 2 or 9; NCBI: National center for biotechnology information; OA: Osteoarthritis; ppm: Parts per million; PRDX2: Periredoxin 2; PTM: Post-translational modification; RA: Rheumatoid arthritis; RGD: Arginine-glycine-aspartate integrin recognition sequence; rpm: Revolutions per minute; TFA: Trifluoroacetic acid; TOF-MS: Time of flight mass spectra; UPGMA: Unweighted pair group method with arithmetic mean; VAS: Visual analogue scale.

Competing interests

The authors declare they have no competing interests.

Authors' contributions

SF and CS carried out the DIGE analysis. JLR performed the mass spectrometry. SF conducted the Western blot analyses and immunohistochemistry. CMcA collated all the patient demographic and clinical data. MR obtained consent from patients and collected tissue biopsies. DSG conceived the study and, along with SRP and MR, participated in its design and coordination. SF, MR and DSG wrote the manuscript. All authors read and approved the final manuscript.

Acknowledgements

DSG and MR would like to acknowledge the funding of this research by Arthritis Research UK in the form of a Project Grant (No. 18748). The UCD Conway Institute and the Proteome Research Centre are funded by the Programme for Research in Third Level Institutions, as administered by the Higher Education Authority of Ireland. SRP acknowledges support for equipment from Science Foundation Ireland.

Author details

[1]Arthritis Research Group, Queen's University Belfast, Centre for Infection and Immunity, Health Sciences Building, 97 Lisburn Road, Belfast BT9 7BL, UK. [2]School of Biological and Biomedical Sciences, Durham University, Durham DH1 3LE, UK. [3]Proteome Research Centre, UCD Conway Institute for Biomolecular and Biomedical Research, University College Dublin, Dublin, Ireland. [4]Pediatric Rheumatology, Withers Ward, Musgrave Park Hospital, 20 Stockman's Lane, Belfast BT9 7JB, UK. [5]Northern Ireland Centre for Stratified Medicine, C-TRIC Building, Altnagelvin Hospital campus, Glenshane Road, Londonderry BT47 6SB, UK.

References

1. Symmons DP, Jones M, Osborne J, Sills J, Southwood TR, Woo P: **Pediatric rheumatology in the United Kingdom: data from the British Pediatric Rheumatology Group National Diagnostic Register.** *J Rheumatol* 1996, **23:**1975–1980.
2. Prakken BJ, Albani S: **Using biology of disease to understand and guide therapy of JIA.** *Best Pract Res Clin Rheumatol* 2009, **23:**599–608.
3. Minden K, Niewerth M, Listing J, Biedermann T, Bollow M, Schöntube M, Zink A: **Long-term outcome in patients with juvenile idiopathic arthritis.** *Arthritis Rheum* 2002, **46:**2392–2401.
4. Petty RE, Southwood TR, Manners P, Baum J, Glass DN, Goldenberg J, He X, Maldonado-Cocco J, Orozco-Alcala J, Prieur AM, Suarez-Almazor ME, Woo P, International League of Associations for Rheumatology: **International League of Associations for Rheumatology classification of juvenile idiopathic arthritis: second revision, Edmonton, 2001.** *J Rheumatol* 2004, **31:**390–392.
5. Petty RE, Southwood TR, Baum J, Bhettay E, Glass DN, Manners P, Maldonado-Cocco J, Suarez-Almazor M, Orozco-Alcala J, Prieur AM: **Revision of the proposed classification criteria for juvenile idiopathic arthritis: Durban, 1997.** *J Rheumatol* 1998, **25:**1991–1994.
6. Sullivan DB, Cassidy JT, Petty RE: **Pathogenic implications of age of onset in juvenile rheumatoid arthritis.** *Arthritis Rheum* 1975, **18:**251–255.
7. Hui-Yuen JS, Imundo LF: **A review guide to oligoarticular and polyarticular juvenile idiopathic arthritis.** *Pediatr Ann* 2012, **41:**1–8.
8. Gattorno M, Gregorio A, Ferlito F, Gerloni V, Parafioriti A, Felici E, Sala E, Gambini C, Picco P, Martini A: **Synovial expression of osteopontin correlates with angiogenesis in juvenile idiopathic arthritis.** *Rheumatology (Oxford)* 2004, **43:**1091–1096.
9. Gregorio A, Gambini C, Gerloni V, Parafioriti A, Sormani MP, Gregorio S, De Marco G, Rossi F, Martini A, Gattorno M: **Lymphoid neogenesis in juvenile idiopathic arthritis correlates with ANA positivity and plasma cells infiltration.** *Rheumatology (Oxford)* 2007, **46:**308–313.
10. Bramlage CP, Kaps C, Ungethüm U, Bramlage P, Koziolek M, Wessels J, Krenn V, Pruss A, Müller GA, Strutz F, Burmester GR, Häupl T: **Modulatory effects of inflammation and therapy on GDF-5 expression in rheumatoid arthritis synovium.** *Scand J Rheumatol* 2008, **37:**401–409.
11. Walker JG, Ahern MJ, Coleman M, Weedon H, Papangelis V, Beroukas D, Roberts-Thomson PJ, Smith MD: **Changes in synovial tissue Jak-STAT expression in rheumatoid arthritis in response to successful DMARD treatment.** *Ann Rheum Dis* 2006, **65:**1558–1564.
12. Koski JM, Helle M: **Ultrasound guided synovial biopsy using portal and forceps.** *Ann Rheum Dis* 2005, **64:**926–929.
13. Gibson DS, Blelock S, Curry J, Finnegan S, Healy A, Scaife C, McAllister C, Pennington S, Dunn M, Rooney M: **Comparative analysis of synovial fluid and plasma proteomes in juvenile arthritis–proteomic patterns of joint inflammation in early stage disease.** *J Proteomics* 2009, **72:**656–676.
14. Gibson DS, Finnegan S, Jordan G, Scaife C, Brockbank S, Curry J, McAllister C, Pennington S, Dunn M, Rooney ME: **Stratification and monitoring of juvenile idiopathic arthritis patients by synovial proteome analysis.** *J Proteome Res* 2009, **8:**5601–5609.
15. Caraux G, Pinloche S: **PermutMatrix: a graphical environment to arrange gene expression profiles in optimal linear order.** *Bioinformatics* 2005, **21:**1280-1281. http://www.atgc-montpellier.fr/permutmatrix/
16. Finnegan S, Clarke S, Gibson D, McAllister C, Rooney M: **Synovial membrane immunohistology in early untreated juvenile idiopathic arthritis: differences between clinical subgroups.** *Ann Rheum Dis* 2011, **70:**1842–1850.
17. Yan X, Zhao Y, Pan J, Fang K, Wang Y, Li Z, Chang X: **Vitamin D-binding protein (group-specific component) has decreased expression in rheumatoid arthritis.** *Clin Exp Rheumatol* 2012, **30:**525–533.
18. Sun S, Fang K, Zhao Y, Yan X, Chang X: **Increased expression of alpha 1-anti-trypsin in the synovial tissues of patients with ankylosing spondylitis.** *Clin Exp Rheumatol* 2012, **30:**39–44.
19. Matsuo K, Xiang Y, Nakamura H, Masuko K, Yudoh K, Noyori K, Nishioka K, Saito T, Kato T: **Identification of novel citrullinated autoantigens of synovium in rheumatoid arthritis using a proteomic approach.** *Arthritis Res Ther* 2006, **8:**R175.
20. Ling XB, Park JL, Carroll T, Nguyen KD, Lau K, Macaubas C, Chen E, Lee T, Sandborg C, Milojevic D, Kanegaye JT, Gao S, Burns J, Schilling J, Mellins ED: **Plasma profiles in active systemic juvenile idiopathic arthritis: biomarkers and biological implications.** *Proteomics* 2010, **10:**4415–4430.
21. Rosenkranz ME, Wilson DC, Marinov AD, Decewicz A, Grof-Tisza P, Kirchner D, Giles B, Reynolds PR, Liebman MN, Kolli VS, Thompson SD, Hirsch R: **Synovial fluid proteins differentiate between the subtypes of juvenile idiopathic arthritis.** *Arthritis Rheum* 2010, **62:**1813–1823.
22. Gibson DS, Blelock S, Brockbank S, Curry J, Healy A, McAllister C, Rooney ME: **Proteomic analysis of recurrent joint inflammation in juvenile idiopathic arthritis.** *J Proteome Res* 2006, **5:**1988–1995.
23. Gibson DS, Newell K, Evans AN, Finnegan S, Manning G, Scaife C, McAllister C, Pennington SR, Duncan MW, Moore TL, Rooney ME: **Vitamin D binding protein isoforms as candidate predictors of disease extension in childhood arthritis.** *J Proteomics* 2012, **75:**5479–5492.
24. Calvete JJ, Henschen A, Gonzalez-Rodriguez J: **Complete localization of the intrachain disulphide bonds and the N-glycosylation points in the alpha-subunit of human platelet glycoprotein IIb.** *Biochem J* 1989, **261:**561–568.
25. Calvete JJ: **On the structure and function of platelet integrin alpha IIb beta 3, the fibrinogen receptor.** *Proc Soc Exp Biol Med* 1995, **208:**346–360.

26. Korkusuz P, Dagdeviren A, Eksioglu F, Ors U: **Immunohistological analysis of normal and osteoarthritic human synovial tissue.** *Bull Hosp Jt Dis* 2005, **63**:63–69.
27. Adam SS, Key NS, Greenberg CS: **D-dimer antigen: current concepts and future prospects.** *Blood* 2009, **113**:2878–2887.
28. Iba T, Kidokoro A, Fukunaga M, Sugiyama K, Sawada T, Kato H: **Association between the severity of sepsis and the changes in hemostatic molecular markers and vascular endothelial damage markers.** *Shock* 2005, **23**:25–29.
29. Ichikawa Y, Yamada C, Horiki T, Hoshina Y, Uchiyama M: **Serum matrix metalloproteinase-3 and fibrin degradation product levels correlate with clinical disease activity in rheumatoid arthritis.** *Clin Exp Rheumatol* 1998, **16**:533–540.
30. Robson SC, Shephard EG, Kirsch RE: **Fibrin degradation product D-dimer induces the synthesis and release of biologically active IL-1 beta, IL-6 and plasminogen activator inhibitors from monocytes *in vitro*.** *Br J Haematol* 1994, **86**:322–326.
31. van Venrooij WJ, van Beers JJ, Pruijn GJ: **Anti-CCP antibodies: the past, the present and the future.** *Nat Rev Rheumatol* 2011, **7**:391–398.
32. Mosesson MW: **Fibrinogen gamma chain functions.** *J Thromb Haemost* 2003, **1**:231–238.
33. Gilliam BE, Reed MR, Chauhan AK, Dehlendorf AB, Moore TL: **Evidence of fibrinogen as a target of citrullination in IgM rheumatoid factor-positive polyarticular juvenile idiopathic arthritis.** *Pediatr Rheumatol Online J* 2011, **9**:8.
34. Quirke AM, Fisher BA, Kinloch AJ, Venables PJ: **Citrullination of autoantigens: upstream of TNFα in the pathogenesis of rheumatoid arthritis.** *FEBS Lett* 2011, **585**:3681–3688.
35. Bathon JM, Hwang JJ, Shin LH, Precht PA, Towns MC, Horton WE Jr: **Type VI collagen-specific messenger RNA is expressed constitutively by cultured human synovial fibroblasts and is suppressed by interleukin-1.** *Arthritis Rheum* 1994, **37**:1350–1356.
36. Alexopoulos LG, Youn I, Bonaldo P, Guilak F: **Developmental and osteoarthritic changes in Col6a1-knockout mice: biomechanics of type VI collagen in the cartilage pericellular matrix.** *Arthritis Rheum* 2009, **60**:771–779.
37. Aidinis V, Carninci P, Armaka M, Witke W, Harokopos V, Pavelka N, Koczan D, Argyropoulos C, Thwin MM, Möller S, Waki K, Gopalakrishnakone P, Ricciardi-Castagnoli P, Thiesen HJ, Hayashizaki Y, Kollias G: **Cytoskeletal rearrangements in synovial fibroblasts as a novel pathophysiological determinant of modeled rheumatoid arthritis.** *PLoS Genet* 2005, **1**:e48.
38. Rhee SG, Chae HZ, Kim K: **Peroxiredoxins: a historical overview and speculative preview of novel mechanisms and emerging concepts in cell signaling.** *Free Radic Biol Med* 2005, **38**:1543–1552.
39. Szabó-Taylor KÉ, Eggleton P, Turner CA, Faro ML, Tarr JM, Tóth S, Whiteman M, Haigh RC, Littlechild JA, Winyard PG: **Lymphocytes from rheumatoid arthritis patients have elevated levels of intracellular peroxiredoxin 2, and a greater frequency of cells with exofacial peroxiredoxin 2, compared with healthy human lymphocytes.** *Int J Biochem Cell Biol* 2012, **44**:1223–1231.
40. Karasawa R, Ozaki S, Nishioka K, Kato T: **Autoantibodies to peroxiredoxin I and IV in patients with systemic autoimmune diseases.** *Microbiol Immunol* 2005, **49**:57–65.
41. Gerlag DM, Borges E, Tak PP, Ellerby HM, Bredesen DE, Pasqualini R, Ruoslahti E, Firestein GS: **Suppression of murine collagen-induced arthritis by targeted apoptosis of synovial neovasculature.** *Arthritis Res* 2001, **3**:357–361.

2

Bone mass and quality in patients with juvenile idiopathic arthritis: longitudinal evaluation of bone-mass determinants by using dual-energy x-ray absorptiometry, peripheral quantitative computed tomography, and quantitative ultrasonography

Stefano Stagi[1†], Loredana Cavalli[2†], Carla Signorini[2], Federico Bertini[3], Marco Matucci Cerinic[3], Maria Luisa Brandi[2†] and Fernanda Falcini[3*†]

Abstract

Introduction: Our objective was to evaluate longitudinally the main bone-mass and quality predictors in young juvenile idiopathic arthritis (JIA) patients by using lumbar spine dual-energy X-ray absorptiometry (DXA) scan, radius peripheral quantitative computed tomography (pQCT), and phalangeal quantitative ultrasonography (QUS) at the same time.

Methods: In total, 245 patients (172 females, 73 males; median age, 15.6 years: 148 oligoarticular, 55 polyarticular, 20 systemic, and 22 enthesitis-related-arthritis (ERA) onset) entered the study. Of these, 166 patients were evaluated longitudinally. Data were compared with two age- and sex-matched control groups.

Results: In comparison with controls, JIA patients, but not with ERA, had a reduced spine bone-mineral apparent density (BMAD) standard deviation score ($P < 0.001$) and musculoskeletal deficits, with significantly lower levels of trabecular bone mineral density (TrabBMD) ($P < 0.0001$), muscle cross-sectional area (CSA) ($P < 0.005$), and density-weighted polar section modulus (SSIp) ($P < 0.05$). In contrast, JIA showed fat CSA significantly higher than controls ($P < 0.0001$). Finally, JIA patients had a significant reduced amplitude-dependent speed of sound (AD-SoS) ($P < 0.001$), and QUS z score ($P < 0.005$).
Longitudinally, we did not find any difference in all JIA patients in comparison with baseline, except for the SSIp value that normalized. Analyzing the treatments, a significant negative correlation among spine BMAD values, TrabBMD, AD-SoS, and systemic and/or intraarticular corticosteroids, and a positive correlation among TNF-α-blocking agents and spine BMAD, TrabBMD, and AD-SoS were observed.

Conclusions: JIA patients have a low bone mass that, after a first increase due to the therapy, does not reach the normal condition over time. The pronounced bone deficits in JIA are greater than would be expected because of reduction in muscle cross-sectional area. Thus, bone alterations in JIA likely represent a mixed defect of bone accrual and lower muscle forces.

* Correspondence: falcini@unifi.it
†Equal contributors
[3]Department of Internal Medicine, Section of Rheumatology, Transition Clinic, University of Florence, Viale Pieraccini 18, 50139 Florence, Italy
Full list of author information is available at the end of the article

Introduction

In juvenile idiopathic arthritis (JIA), a multifactorial reduction of bone mineral accrual with impaired bone mass has been widely reported [1-3]. Chronic inflammation [4-6], delayed pubertal maturation [3], malnutrition [7], muscle weakness [6], limited physical activity [8,9], early onset of JIA [3], and treatments, especially corticosteroids [1,10], influence negatively bone mineral density (BMD) in these subjects. Therefore, although the heredity accounts for a large proportion of variation in BMD, these factors may exert a significant negative influence on the development of peak bone mass (PBM) [3,11,12], with increased fracture risk in adulthood [13,14]. In addition, JIA patients, after a therapy-induced increase of BMD, do not seem to reach a normal condition over time [3].

To assess bone health appropriately, integration between clinical tools and imaging techniques is required [1,2]. Dual-energy x-ray absorptiometry (DXA) bone measures are based on a two-dimensional image that precludes a direct measure of volumetric BMD (vBMD). Because BMD only partly explains bone quality, these abnormalities may be better estimated by a quantitative assessment of macro- and microstructural characteristics [15]. Thus, three-dimensional imaging methods, such as peripheral quantitative computed tomography (pQCT), allow a selective assessment of both trabecular and cortical bone and also estimate bone strength [16]. In addition, quantitative ultrasonography (QUS), increasingly used for its low cost, portability, and lack of exposure to ionizing radiation, is used to evaluate bone density and structure and also permits assessment of changes in trabecular and cortical architecture [16].

Although several studies demonstrated reduced bone mass or quality in JIA patients [3,6,11,17-21], few large cross-sectional or prospective, case–control data exist for children and young adults [3,8,22] and few, in particular, using DXA, pQCT, and QUS scans simultaneously. Thus, the aim of the study was to evaluate bone mass and quality in children, adolescents, and young adults with JIA.

Methods

Patients were recruited consecutively from the Rheumatology Unit of Florence University between January 2008 and July 2011. All underwent forearm pQCT, QUS scans at the phalanges, and DXA at the lumbar spine on the same day.

The study protocol was approved by Hospital Ethics Committee of Careggi University Hospital of Florence, and written informed consent was obtained from all patients and controls or their parents or guardians, as appropriate.

Study population and design

Two hundred forty-five patients (172 female and 73 male patients; median age at study entry, 15.6; range, 9.6 to 28.3 years) fulfilling the criteria for JIA [23] were evaluated. One hundred forty-eight had oligoarticular; 55, polyarticular (rheumatoid factor negative); 20, systemic; and 22, enthesitis-related arthritis (ERA) onset. Of these, 166 patients (132 females, 34 males; 99 oligoarticular, 30 polyarticular, 18 systemic, and 19 ERA) were followed up longitudinally with a second DXA, pQCT, and QUS. Of the oligoarticular patients, 26% had extended arthritis at the first DXA evaluation, whereas an additional 13% were so classified at the second evaluation.

For each patient, clinical and demographic data, including JIA-type onset, age at diagnosis, disease duration, disease course, flares, therapy, height, pubertal stage, weight and body mass index (BMI), and family history of osteoporosis, were recorded from medical charts.

Onset of disease was defined as the date on which arthritis and/or systemic features were documented by a pediatric rheumatologist [3]. The disease subtype and the active JIA assessment were defined according to a previously reported definition [3,23]. Clinical assessment and laboratory evaluation were performed longitudinally to report the disease course and flares [3].

Exclusion criteria for both JIA patients and controls were bone metabolic diseases, hyper-/hypoparathyroidism, hyper-/hypothyroidism, chronic renal failure, cancer, pregnancy, lactation, and osteopenia-inducing drugs, on the basis of the medical history and questionnaires for osteoporosis risk factors.

Study and laboratory methods

Height was measured by using a wall-mounted stadiometer, and weight was measured to the nearest 0.1 kg. Age-related reference values of height and BMI (kg/m^2) were obtained from a wide sample of Italian children [24]. Height and BMI were normalized for chronologic age by conversion to standard deviation scores (SDSs).

Pubertal staging was carried out according to the Tanner and Whitehouse criteria [25], and testicular volume was determined with the Prader orchidometer. The timing of puberty and the comparison between the normal population and JIA patients were assessed [3].

The age at pubertal onset was defined as the age at durable Tanner B2 stage for girls and a testicular volume of more than 4 ml for boys (G2). The age at which the onset of puberty occurred was recorded as the average age between the previous clinic visit, when the child was still prepubertal, and the clinic visit when the child was G2/B2. The duration of puberty was recorded as the time from G2/B2 to G4/B4. The age at G4/B4 was assessed by averaging the ages at the previous clinic visit, when the child was G3/B3, and the clinic visit when the child was G4/B4.

DXA scans

BMD was measured at the lumbar spine by dual-energy x-ray absorptiometry by using the same instrument (Delphi-A 4500 System; Hologic, Inc., Waltham, MA, USA). All BMD results were expressed in terms of g/cm^2 or BMD *Z* scores. Average BMD values for L2 to L4 were used for calculations.

Because the DXA instrument's software does not take into account the actual bone volume strictly related to body size (weight and height), estimation of the respective volumetric density (that is, bone mineral apparent density or BMAD) was determined by using the formula of Kröger *et al.* [26], as previously reported [3]:

$$\mathrm{BMAD} = \mathrm{BMD}_{\mathrm{L2\text{-}L4}} \times (4/(\pi \times \mathrm{width})), \text{expressed in } g/cm^3.$$

The Kröger model was validated by using *in vivo* volumetric data obtained from magnetic resonance imaging of the lumbar vertebrae [27]. The intraobserver coefficient of variation was 1.0%.

Patients' BMAD was expressed as Z scores (that is, the difference between the value of the patient and the normal value for age divided for standard deviation (SD) of the normal patients group) to facilitate comparisons between JIA patients and healthy controls.

Peripheral quantitative computed tomography scan

The left (nondominant) radius was measured by using pQCT by a single, trained investigator, with a Norland-Stratec XCT 3000 scanner (Stratec Medical, Pforzheim, Germany).

Tomographic slices of 2-mm thickness with voxel sizes of 0.4 mm and a scan speed of 25 mm/sec were taken from the shaft and the distal part of the radius (66% and 4% from the distal end plate of the radius, respectively) [28].

Names for end-point variables were chosen according to the Task Force on Standardization of Bone Structure and Density Assessment [29] for high-resolution pQCT.

The 4% (distal) radial site allowed assessment of the trabecular bone to obtain total bone mineral density (TotBMD, mg/cm^3) and trabecular bone mineral density (TrbBMD, mg/cm^3) [28].

For the shaft regions (66%), the analyzed bone traits were cortical bone mineral density (CrtBMD, mg/cm^3), cortical bone area (CBA, mm^2), muscle cross-sectional area (MuscleCSA, mm^2), fat cross-sectional area (FatCSA, cm^2), and density-weighted polar section modulus (SSIp, mm^3, an estimate of bending and torsional bone strength for cortical bone).

Because growth retardation is common in some JIA children and adolescents [1,2], all bone size-dependent parameters (Total, Cortical, and MuscleCSA) were corrected for height.

QUS scans

QUS scans were performed with a DBM Sonic 1200 device (IGEA Bone Profiler, Carpi, Italy), equipped with two probes mounted on an electronic caliper. With this technique, we measured (1) amplitude-dependent speed of sound (AD-SoS, in m/s), the interval between the start time of the transmitted signal and the time the signal received reaches the predetermined minimum amplitude value of 2 mV for the first time); and (b) bone transmission time (BTT, in μsec), the difference between transmission time in phalanx soft tissue and bone and transmission time in phalanx soft tissue. AD-SoS and BTT SDS were automatically generated [16].

Clinical assessment of disease activity

Clinical disease activity was determined as previously described [3]. Documentation of patient data included medical history and physical examination, in particular the number of active joints, number of joints with limited range of motion, physician's global assessment of disease activity, parent's/patient's assessment of overall well-being (visual analogue scale as part of the Childhood Health Assessment Questionnaire [C-HAQ]), and functional ability (disability as measured in eight domains by the C-HAQ). Patients were categorized as having active disease or being in clinical remission for at least 6 consecutive months, as previously described [3]. Relapse was defined according to the preliminary definition of disease flare in JIA [3,29].

Type of treatment

During the cross-sectional and longitudinal evaluations, the following therapies were considered to define the task of these determinants on spine BMAD values: nonsteroidal antiinflammatory drugs (NSAIDs), sulfasalazine, systemic and intraarticular corticosteroids, methotrexate (MTX), and TNF-α-blocking agents [3].

For all drugs, the period of administration was also obtained from the outpatient clinic and hospital records at the time of the first and second evaluations. Moreover, the number of intraarticular glucocorticoids injections and the interval between the injection and DXA assessment were noted. Systemic corticosteroid dosages were converted into a common steroid equivalency (mg/kg body weight per day of prednisolone-equivalent dose).

Healthy control subjects

At the first evaluation, the control group included 80 healthy age- and sex-matched subjects (58 females, 22 males; median age, 14.8 years; range, 8.9 to 26.7 years), observed at our medical units for noninflammatory musculoskeletal complaints. At the time of the second scans, we selected another age- and sex-matched control group with the same characteristics (82 subjects, 59 females, 23 males; median age, 16.9 years; range, 10.9 to 28.4 years). The data for part of these groups were also previously reported [3].

Statistical analysis

Statistical analyses were performed by using SPSSX (SPSSX Inc., Chicago, IL, USA). Summaries of continuous variables were given as the means ± SDs or median and range, depending on whether the data were normally distributed. Differences between patient groups and controls were assessed by using the Student *t* test and Mann–Whitney *U* test, depending on the distribution of the analyzed variable. The χ^2 test and the Fisher Exact test were used as appropriate to examine associations between dichotomous variables. Intergroup comparisons for parameters were conducted by using analysis of variance (ANOVA) or by using repeated-measures analysis of covariance (ANCOVA), as appropriate.

Spearman and Pearson correlation tests were used to determine the correlation coefficients. A multiple stepwise regression was used to determine the variables that correlated independently with lumbar spine BMAD, QUS, and pQCT *z* scores. *P* values <0.05 were considered statistically significant.

Results

The general data of the study population and controls are shown in Table 1.

With respect to exposure to different medications at study entry, 56% of the JIA patients had received NSAIDs. Methotrexate had been prescribed to 44.7% and TNF-α-blocking medications to 22% of patients; 30% had received sulfasalazine, and glucocorticoids were prescribed to 21.7%. High-dose systemic or oral glucocorticoids had been administered only to patients with systemic JIA onset ($P < 0.001$), whereas the dose administered in the other JIA subtypes was low, without significant differences among the different groups. Forty-one percent had taken glucocorticoids during the year before measurements.

With respect to disease activity, at study entry, 46.1% of the JIA patients had disease activity, whereas 53.9% of patients had remission/inactive disease. Our data related

Table 1 Data for the 141 JIA patients longitudinally evaluated in comparison to their respective control groups

	JIA group		Control group	
	Baseline	Second evaluation	Baseline	Second evaluation
Number of subjects	245	166	80	82
Female/male ratio	172:73	132:34	58:22	59:23
Age, years (range)	15.6 (9.6 - 28.3)	17.1 (11.0 - 28.9)	14.8 (8.9 - 26.7)	16.9 (10.9 - 28.4)
Height, *z* score	−0.6 ± 1.1	−0.5 ± 0.9	−0.1 ± 0.9	−0.1 ± 0.7
BMI, *z* score	−0.3 ± 0.8	−0.1 ± 0.6	0.1 ± 0.7	0.2 ± 0.5
Disease duration	5.6 ± 3.2 years	7.2 ± 4.3 years	-	-
C-HAQ DI	0.74 ± 0.63	0.59 ± 0.48	-	-
DXA examination				
BMC, g	45.17 ± 19.13^a	49.04 ± 21.56$^{\circ\circ\circ j}$	51.23 ± 17.90	56.98 ± 16.82^h
BMAD spine, g/cm^2	−0.64 ± 0.80^b	−0.49 ± 1.10$^{\circ\circ\circ}$	0.24 ± 0.21	0.13 ± 0.32
HR-pQCT				
TrbBMD (mg/cm^3)	179.5 ± 34.6^c	181.9 ± 48.8^f	217.7 ± 26.3	244.9 ± 28.5^i
CBA (mm^2)	136.3 ± 122. ^{c}	149.0 ± 87.6^f	209.2 ± 101.3	214.3 ± 74.3
CrtBMD (mg/cm^3)	1,050.2 ± 126.5	1,079.8 ± 82.1^j	1,039.6 ± 79.3	1,078.3 ± 73.1^g
Muscle CSA (mm^2)	2,112.7 ± 732.4^b	2,083.7 ± 697.8^f	2,398.5 ± 773.3	2,579.3 ± 794.5^h
Fat CSA (mm^2)	1,143.1 ± 649.1^c	1,110.1 ± 483.7^e	918.3 ± 382.1	945.8 ± 394.2
SSIp (mm^3)	246.3 ± 140.2^a	306.8 ± 250.7^{d,j}	284.0 ± 127.9	276.7 ± 110.4
Ultrasonography				
-AD-SoS	1,994.5 ± 119.7^b	2,003.0 ± 101.1^e	2,122.3 ± 113.1	2,152.8 ± 118.9
-QUS *z* score	−0.6 ± 1.8^a	−0.5 ± 1.5^e	0.1 ± 1.6	0.2 ± 1.8

JIA versus controls (transversal study): $^aP < 0.05$; $^bP < 0.005$; $^cP < 0.0005$; JIA *versus.* controls (longitudinal study): $^dP < 0.05$; $^eP < 0.005$; $^fP < 0.0005$.
Controls *versus* controls (longitudinal study): $^gP < 0.05$; ^{h}^^ $P < 0.005$; $^iP < 0.0005$; JIA *versus* JIA (longitudinal study): ^{j} $P < 0.05$; $^{\S}j^{\S}P < 0.005$; $^{\S\S\S} < 0.0005$.
AD-SoS, amplitude-dependent speed of sound; BMAD, bone mineral apparent density; BMC, bone mineral content; BMI, body mass index; CBA, cortical bone area; C-HAQ DI, Childhood Health Assessment Questionnaire Disability Index, range, 0–3 (0 = best, 3 = worst); CrtBMD, cortical bone-mineral density; DXA, dual-energy x-ray absorptiometry; FatCSA, fat cross-sectional area; HR-pQCT, high-resolution peripheral quantitative computed tomography; JIA, juvenile idiopathic arthritis; MuscleCSA, muscle cross-sectional area; SSIp, density-weighted polar section modulus; QUS, quantitative ultrasonography; TrbBMD, trabecular bone-mineral density.

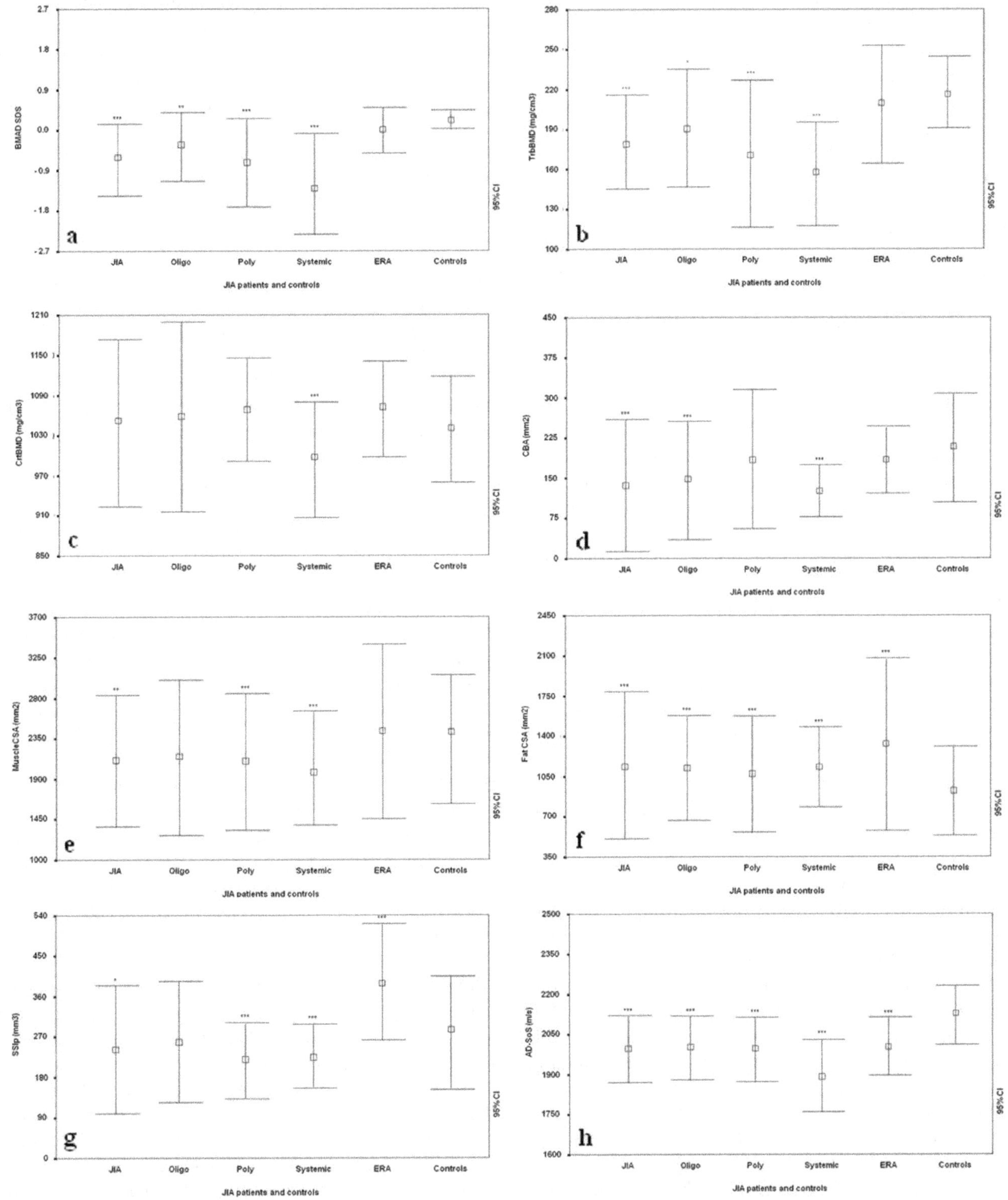

Figure 1 Transversal evaluation. Spine bone mineral apparent density (spine BMAD) SDS **(a)**, trabecular bone mineral density (TrabBMD) **(b)**, cortical bone mineral density (CrtBMD) **(c)**, cortical bone area ([CBA) **(d)**, muscle cross-sectional area (MuscleCSA) **(e)**, fat cross-sectional area (FatCSA) **(f)**, density-weighted polar section modulus (SSIp) **(g)**, and Ad-SoS **(h)** in patients with oligoarticular, polyarticular, systemic, and enthesitis-arthritis (ERA) JIA versus controls. Bars represent means and 95% confidence intervals. $^{**}P < 0.005$; $^{***}P < 0.001$.

to the age at puberty onset, compared with controls, evidenced that age was delayed, but not significantly (years (95% CI)) both in girls (B2, 11.0 ± 2.0 versus 10.5 ± 1.5; B3, 11.8 ± 2.1 versus 11.1 ± 1.7; B4, 12.7 ± 1.9 versus 11.8 ± 1.6) than in boys (G2, 12.2 ± 2.4 versus 11.6 ± 1.8; G3, 13.4 ± 2.3 versus 12.5 ± 2.1; G4, 14.8 ± 1.7 versus 13.6 ± 1.5).

In the first evaluation, the JIA patients showed reduced spine BMAD SDS values in comparison with controls (−0.64 ± 0.80 versus 0.24 ± 0.21; $P < 0.001$); these results were also observed when the subjects were divided into oligoarticular (−0.36 ± 0.80; $P < 0.005$), polyarticular (−0.73 ± 1.01; $P < 0.0001$), and systemic (−1.34 ± 1.20; $P < 0.0001$) onset groups. Conversely, ERA subjects did not show any difference in comparison to controls (0.01 ± 0.52; P = NS) (Figure 1a).

In addition, significant musculoskeletal deficits were observed at the time of the first evaluation. The JIA patients had significantly lower levels of TrbBMD than did controls (179.5 ± 34.6 versus 217.7 ± 26.3 mg/cm^3; $P < 0.0001$). These results were also observed when the subjects were divided into oligoarticular (191.9 ± 43.2, $P < 0.05$), polyarticular (172.5 ± 55.5, $P < 0.0001$), and systemic onset (157.6 ± 39.3, $P < 0.0001$) groups, but not in the ERA group (209.6 ± 44.4, P = NS) (Figure 1b).

In contrast, the JIA patients did not show significant differences in CrtBMD (Figure 1c) in comparison to the controls (1,050.2 ± 126.5 versus 1,039.6 ± 79.3, P = NS), even if we considered the different subtypes (oligoarticular, 1,057.5 ± 142.4; polyarticular, 1,068.1 ± 76.8; ERA, 1070.4 ± 71.2 mg/cm^3), except systemic-onset patients, who had a significant reduction (994.0 ± 87.3 mg/cm^3, $P < 0.0001$). At the same time, cortical bone area, CBA (Figure 1d), appeared significantly reduced in comparison to controls (136.3 ± 122.1 versus 209.2 ± 101.3 mm^2; $P < 0.0001$), even if the subjects were divided into oligoarticular- (148.5 ± 112.0 mm^2, $P < 0.0001$), and systemic-onset (126.3 ± 49.0 mm^2, $P < 0.0001$) groups, but not when comparing the controls with the polyarticular (186.3 ± 131.1 mm^2, P = NS) and ERA (187.5 ± 64.5 mm^2, P = NS) groups.

The JIA patients also showed significantly lower muscle CSA (Figure 1e) than did controls (2,112.7 ± 732.4 versus 2,398.5 ± 773.3 mm^2, $P < 0.005$). These differences relative to the controls were also confirmed in the polyarticular (2,100.5 ± 764.4 mm^2, $P < 0.001$) and systemic-onset (2,023.2 ± 632.8 mm^2, $P < 0.0001$) groups, but not in the oligoarticular (2,167.7 ± 870.2, P = NS) and ERA (2,420.2 ± 973.1 mm^2, P = NS) groups.

Fat CSA (Figure 1f) was significantly increased in the JIA patients relative to the controls (1,143.1 ± 649.1 versus 918.3 ± 382.1 mm^2, $P < 0.0001$), even when the patients were divided into the different subtypes (oligoarticular, 1,129.6 ± 451.0 mm^2; polyarticular, 1,080.9 ± 504.8 mm^2; systemic, 1,139.7 ± 351.9 mm^2; ERA, 1,335.2 ± 748.2 mm^2, $P < 0.0001$).

The JIA patients also had significantly lower SSIp levels (Figure 1g) than controls (246.3 ± 140.2 versus 284.0 ± 127.9 mm^3, $P < 0.05$), even when divided into polyarticular (220.2 ± 82.9, $P < 0.0001$) and systemic-onset groups (228.0 ± 68.6, $P < 0.0001$), but not when controls were compared with the oligoarticular group (261.7 ± 134.5, P = NS). In contrast, subjects with ERA had significantly increased SSIp values with respect to controls (353.1 ± 129.9, $P < 0.05$) (Figure 1g).

Finally, in the JIA patients, AD-SoS (Figure 1h) results were significantly reduced (1,994.5 ± 119.7 versus 2,122.3 ± 113.1 m/s, $P < 0.001$), even when patients were divided into subgroups (oligoarticular: 2,004.7 ± 118.6 m/s; polyarticular: 1,992.2 ± 116.2 m/s; systemic: 1,894.3 ± 133.1 m/s; ERA: 2,003.4 ± 105.8 m/s, $P < 0.0001$). The results were comparable also when QUS z-scores in the JIA patients and controls were evaluated (−0.6 ± 1.8 versus 0.1 ± 1.6, $P = 0.003$) and between the subtypes and the controls (polyarticular: −1.0 ± 1.6; systemic: −2.7 ± 2.0; ERA: −0.8 ± 1.5, $P < 0.0001$), except for the oligoarticular-onset subtype (−0.4 ± 1.7, P = NS).

The correlations among the variables in the transversal study are reported in Tables 2 and 3.

Longitudinal evaluation

At the time of the second evaluation, the median chronologic age was 17.7 years (range, 10.2 to 29.6 years). At this time, disease duration was 7.2 ± 4.3 years, and mean disease activity, 2.8 years. Disease duration was not significantly different among the subgroups of patients (Table 1). Besides, at longitudinal evaluation, 42.2% of the JIA patients had active disease, whereas 57.8% of patients had remission/inactive disease.

The longitudinal evaluation confirmed that the JIA patients had a reduced spine BMAD SDS in comparison with controls (−0.49 ± 1.10 versus 0.13 ± 0.32; $P < 0.001$). These results were still observed when the subjects were divided into oligoarticular (−0.29 ± 1.13; $P < 0.005$), polyarticular (−0.55 ± 1.24; $P < 0.0001$), and systemic subtypes (−1.36 ± 1.33; $P < 0.0001$), but not in the ERA subtype (0.05 ± 0.71; P = NS) (Figure 2a). Evaluating the differences among the JIA subgroups, oligoarticular (−0.36 ± 0.80 versus -0.29 ± 1.11), polyarticular (−0.73 ± 1.01 versus -0.55 ± 1.23), and ERA (0.01 ± 0.52 versus 0.05 ± 0.71; P = NS); no differences with respect to the findings in the first evaluation were noted, except for patients with systemic onset (−1.34 ± 1.20 versus -1.46 ± 1.44; $P < 0.0001$).

The JIA patients were confirmed to have significantly lower levels of TrbBMD (Figure 2b) than controls (181.9 ± 48.8 versus 244.9 ± 28.5 mg/cm^3, $P < 0.0001$). These results were observed also in the oligoarticular (190.6 ± 44.7, $P < 0.0001$), polyarticular (169.9 ± 46.4, $P <$ 0.0001), systemic (158.1 ± 38.1, $P < 0.0001$), and ERA subtypes (210.1 ± 37.4, $P < 0.0001$). With respect to the

Table 2 Correlation coefficients (rho) between the bone traits in the JIA cohort and controls

pQCT phenotypes								DXA Phenotypes			QUS phenotypes		
	TrbBMD	CrtBMD	Total density	CBA	Bone area	Muscle CSA	Fat CSA	SSIp	BMAD	BMD	QUS z-score	AD-SoS	BTT
TrbBMD		0.13 0.19 0.25°	0.60*** 0.59^^^ 0.78°°°	0.10 0.23^ 0.32°°	0.14 0.19 0.24°	0.26* 0.31^^ 0.35°°	0.16 0.29^ −0.10	0.05 0.28^ −0.26°	0.12 0.35^^ 0.39°°	0.12 0.15 0.44°°	- 0.05 0.09 0.17	0.01 0.14 0.12	0.07 0.18 0.31°
CrtBMD			0.34** 0.50^^^ 0.39°°	0.23* 0.52^^^ 0.83°°°	0.14 0.28^ 0.49°°	0.42*** 0.39^^ 0.70°°°	0.09 0.16 - 0.27°	0.36** 0.41^^ 0.39°°	0.49** 0.46^^ 0.63°°°	0.69*** 0.72^^^ 0.80°°°	0.21* 0.22^ 0.61°°°	0.60*** 0.70^^^ 0.72°°°	0.64*** 0.66^^^ 0.82°°°
Tot density				0.11 0.39^^ 0.61°°°	0.19 0.15 0.29°	0.41** 0.38^^ 0.59°°°	0.23 −0.20 0.10	0.22* 0.23^ 0.32°°	0.12 0.36^^ 0.24°	0.46** 0.48^^ 0.56°°°	0.27* 0.24^ 0.18	0.43*** 0.50^^ 0.35°°	0.40*** 0.42^^ 0.43°°
CBA					0.11 0.49^^ 0.82°°°	0.22* 0.81^^^ 0.92°°°	- 0.26* −0.16 0.14	0.25* 0.83^^^ 0.42°°°	- 0.09 0.25^ 0.34°°	0.28** 0.71^^^ 0.89°°°	0.12 0.31^^ 0.57°°°	0.24* 0.48^^ 0.26°	0.25* 0.72^^^ 0.85°°°
Bone area						0.49** 0.49^^ 0.78°°°	0.05 0.11 0.37°°	0.55** 0.66^^ 0.72°°°	0.20 0.31^^ 0.22°	0.18 0.40^^ 0.75°°°	0.05 0.09 0.27°	0.18 0.19 0.47°°	0.30** 0.37^^ 0.71°°°
MuscleCSA							- 0.27* −0.37^^ 0.02	0.47*** 0.63^^^ 0.38°°	0.53*** 0.42^^ 0.34°°	0.66*** 0.61^^^ 0.86°°°	0.15 0.13 0.19	0.48** 0.70^^^ 0.67°°°	0.76*** 0.80^^^ 0.85°°°
FatCSA								−040** −0.48^^ 0.19	0.11 −0.14 0.37°°	0.13 0.38^^ 0.39°°	- 0.19* −0.05 −0.22°°	- 0.11 −0.18 −0.43°°	- 0.14 −0.16 −0.31°°
SSIp									0.25* 0.21^ 0.24°	0.52*** 0.53^^^ 0.69°°°	0.02 0.11 0.16	0.35** 0.31^^ 0.53°°°	0.56*** 0.51^^^ 0.67°°°
BMAD										0.38*** 0.40^^ 0.29°	- 0.01 0.21^ 0.39°°	0.16 0.28^ 0.57°°°	0.02 0.19 0.68°°°
BMD											0.31** 0.28^ 0.71°°	0.78*** 0.76^^^ 0.67°°°	0.87*** 0.72^^^ 0.86°°°
QUS z-score												0.56*** 0.51^^^ 0.54°°°	0.68*** 0.59^^^ 0.65°°°
AD-SoS													0.73*** 0.68^^^ 0.86°°°

The first line of each cell describes the correlation between bone parameters during transversal study of JIA patients; the second line of each cell describes the correlation between bone parameters during longitudinal study of JIA patients; the third line of each cell describes the correlation between bone parameters during transversal study of controls.

*JIA transversal study: $^{*}P < 0.05$; $^{**}P < 0.005$; $^{***}P < 0.0005$; JIA longitudinal study: $^{\wedge}P < 0.05$; $^{\wedge\wedge}P < 0.005$; $^{\wedge\wedge\wedge}P < 0.0005$; °Controls transversal study: $^{\circ}P < 0.05$; $^{\circ\circ}P < 0.005$; $^{\circ\circ\circ}P < 0.0005$. AD-SoS, amplitude-dependent speed of sound; BTT, bone transmission time. CBA, cortical bone area; CrtBMD, cortical bone mineral density; FatCSA, fat cross-sectional area; JIA, juvenile idiopathic arthritis; a; MuscleCSA, muscle cross-sectional area; SSIp, density-weighted polar section modulus; QUS, quantitative ultrasonography; Tot density, total density. TrbBMD, trabecular bone mineral density.

Table 3 Correlation coefficients (rho) between the bone traits and JIA characteristics in the JIA cohort and controls

Bone traits	JIA phenotypes									
	Type at onset	Age at onset	Disease duration	Disease activity	Flares	Chronologic age	MTX	Systemic corticosteroids	Intraarticular corticosteroids	Biological
TrbBMD	- 0.50**	−0.31**	-0.24**	−0.34**	−0.31**	0.05	0.28*	−0.56**	−0.48**	0.48**
	−0.39^^	−0.39^^	−0.43^^	−0.45^^	−0.29^	0.19	0.32^^	−0.61^^	−0.52^^	0.39^^
	-	-	-	-	-	0.74°°°	-	-	-	-
CrtBMD	0.08	0.32**	0.24*	−0.31**	−0.26*	0.64***	−0.28**	0.20	0.26*	0.36**
	0.16	0.37^^	0.28^	−0.28^^	−0.34^^	0.68^^^	−0.31^^	0.24^	0.24^	0.44^^
	-	-	-	-	-	0.89°°°	-	-	-	-
Tot density	−0.11	−0.14	- 0.40***	- 0.44***	- 0.38***	0.28*	−0.24*	−0.29*	−0.26*	0.32**
	−0.25^	−0.18	−0.38^^	−0.36^^	−0.42^^	0.36^^	−0.29^	−0.34^^	−0.28^	0.46^^
	-	-	-	-	-	0.62°°	-	-	-	-
CBA	0.08	−0.04	−0.18	−0.27*	−0.20*	0.46**	−0.22*	0.06	0.16	0.39**
	0.18	−0.16	−0.21^	−0.31^^	−0.24^	0.54^^	−0.31^^	0.14	0.14	0.28^
	-	-	-	-	-	0.79°°°	-	-	-	-
Bone area	−0.09	−0.12	−0.23*	−0.28*	−0.30*	0.09	−0.16	−0.16	−0.14	0.33**
	−0.12	−0.19	−0.27^	−0.21^	−0.34^^	0.10	−0.14	−0.28^	−0.34^^	0.49^^
	-	-	-	-	-	0.73°°°	-	-	-	-
MuscleCSA	−0.26**	−0.18	−0.16	−0.41**	−0.33**	0.35**	−0.17	−0.46**	−0.51***	0.26*
	−0.29^^	−0.24^	−0.25^	−0.46^^	−0.38^^	0.40^^	−0.08	−0.54^^^	−0.56^^^	0.38^^
	-	-	-	-	-	0.73°°°	-	-	-	-
FatCSA	31.9**	0.34**	0.18	0.35*	0.21*	0.04	0.26*	0.42**	0.26*	−0.19
	36.6^^	0.39^^	0.29^	0.28^	0.27^	0.13	0.39^^	0.39^^	0.84^^	−0.31^^
	-	-	-	-	-	0.23°	-	-	-	-
SSIp	0.03	0.09	0.56***	0.45**	0.38**	0.21*	0.36**	0.51***	0..46**	−0.29*
	0.17	0.19	0.48^^	0.49^^	0.32^^	0.23^	0.34^^	0.64^^^	0.39^^	−0.33^^
	-	-	-	-	-	−0.25°	-	-	-	-
BMAD	- 0.25*	0.48***	−0.34**	−0.46***	−0.38**	0.38**	- 0.39**	- 0.45**	- 0.40**	0.43**
	−0.23^	0.52^^^	−0.42^^	−0.51^^^	−0.34^^	0.47^^	−0,41^^	−0.49^^	−0.43^^	0.51^^^
	-	-	-	-	-	0.79°°°	-	-	-	-
BMD	0.16	0.34**	−0.27*	−0.36**	−0.27*	0.38**	−0.36**	−0.53***	−0.41**	0.29*
	0.19	0.36^^	−0.32^^	−0.39^^	−0.31^^	0.58^^	−0.44^^	−0.59^^^	−0.46^^	0.39^^
	-	-	-	-	-	0.88°°°	-	-	-	-
QUS *z*-score	- 0.25*	−0.27*	−0.35**	−0.41**	−0.22*	0.11	0.16	−0.38**	−0.36**	0.21*
	−0.21^	−0.33^^	−0.39^^	−0.33^^	−0.27^	−0.10	0.12	−0.46^^	−0.44^^	0.33^^
	-	-	-	-	-	0.17	-	-	-	-
AD-SoS	−0.18	−0.37**	−0.51***	−0.39**	−0.47**	0.69***	−0.24*	−0.59***	−0.57***	0.61***
	−0.23^	−0.42^^	−0.46^^	−0.31^^	−0.32^^	0.58^^^	−0.38^^	−0.65^^^	−0.51^^^	0.51^^^
	-	-	-	-	-	0.71°°°	-	-	-	-

Table 3 Correlation coefficients (rho) between the bone traits and JIA characteristics in the JIA cohort and controls *(Continued)*

BTT	**−0.57***** **−0.62^^^** -	**−0.51***** **−0.64^^^** -	**−0.67***** **−0.52^^^** -	**−0.47**** **−0.43^^** -	**−0.27*** **−0.32^^** -	**0.43**** **0.66^^** **0.84°°°°**	**−0.36*** **−0.48^^** -	**−0.61***** **−0.72^^^** -	**−0.65***** **−0.78^^^** -	**0.61***** **0.67^^^** -

The first line of each cell describes the correlation between bone parameters and JIA phenotypes during transversal study of JIA patients; the second line of each cell describes the correlation between bone parameters and JIA phenotypes during longitudinal study of JIA patients; the third line of each cell describes the correlation between bone parameters during transversal study of controls.
JIA transversal study: *$P < 0.05$; **$P < 0.005$; ***$P < 0.0005$; JIA longitudinal study: ^$P < 0.05$; ^^$P < 0.005$; ^^^$P < 0.0005$; Controls transversal study: °$P < 0.05$; °°$P < 0.005$; °°°$P < 0.0005$.
AD-SoS, amplitude-dependent speed of sound; BMAD, bone mineral apparent density; BMD, bone mineral density; BTT, bone transmission time; CBA, cortical bone area; CrtBMD, cortical bone mineral density; FatCSA, fat cross-sectional area; JIA, juvenile idiopathic arthritis; MTX, methotrexate; MuscleCSA, muscle cross-sectional area; QUS, quantitative ultrasonography; SSIp, density-weighted polar section modulus; TrbBMD, trabecular bone mineral density; Tot density, total density.

first examination, we did not find any significant differences among the JIA patients (181.9 ± 48.8 versus 179.5 ± 58.6 mg/cm^3, P = NS), even when they were divided into oligoarticular (190.6 ± 44.7 versus 191.9 ± 43.2 mg/cm^3), ERA (210.1 ± 37.4 versus 209.6 ± 44.4 mg/cm^3), polyarticular (169.9 ± 46.4 versus 172.5 ± 55.5 mg/cm^3), and systemic-onset (158.1 ± 38.1 versus 157.6 ± 39.3 mg/cm^3) subtypes. Conversely, the controls showed a significant increase of TrbBMD with age (244.9 ± 28.5 versus 217.7 ± 26.3 mg/cm^3, $P < 0.0001$).

The JIA patients did not show any significant differences in CrtBMD (Figure 2c) with respect to controls (1,079.8 ± 82.1 versus 1,078.3 ± 73.1, P = NS), even when differentiated by subtype (oligoarticular: 1,076.7 ± 86.0; polyarticular: 1,066.7 ± 80.6; ERA: 1,077.1 ± 63.2; systemic onset: 1,068.9 ± 39.6 mg/cm^3, $P < 0.0001$). In comparison to the first examination, a significant increase in CrtBMD for the JIA patients (1,079.8 ± 82.1 versus 1,050.2 ± 126.5 mg/cm^3, $P < 0.05$) was observed, although no differences among the oligoarticular (1,076.7 ± 86.0 versus 1,057.5 ± 142.4 mg/cm^3), polyarticular (1,066.7 ± 80.6 versus 1,068.1 ± 76.8 mg/cm^3), and ERA (1,077.1 ± 63.2 versus 1,070.4 ± 71.2 mg/cm^3) subgroups were detected; a significant difference was noted for the systemic-onset subgroup (1,068.9 ± 39.6 versus. 994.0 ± 87.3 mg/cm^3, $P < 0.0001$). The controls showed a significant increase of CrtBMD with age (1,078.3 ± 73.1 versus 1,039.6 ± 79.3, $P < 0.05$).

However, the JIA patients' CBA values (Figure 2d) were confirmed to be significantly reduced with respect to the controls (149.0 ± 87.6 vs. 214.3 ± 74.3 mm^2, $P < 0.0001$); these results were also observed when the subjects were divided into oligoarticular (149.8 ± 45.0 mm^2; $P < 0.0001$), polyarticular- (139.46 ± 47.50 mm^2, $P < 0.0001$), and systemic-onset subgroups (160.5 ± 49.5 mm^2; $P < 0.005$), but not for the ERA subtype (198.5 ± 69.2 mm^2; P = NS). With respect to the first evaluation, we did not observe significant differences across all JIA patients (149.0 ± 87.6 versus 136.3 ± 122.1 mm^2, P = NS), nor did we observe such differences for the oligoarticular (149.8 ± 45.0 versus 148.5 ± 112.0 mm^2; P = NS), ERA (198.5 ± 69.2 versus 187.5 ± 64.5 mm^2, P = NS), and polyarticular (186.3 ± 131.1 versus 139.5 ± 47.5 mm^2, P = NS) subgroups; however, the systemic-onset patients (160.5 ± 49.5 versus 126.3 ± 49.0 mm^2; $P < 0.05$) had significantly increased values.

Muscle CSA (Figure 2e) was confirmed to be significantly reduced in JIA with respect to controls (2,083.7 ± 697.8 versus 2579.3 ± 794.5 mm^2, $P < 0.0001$). When the patients were divided into subgroups, we observed a significant difference in the oligoarticular (2,126.5 ± 711.9, $P < 0.0001$), polyarticular (2,146.7 ± 670.7 mm^2, $P < 0.001$), and systemic (2,056.9 ± 401.0 mm^2, $P < 0.0001$) subtypes but not in the ERA subtype (2,281.2 ± 887.9 mm^2, P = NS). In comparison to the first examination, we did not observe significant differences in the whole group of JIA patients (2,112.7 ± 732.4 versus 2,083.7 ± 697.8 mm^2, P = NS) nor in the oligoarticular (2,126.5 ± 711.9 versus 2,167.7 ± 870, P = NS), polyarticular (2,146.7 ± 670.7 versus 2,100.5 ± 764.4 mm^2, P = NS), systemic-onset (2,056.9 ± 401.0 versus 2,023.2 ± 632.8 mm^2, P = NS), and ERA (2,420.2 ± 973.1 mm^2, P = NS) subgroups. Conversely, for the controls, we observed a significant increase with age (2,579.3 ± 794.5 versus 2,398.5 ± 773.3 mm^2, $P < 0.001$).

Fat CSA (Figure 2f) was still significantly increased in the JIA patients compared with controls (1,110.1 ± 483.7 versus 945.8 ± 394.2 mm^2, $P < 0.005$), a finding that was similar for all subtypes (oligoarticular: 1,103.2 ± 489.3 mm^2, $P < 0.005$; polyarticular: 1,099.0 ± 565.2 mm^2, $P < 0.0001$; systemic: 1,255.5 ± 423.1 mm^2, $P < 0.0001$; ERA: 1,289.7 ± 766.8 mm^2, $P < 0.0001$). With respect to the first examination, we did not find any significant difference for the whole group of JIA patients (1,110.1 ± 483.7 versus 1,143.1 ± 649.1 mm^2, P = NS) nor for any subtype (oligoarticular: 1,103.2 ± 489.3 versus 1,129.6 ± 451.0, P = NS; polyarticular: 1,099.0 ± 565.2 versus 1,080.9 ± 504.8 mm^2, P = NS; systemic onset: 1,255.5 ± 423.1 versus 1,139.7 ± 351.9 mm^2, P = NS; ERA: 1,289.7 ± 766.8 versus 1,335.2 ± 748.2 mm^2, P = NS).

The SSIp longitudinal evaluation (Figure 2g) showed that the JIA patients had slightly significant lower levels than the controls (306.8 ± 200.7 versus 276.7 ± 110.4 mm^3, $P < 0.05$), which was also found in the oligoarticular (287.6 ± 178.4, P = NS) and polyarticular subsets (316.1 ± 209.4,

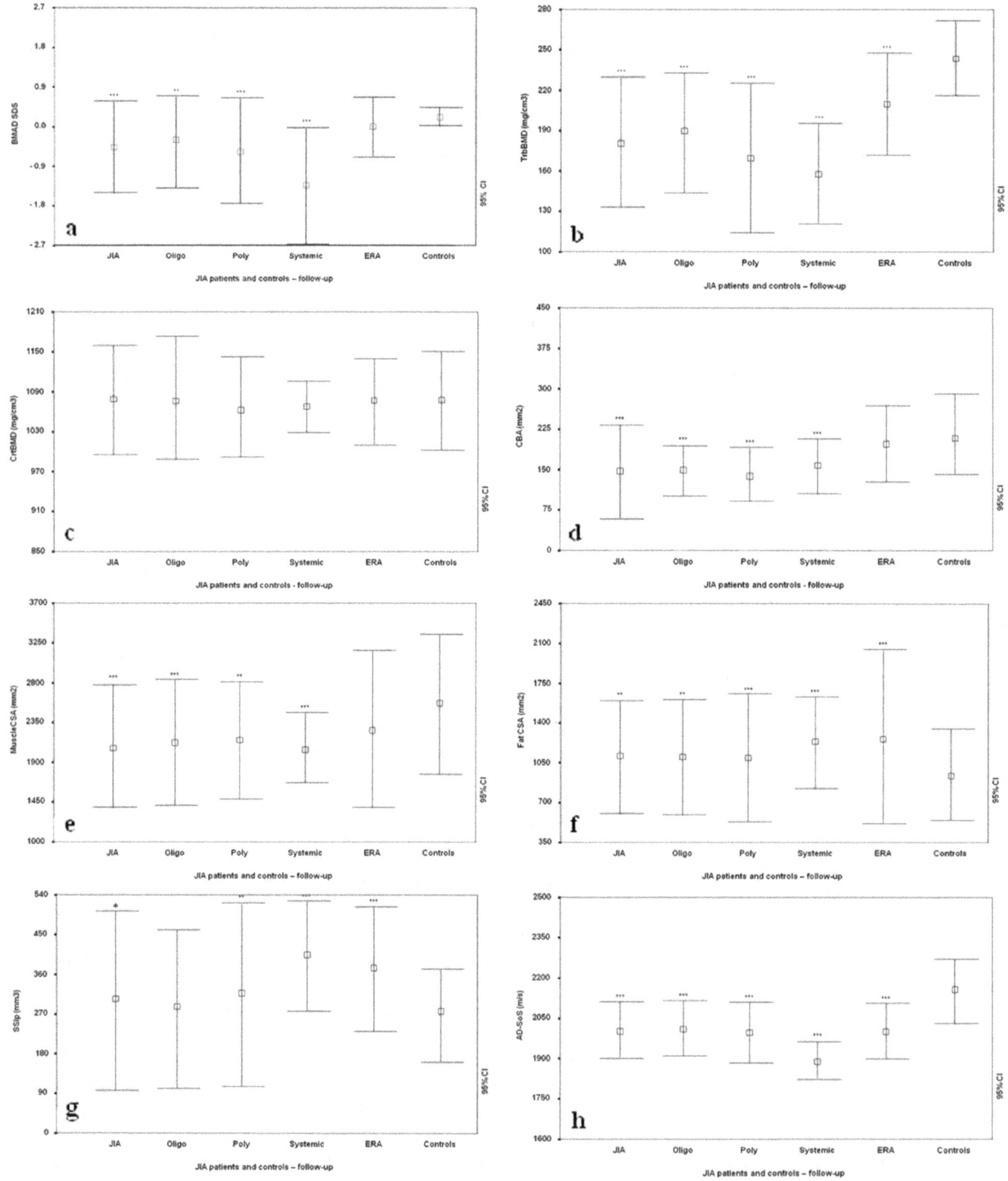

Figure 2 Longitudinal evaluation. Spine bone mineral apparent density (spine BMAD) SDS **(a),** trabecular bone mineral density (TrabBMD) **(b),** cortical bone mineral density (CrtBMD) **(c),** cortical bone area (CBA) **(d),** muscle cross-sectional area (MuscleCSA) **(e),** fat cross-sectional area (FatCSA) **(f),** density-weighted polar section modulus [SSIp] **(g),** and Ad-SoS **(h)** in patients with oligoarticular, polyarticular, systemic, and enthesitis-arthritis (ERA) JIA versus controls. Bars represent means and 95% confidence intervals. $^{**}P < 0.005$; $^{***}P < 0.001$.

$P < 0.005$). In contrast, the subjects with systemic onset (410.4 ± 132.1, $P < 0.001$) and ERA (374.1 ± 139.1, $P < 0.001$) had SSIp values significantly increased above those of the controls (Figure 2). At follow-up, we detected significant differences in the JIA patients (306.8 ± 250.7 versus 246.3 ± 140.2 mm^3, $P < 0.05$), but not in the controls (276.7 ± 110.4 versus 284.0 ± 127.9 mm^3, P = NS). The results were replicated when JIA patients were divided into oligoarticular (251.7 ± 144.5 versus 287.6 ± 178.4 mm^3, P = NS) and ERA (374.1 ± 139.1 versus 403.1 ± 189.9 mm^3, P = NS) subgroups, whereas SSIp was significantly increased in the polyarticular- (314.1 ± 329.4 versus 220.2 ± 82.9 mm^3, $P < 0.05$) and systemic-onset (400.4 ± 157.1 versus 228.0 ± 68.6 mm^3, $P < 0.001$) subgroups.

Finally, longitudinal follow-up showed that AD-SoS (Figure 2h) remained significantly reduced (2,003.0 ± 101.1 versus 2152.8 ± 118.9 m/s, $P < 0.001$) in all subtypes of the JIA patients (oligoarticular: 2,016.1 ± 95.3 m/s; polyarticular: 1,993.3 ± 108.0 m/s; systemic: 1,897.0 ± 67.7 m/s; ERA: 2,000.4 ± 100.1 m/s, $P < 0.0001$). With respect to the first examination, we did not find significant differences for any JIA subgroups. The results remained comparable when we evaluated QUS z-scores between the JIA patients and controls (−0.5 ± 1.5 versus 0.2 ± 1.8, $P < 0.005$) and between the subtypes and controls (polyarticular: −0.7 ± 1.5; systemic: −3.3 ± 1.0; ERA: −0.7 ± 1.4, $P < 0.0001$); this finding was not replicated for the oligoarticular-onset subgroup (−0.2 ± 1.3, P = NS). Analyzing the first examination, we did not find significant differences for any subset of JIA patients.

The correlations among the variables in the longitudinal study are reported in Tables 2 and 3.

Discussion

This study confirms our previously published data and further emphasizes that patients with JIA, although currently effective therapies are available, still manifest impaired bone mass and architecture. In addition, these patients seem not to reach a normal condition over time, potentially having a high risk of osteoporosis in early adulthood [3]. This characteristic is especially notable for children with polyarticular or systemic onset, whereas those with the oligoarticular and ERA subtypes do not show low values of BMAD SDS and other bone-density and quality determinants.

Furthermore, our results show remarkable evidence for significant musculoskeletal deficits in JIA patients and persistent impaired bone accrual over a period of years, thereby leading to further reductions of bone mass, in agreement with previously reported data [1,30,31]. Our baseline results using pQCT elucidate substantial muscle-skeletal deficits, partially due to the underlying inflammation typical of JIA. Nevertheless, our longitudinal data show that this pattern likely represents the combined effects of decreased biomechanical loading by muscle forces and increased inflammatory cytokines, because only patients with systemic onset experienced significant amelioration from antiinflammatory treatments.

Indeed, as muscles increase during growth, bones adjust by increasing in their dimensions and strength. The capacity of bone to respond to mechanical loading with increased bone strength is at its maximum during childhood [1]. Numerous studies have demonstrated that physical activity during childhood promotes cortical bone acquisition, either because of greater periosteal expansion or greater endosteal contraction [1,30].

In the last decades, new antirheumatic drugs, such as methotrexate and anti-TNF-α agents, have radically altered the course and outcome of JIA [32]. Despite these changes, numerous studies have documented persistent impaired bone mass and density in the majority of JIA patients [1,3]. This may suggest that current therapies, despite improving overall skeletal health, do not support adequate bone mass with respect to controls across nearly all JIA subgroups, thereby causing subsequent osteopenia and osteoporosis [3]. This hypothesis may be confirmed by the fact that many patients in our study did not have active arthritis at the time of evaluation.

Thus, bone alterations in JIA likely represent a mixed defect of bone development and lower muscle strength [6]. Our data show that young adults with a history of JIA may be susceptible to deleterious alterations in cortical bone strength and trabecular bone density, placing them at greater risk of fracture in the future. To reduce the risk, close monitoring of BMD, better control of disease activity, dietary intake of calcium and vitamin D, and especially greater physical activity may be advocated to support greater bone mass [3]. Thus, interventions aimed to improve muscle mass and strength may optimize bone health, resulting in a better PBM.

However, our data provide evidence that children and adolescents with ERA seem not to have significant reductions in bone mass with respect to controls, although these patients may have lower levels of physical activity, poorer physical health, and more bodily pain compared with oligoarticular or polyarticular subtypes of patients and controls [33]. So reduced physical activity and reduction of muscular mass may not completely explain these differences between JIA patients and controls and between patients with ERA and other JIA subgroups. It is possible that the reduced physical activity may be critical in conditioning the missed or reduced bone accrual, whereas the reduction of BMAD, which is frequently present at diagnosis, may be more related to inflammation. Limited data are available in the literature regarding bone status in patients with ERA. Burnham *et al.* [6], by using pQCT of the left tibia, observed reduced trabecular vBMD z-scores in this subtype of JIA.

The observation that loss of bone mass in ankylosing spondylitis (AS) seems to occur only in patients with persistent active disease, strongly suggests that the inflammatory activity of the disease itself plays a major role in the pathophysiology of the early bone mineral disorders observed in these patients [34]. Disease duration may also have a role in contributing to impaired BMD in these patients.

Another concern of our study is the high values of fatCSA detected in the JIA patients with respect to controls. The link between fat area and BMD remains unclear. However, recent studies led researchers to hypothesize a strong relation among leptin, metabolic state, and immunologic self-tolerance [35]. Moreover, chronic systemic inflammation, present in chronic arthritis, has been shown to increase lipogenesis in nonadipose tissues and lipolysis in white adipose tissue, resulting in ectopic lipid deposition in nonadipose tissues, such as muscle and liver [36]. The production of proinflammatory cytokines, characterizing an autoimmune disorder such as SLE, could be associated with an increased secretion of leptin and ectopic lipid accumulation in skeletal muscles, and, conversely, with higher rates of bone turnover and consequent loss of bone mass.

Our data also suggest that JIA patients, except for those with oligoarticular onset, do not experience improvements in their QUS *z*-scores with respect to baseline. It has been postulated that QUS may reflect qualitative aspects of bone, such as elasticity and microarchitectural characteristics [37] and may potentially be suitable for measuring several of the various determinants of bone strength [38]. Therefore, although during the follow-up, DXA may show stable values, the other methods may indicate the contrary: a decrease of bone parameters in some JIA subgroups, thus better reflecting the evaluation of skeletal status.

Conclusions

Children with JIA are at risk for deleterious alterations in cortical bone strength and trabecular bone density, and consequently, for fractures. In contrast to other studies, our study demonstrated that the pronounced bone deficits in JIA are possibly also related to reductions in muscle cross-sectional area. Thus, bone alterations in JIA likely represent a mixed defect of bone remodeling and, in some cases, lower muscle forces. Future clinical trials assessing bone-active therapies and mechanical-loading interventions are required.

Abbreviations

AD-SoS: Amplitude-dependent speed of sound; BMAD: bone mineral apparent density; BMD: bone mineral density; BMI: body mass index; BTT: bone transmission time; CBA: cortical bone area; C-HAQ: Childhood Health Assessment Questionnaire; CrtBMD: cortical bone mineral density; DXA: dual-energy x-ray absorptiometry; ERA: enthesitis-related arthritis; FatCSA: fat cross-sectional area; JIA: juvenile idiopathic arthritis; MuscleCSA: muscle cross-sectional area; NSAIDs: nonsteroidal antiinflammatory drugs; PBM: peak bone mass; pQCT: peripheral quantitative computed tomography; QUS: quantitative ultrasonography; SDS: standard deviation score; SSIp: density-weighted polar-section modulus; TotBMD: total bone mineral density; TrbBMD: trabecular bone mineral density; vBMD: volumetric BMD.

Competing interests

The authors declare that no conflicts of interest could be perceived as prejudicing the impartiality of the research reported.

Authors' contributions

SS: conception and design, endocrinologic evaluation, manuscript writing, and final approval of the manuscript. LC: conception and design, data collection and analysis, manuscript writing, and final approval of the manuscript. FB: rheumatologic evaluation, data collection and analysis, manuscript writing, and final approval of the manuscript. CS: data collection and analysis, critical revision, and final approval of the manuscript. MMC: rheumatologic evaluation, critical revision, and final approval of the manuscript. MLB: endocrinologic evaluation, critical revision, and final approval of the manuscript. FF: rheumatologic evaluation, data collection, manuscript writing, critical revision, and final approval of the manuscript. All authors read and approved the final manuscript.

Funding

This research did not receive any specific grant from any funding agency in the public, commercial, or not-for-profit sectors.

Author details

[1]Health's Sciences Department, University of Florence, Florence, Italy. [2]Department of Internal Medicine, Endocrinology Unit, University of Florence, Florence, Italy. [3]Department of Internal Medicine, Section of Rheumatology, Transition Clinic, University of Florence, Viale Pieraccini 18, 50139 Florence, Italy.

References

1. Roth J, Bechtold S, Borte G, Dressler F, Girschick HJ, Borte M: **Osteoporosis in juvenile idiopathic arthritis: a practical approach to diagnosis and therapy.** *Eur J Pediatr* 2007, **166:**775–784.
2. Pepmueller PH, Cassidy JT, Allen SH, Hillman LS: **Bone mineralization and bone mineral metabolism in children with juvenile rheumatoid arthritis.** *Arthritis Rheum* 1996, **39:**746–757.
3. Stagi S, Masi L, Capannini S, Cimaz R, Tonini G, Matucci-Cerinic M, de Martino M, Falcini F: **Cross-sectional and longitudinal evaluation of bone mass in children and young adults with juvenile idiopathic arthritis: the role of bone mass determinants in a large cohort of patients.** *J Rheumatol* 2010, **37:**1935–1943.
4. Gravallese EM: **Bone destruction in arthritis.** *Ann Rheum Dis* 2002, **61:**84–86.
5. Strand V, Kavanaugh AF: **The role of interleukin-1 in bone resorption in rheumatoid arthritis.** *Rheumatology (Oxford)* 2004, **43:**10–16.
6. Burnham JM, Shults J, Dubner SE, Sembhi H, Zemel BS, Leonard MB: **Bone density, structure, and strength in juvenile idiopathic arthritis: importance of disease severity and muscle deficits.** *Arthritis Rheum* 2008, **58:**2518–2527.
7. Cleary AG, Lancaster GA, Annan F, Sills JA, Davidson JE: **Nutritional impairment in juvenile idiopathic arthritis.** *Rheumatology (Oxford)* 2004, **43:**1569–1573.
8. Roth J, Linge M, Tzaribachev N, Schweizer R, Kuemmerle-Deschner J: **Musculoskeletal abnormalities in juvenile idiopathic arthritis: a 4-year longitudinal study.** *Rheumatology (Oxford)* 2007, **46:**1180–1184.
9. Häkkinen A, Sokka T, Kautiainen H, Kotaniemi A, Hannonen P: **Sustained maintenance of exercise induced muscle strength gains and normal bone mineral density in patients with early rheumatoid arthritis: a 5 year follow up.** *Ann Rheum Dis* 2004, **63:**910–916.
10. Falcini F, Trapani S, Civinini R, Capone A, Ermini M, Bartolozzi G: **The primary role of steroids on the osteoporosis in juvenile rheumatoid arthritis patients evaluated by dual energy X-ray absorptiometry.** *J Endocrinol Invest* 1996, **19:**165–169.

11. Celiker R, Bal S, Bakkaloğlu A, Ozaydin E, Coskun T, Cetin A, Dinçer F: **Factors playing a role in the development of decreased bone mineral density in juvenile chronic arthritis.** *Rheumatol Int* 2003, **23**:127–129.
12. Bonjour JP, Chevalley T, Ferrari S, Rizzoli R: **The importance and relevance of peak bone mass in the prevalence of osteoporosis.** *Salud Publica Mex* 2009, **51**:S5–S17.
13. Varonos S, Ansell BM, Reeve J: **Vertebral collapse in juvenile chronic arthritis: its relationship with glucocorticoid therapy.** *Calcif Tissue Int* 1987, **41**:75–78.
14. Henderson CJ, Panush RS: **Diets, dietary supplements, and nutritional therapies in rheumatic diseases.** *Rheum Dis Clin North Am* 1999, **25**:937–968. ix.
15. Wey HE, Binkley TL, Beare TM, Wey CL, Specker BL: **Cross-sectional versus longitudinal associations of lean and fat mass with pQCT bone outcomes in children.** *J Clin Endocrinol Metab* 2011, **96**:106–114.
16. Baroncelli GI, Federico G, Vignolo M, Valerio G, del Puente A, Maghnie M, Baserga M, Farello G, Saggese G, Phalangeal Quantitative Ultrasound Group: **Cross-sectional reference data for phalangeal quantitative ultrasound from early childhood to young-adulthood according to gender, age, skeletal growth, and pubertal development.** *Bone* 2006, **39**:159–173.
17. Falcini F, Bindi G, Ermini M, Galluzzi F, Poggi G, Rossi S, Masi L, Cimaz R, Brandi ML: **Comparison of quantitative calcaneal ultrasound and dual energy X-ray absorptiometry in the evaluation of osteoporotic risk in children with chronic rheumatic diseases.** *Calcif Tissue Int* 2000, **67**:19–23.
18. Górska A, Urban M, Bartnicka M, Zelazowska-Rutkowska B, Wysocka J: **Bone mineral metabolism in children with juvenile idiopathic arthritis: preliminary report.** *Ortop Traumatol Rehabil* 2008, **10**:54–62.
19. Kotaniemi A, Savolainen A, Kröger H, Kautiainen H, Isomäki H: **Weight-bearing physical activity, calcium intake, systemic glucocorticoids, chronic inflammation, and body constitution as determinants of lumbar and femoral bone mineral in juvenile chronic arthritis.** *Scand J Rheumatol* 1999, **28**:19–26.
20. Lurati A, Cimaz R, Gattinara M, Gerloni V, Teruzzi B, Salmaso A, Fantini F: **Skeletal mineralization in a prepubertal female population affected by juvenile idiopathic arthritis.** *Reumatismo* 2008, **60**:224–229.
21. Pereira RM, Corrente JE, Chahade WH, Yoshinari NH: **Evaluation by dual X-ray absorptiometry (DXA) of bone mineral density in children with juvenile chronic arthritis.** *Clin Exp Rheumatol* 1998, **16**:495–501.
22. Lien G, Selvaag AM, Flatø B, Haugen M, Vinje O, Sørskaar D, Dale K, Egeland T, Førre Ø: **A two-year prospective controlled study of bone mass and bone turnover in children with early juvenile idiopathic arthritis.** *Arthritis Rheum* 2005, **52**:833–840.
23. Petty RE, Southwood TR, Manners P, Baum J, Glass DN, Goldenberg J, He X, Maldonado-Cocco J, Orozco-Alcala J, Prieur AM, Suarez-Almazor ME, Woo P, International League of Associations for Rheumatology: **International League of Associations for Rheumatology classification of juvenile idiopathic arthritis: second revision, Edmonton, 2001.** *J Rheumatol* 2004, **31**:390–392.
24. Cacciari E, Milani S, Balsamo A, Spada E, Bona G, Cavallo L, Cerutti F, Gargantini L, Greggio N, Tonini G, Cicognani A: **Italian cross-sectional growth charts for height, weight and BMI (2 to 20 yr).** *J Endocrinol Invest* 2006, **29**:581–593.
25. Tanner JM, Whitehouse RH: **Clinical longitudinal standards for height, weight, height velocity, weight velocity, and stages of puberty.** *Arch Dis Child* 1976, **51**:170–179.
26. Kröger H, Kotaniemi A, Vainio P, Alhava E: **Bone densitometry of the spine and femur in children by dual-energy x-ray absorptiometry.** *Bone Miner* 1992, **17**:75–85.
27. Kröger H, Vainio P, Nieminen J, Kotaniemi A: **Comparison of different models for interpreting bone mineral density measurements using DXA and MRI technology.** *Bone* 1995, **17**:157–159.
28. D'Elia G, Caracchini G, Cavalli L, Innocenti P: **Bone fragility and imaging techniques.** *Clin Cases Miner Bone Metab* 2009, **6**:234–246.
29. Brunner HI, Lovell DJ, Finck BK, Giannini EH: **Preliminary definition of disease flare in juvenile rheumatoid arthritis.** *J Rheumatol* 2002, **29**:1058–1064.
30. Roth J, Palm C, Scheunemann I, Ranke MB, Schweizer R, Dannecker GE: **Musculoskeletal abnormalities of the forearm in patients with juvenile idiopathic arthritis relate mainly to bone geometry.** *Arthritis Rheum* 2004, **50**:1277–1285.
31. Felin EM, Prahalad S, Askew EW, Moyer-Mileur LJ: **Musculoskeletal abnormalities of the tibia in juvenile rheumatoid arthritis.** *Arthritis Rheum* 2007, **56**:984–994.
32. Simonini G, Giani T, Stagi S, de Martino M, Falcini F: **Bone status over 1 yr of etanercept treatment in juvenile idiopathic arthritis.** *Rheumatology (Oxford)* 2005, **44**:777–780.
33. Flatø B, Hoffmann-Vold AM, Reiff A, Førre Ø, Lien G, Vinje O: **Long-term outcome and prognostic factors in enthesitis-related arthritis: a case-control study.** *Arthritis Rheum* 2006, **54**:3573–3582.
34. Gratacós J, Collado A, Pons F, Osaba M, Sanmartí R, Roqué M, Larrosa M, Múñoz-Gómez J: **Significant loss of bone mass in patients with early, active ankylosing spondylitis: a followup study.** *Arthritis Rheum* 1999, **42**:2319–2324.
35. Matarese G, Procaccini C, De Rosa V: **At the crossroad of T cells, adipose tissue, and diabetes.** *Immunol Rev* 2012, **249**:116–134.
36. Mei M, Zhao L, Li Q, Chen Y, Huang A, Varghese Z, Moorhead JF, Zhang S, Powis SH, Li Q, Ruan XZ: **Inflammatory stress exacerbates ectopic lipid deposition in C57BL/6 J mice.** *Lipids Health Dis* 2011, **10**:110.
37. Glüer C, Wu C, Jergas M, Goldstein S, Genant H: **Three quantitative ultrasound parameters reflect bone structure.** *Calcif Tissue Int* 1994, **55**:45–52.
38. Faulkner KG, Glüer CC, Majumdar S, Lang P, Engelke K, Genant HK: **Noninvasive measurements of bone mass, structure, and strength: current methods and experimental techniques.** *AJR Am J Roentgenol* 1991, **157**:1229–1237.

3

Network analysis identifies protein clusters of functional importance in juvenile idiopathic arthritis

Adam Stevens[1], Stefan Meyer[1,2], Daniel Hanson[1], Peter Clayton[1*] and Rachelle Donn[3*]

Abstract

Introduction: Our objective was to utilise network analysis to identify protein clusters of greatest potential functional relevance in the pathogenesis of oligoarticular and rheumatoid factor negative (RF-ve) polyarticular juvenile idiopathic arthritis (JIA).

Methods: JIA genetic association data were used to build an interactome network model in BioGRID 3.2.99. The top 10% of this protein:protein JIA Interactome was used to generate a minimal essential network (MEN). Reactome FI Cytoscape 2.83 Plugin and the Disease Association Protein-Protein Link Evaluator (Dapple) algorithm were used to assess the functionality of the biological pathways within the MEN and to statistically rank the proteins. JIA gene expression data were integrated with the MEN and clusters of functionally important proteins derived using MCODE.

Results: A JIA interactome of 2,479 proteins was built from 348 JIA associated genes. The MEN, representing the most functionally related components of the network, comprised of seven clusters, with distinct functional characteristics. Four gene expression datasets from peripheral blood mononuclear cells (PBMC), neutrophils and synovial fluid monocytes, were mapped onto the MEN and a list of genes enriched for functional significance identified. This analysis revealed the genes of greatest potential functional importance to be *PTPN2* and *STAT1* for oligoarticular JIA and *KSR1* for RF-ve polyarticular JIA. Clusters of 23 and 14 related proteins were derived for oligoarticular and RF-ve polyarticular JIA respectively.

Conclusions: This first report of the application of network biology to JIA, integrating genetic association findings and gene expression data, has prioritised protein clusters for functional validation and identified new pathways for targeted pharmacological intervention.

Introduction

Juvenile idiopathic arthritis (JIA) is a common chronic disease of childhood. It is not a single disease, but a term that encompasses all forms of arthritis, of unknown origin, that begin before the age of 16 years and persist for longer than 6 weeks. It is the commonest form of chronic arthritis in children and the cause of substantial morbidity. JIA is a complex disease with both environmental factors, currently unknown, and genetic contributions to its aetiopathogenesis. Of the clinical subtypes defined by the International League Against Rheumatism (ILAR) classification of JIA [1] oligoarticular (both persistent and extended forms) and rheumatoid factor (RF)-negative (RF-ve) polyarticular arthritis are the predominant forms, accounting for approximately half of all presenting cases in the UK [2]. Factors that influence the susceptibility to, and progression of, these major phenotypic forms are currently unknown. Similarly, treatment options remain limited with steroid joint injections and methotrexate being most frequently employed. However, the relapse rate is often high and over 40% of individuals continue to have active disease as adults [3,4].

Replicated genetic loci from JIA candidate gene, genome-wide association studies (GWAS) and fine

* Correspondence: Peter.clayton@manchester.ac.uk; Rachelle.donn@manchester.ac.uk
[1]Manchester Academic Health Sciences Centre, Royal Manchester Children's Hospital, Manchester M13 9WL, UK
[3]Centre for Musculoskeletal Research, University of Manchester, Manchester M13 9PT, UK
Full list of author information is available at the end of the article

mapping genotyping are emerging [5-7]. In addition, a limited number of gene expression studies have attempted to establish changes in gene expression patterns with oligoarticular or with RF-ve polyarticular JIA subtypes [8-10]. Single nucleotide polymorphism (SNP) association studies, be it by a candidate gene or a GWAS approach, can identify variations that are associated with a particular complex trait. However, multiple constraints exist in extrapolating these observations forwards to any biological significance. SNP analysis, in the main, is done only at the single locus level. The associated variant may not be the functional polymorphism. Furthermore, SNPs associated with complex traits such as JIA, typically have small effect sizes and account for only a very small fraction of the genetic risk [11]. Thus, for most complex diseases, including JIA, an understanding of the underlying biology, leading to better diagnosis and treatment, is unlikely to arise by detailing the functional consequence of individual SNPs. Therefore, a major challenge for JIA, as for other complex diseases, is the integration of high-throughput omic datasets and subsequent identification and prioritisation of disease-associated loci for additional investigation.

JIA, most likely, arises as a result of abnormalities in genes, but more specifically, via the manifestation of perturbations in multiple protein networks that integrate cellular processes, and those that also link cells within tissues, and tissues within organ systems. An innovative approach to identifying key contributing genetic loci, and potential mechanisms of disease in patients with JIA, is the use of network biology. Network analysis (see Table 1) can allow the summation of various interactions and interdependencies between SNP associations and gene expression data [12]. Defining such a network structure is relevant for biological function. Topologically derived networks have interacting proteins that tend to be co-evolving [13], co-functional [14], and co-expressed [15,16].

It is recognised that for the majority of SNPs with a potential functional role in disease the genome-wide significance threshold for disease association ($P < 1 \times 10^{-8}$) may not be reached [17]. Therefore, despite not individually reaching genome-wide statistical significance, SNPs that cluster in networks can inform the underlying biology of a complex genetic disease such as JIA. Studies now describe how network biology place signature changes within the human interactome, uncovering some of the complexities of human diseases [12,18,19]. Furthermore, network analysis can inform drug discovery and drug targeting for complex genetic diseases such as JIA [20,21].

In this present study we have performed network analysis focussed on oligoarticular and RF-ve polyarticular arthritis, integrating genetic association data with gene expression data. This has been used to derive a JIA interactome, and clusters of proteins of functional relevance.

Table 1 Glossary

Term	Definition[a]
Bottleneck	A network position that limits the performance of the system. Described by the mathematical idea of *betweeness centrality* - a description of the number of paths travelling through a node in a network. An example would be a rate-limiting enzymatic reaction.
Cluster	A measure of the tendency of network nodes to form groups. It manifests from a high density of edges between nodes. In biological networks a cluster could represent a protein complex.
Connectivity/degree	The number of connections (see edge) made by any node within a network.
Edge	An interaction between two nodes. Commonly represents a protein:protein interaction but can also be representative of other biological phenomena such as co-expression.
Interactome	A network representing a whole set of direct and/or indirect interactions related to a specific biological phenomenon.
Minimal Essential Network (MEN)	Top 10% of network protein nodes, as scored by connectivity and bottleneck network properties. Corresponds to highly functionally related positions within the network.
Network analysis	Analysis that relates the structural and mathematical properties of a network to its function.
Node	A vertex within a network. In biological networks a node will usually be a gene, protein or metabolite.
Seed genes	A starting set of genes or metabolites of interest that are used to generate an interactome model by inferring joining interactions algorithmically.

[a]Further technical references are given in Stevens *et al.*, [33].

Methods

An overview of the approach taken is shown in Figure 1, and the sections below are labelled in correspondence with this figure. These sections detail the key processes and stages in the work flow for the formulation of the JIA subgroup specific network clusters of functional importance.

Genetic association data

Initially, PubMed [22] and Web of Science [23] searches were conducted and only validated SNP associations from studies of oligoarticular and RF-ve polyarticular JIA were selected. These included multiple well-replicated loci initially associated with adult rheumatoid arthritis found to be significantly associated with JIA [24-30]. In addition, the top findings ($P \leq 1 \times 10^{-4}$) from the largest GWAS study in JIA have been used [6], together with loci replicated by dense genotyping of immune-related disease regions in JIA [7]. SNPs were assigned to genes using an algorithm within Gene Relationships Across Implicated Loci (GRAIL) [31,32] (Additional file 1: Table S1A). This identified a total of 348 JIA-associated genes (Figure 1A).

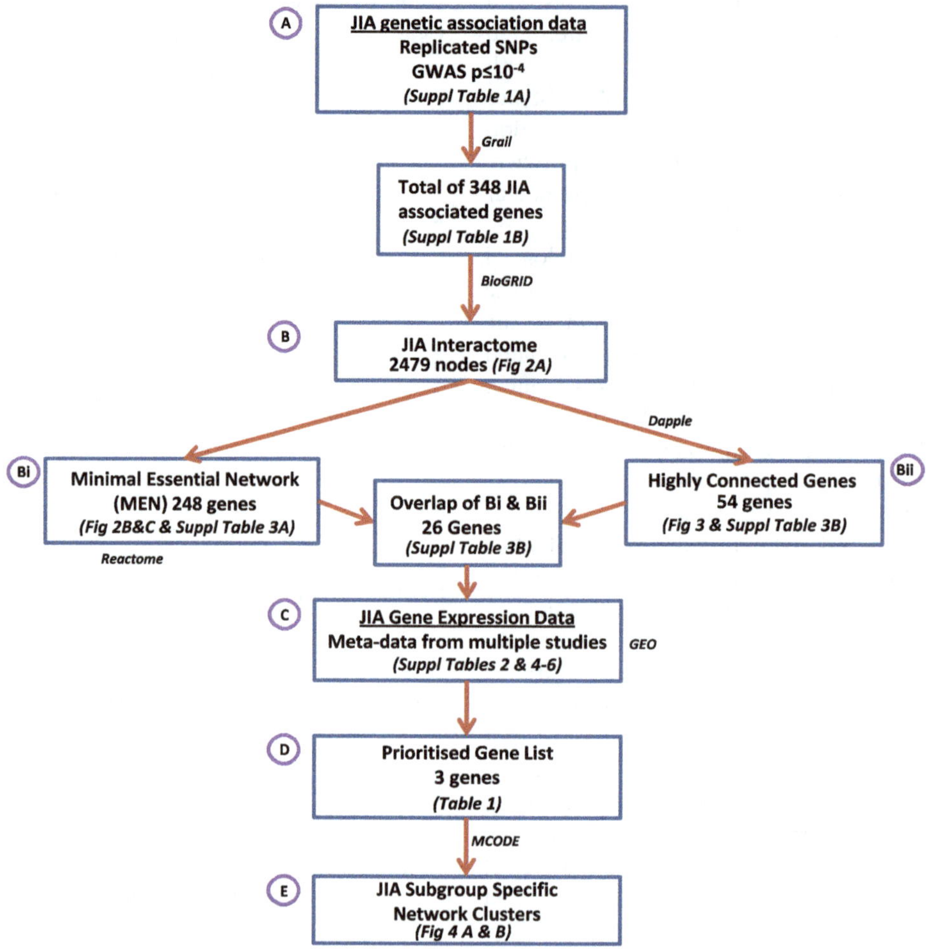

Figure 1 Overview of the workflow used to identify protein clusters of functional importance in rheumatoid factor-negative (RF-ve) polyarticular and oligoarticular juvenile idiopathic arthritis (JIA). This figure outlines each of the steps taken and gives cross references to the specific tables and figures that provide further details of that particular step in the process. **(A)** JIA genetic association data of replicated single nucleotide polymorphisms (SNPs) associated with RF-ve polyarticular JIA or oligoarticular JIA and JIA genome-wide association data findings were ascertained. SNPs were mapped to genes using Gene Relationships Across Implicated Loci (GRAIL) software (n = 348) (Additional file 1: Table S1A and B). **(B)** A JIA interactome network model (JIA Interactome) was inferred from JIA-associated genes using the BioGRID database (Figure 2A). **(Bi)** The top 10% of nodes, ranked by connectivity and bottlenecks, were used to derive a minimal essential network (MEN) of 248 genes (Figure 2B and Additional file 3: Table S3A). The Reactome database and spectral partition clustering was used to determine clusters of genes within the MEN (Figure 2C). **(Bii)** The Disease Association Protein-Protein Link Evaluator (Dapple) algorithm was used to identify Highly Connected Genes (Figure 3 and Additional file 3: Table S3B). The overlap of genes between **Bi** and **Bii** was determined (n = 26 genes) (Additional file 3: Table S3B). **(C)** JIA gene expression data from published sources, collated from the Gene Expression Omnibus database (GEO) (Additional file 2: Table S2 and Additional file 4: Table S4, Additional file 5: Table S5, Additional file 6: Table S6), was integrated with the overlap of the genes from **Bi** and **Bii**. **(D)** A prioritised list of JIA-associated genes with functionally associated network properties was identified from the integration of JIA genetic association and gene expression data (n = 3 genes) (Table 2). **(E)** MCODE was used to determine RF-ve polyarticular and oligoarticular JI-specific network clusters, protein:protein interactions of functional relevance (Figure 4A and B). GWAS, genome-wide association studies.

These 348 JIA-associated genes were the seed genes, that is, known genes that are used to generate an interactome model from all known protein-protein interactions (Additional file 1: Table S1B).

Building the JIA interactome

A JIA interactome was derived from the genetic association data using two independent methods (Figure 1Bi and Bii). Interactome modelling uses seed genes, in this case JIA-associated genes, to infer a network of protein: protein interactions, which are derived from known interactions between the seed genes and their near neighbours [33].

Bi: the first approach used the BioGRID Cytoscape Plugin [34] to create a filter for the BioGRID human interactome model (3.2.99), based on the JIA-associated genes. The resultant JIA interactome was visualised in Cytoscape (version 2.8.3). The Cytohubba Cytoscape Plugin was used to provide topological analysis of this network and connectivity and bottlenecks were calculated. The JIA interactome was then ranked for both connectivity and bottleneck properties and these were used to evaluate the relative importance of each node [35,36], and to generate a minimal essential network (MEN) [33,37,38]. The top 10% of network nodes was chosen to define the MEN (Figure 1Bi), as this represents the most functional elements of the network [33,37]. The Reactome FI Cytoscape 2.8.3 Plugin [39,40] was then used to determine clusters - distinct groups of protein:protein interactions [41] and to analyse the functional enrichment of biological pathways within the MEN.

Bii: the second approach utilised the Disease Association Protein-Protein Link Evaluator (Dapple) algorithm [42,43] and InWeb database [44]. This approach revealed highly connected genes within the JIA interactome by testing the significance of biological networks using a permutation method (10,000 permutations). The overlap of genes from Bi and Bii was determined using a Venn diagram (Partek Genomics Suite).

Gene expression data was integrated with the JIA interactome

Gene expression analysis was conducted on a library of gene expression datasets from children with JIA collated from the NCBI Gene Expression Omnibus (GEO) database (Additional file 2: Table S2). Selection was made based on the phenotypic criteria of oligoarticular or RF-ve polyarticular JIA and on control data being accessible.

Gene expression studies were downloaded from GEO [45] and annotation was assessed using QlucoreOmics Explorer 2.2 (Lund, Sweden). Sample comparisons were grouped for disease versus controls, or disease versus disease, using the data in the original peer-reviewed study. Available covariates (confounding factors) as provided in the published data were used. Four separate gene expression datasets were utilised [GEO:GDS711 [9], GSE:11083 [10], GSE:20307 [8], GSE:17755] [46]. The full details of these datasets are given in Additional file 2: Table S2.

Probe-to-gene assignment was made using the appropriate Affymetrix annotation file (Netaffx.com). Dimensional scaling using principal components analysis (PCA) and Iso-map multidimensional scaling [47,48] were used to demonstrate data homogeneity (Qlucore Omics Explorer 2.2) and to identify outliers using cross-validation. Analysis of variance (ANOVA) was used to determine differential gene expression between groups ($P \leq 0.05$) and functional associations were cross-referenced using Ingenuity Pathway Analysis software (IPA). Overlap of gene expression data sets was performed separately for both up- and down-regulated genes using Venn diagrams (Partek).

Deriving a list of prioritised genes of functional relevance

Genes identified within the MEN by network topology (Figure 1Bi) were overlapped with highly connected genes defined using Dapple ($P \leq 0.05$) (Figure 1Bii). This step identified network positions with putative functional importance using two semi-independent analytical approaches. This overlap was then combined with gene expression data (Figure 1C) to derive a prioritised list of genes of functional relevance.

Identification of JIA subgroup-specific network clusters

RF-ve polyarticular JIA and oligoarticular JIA clusters were identified from the JIA interactome using the MCODE algorithm plugin for Cytoscape [49]. These clusters identify the most highly related RF-ve polyarticular and oligoarticular JIA subgroup-specific genetic and transcriptomic data within the JIA interactome.

Statistics

Assessment of pathway associations was performed by the hypergeometric test using the Benjamini-Hochberg false discovery rate (FDR) correction (FDR correction-modified P-value ≤ 0.05) [50].

Results

Deriving a minimal essential network of biologically relevant JIA genes

A collated list of 348 JIA-associated seed genes was used to derive a JIA interactome inferred from the BioGRID human interactome database (3.2.99). This consisted of the 348 seed genes (marked red in Figure 2A) along with their immediate inferred interaction partners (protein: protein interactions - purple in Figure 2A). This gave a network of 2,479 proteins and 4,147 edges (Figure 2A). The top 10% of nodes, ranked by connectivity and bottleneck properties were selected to generate a minimal essential network (MEN) (Figure 2B, Additional file 3: Table S3A). The MEN represents the most functionally related components of a network [33,37].

The JIA-associated clusters (same colour code in Figure 2B and C; listed in Additional file 3: Table S3A) within the MEN were mapped onto biological pathways using the Reactome Cytoscape plugin to ascertain function. Six clusters were identified within the MEN, which had clear associated biological pathways (FDR, $p \leq 0.05$). These include pathways related to growth factor signalling and antigen presentation, regulation of the cell cycle and cytokine signalling (Figure 2C).

Permutation analysis of network topology

Network analysis of the JIA-associated genes was also performed using the Dapple algorithm [42]. This was done to calculate changes in connectivity in the inferred network greater than those expected by chance. First an inferred

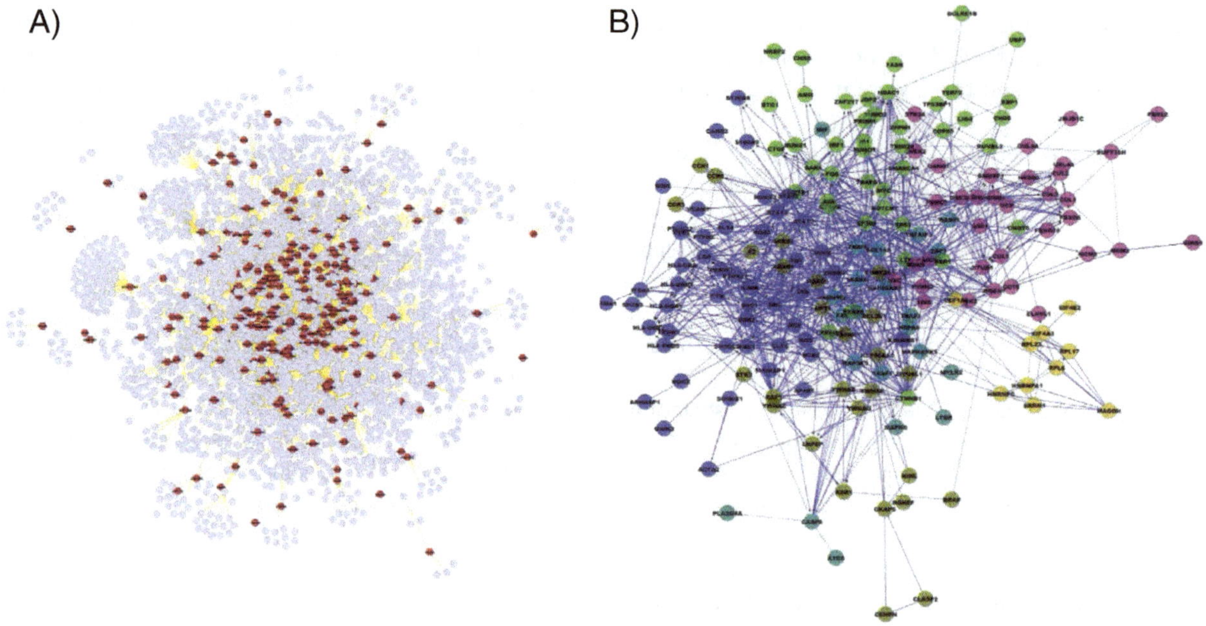

C)

Functional Group	Module	Pathway	FDR
Growth Factor Signalling & Antigen Presentation	1.	Angiogenesis	1.82E-05
		MHC class II antigen presentation	1.92E-05
		FGF signaling pathway	2.63E-05
		Signaling by PDGF	2.94E-05
		IGF1 pathway	5.56E-05
Signalling pathways	2.	Signaling by NOTCH	8.33E-05
		Wnt signaling pathway	9.09E-05
		TGF-beta signaling pathway	2.00E-04
		Regulation of Telomerase	2.50E-04
		Glucocorticoid receptor regulatory network	3.33E-04
Cell Cyle Regulation	3.	Regulation of DNA replication	1.11E-04
		Cell cycle	1.43E-04
		p53 pathway	5.00E-04
		Cellular responses to stress	7.50E-04
		Ubiquitin mediated proteolysis	1.00E-03
Cytokine Signalling	4.	IL2 signaling events mediated by PI3K	4.76E-05
		Chemokine signaling pathway	6.25E-05
		IL8- and CXCR1-mediated signaling events	2.00E-04
		IL8- and CXCR2-mediated signaling events	3.50E-04
		Class I PI3K signaling events mediated by Akt	1.00E-03
Immune response	5.	Toll-like receptor signaling pathway	6.67E-05
		FAS (CD95) signaling pathway	7.69E-05
		MAPK signaling pathway	1.25E-04
		TNF receptor signaling pathway	1.43E-04
		NF-kappa B signaling pathway	1.67E-04
RNA Splicing	6.	Translation	2.00E-04
		Spliceosome	3.33E-04
		RNA transport	5.00E-04

Figure 2 Network analysis of juvenile idiopathic arthritis (JIA)-associated genes. (A) A collated list of 348 JIA-associated genes was used to derive an interaction network inferred from the BioGRID model of the human interactome (3.2.99); red = JIA-associated gene, blue = inferred interaction (Figure 1B). **(B)** Minimal essential network of top 10% of the genes from the JIA interactome, ranked by connectivity and bottleneck, colours represent clusters of related genes calculated by spectral partition clustering [41] (Figure 1Bi). **(C)** Biological pathways associated with minimal essential network (MEN) clusters (colour of cluster relates to Figure 2B), false discovery rate (FDR) *P*-value of hypergeometric test ($P \leq 0.05$) (Figure 1Bi). *MHC* Major histocompatibility complex, *FGF* Fibroblast growth factor, *PDGF* Platelet-derived growth factor *IGF-1* Insulin-like growth factor 1, *TGF* beta Transforming growth factor beta, *IL-2* Interleukin 2, *IL-8* Interleukin 8 *PI3K* Phosphoinositide 3-kinase, *TNF* Tumour necrosis factor, *CXCR1* chemokine (C-X-C motif) receptor 1, *CXCR2* chemokine (C-X-C motif) receptor 2.

interaction network was derived using the JIA genetic associations as seed genes (Figure 1B). Permutation analysis of this inferred network demonstrated an increase of seed gene connectivity ($P < 0.002$). The seed genes were ranked, by *P*-value of increased connectivity (colour scale of ranking, Figure 3; all seed genes listed in Additional file 3: Table S3B).

Prioritisation of JIA-associated genes by integration of the JIA interactome with gene expression data

The overlap between the genes present within the MEN and the highly connected loci, identified by Dapple (Figure 1Bi and Bii) was established. This identified 26 genes of the 248 genes that occur in the MEN, that are ranked by Dapple with a *P*-value ≤0.05 (coloured orange

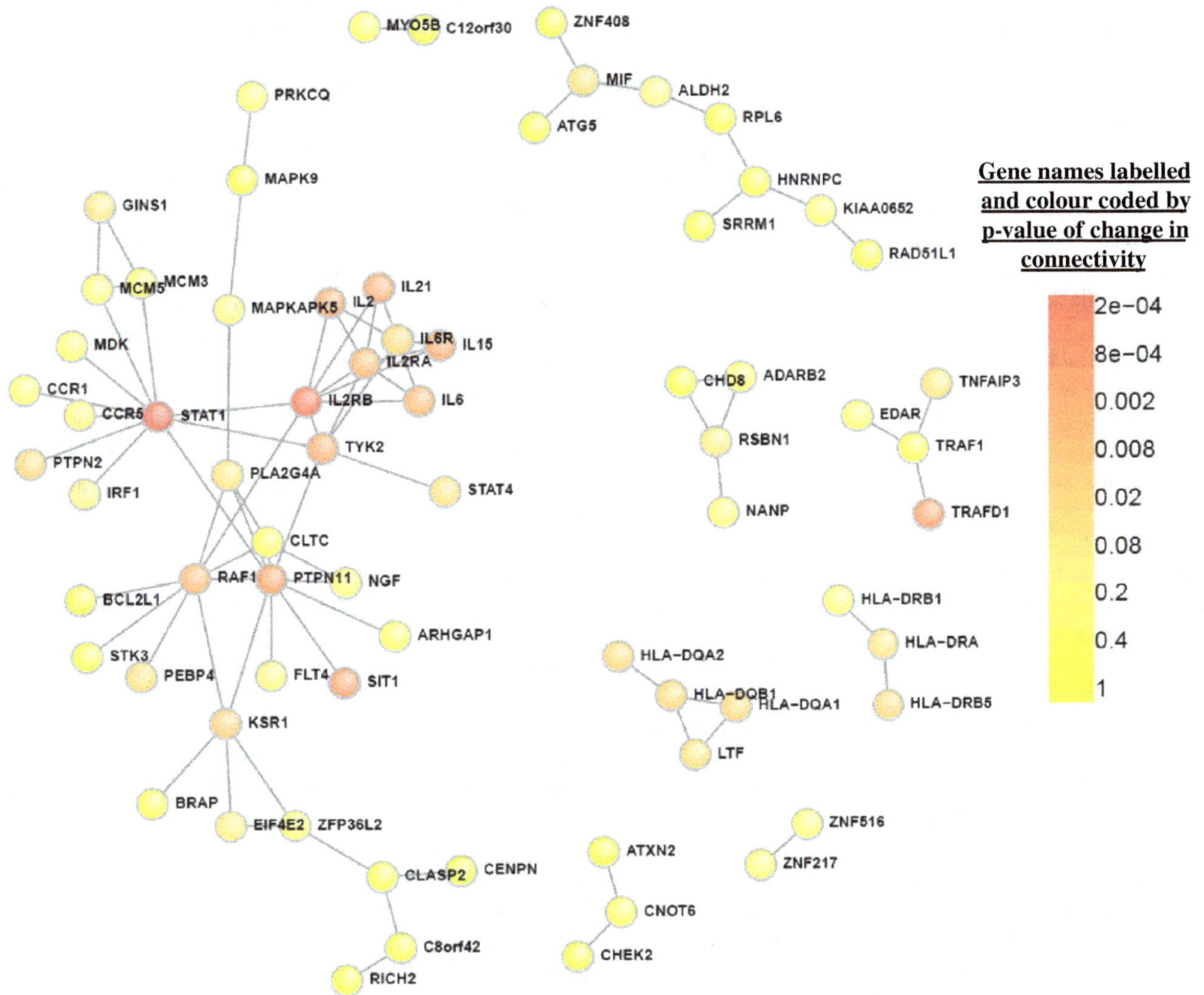

Figure 3 Changes in connectivity of juvenile idiopathic arthritis (JIA)-associated genes. The Disease Association Protein-Protein Link Evaluator (Dapple) algorithm was used to generate an inferred interactome network from the 348 JIA-associated genes, an iterative process was then used to generate random networks and significant changes in seed gene connectivity were calculated. The JIA-associated seed genes are shown coloured by significance of deviation of observed network connectivity from expected (red = highly significant to green = not significant) (Figure 1Bii).

in Additional file 3: Table S3B). These 26 genes represent the most highly connected, and therefore, potentially most functionally important loci, derived from the genetic association findings. Then, in order to prioritise these JIA-associated genes for future functional investigation, gene expression data were aligned (Figure 1C, Figure 2A - red nodes). Four different gene expression series were identified that provided data from RF-ve polyarticular, oligoarticular JIA and controls in previously published studies (GEO). These datasets allowed comparison between gene expression in peripheral blood mononuclear cells (PBMCs), neutrophils or synovial fluid monocytes (SFM) (Additional file 2: Table S2).

RF-ve polyarticular JIA versus controls

RF-ve polyarticular JIA gene expression data were compared with controls. Four comparisons were made using PBMC data and one using neutrophils (Additional file 2: Table S2). Comparisons were made separately between up-regulated and down-regulated genes. To increase confidence in the statistical interpretation of the data, and to reduce confounding effects, only genes with significant differential expression in at least three out of the five of these comparisons (Additional file 4: Table S4) were mapped onto JIA-associated genes ranked by network properties. In total this comprised 325 genes; 138 up-regulated and 187 down-regulated (Additional file 4: Table S4).

Oligoarticular JIA versus controls

Oligoarticular JIA gene expression was compared with controls using PBMC expression data (Additional file 2: Table S2). Comparisons were made separately between up-regulated and down-regulated genes. Genes with significant differential expression in both comparisons (Additional file 5: Table S5) were then mapped onto the list of JIA-associated genes ranked by network properties. There were a total of 150 genes with altered gene expression, 46 being up-regulated and 104 down-regulated (Additional file 5: Table S5).

Oligoarticular JIA versus RF-ve polyarticular JIA

Oligoarticular was compared to RF-ve polyarticular JIA gene expression data. Two PBMC and one synovial fluid mononuclear cell expression data set were utilised (Additional file 2: Table S2). Comparisons were made separately between up-regulated and down-regulated genes. Genes with significant differential expression in all three comparisons (Additional file 6: Table S6) were then mapped onto the list of JIA associated genes ranked by network properties. A total of 108 genes were changed, 88 were up-regulated and 20 were down-regulated (Additional file 6: Table S6).

JIA subgroup-specific loci of greatest functional relevance

The JIA subgroup specific loci of greatest functional relevance were identified as those loci that were present within the overlap of the MEN and highly connected genes (Figure 1Bi and Bii) with concomitant variation in gene expression (Figure 1C). These loci are listed in Table 2.

The network analysis identified *KSR1* as the locus of greatest potential functional relevance in RF-ve polyarticular JIA, and *PTPN2* for oligoarticular JIA (Table 2). *Signal transducer and activator of transcription 1* (*STAT1*) is differentially involved in oligoarticular versus the polyarticular subgroup. It has increased connectivity, indicating a primary functional role, in oligoarticular JIA compared with RF-ve polyarticular disease (Table 2).

Prioritised genes form JIA subgroup-specific functional clusters

In order to determine functional clusters, that is, distinct groups of protein:protein interactions in relation to the key prioritised genes, KSR1 for RF-ve polyarticular JIA and Protein tyrosine phosphatase, non-receptor type 2 (PTPN2) for oligoarticular JIA the MCODE algorithm was applied to the JIA interactome (Figure 1E). The MCODE algorithm identifies highly connected regions of biological networks representing clusters of related function that include protein:protein interaction complexes [49]. This approach identified two high scoring clusters each containing <25 proteins. High-scoring clusters have a high density of local connections and thus they represent a network region with related function [33,51,52]. The cluster score generated by an algorithm such as the MCODE algorithm used in this case, ranks network clusters as a way of prioritising function.

A cluster of 23 proteins contained PTPN2 and STAT1 (Figure 4A). Both *PTPN2* and *STAT1* are JIA-associated genes (Additional file 1: Table S1) with concomitant significant changes in gene expression in oligoarticular JIA patients. *PTPN2* was significantly down-regulated in oligoarticular JIA compared with controls; *STAT1* significantly increased in expression in oligoarticular compared to RF-ve polyarticular JIA cases (Additional file 6: Table S6). The main biological pathways associated with this cluster are cytokine signalling ($P < 1.8 \times 10^{-4}$) and DNA repair ($P < 1.4 \times 10^{-3}$).

A second functional cluster of 14 proteins was identified that contained KSR1 (Figure 4B). *KSR1* is a JIA-associated gene (Additional file 1: Table S1) with significant increased expression in RF-ve polyarticular JIA patients (Additional file 4: Table S4). The main biological pathways found to be associated with the KSR1-related cluster are the RAF/MAP kinase cascade ($P < 8.9 \times 10^{-5}$), cell cycle checkpoints ($P < 5.6 \times 10^{-4}$), DNA replication ($P < 1.3 \times 10^{-4}$) and cytokine signalling ($P < 1.2 \times 10^{-2}$).

Discussion

Recognising the necessity to move away from an approach focussed around the determination of SNP function *per se* we have utilised network biology approaches to reveal highly connected regions within a derived JIA interactome in order to identify the interplay of molecular elements that leads to the phenotypic expression of RF-ve polyarticular JIA or to oligoarticular JIA.

Table 2 Genes of greatest potential functional relevance determined by network analysis

	JIA-associated genes with correlated expression data that lie within the minimal essential network (MEN)	Dapple *P*-value
RF-ve polyarticular JIA compared with controls	*KSR1*	0.0088
Oligoarticular JIA compared with controls	*PTPN2*	0.0112
Oligoarticular compared with RF-ve polyarticular JIA	*STAT1*	0.0002

Genes present within the MEN which also show altered gene expression in either rheumatoid-negative (RF-ve) polyarticular juvenile idiopathic arthritis (JIA) compared with controls, oligoarticular JIA compared with controls, or between oligoarticular compared with RF-ve polyarticular JIA are listed. Presence in the MEN indicates functional priority and the Disease association protein-protein link evaluator (Dapple) *P*-value assesses the statistical significance of network connectivity compared to what would be expected by chance.

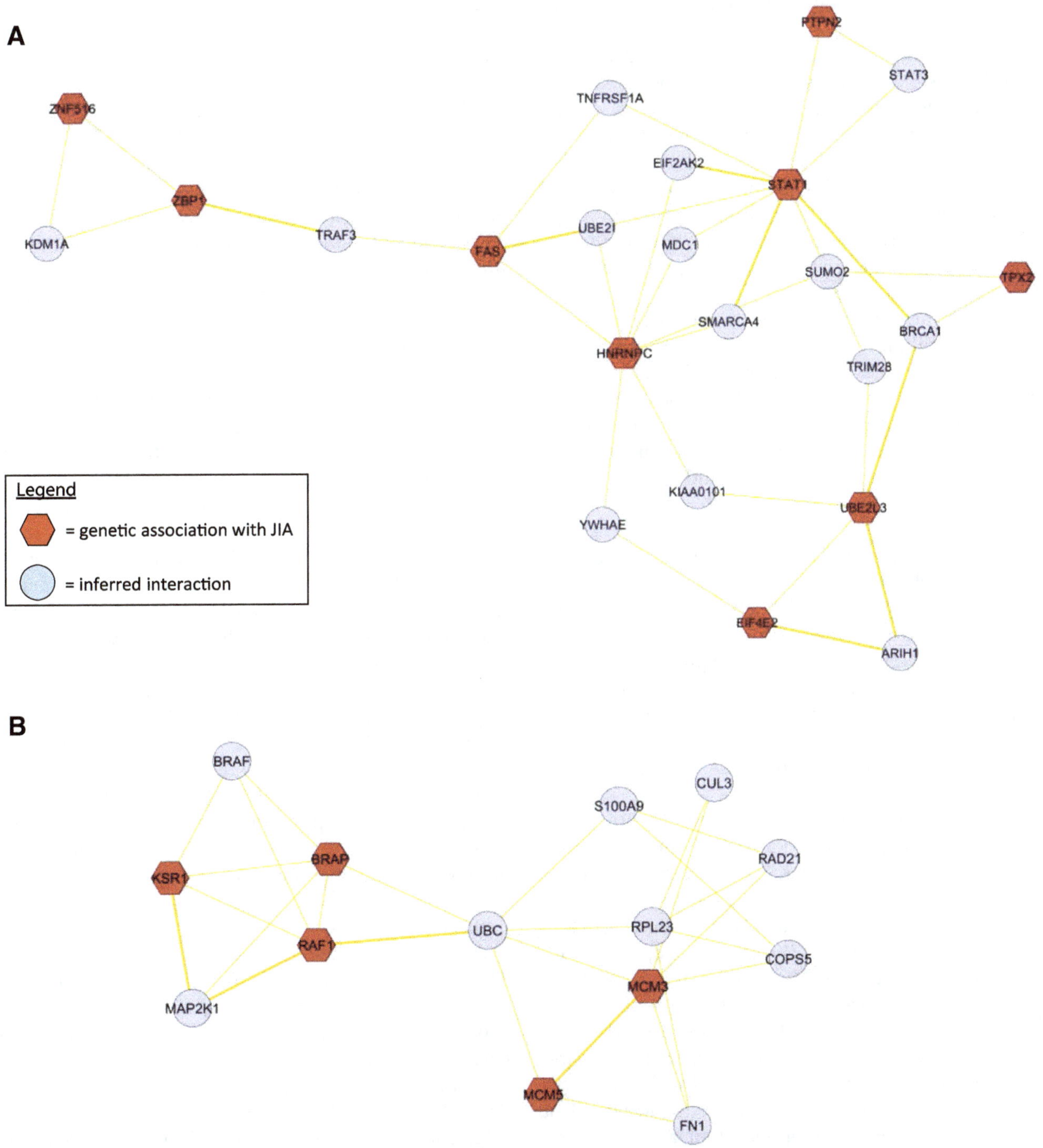

Figure 4 Identification of clusters of highly connected nodes within the juvenile idiopathic arthritis (JIA) interactome. Two clusters were identified using the MCODE clustering algorithm. **(A)** The oligoarticular JIA cluster includes PTPN2 and STAT1; **(B)** the RF-ve polyarticular related cluster contains KSR1. JIA-associated genes = red hexagons, blue circles = inferred genes within the JIA interactome (Figure 1E).

We have used a comprehensive set of genetic loci as the starting point to build the network. These loci are replicated SNP associations from candidate genes and the top statistical associations from recent GWAS and fine-mapping studies. There are limited collections of JIA patients worldwide to allow for subsequent GWAS or future GWAS meta-analysis. Given the premise that gene-gene interactions contribute to complex diseases, combining modest association signals from GWAS analysis with biological data to build networks can help to detect the joint effects of multiple genes [53]. Also, Hua *et al.* recently described the relevance of incorporating

GWAS SNPs with a *P*-value of lower than 0.01 in network analysis [54].

The genetic network was initially built using the BioGRID database. Subsequently, a MEN, representing the core genetic clusters related to the JIA phenotype, was derived using both connectivity and bottleneck network properties [12,33,36-38,55]. Six biological groupings were associated with the MEN, with a predominance of immune-related and cellular signalling pathways being represented (Figure 2). In addition, we utilised the approach described by Rossin *et al.* [42] to provide a statistical measure to the MEN.

The value of network biology is the inter-relational display of multiple omic datasets [56]. An integrated, multi-omic approach reduces noise in the statistical interpretation [57]. Furthermore, network biology focuses on the importance of clusters [58-61] as a measure of similarity rather than simply an overlap of gene sets. It is also an approach that is robust to random variation in the data [62] and to variation over different sizes of networks [60].

Our strategy has been to build the network from genetic association findings and to refine and validate the SNP data by overlaying stringently derived gene expression data. In order to have the most stringent refinement of the network we integrated the gene expression data with the MEN [33,37,38], and then the Dapple algorithm [42] was again employed to rank the gene expression loci that aligned to the MEN, to provide a further level of statistical robustness. This analysis identified JIA subgroup-specific loci.

The key seed gene for RF-ve polyarticular JIA is the scaffold kinase suppressor of Ras (*KSR1*). In three of the five gene expression datasets *KSR1* was over-expressed in RF-ve polyarticular JIA (Additional file 4: Table S4). KSR1 acts as a location-regulated scaffolding protein connecting MEK to RAF. It promotes MEK and RAF phosphorylation and activity through assembly of an activated signalling complex. By itself, however, it has not been demonstrated to have kinase activity. Importantly, Fusello *et al.* established that KSR1 knockout mice have reduced susceptibility to rheumatoid arthritis [63]. As KSR1-deficient T cells are functionally impaired [64] Fusello tested *Ksr*-deficient mice using a passive transfer model of arthritis. Their findings showed that the induction of arthritis is impaired in the absence of KSR1 and that this gene plays a role in ERK activation during inflammatory and stress responses both *in vitro* and *in vivo*. Using the MCODE algorithm, KSR1 interacts with a sub-cluster of 14 other proteins including a functional relationship with RAF1 (Figure 4B). We propose that this sub-cluster is of key functional relevance to the pathogenesis of RF-ve polyarticular JIA.

For oligoarticular JIA *PTPN2* was the seed gene of importance. *PTPN2* was significantly altered (down-regulated) in expression and mapped to the MEN (Additional file 5: Table S5). The cluster in relation to PTPN2 is shown, (Figure 4A), and consists of 23 proteins, the majority of which have a role in cytokine signalling and DNA repair.

PTPN2 encodes for the ubiquitously expressed T cell protein tyrosine phosphatase (TCPTP), a JAK/STAT and growth factor receptor phosphatase that has been linked with the pathogenesis of type 1 diabetes mellitus, rheumatoid arthritis and Crohn's disease by GWAS findings of non-coding SNP associations. Mouse and human studies have shown that reduced expression of TCPTP may drive autoimmune pathologies by enhancing signalling downstream of the T cell receptor (TCR), cytokines, or growth factors to produce a pro-inflammatory cytokine milieu [65].

Hinks *et al.* reported the *C5orf56-IRF1* region to show differential association between oligoarticular and RF-ve polyarticular JIA [7]. IRF1 is present in the MEN (Figure 2B & Additional file 3: Table S3A) and *IRF1* gene expression is significantly increased in oligoarticular compared to RF-ve polyarticular JIA (Additional file 6: Table S6). It has borderline significance in post iterative modelling (Dapple) ($P = 0.07$). *STAT1*, a signal transducer and transcription activator that mediates cytokine activity and growth factor, mapped within the MEN, was differentially expressed, with higher expression occurring in oligoarticular compared to RF-ve polyarticular disease, and met the FDR cut off for Dapple assignment of $P \leq 0.05$. STAT1 is present in the oligoarticular JIA but not the RF-ve polyarticular JIA sub-cluster. It appears, therefore, to represent a gene that differentiates between the oligoarticular and RF-ve polyarticular clinical subtypes. Further evaluation of IRF1 and STAT1 in persistent versus extended oligoarticular JIA is not possible as neither the genetic association nor the gene expression studies have classified oligoarticular JIA cases in this way.

The main observations from the GWAS analysis by Thompson *et al.* [6] relate to the *C3orf1* and *JMJD1C* genes. We find the proteins for these loci to be peripheral within our interactome network and they are not prioritised by Dapple. This implies that although these loci may have a role in JIA pathogenesis their lack of connectivity limits their druggable potential (reviewed in [66]).

Functional assessment of the RF-ve polyarticular and oligoarticular clusters needs to be determined. Mounting evidence indicates that biological systems are organised as modular networks, in which genes, proteins, metabolites and other factors operate in groups rather than as single entities. There is increasing recognition that transcription factors, micro RNAs, DNA methylation and chromatin remodelling regulate the expression of large numbers of genes in concert [67].

It is intriguing that preliminary analysis using the TargetScan human database [68] shows that the three candidate genes prioritised by this study (*KSR1, PTPN2* and *STAT1*) are co-regulated by miR-30a-5p ($P = 5.3 \times 10^{-4}$). Whilst hundreds of miRNAs have been identified to be dysregulated in various disease tissues, only a fraction have been functionally characterised. mIR 30a-5p been shown to be differentially expressed and to have biological function regulating expression of genes in a number of diseases including systemic lupus erythematosus (SLE) [69], rodent models of diabetes mellitus [70] glioma growth [71] and carcinoma of the colon [72]. Individual miRNAs can regulate several hundered transcripts with effector molecules that function at various sites within cellular pathways and networks, making them master regulators of the genome. miRNA-based therapy is progressing [73]. miRNAs of potential therapeutic value are those that yield satisfactory efficacy in disease model systems and mechanistic data to allow accurate placement of the miRNA into disease-related pathways. The network analysis we have conducted so far allows us to begin to investigate the capacity of mIR 30a-5p in a targeted way in JIA.

Repositioning of drugs is another important therapeutic advantage that can be maximised from network analysis [20,21]. The KSR1 sub-cluster (Figure 4B) could be therapeutically targeted in RF-ve polyarticular JIA patients, using small-molecule inhibitors of RAF1. Repurposing a drug such as sorafenib (nexavar), currently licensed for the treatment of renal and hepatocellular carcinoma, for the management of RF-ve polyarticular JIA could therefore be considered.

There are limitations to the present analysis. First, we have utilised data from a single GWAS, that is, the only one that currently exists for JIA, and included SNP associations of $P \leq 1 \times 10^{-4}$. The widening of input data for the generation of initial interactome networks is, however, acceptable and valid [53,54]. In addition, we have used the data from dense genotyping of immune-related loci [7]. Although only a proportion of the genes potentially involved in JIA pathogenesis may be immune-related, such pathways were highly significant within our network (Figure 2C). Interactome network models can be used to map associated biological function in a sensitive and robust manner via network clusters using stringent downstream analysis [33]. This is the strategy we have applied. Furthermore, if subsequent JIA GWAS or replication of new candidate gene associations do emerge, our network model can readily be adapted to incorporate the additional findings.

Second, there were only four gene expression studies suitable for inclusion. However, these four studies allowed comparisons across different cell populations (PBMCs, neutrophils, synovial fluid monocytes). Including gene expression data, significant across these sites, with the genetic association data and network analysis is a robust approach to identifying major contributing loci to the disease phenotype. Such integrative approaches have improved statistical power [56,57].

Third, the functional significance of the protein clusters remains to be established. The collection of biological material from oligoarticular and RF-ve polyarticular JIA patients is now underway to facilitate this.

Conclusions

To our knowledge this is the first use of network analysis to integrate JIA genetic and expression data for the prioritisation of loci for further functional assessment. The value of the use of network biology is to increase confidence in the observations of differentially expressed genes, and genetic findings, by correlation with functionally related network structure. This enhances the identification of functional units or clusters and, critically, can inform the targeting of new therapies. We have used different software-based methods (BioGRID, Ingenuity, Reactome) to infer relationships of differentially expressed genes and genetic association data with known interactions in the literature or protein databases. Dapple has been used at two stages in the analysis to add statistical robustness to our findings.

Deciphering the basis of complex pathologies such as JIA is challenging and although certain progress has been made, much remains to be understood. Deriving a JIA interactome model and sub-clusters, as described herein, offers the potential for a new era in addressing the mechanisms and future interventions for this chronic, disabling condition.

Additional files

Additional file 1: Table S1. Single nucleotide polymorphism (SNP) datasets: replicated loci showing association with oligoarticular and rheumatoid factor-negative (RF-ve) polyarticular juvenile idiopathic arthritis (JIA) were identified from published literature and collated with top genome-wide association studies (GWAS) findings **(A)**. The collated list of genes **(B)** was used as the seed genes for the network analysis and the generation of the JIA interactome (Figure 1).

Additional file 2: Table S2. Gene expression data: juvenile idiopathic arthritis (JIA) gene expression datasets were identified from the Gene Expression Omnibus (GEO). Details of the datasets include sample and control numbers, comparisons made, number of probe sets identified by analysis of variance (ANOVA) as significant (P <0.05), number of individual genes with a gene expression change, confounding factors included as covariants in the ANOVA and type of Affymetrix Chip. PBMC, peripheral blood mononuclear cells: SFM, synovial fluid mononuclear cells; Neut, neutrophils. Overlap groups used for comparisons are colour coded.

Additional file 3: Table S3. Network topology of the juvenile idiopathic arthritis (JIA) interactome: **(A)** Genes from the minimal essential network (MEN), that is, the top 10% of genes from the JIA interactome (ranked by degree (Deg) and bottleneck score (BN)). **(B)** JIA seed genes from the JIA interactome ranked by significance of deviation of observed network connectivity from expected (Disease Association Protein-Protein Link Evaluator (Dapple) algorithm, P ≤0.05). Orange = also present in minimal essential network (Figure 2B).

Additional file 4: Table S4. Rheumatoid factor-negative (RF-ve) polyarticular juvenile idiopathic arthritis (JIA) versus control gene expression: overlap of genes in RF-ve polyarticular JIA compared to controls present in three of the five gene expression datasets analysed. Datasets described in Additional file 2: Table S2. Red = up-regulated in JIA, green = down-regulated in JIA.

Additional file 5: Table S5. Oligoarticular versus control gene expression: overlap of genes in oligoarticular juvenile idiopathic arthritis (JIA) compared to controls present in both gene expression datasets analysed. Datasets described in Additional file 2: Table S2. Red = up-regulated in JIA, green = down-regulated in JIA.

Additional file 6: Table S6. Oligoarticular versus rheumatoid factor-negative (RF-ve) polyarticular juvenile idiopathic arthritis (JIA) gene expression: overlap of genes in oligoarticular JIA compared to RF-ve polyarticular JIA present in both gene expression datasets analysed. Datasets described in Additional file 2: Table S2. Red = up-regulated in JIA, green = down-regulated in JIA.

Abbreviations

ANOVA: analysis of variance; C3orf1: Chromosome 3 open reading frame 1; C5orf56: Chromosome 5 open reading frame 56; Dapple: Disease Association Protein-Protein Link Evaluator; FDR: false discovery rate; GEO: Gene Expression Omnibus; Grail: Gene Relationships Across Implicated Loci; GWAS: genome-wide association studies; ILAR: International League Against Rheumatism; IPA: Ingenuity pathway analysis; IRF1: Interferon regulatory factor 1; JIA: juvenile idiopathic arthritis; JMJD1C: Jumonji domain containing 1C; KSR1: Kinase suppressor of Ras; MEN: minimal essential network; PBMC: peripheral blood mononuclear cell; PCA: principal components analysis; PTPN2: Protein tyrosine phosphatase, non-receptor type 2; RF: rheumatoid factor; SFM: synovial fluid monocytes; SNP: single nucleotide polymorphism; STAT1: Signal transducer and activator of transcription 1.

Competing interests

The authors declare that they have no competing interests.

Authors' contributions

AS and RD conceived the idea for integrating genetic and transcriptomic datasets to investigate JIA. AS performed the analyses and developed the minimal essential network as a study tool. DH contributed to and supported network analysis of data. AS, RD, SM and PC designed the analysis plan and the presentation of the data. AS and RD led the writing of the manuscript with input from all authors. All authors read and approved the final manuscript.

Acknowledgements

AS is funded in part by a grant from Merck Serono SA, Geneva, Switzerland to assess the Pharmacogenomics of human growth disorders. DH is funded by the University of Manchester Wellcome Trust Institutional Strategic Support Fund. SM is supported by Leukaemia Lymphoma Research, UK, and the Kay Kendall Leukaemia Fund.

Author details

[1]Manchester Academic Health Sciences Centre, Royal Manchester Children's Hospital, Manchester M13 9WL, UK. [2]Stem Cell and Leukaemia Proteomics Laboratory, School of Cancer and Imaging Sciences, University of Manchester, Manchester, UK. [3]Centre for Musculoskeletal Research, University of Manchester, Manchester M13 9PT, UK.

References

1. Petty RE, Southwood TR, Manners P, Baum J, Glass DN, Goldenberg J, He X, Maldonado-Cocco J, Orozco-Alcala J, Prieur AM, Suarez-Almazor ME, Woo P: **International League of Associations for Rheumatology classification of juvenile idiopathic arthritis: second revision, Edmonton, 2001.** *J Rheumatol* 2004, **31:**390–392.
2. Hyrich KL, Lal SD, Foster HE, Thornton J, Adib N, Baildam E, Gardner-Medwin J, Wedderburn LR, Chieng A, Davidson J, Thomson W: **Disease activity and disability in children with juvenile idiopathic arthritis one year following presentation to paediatric rheumatology. Results from the Childhood Arthritis Prospective Study.** *Rheumatology (Oxford)* 2010, **49:**116–122.
3. Ravelli A, Martini A: **Juvenile idiopathic arthritis.** *Lancet* 2007, **369:**767–778.
4. Bertilsson L, Andersson-Gare B, Fasth A, Petersson IF, Forsblad-d'Elia H: **Disease course, outcome, and predictors of outcome in a population-based juvenile chronic arthritis cohort followed for 17 years.** *J Rheumatol* 2013, **40:**715–724.
5. Prahalad S, Glass DN: **A comprehensive review of the genetics of juvenile idiopathic arthritis.** *Pediatr Rheumatol Online J* 2008, **6:**11.
6. Thompson SD, Marion MC, Sudman M, Ryan M, Tsoras M, Howard TD, Barnes MG, Ramos PS, Thomson W, Hinks A, Haas JP, Prahalad S, Bohnsack JF, Wise CA, Punaro M, Rosé CD, Pajewski NM, Spigarelli M, Keddache M, Wagner M, Langefeld CD, Glass DN: **Genome-wide association analysis of juvenile idiopathic arthritis identifies a new susceptibility locus at chromosomal region 3q13.** *Arthritis Rheum* 2012, **64:**2781–2791.
7. Hinks A, Cobb J, Marion MC, Prahalad S, Sudman M, Bowes J, Martin P, Comeau ME, Sajuthi S, Andrews R, Brown M, Chen WM, Concannon P, Deloukas P, Edkins S, Eyre S, Gaffney PM, Guthery SL, Guthridge JM, Hunt SE, James JA, Keddache M, Moser KL, Nigrovic PA, Onengut-Gumuscu S, Onslow ML, Rosé CD, Rich SS, Steel KJ, Wakeland EK, *et al*: **Dense genotyping of immune-related disease regions identifies 14 new susceptibility loci for juvenile idiopathic arthritis.** *Nat Genet* 2013, **45:**664–669.
8. Barnes MG, Grom AA, Thompson SD, Griffin TA, Luyrink LK, Colbert RA, Glass DN: **Biologic similarities based on age at onset in oligoarticular and polyarticular subtypes of juvenile idiopathic arthritis.** *Arthritis Rheum* 2010, **62:**3249–3258.
9. Barnes MG, Aronow BJ, Luyrink LK, Moroldo MB, Pavlidis P, Passo MH, Grom AA, Hirsch R, Giannini EH, Colbert RA, Glass DN, Thompson SD: **Gene expression in juvenile arthritis and spondyloarthropathy: pro-angiogenic ELR + chemokine genes relate to course of arthritis.** *Rheumatology (Oxford)* 2004, **43:**973–979.
10. Frank MB, Wang S, Aggarwal A, Knowlton N, Jiang K, Chen Y, McKee R, Chaser B, McGhee T, Osban J, Jarvis JN: **Disease-associated pathophysiologic structures in pediatric rheumatic diseases show characteristics of scale-free networks seen in physiologic systems: implications for pathogenesis and treatment.** *BMC Med Genomics* 2009, **2:**9.
11. Chang D, Keinan A: **Predicting signatures of "synthetic associations" and "natural associations" from empirical patterns of human genetic variation.** *PLoS Comput Biol* 2012, **8:**e1002600.
12. Lee Y, Li H, Li J, Rebman E, Achour I, Regan KE, Gamazon ER, Chen JL, Yang XH, Cox NJ, Lussier YA: **Network models of genome-wide association studies uncover the topological centrality of protein interactions in complex diseases.** *J Am Med Inform Assoc* 2013, **20:**619–629.
13. Yeang CH, Haussler D: **Detecting coevolution in and among protein domains.** *PLoS Comput Biol* 2007, **3:**e211.
14. Agarwal S, Deane CM, Porter MA, Jones NS: **Revisiting date and party hubs: novel approaches to role assignment in protein interaction networks.** *PLoS Comput Biol* 2010, **6:**e1000817.
15. Han JD, Bertin N, Hao T, Goldberg DS, Berriz GF, Zhang LV, Dupuy D, Walhout AJ, Cusick ME, Roth FP, Vidal M: **Evidence for dynamically organized modularity in the yeast protein-protein interaction network.** *Nature* 2004, **430:**88–93.
16. Lemos B, Meiklejohn CD, Hartl DL: **Regulatory evolution across the protein interaction network.** *Nat Genet* 2004, **36:**1059–1060.
17. Duan S, Luo X, Dong C: **Identification of susceptibility modules for coronary artery disease using a genome wide integrated network analysis.** *Gene* 2013, **531:**347–354.
18. Vidal M, Cusick ME, Barabasi AL: **Interactome networks and human disease.** *Cell* 2011, **144:**986–998.
19. Goh KI, Cusick ME, Valle D, Childs B, Vidal M, Barabasi AL: **The human disease network.** *Proc Natl Acad Sci USA* 2007, **104:**8685–8690.
20. Randhawa V, Bagler G: **Identification of SRC as a potent drug target for asthma, using an integrative approach of protein interactome analysis and in silico drug discovery.** *OMICS* 2012, **16:**513–526.
21. Zhao S, Iyengar R: **Systems pharmacology: network analysis to identify multiscale mechanisms of drug action.** *Annu Rev Pharmacol Toxicol* 2012, **52:**505–521.
22. **PubMed.** [http://www.ncbi.nlm.nih.gov/pubmed]
23. **Web of Science.** [www.webofknowledge.com]
24. Donn R, Alourfi Z, Zeggini E, Lamb R, Jury F, Lunt M, Meazza C, De BF, Thomson W, Ray D: **A functional promoter haplotype of macrophage migration inhibitory factor is linked and associated with juvenile idiopathic arthritis.** *Arthritis Rheum* 2004, **50:**1604–1610.

25. Lamb R, Thomson W, Ogilvie E, Donn R: **Wnt-1-inducible signaling pathway protein 3 and susceptibility to juvenile idiopathic arthritis.** *Arthritis Rheum* 2005, **52**:3548–3553.
26. Hinks A, Eyre S, Ke X, Barton A, Martin P, Flynn E, Packham J, Worthington J, Thomson W: **Overlap of disease susceptibility loci for rheumatoid arthritis and juvenile idiopathic arthritis.** *Ann Rheum Dis* 2010, **69**:1049–1053.
27. Thompson SD, Sudman M, Ramos PS, Marion MC, Ryan M, Tsoras M, Weiler T, Wagner M, Keddache M, Haas JP, Mueller C, Prahalad S, Bohnsack J, Wise CA, Punaro M, Zhang D, Rosé CD, Comeau ME, Divers J, Glass DN, Langefeld CD: **The susceptibility loci Juvenile Idiopathic Arthritis shares with other autoimmune diseases extend to PTPN2, COG6 and ANGPT1.** *Arthritis Rheum* 2010, **62**:3265–3276.
28. Hinks A, Barton A, John S, Bruce I, Hawkins C, Griffiths CE, Donn R, Thomson W, Silman A, Worthington J: **Association between the PTPN22 gene and rheumatoid arthritis and juvenile idiopathic arthritis in a UK population: further support that PTPN22 is an autoimmunity gene.** *Arthritis Rheum* 2005, **52**:1694–1699.
29. Hinks A, Cobb J, Sudman M, Eyre S, Martin P, Flynn E, Packham J, Childhood Arthritis Prospective Study (CAPS); UK RA Genetics (UKRAG) Consortium; British Society of Paediatric and Adolescent Rheumatology (BSPAR) Study Group, Barton A, Worthington J, Langefeld CD, Glass DN, Thompson SD, Thomson W: **Investigation of rheumatoid arthritis susceptibility loci in juvenile idiopathic arthritis confirms high degree of overlap.** *Ann Rheum Dis* 2012, **71**:1117–1121.
30. Hinks A, Barton A, Shephard N, Eyre S, Bowes J, Cargill M, Wang E, Ke X, Kennedy GC, John S, Worthington J, Thomson W, British Society of Paediatric and Adolescent Rheumatology Study Group: **Identification of a novel susceptibility locus for juvenile idiopathic arthritis by genome-wide association analysis.** *Arthritis Rheum* 2009, **60**:258–263.
31. Raychaudhuri S, Plenge RM, Rossin EJ, Ng AC, Purcell SM, Sklar P, Scolnick EM, Xavier RJ, Altshuler D, Daly MJ: **Identifying relationships among genomic disease regions: predicting genes at pathogenic SNP associations and rare deletions.** *PLoS Genet* 2009, **5**:e1000534.
32. **GRAIL: Gene Relationships Across Implicated Loci.** [www.broadinstitute.org/mpg/grail/]
33. Stevens A, De Leonibus C, Hanson D, Dowsey AW, Whatmore A, Meyer S, Donn RP, Chatelain P, Banerjee I, Cosgrove KE, Clayton PE, Dunne MJ: **Network analysis: a new approach to study endocrine disorders.** *J Mol Endocrinol* 2013, **52**:R79–R93.
34. Chatr-Aryamontri A, Breitkreutz BJ, Heinicke S, Boucher L, Winter A, Stark C, Nixon J, Ramage L, Kolas N, O'Donnell L, Reguly T, Breitkreutz A, Sellam A, Chen D, Chang C, Rust J, Livstone M, Oughtred R, Dolinski K, Tyers M: **The BioGRID interaction database: 2013 update.** *Nucleic Acids Res* 2013, **41**:D816–D823.
35. Lin CY, Chin CH, Wu HH, Chen SH, Ho CW, Ko MT: **Hubba: hub objects analyzer–a framework of interactome hubs identification for network biology.** *Nucleic Acids Res* 2008, **36**:W438–W443.
36. Yu H, Kim PM, Sprecher E, Trifonov V, Gerstein M: **The importance of bottlenecks in protein networks: correlation with gene essentiality and expression dynamics.** *PLoS Comput Biol* 2007, **3**:e59.
37. Stevens A, Hanson D, Whatmore A, Destenaves B, Chatelain P, Clayton P: **Human growth is associated with distinct patterns of gene expression in evolutionarily conserved networks.** *BMC Genomics* 2013, **14**:547.
38. Stevens A, Clayton P, Tatò L, Yoo HW, Rodriguez-Arnao MD, Skorodok J, Ambler GR, Zignani M, Zieschang J, Della Corte G, Destenaves B, Champigneulle A, Raelson J, Chatelain P: **Pharmacogenomics of insulin-like growth factor-I generation during GH treatment in children with GH deficiency or Turner syndrome.** *Pharmacogenomics J* 2013, **14**:54–62.
39. Smoot ME, Ono K, Ruscheinski J, Wang PL, Ideker T: **Cytoscape 2.8: new features for data integration and network visualization.** *Bioinformatics* 2011, **27**:431–432.
40. Cline MS, Smoot M, Cerami E, Kuchinsky A, Landys N, Workman C, Christmas R, Avila-Campilo I, Creech M, Gross B, Hanspers K, Isserlin R, Kelley R, Killcoyne S, Lotia S, Maere S, Morris J, Ono K, Pavlovic V, Pico AR, Vailaya A, Wang PL, Adler A, Conklin BR, Hood L, Kuiper M, Sander C, Schmulevich I, Schwikowski B, Warner GJ, *et al*: **Integration of biological networks and gene expression data using Cytoscape.** *Nat Protoc* 2007, **2**:2366–2382.
41. Newman ME: **Modularity and community structure in networks.** *Proc Natl Acad Sci USA* 2006, **103**:8577–8582.
42. Rossin EJ, Lage K, Raychaudhuri S, Xavier RJ, Tatar D, Benita Y, Cotsapas C, Daly MJ: **Proteins encoded in genomic regions associated with immune-mediated disease physically interact and suggest underlying biology.** *PLoS Genet* 2011, **7**:e1001273.
43. **The DAPPLE algorithm.** [www.broadinstitute.org/mpg/dapple/dapple.php]
44. **InWeb Database.** [www.cbs.dtu.dk/suppl/dgf/]
45. **Gene Expression Omnibus.** [www.ncbi.nlm.nih.gov/geo/]
46. Lee HM, Sugino H, Aoki C, Nishimoto N: **Underexpression of mitochondrial-DNA encoded ATP synthesis-related genes and DNA repair genes in systemic lupus erythematosus.** *Arthritis Res Ther* 2011, **13**:R63.
47. Tenenbaum JB, De SV, Langford JC: **A global geometric framework for nonlinear dimensionality reduction.** *Science* 2000, **290**:2319–2323.
48. Nilsson J, Fioretos T, Hoglund M, Fontes M: **Approximate geodesic distances reveal biologically relevant structures in microarray data.** *Bioinformatics* 2004, **20**:874–880.
49. Bader GD, Hogue CW: **An automated method for finding molecular complexes in large protein interaction networks.** *BMC Bioinforma* 2003, **4**:2.
50. Benjamini YHY: **Controlling the false discovery rate: a practical and powerful approach to multiple testing.** *J R Stat Soc Se B Methodological* 1995, **57**:289–300.
51. Ravasz E, Barabasi AL: **Hierarchical organization in complex networks.** *Phys Rev E Stat Nonlin Soft Matter Phys* 2003, **67**:026112.
52. van Dongen S, Breu-Goodger C: **Using MCL to extract clusters from networks.** *Methods Mol Biol* 2012, **804**:281–295.
53. Pedroso I: **Gaining a pathway insight into genetic association data.** *Methods Mol Biol* 2010, **628**:373–382.
54. Hua L, Zhou P, Liu H, Li L, Yang Z, Liu ZC: **Mining susceptibility gene modules and disease risk genes from SNP data by combining network topological properties with support vector regression.** *J Theor Biol* 2011, **289**:225–236.
55. Sun YV: **Integration of biological networks and pathways with genetic association studies.** *Hum Genet* 2012, **131**:1677–1686.
56. Choi H, Pavelka N: **When one and one gives more than two: challenges and opportunities of integrative omics.** *Front Genet* 2011, **2**:105.
57. Ideker T, Dutkowski J, Hood L: **Boosting signal-to-noise in complex biology: prior knowledge is power.** *Cell* 2011, **144**:860–863.
58. Aloy P, Russell RB: **Taking the mystery out of biological networks.** *EMBO Rep* 2004, **5**:349–350.
59. Arrell DK, Terzic A: **Interpreting networks in systems biology.** *Clin Pharmacol Ther* 2013, **93**:389–392.
60. Barabasi AL, Albert R: **Emergence of scaling in random networks.** *Science* 1999, **286**:509–512.
61. Barabasi AL: **Scale-free networks: a decade and beyond.** *Science* 2009, **325**:412–413.
62. Albert R, Jeong H, Barabasi AL: **Error and attack tolerance of complex networks.** *Nature* 2000, **406**:378–382.
63. Fusello AM, Mandik-Nayak L, Shih F, Lewis RE, Allen PM, Shaw AS: **The MAPK scaffold kinase suppressor of Ras is involved in ERK activation by stress and proinflammatory cytokines and induction of arthritis.** *J Immunol* 2006, **177**:6152–6158.
64. Nguyen A, Burack WR, Stock JL, Kortum R, Chaika OV, Afkarian M, Muller WJ, Murphy KM, Morrison DK, Lewis RE, McNeish J, Shaw AS: **Kinase suppressor of Ras (KSR) is a scaffold which facilitates mitogen-activated protein kinase activation in vivo.** *Mol Cell Biol* 2002, **22**:3035–3045.
65. Zikherman J, Weiss A: **Unraveling the functional implications of GWAS: how T cell protein tyrosine phosphatase drives autoimmune disease.** *J Clin Invest* 2011, **121**:4618–4621.
66. Csermely P, Korcsmaros T, Kiss HJ, London G, Nussinov R: **Structure and dynamics of molecular networks: A novel paradigm of drug discovery: A comprehensive review.** *Pharmacol Ther* 2013, **138**:333–408.
67. Weiss JN, Karma A, MacLellan WR, Deng M, Rau CD, Rees CM, Wang J, Wisniewski N, Eskin E, Horvath S, Qu Z, Wang Y, Lusis AJ: **"Good enough solutions" and the genetics of complex diseases.** *Circ Res* 2012, **111**:493–504.
68. **TargetScan human database.** [http://www.targetscan.org/]
69. Dai Y, Sui W, Lan H, Yan Q, Huang H, Huang Y: **Comprehensive analysis of microRNA expression patterns in renal biopsies of lupus nephritis patients.** *Rheumatol Int* 2009, **29**:749–754.
70. Kim JW, You YH, Jung S, Suh-Kim H, Lee IK, Cho JH, Yoon KH: **miRNA-30a-5p-mediated silencing of Beta2/NeuroD expression is an important initial event of glucotoxicity-induced beta cell dysfunction in rodent models.** *Diabetologia* 2013, **56**:847–855.

71. Wang X, Wang K, Han L, Zhang A, Shi Z, Zhang K, Zhang H, Yang S, Pu P, Shen C, Yu C, Kang C: **PRDM1 is directly targeted by miR-30a-5p and modulates the Wnt/beta-catenin pathway in a Dkk1-dependent manner during glioma growth.** *Cancer Lett* 2013, **331**:211–219.
72. Baraniskin A, Birkenkamp-Demtroder K, Maghnouj A, Zollner H, Munding J, Klein-Scory S, Reinacher-Schick A, Schwarte-Waldhoff I, Schmiegel W, Hahn SA: **MiR-30a-5p suppresses tumor growth in colon carcinoma by targeting DTL.** *Carcinogenesis* 2012, **33**:732–739.
73. Wu Y, Crawford M, Mao Y, Lee RJ, Davis IC, Elton TS, Lee LJ, Nana-Sinkam SP: **Therapeutic delivery of microRNA-29b by cationic lipoplexes for lung cancer.** *Mol Ther Nucleic Acids* 2013, **2**:e84.

4

Automated determination of bone age and bone mineral density in patients with juvenile idiopathic arthritis

Janneke Anink[1†], Charlotte M Nusman[2,3*†], Lisette WA van Suijlekom-Smit[1], Rick R van Rijn[2], Mario Maas[2] and Marion AJ van Rossum[3,4]

Abstract

Introduction: Chronic inflammation combined with glucocorticoid treatment and immobilization puts juvenile idiopathic arthritis (JIA) patients at risk of impaired growth and reduced bone mineral density (BMD). Conventional methods for evaluating bone age and BMD are time-consuming or come with additional costs and radiation exposure. In addition, an automated measurement of bone age and BMD is likely to be more consistent than visual evaluation. In this study, we aimed to evaluate the feasibility of an automated method for determination of bone age and (cortical) bone mineral density (cBMD) in severely affected JIA patients. A secondary objective was to describe bone age and cBMD in this specific JIA population eligible for biologic treatment.

Methods: In total, 69 patients with standard hand radiographs at the start of etanercept treatment and of calendar age within the reliability ranges (2.5 to 17 years for boys and 2 to 15 years for girls) were extracted from the Dutch Arthritis and Biologicals in Children register. Radiographs were analyzed using the BoneXpert method, thus automatically determining bone age and cBMD expressed as bone health index (BHI). Agreement between measurements of the left- and right-hand radiographs and a repeated measurement of the left hand were assessed with the intraclass correlation coefficient (ICC). Regression analysis was used to identify variables associated with Z-scores of bone age and BHI.

Results: The BoneXpert method was reliable in the evaluation of radiographs of 67 patients (radiographs of 2 patients were rejected because of poor image quality). Agreement between left- and right-hand radiographs (ICC = 0.838 to 0.996) and repeated measurements (ICC = 0.999 to 1.000) was good. Mean Z-scores of bone age (−0.36, $P = 0.051$) and BHI (−0.85, $P < 0.001$) were lower compared to the healthy population. Glucocorticoid use was associated with delayed bone age (0.79 standard deviation (SD), $P = 0.028$), and male gender was associated with a lower Z-score of BHI (0.65 SD, $P = 0.021$).

Conclusions: BoneXpert is an easy-to-use method for assessing bone age and cBMD in patients with JIA, provided that radiographs are of reasonable quality and patients' bone age lies within the age ranges of the program. The population investigated had delayed bone maturation and lower cBMD than healthy children.

* Correspondence: c.m.nusman@amc.uva.nl
†Equal contributors
[2]Department of Radiology, Academic Medical Center, Meibergdreef 9, 1105 AZ Amsterdam, The Netherlands
[3]Department of Pediatric Hematology, Immunology, Rheumatology and Infectious Disease, Emma Children's Hospital, Academic Medical Center, Meibergdreef 9, 1105 AZ Amsterdam, The Netherlands
Full list of author information is available at the end of the article

Introduction

Chronic inflammatory diseases such as juvenile idiopathic arthritis (JIA) can influence bone development. Continuous exposure to inflammatory cytokines, together with glucocorticoid therapy, affects bone formation. This combined with decreased physical activity and pubertal delay puts JIA patients at risk of impaired growth and reduced bone mineral density (BMD) [1,2]. The pediatric rheumatologist needs to be aware of both the bone age and the BMD of JIA patients in order to take this into account in choosing the best therapy.

The assessment of bone age is usually made using the Greulich and Pyle atlas [3]. Dual-energy X-ray densitometry (DXA) is the most commonly used method of assessing BMD [4]. Recently, BoneXpert was developed, bringing back the use of radiogrammetry, one of the oldest methods for assessing BMD [5]. This new digital X-ray radiogrammetry (DXR) method combines the assessment of bone age with a radiogrammetric measurement of (cortical) BMD (cBMD) of the second to fourth metacarpal joints. The cBMD is expressed by BoneXpert as a Bone Health Index (BHI), in which cBMD is corrected for size. The BoneXpert method makes use of conventional radiographs of the hand, thereby making it attractive for pediatric use because of its simple application, relatively low costs [6]) and lower effective radiation dose compared with other methods. Normative data are available because the method was validated in a healthy pediatric population [7,8]. The application has not been tested in JIA patients, in whom long-standing inflammation of the wrist can lead to growth abnormalities and destruction of the bone, thereby possibly complicating the assessment of bone age and bone health. Utilization of the Dutch Arthritis and Biologicals in Children (ABC) register provides a unique way to evaluate this method in a severely affected JIA population eligible for biologic treatment.

Our objective in this study was to evaluate the feasibility of an automated method for the determination of bone age and cBMD in severely affected JIA patients. A secondary objective was to describe bone age and cBMD in this specific JIA population eligible for biologic therapy.

Methods

Patient selection

Patients from two centers participating in the Dutch ABC register who were prospectively enrolled between 1999 and 2012 were eligible for this study. Biologic-naïve patients were selected, starting etanercept, of whom a standard radiograph of both hands and wrist in the posteroanterior view was made at the start of treatment (that is, 1 year before to 3 months after starting etanercept). The participants' calendar age had to be within the reliability range of the BoneXpert method (that is, 2.5 to 17 years for boys and 2 to 15 years for girls). Ultimately, the radiographs of 69 patients were eligible for automatic analysis by BoneXpert. A flowchart of the patient selection is provided in Additional file 1.

Clinical data collection

The ABC register, a multicenter, prospective, observational study, aimed to include all children diagnosed with JIA in whom biologic treatment was being initiated. Informed consent was obtained from all patients older than 12 years of age, in addition to the parents or guardians of all patients younger than 16 years of age. The study protocol was centrally approved by the Medical Ethics Committee of the Erasmus MC, and local permission was obtained from the ethical bodies in the two other participating hospitals (Academic Medical Center and Reade). From the ABC register, patient and disease characteristics were collected at baseline, including data on disease activity from the following sources: physician's global assessment of disease activity on a visual analogue scale (VAS) (range from 0 to 10 cm, with 0 being the best score); Childhood Health Assessment Questionnaire (CHAQ) (range from 0 to 3, with 0 being the best score) by patients and/or their parents, including global assessment of well-being and pain on a VAS (range from 0 to 10 cm, with 0 being the best score); number of joints with active arthritis and joints with limited motion; and erythrocyte sedimentation rate (ESR). Using these variables, the Juvenile Arthritis Disease Activity Score in 10 active joints (JADAS-10) was calculated. The scale from 0 to 40 represents the simple linear sum of the scores of the physician and parent and/or patient global assessment, an active joint count (up to 10 joints) and a normalized value of ESR to a 0 to 10 scale [9].

Image analysis

The stand-alone Windows product of BoneXpert (BoneXpert Version 2.1.0.12; Visiana, Holte, Denmark) was used to analyze the hand radiographs. BoneXpert automatically generates the following outcome variables: (calendar) age, bone age based on Greulich and Pyle, Z-scores of bone age (compared with a healthy reference population) [10], BHI and Z-scores of BHI [5]. BHI is based on the cortical thickness (T) of the three middle metacarpals. In the construction of BHI, metacarpal width (W) and length (L) are also incorporated to compensate for the high variation in stature of growing children, as expressed in the following formula [5]:

$$\mathrm{BHI} = \pi \mathrm{T}(1 - \mathrm{T}/\mathrm{W})/(\mathrm{LW})^{0.33}$$

The radiographs included the complete hand and wrist joints of both the left and right sides. All images were collected as a DICOM files from three different centers. If the radiographs were available only on conventional films, they were digitized with a Sierra Plus scanner (VIDAR Systems, Herndon, VA, USA) and converted to a 300-dpi DICOM file. During the analytical process in BoneXpert, possible error messages were noted. The left-hand radiograph was uploaded and analyzed in BoneXpert a second time in order to be able to determine its test–retest reliability.

Statistical analysis

Descriptive statistics are reported in terms of absolute numbers, median and interquartile range (IQR) or mean and standard deviation (SD). The single measure intraclass correlation coefficient (ICC) and Bland-Altman plots were used to determine the agreement of the outcome variables of the BoneXpert method.

To determine whether the Z-score of bone age and the Z-score of BHI were different from those in the healthy population, a one sample *t*-test was used. Univariate linear regression analysis was performed to identify variables associated with the Z-score of bone age and the Z-score of BHI. Because of the small sample size, only a limited number of variables could be tested. The prespecified variables entered into the univariate model were age, sex, JADAS-10, disease duration and use of systemic glucocorticoids, defined as "ever use" or "never use." All analyses were performed with SPSS version 20 software (SPSS, Chicago, IL, USA).

Results

Feasibility

A standard hand radiograph of both hands was available for 69 patients starting etanercept treatment. The calculations of bone age and BMD by BoneXpert took a few seconds. BoneXpert rejected the radiographs of two patients because of poor image quality, resulting in available BoneXpert outcomes of 67 patients. In three patients, an error message indicating uncertainty of bone age was given by BoneXpert; these patients had calendar ages within the BoneXpert age ranges (2.5 to 17 years for boys and 2 to 15 years for girls), but their bone age came out of the analysis to be outside these age ranges, resulting in an error message. However, BoneXpert produced all outcome variables in these three patients, except for a missing Z-score of BHI in one patient.

The ICC of the agreement of all outcome variables between the left and right hand radiographs varied from 0.838 to 0.996. Bland-Altman plots of the agreement between left- and right-hand radiographs are provided in Additional file 2. The ICC of the agreement of repeated measurements of all left-hand radiographs on Z-scores of bone age and BHI varied from 0.999 to 1.000.

Patient and disease characteristics

Patient and disease characteristics of the 67 patients who could be evaluated with BoneXpert are presented in Table 1. Disease activity of these patients was moderate to severe at the time the hand radiographs were made (mean JADAS-10 score = 21 ± 5).

Table 1 Patient and disease characteristics at start of etanercept therapy[a]

Baseline characteristics	*N* = 67 patients
Females, *n* (%)	36 (54)
Age at onset JIA in years, mean (±SD)	8.5 (±3.8)
Age at start etanercept in years, mean (±SD)	11.0 (±3.1)
JIA disease duration before start etanercept in years, median (IQR)	1.8 (1.1 to 3.8)
ANA-positive, *n* (%)	14 (21)
Category JIA, *n* (%)	
Systemic JIA	4 (6)
Polyarticular RF-negative	27 (40)
Polyarticular RF-positive	9 (13)
Oligoarticular extended	18 (27)
Psoriatic arthritis	5 (8)
Enthesitis-related arthritis	4 (6)
Previously used medications, *n* (%)	
Systemic prednisone	32 (48)
Methotrexate	66 (99)
DMARD other than MTX	14 (21)
Concomitant comedication at start of biologic therapy, *n* (%)	
Systemic prednisone	26 (39)
Methotrexate	64 (96)
DMARD other than MTX	2 (3)
Disease activity parameters at baseline, median (IQR)	
Physician-rated VAS (0 to 10 cm; best score = 0)	6.5 (5.0 to 7.4)
CHAQ total (0 to 3; best score = 0)	1.50 (0.90 to 2.10)
VAS pain (0 to 10 cm; best score = 0)	6.3 (2.4 to 7.7)
VAS well-being (0 to 10 cm; best score = 0)	6.1 (3.2 to 7.4)
Active joints	11 (7 to 18)
Limited joints	6 (3 to 13)
ESR	11 (5 to 29)
JADAS-10 (0 to 40), mean (±SD)	21 (±5)
Ever hand or wrist involvement, *n* (%)	64 (96)
Z-score of BA, mean (±SD)	−0.36 (±1.44)
Z-score of BHI, mean (±SD)	−0.85 (±1.15)[b]

[a]ANA, Antinuclear antibody; BA, Bone age; BHI, Bone Health Index; CHAQ, Child Health Assessment Questionnaire; DMARD, Disease-modifying antirheumatic drug; ESR, Erythrocyte sedimentation rate; JADAS, Juvenile Arthritis Disease Activity Score; JIA, Juvenile idiopathic arthritis; MTX, Methotrexate; RF, Rheumatoid factor; VAS, Visual analogue scale; Z-score, Standard deviation compared with healthy population. [b]Significantly different from 0 at the $P < 0.05$ level.

Bone maturation was delayed compared with the normal population, but not significantly (mean Z-score of bone age = −0.36 (±1.44), $P = 0.051$). Bone maturation was greatly impaired (below −2 standard deviations (SD)) in eight patients, and three patients had highly accelerated bone maturation (above +2 SD). The mean Z-score of bone age was strongly influenced by one patient with a very high bone age (+5 SD), who had long-standing severe polyarticular enthesitis-related arthritis. When this patient was left out of the analysis, the mean bone maturation of the remaining patients was significantly delayed (mean Z-score of bone age = −0.45 (±1.28), $P = 0.008$). Compared with the normal population, the cBMD was lower (mean Z-score of BHI = −0.85 (±1.15), $P < 0.001$). Ten patients had a Z-score of BHI less than −2 SD.

Regression analysis

A univariate linear regression analysis of bone age and BHI was performed to investigate which variables were associated with the Z-score of bone age and the Z-score of BHI (Tables 2 and 3). Glucocorticoid use was associated with a lower Z-score of bone age (0.79 SD, $P = 0.028$). Only male gender was significantly associated with the Z-score of BHI; being a boy lowered the Z-score of BHI of 0.65 points ($P = 0.021$).

Discussion

Application of the BoneXpert automated method for assessing bone age and cBMD in JIA patients proved to be feasible. Its use was easy and fast, and the program rejected few radiographs. The Z-scores of bone age and BHI were found to be impaired in the population of JIA patients evaluated in this study compared with a healthy population.

In addition to its validation in a healthy pediatric population [7,8], bone age measurement using BoneXpert has been evaluated in pediatric patients of short stature, children with precocious puberty and patients with congenital adrenal hyperplasia [11-13]. In these patient groups, in whom bone maturation is likely to be affected, the BoneXpert bone measurement method proved feasible. We had anticipated a higher number of rejections by the BoneXpert program relating to growth abnormalities, periarticular abnormalities and deviation of bone age commonly found in severely affected JIA patients [14-17]. Unexpectedly, BoneXpert rejected no radiographs because of these abnormalities. Besides the two rejections due to poor image quality, only one radiograph with extremely accelerated bone maturation resulted in absence of a Z-score of BHI. The low rejection rate is advantageous; however, one has to take into account that patients outside the age ranges of the program had to be excluded, who were composed mostly of older patients (older than 15 years of age for girls and older than age 17 years for boys). For follow-up of patients, it would be useful if a BHI reference existed for children who have reached skeletal maturity. Besides a low rejection rate, the method also showed a very good agreement between left- and right-hand assessment and two repeated measurements of the left-hand radiograph. The excellent agreement of the repeated measurement of one radiograph is to be expected, whereas BoneXpert is an automated computer technique. Other methods used to determine reliability, such as analysis of two radiographs of the same hand of the same patient at one time point, could not be performed, because these radiographs were not available. Bone maturation and cBMD were found to be impaired, as was expected for this group of JIA patients [1,2,17]. A regression analysis showed that delayed bone age was associated with glucocorticoid use and that lower BHI was associated with male gender. The association between delayed bone age and glucocorticoid use was not unexpected, as numerous studies have shown that glucocorticoid use may slow longitudinal bone growth and growth plate senescence [18,19]. In other earlier studies, not only bone age but also impaired BMD has been associated with the use of glucocorticoids [1,20,21]. In the present study, this was not the case; the only variable in the regression analysis significantly associated with cBMD was male gender. The lack of association between glucocorticoid use and cBMD could be due to the broad definition of glucocorticoid use (that is, cumulative dose was not taken into account) and the relatively small size of our study

Table 2 Univariate regression coefficients of baseline variables with Z-scores of bone age[a]

Baseline variable	Estimated β	95% CI	*P*-value
Age	0.024	−0.116 to 0.164	0.736
Male gender	−0.190	−0.921 to 0.541	0.605
Disease duration	−0.030	−0.184 to 0.1234	0.694
CHAQ	−0.021	−0.577 to 0.534	0.940
JADAS-10	0.008	−0.065 to 0.081	0.830
Ever use of systemic glucocorticoids	−0.790	−1.492 to −0.088	0.028

[a]CHAQ, Child Health Assessment Questionnaire; JADAS, Juvenile Arthritis Disease Activity Score; Z-score, Standard deviation score compared with healthy population.

Table 3 Univariate regression coefficients of baseline variables with the Z-score of Bone Health Index[a]

Baseline variable	Estimated β	95% CI	*P*-value
Age	0.067	−0.024 to 0.159	0.147
Male gender	−0.649	−1.197 to −0.102	0.021
Disease duration	0.040	−0.080 to 0.160	0.505
CHAQ	0.008	−0.420 to 0.436	0.971
JADAS-10	−0.036	−0.094 to 0.023	0.224
Ever use of systemic glucocorticoids	−0.340	−0.904 to 0.224	0.233

[a]CHAQ, Child Health Assessment Questionnaire; JADAS, Juvenile Arthritis Disease Activity Score; Z-score, Standard deviation score compared with the healthy population.

population. On the other hand, several randomized trials in adults with rheumatoid arthritis have shown that glucocorticoids can decelerate the loss of hand BMD [22,23]. Although rheumatoid arthritis and JIA are two different entities, a similar protective effect of glucocorticoids on hand BMD may have played a role in our population. The association with male gender is less easy to interpret. It was previously shown that differences exist between healthy boys and girls in BMD of the forearm, with boys having higher BMD of the forearm than girls [24]. This difference is not associated with body mass index, but is likely to be associated with other factors. The same group also found an association between physical activity and BMD of the forearm, combined with the finding that boys are more physically active than girls [25]. The difference in BHI between boys and girls in the current studies might therefore be explained by low physical activity due to disease activity and by boys being relatively less physically active compared to their healthy peers than girls. The link between physical activity and lower cortical thickness of the forearm was also hinted at in a study in pediatric Crohn's disease patients. In that study, a lower cortical thickness was also found in boys, which improved with treatment, possibly because patients also increased their daily physical activities with their response to treatment [26].

The BoneXpert method is used to measure bone age and BHI. With respect to bone age, the method can be considered feasible for future use in multicenter or longitudinal follow-up studies in JIA patients, because of its easy use, high precision and small differences between left- and right-hand radiographs [8]. Besides its application in research, the BoneXpert method can also potentially be of use in clinical practice. The automatic determination of bone age and cBMD is less costly than other methods and is time-saving for both pediatric rheumatologists and radiologists. Moreover, only one hand—either right or left—needs to be analyzed, which increases the feasibility of use in daily practice (unless there is an extreme clinical discrepancy between left and right).

The other major outcome variable, the BHI, needs more validation studies before it can be used in research and clinical practice. The DXR method for the assessment of cBMD, used by BoneXpert, has been compared to DXA in several patient groups, including patients with inflammatory bowel disease [27]. In these patients, the correlation between DXR and DXA was found to be moderate to good. In JIA patients, however, cBMD of the hand may be influenced by local inflammation, possibly resulting in a lower correlation with generalized BMD, as shown in adult patients with rheumatoid arthritis [28]. If BHI can be used as a proxy for generalized BMD in JIA patients, further validation in this population is needed, including a comparison with other BMD measurement techniques. This is complicated by the fact that there are different methods used to determine BMD without consensus on the gold standard, although DXA is the most widely utilized technique.

Limitations

This study is limited by its observational design and the very specific population derived from the ABC register. These factors introduce a selection bias, which limits generalization to the full JIA population. However, patients included in the ABC register are considered to be the most severely affected patients because of their eligibility for biologic treatment; therefore, these patients are most likely to have structural bone damage. It can be assumed that if the BoneXpert method can be applied in these patients, it can be used in all JIA patients. Most radiographs used in this study were digital; however, some conventional radiographs were included. BoneXpert works less well with these digitized images, as demonstrated by the two radiographs that were rejected by the program. Given the widespread use of digital radiology throughout Europe, this will not be a problem in future studies.

Conclusions

To our knowledge, this study is the first in which the BoneXpert automated determination of bone age and cBMD has been evaluated in JIA patients. The method proved feasible and easy to use, even in severely affected JIA patients, provided that radiographs were of reasonable quality and patients were within the age ranges of the BoneXpert program. This method can be implemented in clinical practice for the determination of bone age in JIA patients. It needs further validation for the determination of bone health, including comparison with existing methods for the determination of BMD.

Abbreviations

BA: Bone age; BHI: Bone Health Index; (c)BMD: (Cortical) bone mineral density; CHAQ: Child Health Assessment Questionnaire; DMARD: Disease-modifying antirheumatic drug; DXA: Dual-energy X-ray absorptiometry; DXR: Digital X-ray radiogrammetry; ESR: Erythrocyte sedimentation rate; ICC: Intraclass correlation coefficient; JADAS: Juvenile Arthritis Disease Activity Score; JIA: Juvenile idiopathic arthritis; MTX: Methotrexate; VAS: Visual analogue scale.

Competing interests

LvS has received research grants and/or research support from the Dutch Board of Health Insurances, Pfizer and AbbVie for the submitted work and grants outside the submitted work from the Dutch Arthritis Association; consultancy fees from Pfizer, Roche and Novartis; and travel grants from Pfizer and Bristol-Myers Squibb. JA and MvR have received travel grants from Pfizer. CN, RvR and MM declare that they have no competing interests.

Authors' contributions

JA and CN participated in the design of the study and performed data acquisition and data analysis. LvS RvR, MM and MvR participated in the study design and data interpretation. All authors read and approved the manuscript.

Acknowledgements

The authors acknowledge Hans Henrik Thodberg for his support with and the free use of BoneXpert. For maintenance and design of the ABC register, we received unconditional support from the Dutch Board of Health Insurances (2003–2006), unconditional support from Pfizer (formerly Wyeth International, since 2007) and unconditional support from AbbVie (formerly Abbott, 2010–2012).

Author details

[1]Department of Pediatrics/Pediatric Rheumatology, Sophia Children's Hospital, ErasmusMC, Wytemaweg 80, 3015 CN Rotterdam, The Netherlands. [2]Department of Radiology, Academic Medical Center, Meibergdreef 9, 1105 AZ Amsterdam, The Netherlands. [3]Department of Pediatric Hematology, Immunology, Rheumatology and Infectious Disease, Emma Children's Hospital, Academic Medical Center, Meibergdreef 9, 1105 AZ Amsterdam, The Netherlands. [4]Department of Pediatric Rheumatology, Reade location Jan van Breemen, Dr. Jan van Breeemenstraat 2, 1056 AB Amsterdam, The Netherlands.

References

1. Thornton J, Pye SR, O'Neill TW, Rawlings D, Francis RM, Symmons DP, Ashcroft DM, Foster HE: **Bone health in adult men and women with a history of juvenile idiopathic arthritis.** *J Rheumatol* 2011, **38:**1689–1693.
2. Burnham JM: **Inflammatory diseases and bone health in children.** *Curr Opin Rheumatol* 2012, **24:**548–553.
3. Greulich W, Pyle S: *Radiographic Atlas of the Skeletal Development of the Hand and Wrist.* 2nd edition. Stanford, CA: Stanford University Press; 1959.
4. van Rijn RR, van Kuijk C: **Of small bones and big mistakes: bone densitometry in children revisited.** *Eur J Radiol* 2009, **71:**432–439.
5. Thodberg HH, van Rijn RR, Tanaka T, Martin DD, Kreiborg S: **A paediatric bone index derived by automated radiogrammetry.** *Osteoporos Int* 2010, **21:**1391–1400.
6. **BoneXpert.** [www.bonexpert.com/the-bonexpert-product]
7. van Rijn RR, Lequin MH, Thodberg HH: **Automatic determination of Greulich and Pyle bone age in healthy Dutch children.** *Pediatr Radiol* 2009, **39:**591–597.
8. Thodberg HH, Sävendahl L: **Validation and reference values of automated bone age determination for four ethnicities.** *Acad Radiol* 2010, **17:**1425–1432.
9. Consolaro A, Ruperto N, Bazso A, Pistorio A, Magni-Manzoni S, Filocamo G, Malattia C, Viola S, Martini A, Ravelli A: **Development and validation of a composite disease activity score for juvenile idiopathic arthritis.** *Arthritis Rheum* 2009, **61:**658–666.
10. Thodberg HH, Kreiborg S, Juul A, Pedersen KD: **The BoneXpert method for automated determination of skeletal maturity.** *IEEE Trans Med Imaging* 2009, **28:**52–66.
11. Martin DD, Deusch D, Schweizer R, Binder G, Thodberg HH, Ranke MB: **Clinical application of automated Greulich-Pyle bone age determination in children with short stature.** *Pediatr Radiol* 2009, **39:**598–607.
12. Martin DD, Heil K, Heckmann C, Zierl A, Schaefer J, Ranke MB, Binder G: **Validation of automatic bone age determination in children with congenital adrenal hyperplasia.** *Pediatr Radiol* 2013, **43:**1615–1621.
13. Martin DD, Meister K, Schweizer R, Ranke MB, Thodberg HH, Binder G: **Validation of automatic bone age rating in children with precocious and early puberty.** *J Pediatr Endocrinol Metab* 2011, **24:**1009–1014.
14. Mason T, Reed AM, Nelson AM, Thomas KB, Patton A, Hoffman AD, Achenbach S, O'Fallon WM: **Frequency of abnormal hand and wrist radiographs at time of diagnosis of polyarticular juvenile rheumatoid arthritis.** *J Rheumatol* 2002, **29:**2214–2218.
15. Oen K, Reed M, Malleson PN, Cabral DA, Petty RE, Rosenberg AM, Cheang M: **Radiologic outcome and its relationship to functional disability in juvenile rheumatoid arthritis.** *J Rheumatol* 2003, **30:**832–840.
16. van Rossum MA, Zwinderman AH, Boers M, Dijkmans BA, van Soesbergen RM, Fiselier TJ, Franssen MJ, ten Cate R, van Suijlekom-Smit LW, Wulffraat NM, Kuis W, van Luijk WH, Oostveen JC, Dijkstra PF, Dutch Juvenile Idiopathic Arthritis Study Group: **Radiologic features in juvenile idiopathic arthritis: a first step in the development of a standardized assessment method.** *Arthritis Rheum* 2003, **48:**507–515.
17. Cassidy JT, Hillman LS: **Abnormalities in skeletal growth in children with juvenile rheumatoid arthritis.** *Rheum Dis Clin North Am* 1997, **23:**499–522.
18. Gupta N, Lustig RH, Kohn MA, Vittinghoff E: **Determination of bone age in pediatric patients with Crohn's disease should become part of routine care.** *Inflamm Bowel Dis* 2013, **19:**61–65.
19. Lui JC, Nilsson O, Baron J: **Growth plate senescence and catch-up growth.** *Endocr Dev* 2011, **21:**23–29.
20. Stagi S, Masi L, Capannini S, Cimaz R, Tonini G, Matucci-Cerinic M, de Martino M, Falcini F: **Cross-sectional and longitudinal evaluation of bone mass in children and young adults with juvenile idiopathic arthritis: the role of bone mass determinants in a large cohort of patients.** *J Rheumatol* 2010, **37:**1935–1943.
21. Mul D, van Suijlekom-Smit LW, ten Cate R, Bekkering WP, de Muinck Keizer-Schrama SM: **Bone mineral density and body composition and influencing factors in children with rheumatic diseases treated with corticosteroids.** *J Pediatr Endocrinol Metab* 2002, **15:**187–192.
22. Haugeberg G, Strand A, Kvien TK, Kirwan JR: **Reduced loss of hand bone density with prednisolone in early rheumatoid arthritis: results from a randomized placebo-controlled trial.** *Arch Intern Med* 2005, **165:**1293–1297.
23. Forslind K, Boonen A, Albertsson K, Hafström I, Svensson B, the BARFOT Study Group: **Hand bone loss measured by digital X-ray radiogrammetry is a predictor of joint damage in early rheumatoid arthritis.** *Scand J Rheumatol* 2009, **38:**431–438.
24. Hasselstrøm H, Karlsson KM, Hansen SE, Grønfeldt V, Froberg K, Andersen LB: **Sex differences in bone size and bone mineral density exist before puberty: the Copenhagen School Child Intervention Study (CoSCIS).** *Calcif Tissue Int* 2006, **79:**7–14.
25. Hasselstrøm H, Karlsson KM, Hansen SE, Grønfeldt V, Froberg K, Andersen LB: **Peripheral bone mineral density and different intensities of physical activity in children 6–8 years old: the Copenhagen School Child Intervention study.** *Calcif Tissue Int* 2007, **80:**31–38.
26. Werkstetter KJ, Pozza SB, Filipiak-Pittroff B, Schatz SB, Prell C, Bufler P, Koletzko B, Koletzko S: **Long-term development of bone geometry and muscle in pediatric inflammatory bowel disease.** *Am J Gastroenterol* 2011, **106:**988–998.
27. Mentzel HJ, Blume J, Boettcher J, Lehmann G, Tuchscherer D, Pfeil A, Kramer A, Malich A, Kauf E, Hein G, Kaiser WA: **The potential of digital X-ray radiogrammetry (DXR) in the assessment of osteopenia in children with chronic inflammatory bowel disease.** *Pediatr Radiol* 2006, **36:**415–420.

5

Transcription factor motif enrichment in whole transcriptome analysis identifies STAT4 and BCL6 as the most prominent binding motif in systemic juvenile idiopathic arthritis

Boris Hügle[1*], Anastasia Schippers[2], Nadine Fischer[1], Kim Ohl[2], Bernd Denecke[2], Fabio Ticconi[3], Bas Vastert[4], Ivan G. Costa[3], Johannes-Peter Haas[1] and Klaus Tenbrock[2]

Abstract

Background: The term systemic juvenile idiopathic arthritis (sJIA) describes an autoinflammatory condition characterized by arthritis and severe systemic inflammation, which in later stages can transform into interleukin (IL)-17-driven autoimmune arthritis. IL-1 antagonists have been used with good efficacy in the early stages of sJIA.

Methods: A whole transcriptome analysis of peripheral blood RNA samples was performed in six patients with sJIA and active systemic disease, before initiating treatment with the IL-1β receptor antagonist anakinra, and after induction of inactive disease, compared with a single-sample control cohort of 21 patients in several clinical stages of sJIA activity. Whole transcriptomes were compared longitudinally and interindividually including gene ontology and motif enrichment analysis of differentially expressed genes.

Results: There were 741 transcripts were identified using a threshold with a p value <0.01 and a fold change > 2. HLADRB1 and CD74 were identified as the most strongly upregulated genes in inactive compared to active disease; CD177 expression was significantly enhanced in active disease compared to inactive disease. Motif enrichment analysis revealed STAT4, BCL6, and STAT3 as the most prominent transcription factors that were present during active disease. In addition, strong upregulation of the major histocompatability complex II (MHCII) ligand CD74 was found in both active and inactive sJIA compared to healthy controls.

Conclusion: Using transcription factor motif enrichment, this study identifies novel putative pathways in sJIA (STAT4, BCL6) implicating B cell activation at an earlier stage than predicted in refractory disease. The implication of BCL-6 dependent pathways argues for occurrence of autoimmunity early within the process of sJIA chronification. Transcriptional regulation of HLA-DRB1, a recently described independent genetic risk factor, in combination with its cooperating partner CD74 in patients where sJIA is confirmed, supports pathogenic involvement in alterations in antigen presentation during sJIA.

Keywords: Juvenile systemic arthritis, Juvenile idiopathic arthritis, RNA expression, HLA-DRB1, CD74, CD177

* Correspondence: huegle.boris@rheuma-kinderklinik.de
[1]German Center for Pediatric and Adolescent Rheumatology, Gehfeldstrasse 24, 82467 Garmisch-Partenkirchen, Germany
Full list of author information is available at the end of the article

Background

Systemic juvenile idiopathic arthritis (sJIA) is an inflammatory disease with severe systemic inflammation leading to marked morbidity and mortality. Children with sJIA usually present with fever, arthritis, and a typical rash and can have a highly variable outcome [1]. Despite sJIA being listed as a subtype of juvenile idiopathic arthritis, it is currently considered to be of autoinflammatory rather than autoimmune origin [2, 3]. At least two phenotypes of sJIA can be identified by their clinical course: patients with monocyclic sJIA with only a single phase of severe systemic inflammation and concomitant arthritis, and patients developing chronic disease with recurrent flares of autoinflammation and severe arthritis [1].

Peripheral blood mononuclear cells (PBMC) and monocytic cells from patients with active sJIA have been analyzed in gene expression studies and have been shown to have a variable RNA expression pattern in patients with sJIA compared to healthy controls, patients with other autoimmune diseases, and patients with other subtypes of JIA, with uneven results [4, 5]. With the exception of a recent study looking at RNA expression in patient samples from two clinical trials of canakinumab, these studies have so far only used a cross-sectional approach, and patients with sJIA were not stratified according to their disease activity [6].

The objective of this study was to perform longitudinal whole transcriptome analysis of children with sJIA refractory to conventional, non-biological therapy before treatment with IL-1 antagonists and after achieving inactive disease, to identify transcriptional patterns and possible novel markers involved in the pathogenesis of the disease.

Methods

Patients

Clinical data and patient samples were acquired from the AID-Net database, a German registry and biobank that prospectively collects information and biomaterials from patients with autoinflammatory syndromes including periodic fever syndromes and sJIA. Written informed consent was obtained from the patients prior to inclusion. Healthy aged-matched controls undergoing elective surgery were recruited from the pediatric department of the university hospital RWTH Aachen. Further information on data safety and pseudonymization has been published previously [7]. A single-center sample of all patients with sJIA at the German Center for Pediatric and Adolescent Rheumatology was obtained between January 2010 and March 2015. All patients who met the following criteria were included in cohort I, which was set up for longitudinal analysis: (1) confirmed diagnosis of sJIA according to International League of Associations for Rheumatology (ILAR) criteria [3], (2) initial treatment with IL-1 antagonists after persistence of symptoms while taking non-steroidal antirheumatic drugs and/or corticosteroids, (3) achievement of subsequent inactive disease, and (4) available samples from at least two time points, i.e. at initial manifestation prior to treatment with IL-1 antagonists, and at a point of inactive disease on treatment with IL-1 antagonists. Additional samples from recurring disease flares and subsequent periods of inactivity were also acquired, where available.

A second cohort, cohort II, was set up for verification purposes. These were patients with only a single sample available, who had active systemic disease, active polyarticular disease without systemic activity or inactive disease.

Inactive disease was defined according to the American College of Rheumatology provisional criteria [8]. Active systemic disease was defined as presence of fever, rash, serositis, splenomegaly, or generalized lymphadenopathy attributable to JIA, with or without concurrent arthritis at that time. Active polyarticular disease was defined as presence of arthritis without fever, rash, serositis, splenomegaly, or generalized lymphadenopathy.

Data collection

A retrospective chart survey was used to extract demographic data, including date of first manifestation, date of diagnosis, total joint count at diagnosis, laboratory parameters at diagnosis including C-reactive protein, ferritin and thrombocyte count and the initial dose of prednisolone and anakinra.

Sample preparation

Whole blood was drawn during active disease before start of treatment with anakinra, after achievement of inactive disease and on subsequent visits. Peripheral blood was collected using PAXgene Blood RNA tubes (Qiagen, Valencia, CA, USA). RNA was extracted at the collection site using RNeasy columns (Qiagen, Valencia, CA, USA), then stored at − 20 °C. RNA quantity and quality was assessed using a Pico100 Picodrop ul Spectrophotometer (Picodrop, Saffron Walden, UK).

Expression analysis

Genome-wide transcriptome analyses were performed in cohort I using Gene Chip® Human HTA 2.0 arrays (Affymetrix, Santa Clara, CA, USA). Prior to analysis, RNA quality was assessed using the RNA 6000 Nano Assay with the 2100 Bioanalyzer (Agilent, Santa Clara, CA, USA). Samples for the HTA 2.0 arrays were prepared and hybridized to the arrays according to the Affymetrix WT Plus Kit manual. Briefly, for each sample, 100 ng of total RNA was reverse transcribed into complementary DNA (cDNA) using a random hexamer oligonucleotide tagged with a T7 promoter sequence. After second-strand synthesis, double-strand cDNA was used as a template for amplification with T7 RNA polymerase to obtain antisense cRNA. Random hexamers and deoxyribose adenine triphosphates (dNTPs) spiked out with deoxyuridine triphosphate (dUTP) were then used to reverse transcribe the cRNA into single-stranded sense strand cDNA. The cDNA was then fragmented with uracil DNA glycosylase and apurinic/apyrimidic endonuclease 1. Fragment size was checked using the 2100 Bioanalyzer and ranged from 50 to 200 bp. Fragmented sense cDNA was biotin-end-labeled with terminal deoxynucleotidyl transferase (TdT) and probes were hybridized to the Gene 2.0 arrays at 45 °C for 16 h with 60 rpms. Hybridized arrays were washed and stained on a Fluidics Station 450 (program FS450 0002) and scanned on a GeneChip® Scanner 3000 7G (both Affymetrix). Raw image data were analyzed with Affymetrix® Expression ConsoleTM Software (Affymetrix, USA), and gene expression intensities were normalized and summarized with a robust multiarray average algorithm [9]. Transcripts that were expressed differently more than twofold with a raw p value <0.01 between the sample groups were categorized as regulated. Enrichment analysis for Wiki pathways was performed using WebGestalt [10]. For the enrichment analysis only genes that changed at least twofold with a p value <0.01 between patients with active disease and those with inactive disease were taken into consideration.

Reverse transcription-polymerase chain reaction (RT-PCR)

For verification purposes, RT-PCR for several genes was performed in cohort I and II. The genes selected were chosen both due to the results of the expression analysis and previous descriptions in the literature [6, 11]. cDNA was generated from RNA using RevertAid H Minus First Strand cDNA Synthesis Kit (Thermo Fisher Scientific, USA) according to the manufacturer's instructions. Standard real-time PCR was carried out on TaqMan with the ABI prism 7300 real-time PCR systems (Applied Biosystems by Life Technologies, Germany) using the DNA intercalating dye SYBR Green Kit (Eurogentec, Germany). The housekeeping gene used was ribosomal protein L (RPL). The following primer sequences were used: for HLA-DRB1, TTC TTC AAT GGG ACG GAG CG (forward) and TTC CAG TAC TCA GCG TCA GG (reverse); for CD74, TTA TCT CCA ACA ATG AGC AAC T (forward) and ACA GGA AGT AGG CGG TGG T (reverse); for CD177, CAT GTG TGG AAG GTG TCC GA (forward) and CTT GGG GTC CGC TCT CAA TG (reverse); and for RPL, AGGTATGCTGCCC CACAAAAC (forward), TGTAGGCTTCAGACGCAC GAC (reverse).

The relative quantification method was applied and delta cycle threshold (ΔCt) values were determined by subtracting the Ct of the housekeeping gene (RPL) from the Ct of the target gene for each sample, respectively. Fold change was compared in active disease and inactive disease in the same individual using the ΔCt method.

Statistical analysis

Clinical data were analyzed using descriptive statistics. Statistical analysis was performed using SPSS version 21.0 (SPSS Inc., Chicago, USA). Microarray data were imported into GeneSpring GX 7.3.1 software (Agilent Technologies, Santa Clara, USA) and preprocessed using robust multichip analysis (RMA), followed by normalization of each probe to the median of all samples. Distance-weighted discrimination was used to align the centroids of predefined groups (12–16) to control for batch-to-batch variation.

Gene Ontology (GO)-based analysis of biological process was performed using AltAnalyze 2.1.0 software (altanalyze.org); significance values were between an adjusted p-value of 3.17e-08 and 0.0005.

Motif enrichment analysis

Transcription factor motif enrichment on upregulated/downregulated genes was performed using MotifMatch (www.regulatory-genomics.org). In short, this software searches for binding sites on the promoter region of all candidate genes (1 kbp upstream). Motifs were obtained from the Jaspar database. It then performs a Fisher exact test to evaluate if the proportion of binding sites in the gene sets is higher than expected by chance. The p-values were adjusted for multiple testing using the Benjamini-Hochberg method.

Results

Study population

Cohort I included longitudinal samples of six children with sJIA, with all patients having at least a sample pair prior to treatment with anakinra and with inactive disease on anakinra; samples were also available from two patients during a flare after withdrawal of anakinra. Cohort II consisted of single samples from eight patients with systemically active sJIA, five patients with sJIA with a polyarticular flare but no clinical signs of systemic activity, and eight patients with inactive sJIA. The clinical and demographic data at time of diagnosis in both cohorts are given in Table 1. All patients were of Caucasian origin and initially showed a typical clinical picture of sJIA with rash, fever, and arthritis, and typical bloodwork with elevated inflammatory markers. All patients in cohort I reacted rapidly to treatment with IL-1 antagonists, achieving an inactive disease state within days to weeks.

Patients with sJIA and inactive disease have differences in RNA expression profiles compared to patients with active disease and disease flares

Using a p value <0.01 and fold change > 2, 741 transcripts encoding for 481 known genes were identified (Additional file 1: Table S1) that were significantly differently expressed in inactive disease compared to active disease (both on initial presentation and during disease

Table 1 Demographic, clinical and laboratory characteristics of the study cohorts

Patient	Cohort I ($n = 6$)	Cohort II ($n = 8$) Active disease, systemic	Cohort II ($n = 5$) Active disease, polyarticular	Cohort II (n = 8) Inactive disease
Gender	5 male, 1 female	5 male, 3 female	2 male, 3 female	5 male, 3 female
Age at diagnosis, years (median, range)	5.3 (1.8–12.9)	6.8 (0.4–17.4)	6.0 (0.5–15.3)	3.5 (0.4–9.7)
Time since first symptoms (median, range)	71 days (47–107 days)	18.6 months (1.6–109.7 months)	86.9 months (7.4–198.3 months)	105.1 months (52.6–195.8 months)
Number of active joints (median, range)	2 (1–18)	3.5 (0–10)	3 (2–4)	0 (0–0)
Platelet count (median, range)	520,500/mm^3 (474,000–557,000/mm^3)	352,000/mm^3 (151,000–649,000/mm^3)	276,000/mm^3 (195,000–395,000/mm^3)	306,500/mm^3 (208,000–394,000/mm^3)
Rheumatoid factor, negative	6/6 (100%)	8/8 (100%)	5/5 (100%)	8/8 (100%)
Ferritin, μg/l (median, range)	414 (32–1785)	754 (234–9980 μg/l)	n.d.	n.d.
C-reactive protein, mg/dl (median, range)	11.84 (4.87–25.6)	3.65 (1.10–26.4)	0.07 (0.03–6.57)	0.11 (0.03–0.63)
Initial prednisolone dose, mg/kg (median, range)	1.6 (0–2.08)	n.a.	n.a.	n.a.
Initial anakinra dose, mg/kg (median, range)	1.63 (1.02–2.5)	n.a.	n.a.	n.a.

***n.a.* not applicable, *n.d.* not determined**

Table 2 Ontology-based analysis of the most significantly regulated genes

Inflammatory response (GO:0006954)
Regulation of T cell differentiation (GO:0045580)
Acute inflammatory response (GO:0002526)
Positive regulation of T cell differentiation in thymus (GO:0033089)
Response to molecule of bacterial origin (GO:0002237)
Regulation of lymphocyte differentiation (GO:0045619)
Regulation of T cell activation (GO:0050863)
Regulation of syncytium formation by plasma membrane fusion (GO:0060142)
Positive regulation of leukocyte activation (GO:0002696)
Positive regulation of cell activation (GO:0050867)
Activation of innate immune response (GO:0002218)
Response to lipopolysaccharide (GO:0032496)
Detection of external biotic stimulus (GO:0098581)
Activation of immune response (GO:0002253)
Negative regulation of immune response (GO:0050777)

Shown are the 15 biological processes that are the most stringent according to the *p* value in the Gene Ontology (GO) analysis

flare), of which most were associated with immune- mediated processes (Table 2, Figs. 1 and 2). Of these, genes, 239 were downregulated while 242 were upregulated in active disease. Using fold change > 3 as a more stringent criterion, more than 100 genes still remained. Gene Ontology (GO)-based analysis favored pathways of the innate immune response as the most significantly represented pathways in active disease (Table 2). Some of the highly regulated genes (HLA-DRB1, CD74, CD177) were confirmed using RT-PCR, as described below. Additional data on ANXA3/annexin A 3, a gene locus where a SNP within the gene has been identified as a risk factor in rheumatoid arthritis, and IL-1 receptor associated kinase 3 (IRAK3), are presented in Additional file 2: Figures S1 and S2 [12].

Of note, patient 5 had a markedly different expression pattern in active disease, and patients 2 and 5 had a different expression pattern in inactive disease (Fig. 1). Patient 5 differs to the other patients in being the only female patient. The marked difference in gene expression patterns is, however, more likely due to the fact that patient 5 received three methylprednisolone pulses prior to the RNA sample being drawn. Patient 2 also received

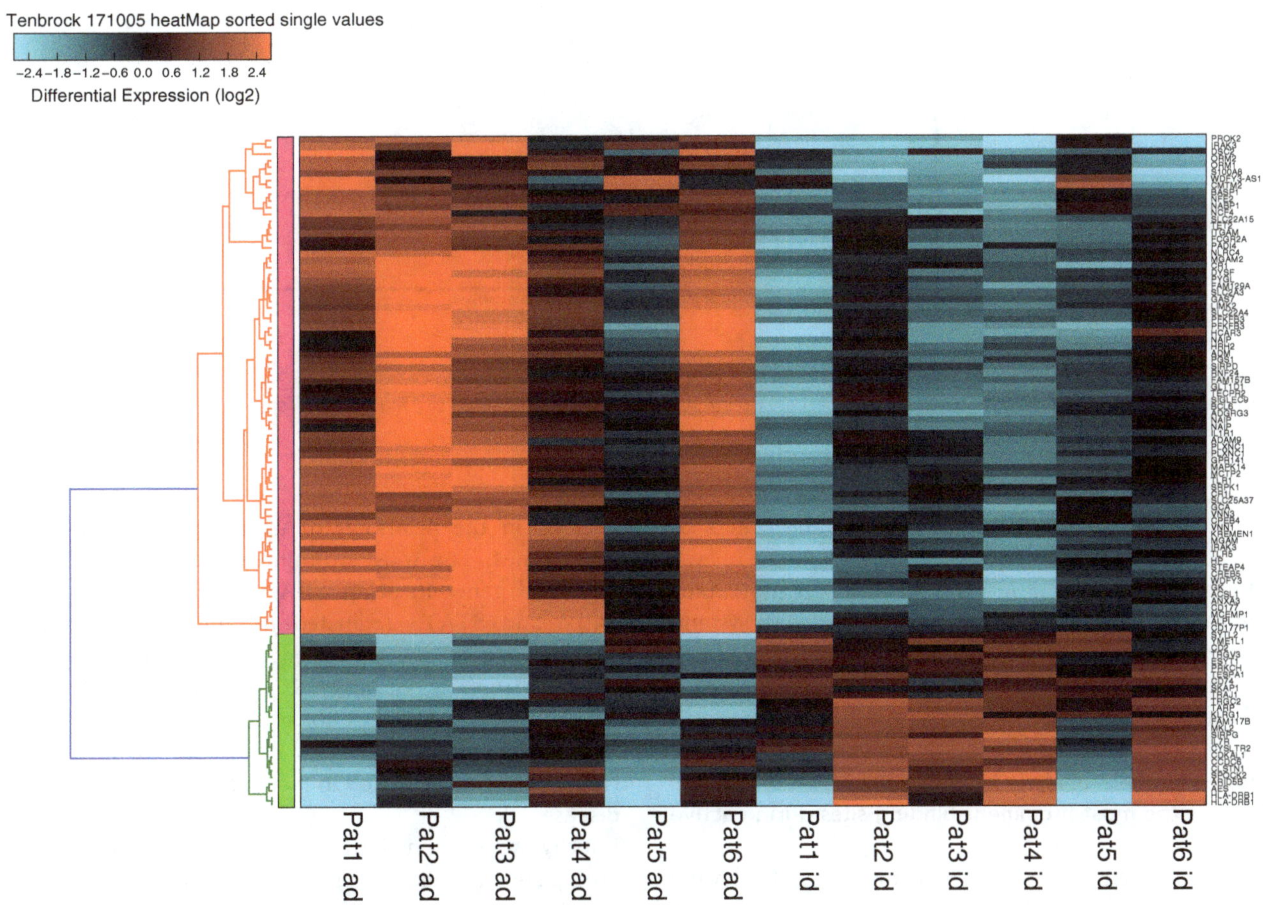

Fig. 1 Heatmap with hierarchical clustering of patients (Pat) with active disease (ad) and inactive disease (id). Shown are all genes with fold change > 3

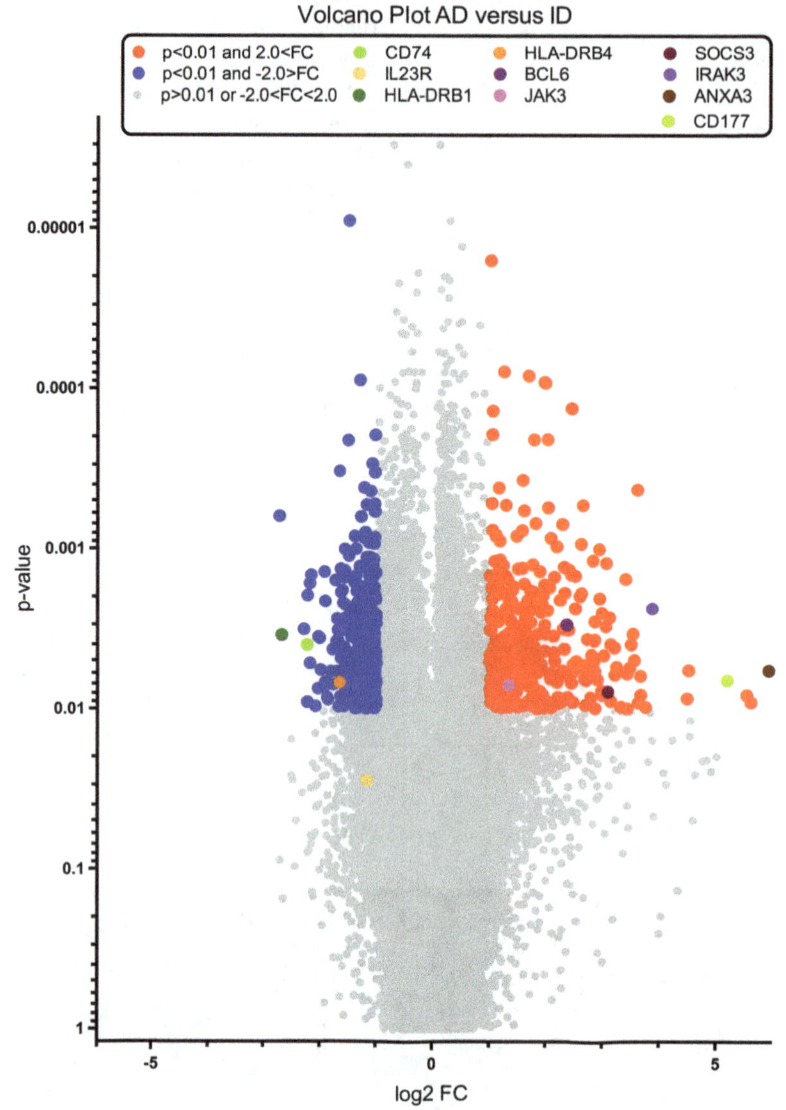

Fig. 2 Regulated genes in patients with active disease (ad) versus inactive disease (id) using fold change (FC) > 2 and a p value <0.01. Red dots include genes with fold change > 2 in active disease, blue dots with a fold change <− 2. Names of highly regulated and significant genes are depicted in the graph using different colors

one pulse of methylprednisolone, which the others did not.

As for the changes in inactive disease, patients 1 and 5 required ongoing IL-1 blockade and reacted with systemic signs to withdrawal, while the other patients were able to taper and discontinue the IL-1 antagonists (both anakinra and canakinumab) over the course of the next year.

Motif enrichment analysis identifies STAT4, BCL6 and STAT3 as the most prominent binding sites during active disease

In order to identify pathways that might be of relevance in sJIA, we performed transcription factor (TF) motif enrichment analysis to evaluate which TFs are preferably binding in the promoter of upregulated or downregulated genes. The most prominent binding motif in upregulated genes in active sJIA was STAT4, followed by BCL6 and STAT3 (adjusted p value <0.005) (Fig. 3). Moreover BCL6 was also upregulated on the array in active disease (fold change 5.15, $p = 0.002$, Fig. 2), while STAT4 and STAT3 were not.

HLA-DRB1 is upregulated in inactive compared to active disease

Initially we examined transcripts shown to be regulated during sJIA, to validate that the patients under study exhibited the features described previously for this condition. For example, there was a fold change of 4.76 ($p = 0.006$) in

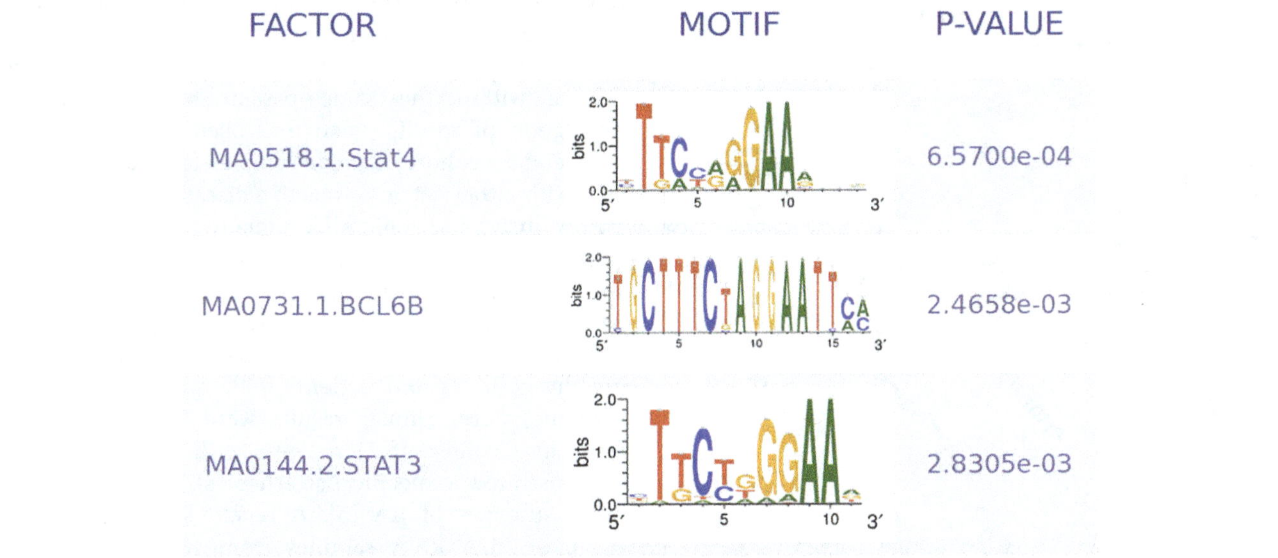

Fig. 3 Motifs of the most regulated transcription factor binding sites in the whole transcriptome of patients with active systemic juvenile idiopathic arthritis (sJIA) compared to inactive sJIA, analyzed using MotifMatch

S100A8 in our patients, as expected [13, 14]. Our analysis revealed HLA-DRB1 as the most strongly upregulated gene in inactive compared to active disease (fold change 6.8, $p =$ 0.003, Fig. 2). This observation was confirmed using RT-PCR in the longitudinal per-patient sample analysis, while we did not find upregulation in cohort II compared to healthy controls due to high individual expression differences (Fig. 4). Other HLA class II genes, for example HLA-DRB4 (fold change − 2.92, $p = 0.008$, Fig. 2), HLA-DRB3 and HLA-DRB6, were found to be downregulated.

CD74 is regulated in sJIA irrespective of disease activity

CD74 was also upregulated in inactive compared to active disease on an individual per patient base (fold change 4.73, $p = 0.036$, Fig. 2). However, and more strikingly, in cohort II CD74 was much higher expressed in patients with systemic activity as well as inactive disease compared to age-matched healthy controls using RT-PCR (Fig. 5). The protein encoded by this gene is the invariant chain of the HLA-DR complex, which is associated with class II major histocompatibility complex (MHC) including HLADRB1 and is an important chaperone that regulates antigen presentation for immune response.

CD177 is strongly upregulated in active disease

CD177 was upregulated in patients with active disease compared to those with inactive disease or healthy controls (fold change 37, $p = 0.007$, Fig. 2), which has recently

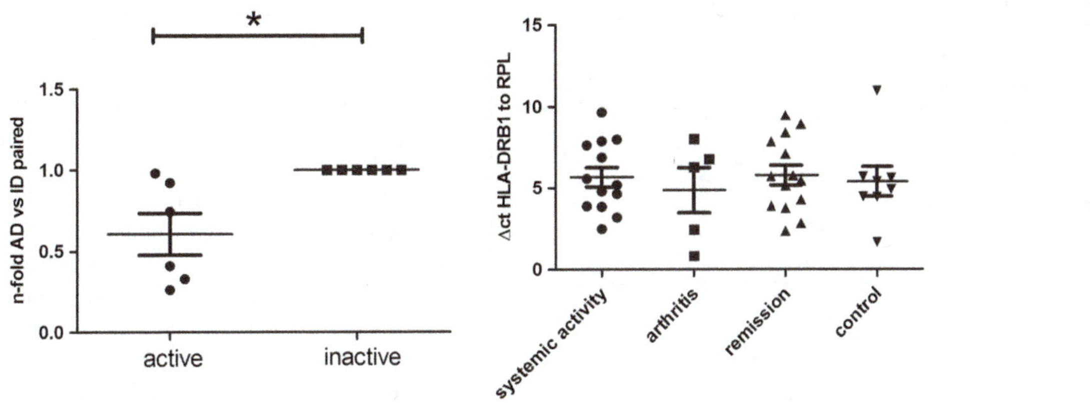

Fig. 4 Expression of HLA-DRB1 in active (AD) versus inactive (ID) systemic juvenile idiopathic arthritis using reverse transcription PCR. Left graph, fold change (*n*-fold) of longitudinal samples before and after treatment with anakinra, with inactive disease set to level 1 (*$p < 0.05$). Right graph, delta cycle threshold (ΔCt) values (relative expression values related to ribosomal protein L (RPL)) in active systemic disease (cohorts I and II), active polyarticular disease, and inactive disease/remission, and controls (all cohort II)

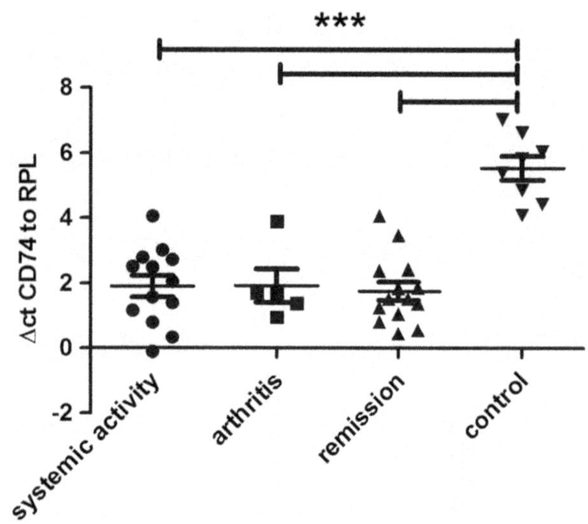

Fig. 5 Expression of CD74 using reverse transcription PCR: delta cycle threshold (ΔCt) values (relative expression values related to ribosomal protein L) in controls, active systemic disease, active polyarticular, and inactive disease (all ***$p < 0.001$)

been described in the study by Brachat et al. and confirms their findings using RT-PCR (Fig. 6) [6]. This gene encodes a glycosyl-phosphatidylinositol-linked cell surface glycoprotein that plays a role in neutrophil activation. The protein can bind platelet endothelial cell adhesion molecule-1 and function in neutrophil transmigration.

Discussion

By using comparative array analysis of RNA expression in a cohort of sJIA patients in different stages of disease refractory to conventional therapy, we were able to show differential regulation of a variety of genes, comparing inactive disease on IL-1 antagonist treatment with active disease within the same patient before treatment. Regulation of specific genes has been confirmed in an independent cohort of single samples from patients with sJIA with either active or inactive disease.

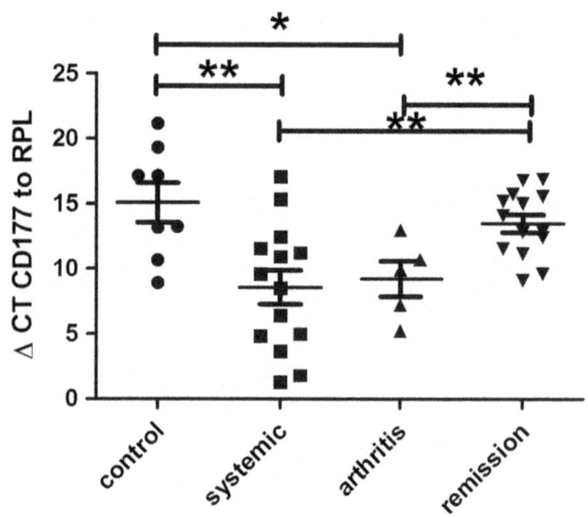

Fig. 6 Expression of CD177 using reverse transcription PCR: delta cycle threshold (ΔCt) values (relative expression values related to ribosomal protein L) in controls, active disease, and inactive disease (***$p < 0.001$)

Previously, a specific sJIA signature of RNA expression has been described in 44 patients with sJIA in various stages of the disease [4]. In this study, 12 patients with systemic and arthritic symptoms displayed a specific expression pattern compared to healthy controls and patients with polyarticular (non-systemic) flare. Similar results were found by Barnes et al. in a cohort of 21 patients with sJIA, which also demonstrated a specific pattern of sJIA different from other subtypes of JIA [5]. A recent study by Brachat et al. on sJIA RNA samples from two studies using canakinumab also demonstrated a large number of differentially expressed genes in patients prior to and after initiation of anti-IL-1 treatment [6]. Similar to these preceding studies, the overall specific sJIA signature consists of regulation of the inflammatory response and innate immune pathways including the IL-1 pathway, IL-6 and toll-like receptor 1, but also modulation of lymphocyte differentiation and response, with an emphasis on T cells (Table 2). A recent large genome-wide association study also demonstrated a framework of pathophysiological pathways that appears to be specific for sJIA [15].

Transcription factor motif enrichment analysis in patients with active and inactive disease identified STAT4, BCL6, and STAT3 as the most prominent motifs within the regulated genes. STAT4 is mainly expressed in myeloid cells and is the transcription factor downstream of IL-12, which has been identified as a potential biomarker in sJIA, but has not been discussed as a potential therapeutic target so far [16–18]. We have previously shown that the likelihood of the occurrence of a polymorphism enhancing IL-12 expression was somewhat higher in patients with sJIA compared to other forms of JIA, which points toward IL-12 being more prominent in sJIA than previously thought [19]. In our array analysis, IL-12 was not differentially expressed; however, the IL-23 receptor, which is involved in IL-12 downstream signaling was downregulated in active disease (fold change 2.5, $p = 0.012$, Fig. 2), which suggests a physiological reaction towards the proinflammatory state.

The identification of BCL6 as the second most prominent binding motif is more striking: BCL6 is a lineage transcription factor for follicular T helper (Tfh) cells, a cell type that is important for B cellular responses. This cell type is especially important for autoimmune arthritis mediated by gut bacteria [20]. BCL6 expression has been shown to be sustained by IL-6 signaling in patients with rheumatoid arthritis (RA), and specific targeting of IL-6 using tocilizumab in patients with RA results in a significant reduction of circulating Tfh cells; IL-21 production by Tfh cells was also correlated with reduced expression of antibody-producing plasmablasts [21]. BCL6 was also directly upregulated on the array, which supports the hypothesis that this TF is of major importance (fold change 5.15, $p = 0.002$, Fig. 2), and would also argue for even earlier involvement of autoimmunity with B cell responses in the course of the disease [22]. There is some evidence of B cell-driven autoimmunity in the later phases of sJIA, in which autoantibody production has been demonstrated [23]. Our findings here indicate that B cell activation might already be present during the first phase of disease where autoinflammation is the most prominent feature. This might potentially determine whether the patients develop a polyarticular course later. In contrast, finding STAT3 as the third most prominent transcription factor is unsurprising, since STAT3 signals downstream of IL-6, a well-known therapeutic target using tocilizumab in sJIA [24, 25]. In the study by Brachat et al., where canakinumab was used for IL-1ß blockade, IL-6 declined by day 3 and remained suppressed over time [6]. STAT3 was not differentially expressed on the array; however, STAT3 is usually activated by phosphorylation and not by transcriptional regulation. Nevertheless, IL-6 signals via JAK3, which then activates STAT3 and is downstream of the IL-6 receptor, and it was found to be enhanced (fold change 2. 5, $p = 0.006$). Vice versa, the antagonist of STAT3 signaling is the suppressor of cytokine signaling 3 (SOCS3), which was highly induced in active disease (fold change 8.5, $p = 0.012$, Fig. 2), probably to counterbalance the overwhelming immune stimulation.

HLA-DRB1 and its cooperation partner CD74 were upregulated in the active disease stage, and CD74 was upregulated in the inactive disease stage in patients with sJIA in this study. Certain genotypes of HLA-DRB1, most notably HLA-DRB1*11, have been found to be strongly associated with sJIA in a large recent study of 982 patients across nine different populations, and also in a fine-mapping study of the HLA locus comparing it to other forms of JIA [11, 15, 26]. However, no expression studies of HLA-DRB1 in sJIA have been performed to date. HLA-DRB1 has also previously been demonstrated to be strongly associated with early, severe RA [27]. RA-associated HLA-DRB1 alleles have conserved amino acid sequences in position 70–74 of the molecule. This molecular structure is termed the shared epitope, with a variety of hypotheses explaining its function [28]. An association with the shared epitope has also been found in children with rheumatoid-factor positive JIA [29]. However, RNA expression patterns of the shared epitope are variable, and apparently dependent on the copy number [27].

CD74 is the invariant chain of HLA-DR and therefore a cooperation partner on the cell surface, where it critically regulates antigen presentation. It also serves as a cell surface receptor for the cytokine macrophage migration inhibitory factor (MIF) which, when bound to the encoded protein, initiates survival pathways and cell proliferation. In cooperation with IL-12, MIF is important for survival in children with malaria and trypanosoma infection [30, 31]. CD74 also interacts with amyloid precursor protein and suppresses the production of beta amyloid [32]. The high expression of CD74 even in an inactive disease state could serve as a possible candidate for disease markers for sJIA, and possibly - in the context of MIF - even for therapeutic intervention.

An additional gene that was highly upregulated in the active stages of sJIA was CD177, confirming recent results [6]. CD177 codes for human neutrophil antigen 2 (HNA-2), also called NB1, a cell surface glycoprotein [33]. HNA-2 expression is highly variable in humans and is lacking in approximately 3–5% of the North American population [34]. HNA-2 plays an important role in myeloid cell proliferation and function of neutrophils, including transendothelial migration [35]. It has also been associated with anti-neutrophil-cytoplasmic antibody (ANCA)-associated vasculitides, where CD177 has been proposed as a receptor of mPR3 on the neutrophil surface [36]. Interestingly, CD177 has also been observed as the most upregulated parameter in a microarray study of purified neutrophils from patients with septic shock. However, since we performed our analysis in whole blood, the numbers of neutrophils could also have had a considerable effect on our findings. There was, however, no difference in CD177 transcription between active systemic and active polyarticular disease, while neutrophil counts were significantly lower in polyarticular disease than in systemic flares (data not shown). Nevertheless, in light of the large variations in CD177 expression in controls and throughout the patient cohorts, these data have to be interpreted with caution.

This is a small study with a limited number of patients examined longitudinally, even if the results are confirmed in a second cohort. As RNA was extracted from whole blood rather than sorted cells due to the constraints of a biobank, and given that a number of genes discussed, especially CD177, are expressed by neutrophils, changes in neutrophil numbers could have significantly impacted the results. However, not all genes described here are predominantly expressed in neutrophils and CD177 was also consistently upregulated in patients with polyarticular flares and low neutrophil numbers. As variable cell numbers are a valid point of criticism of preceding studies as well, confirmation using sorted cells is a logical next step in researching gene expression patterns in sJIA [4–6]. The strength of this study is the longitudinal examination of patients who have undergone a consistent institutional treatment protocol with IL-1 agonists in different stages of their disease.

Conclusions

By using this longitudinal analysis, our study identifies novel pathways (STAT4 and BCL6) that might be of relevance in sJIA and indicates strong upregulation of HLA-DRB1 in cooperation with CD74 in patients with sJIA in inactive disease upon treatment with IL-1 antagonists. This provides the first functional confirmation of a previous study, which identified HLA-DRB1 as a risk factor in sJIA. Additionally CD177 was confirmed as a new marker in sJIA. Studies with larger patient cohorts using flow cytometry for protein expression are necessary to confirm these results.

Additional files

Additional file 1: Table S1. List of regulated genes with fold change (FC) > 2 in patients with active disease (ad) versus inactive disease (id) showing signal intensity in both disease states, gene symbol and description. (XLSX 60 kb)

Additional file 2: Figure S1. Expression of ANXA3 using RT-PCR: delta Ct values (relative expression values related to RPL) in controls, active systemic or polyarticular disease and inactive disease (***$p < 0.001$, ****$p < 0.0001$). **Figure S2.** Expression of IRAK3 using RT-PCR: delta Ct values (relative expression values related to RPL) in controls, active systemic or polyarticular disease and inactive disease (**$p < 0.01$). (DOCX 619 kb)

Abbreviations

bp: Base pairs; cDNA: Complementary DNA; Ct: Cycle threshold; HNA-2: Human neutrophil antigen 2; GO: Gene Ontology; IRAK: IL-1 receptor associated kinase; IL: Interleukin; ILAR: International League of Associations for Rheumatology; MHC: Major histocompatibility complex; MIF: Macrophage migration inhibitory factor; PBMC: Peripheral blood mononuclear cells; RA: Rheumatoid arthritis; RPL: Ribosomal protein L; RT-PCR: Reverse transcription PCR; sJIA: Systemic juvenile idiopathic arthritis; TF: Transcription factor; Tfh: Follicular T helper (cells)

Acknowledgements

We thank Nienke Ter Haar for careful review of the manuscript.

Funding

This study was supported by the Interdisciplinary Center for Clinical Research (IZKF) Aachen and UCAN-AC (Understanding Childhood Arthritis Network Aachen) and an unrestricted grant from Novartis AG to the German Center for Pediatric and Adolescent Rheumatology. The AID-Net database is supported by the Federal Ministry of Education and Research (BMBF project 01GM08104, 01GM1112D).

Authors' contributions

BH, JPH, and KT conceived of the study and drafted the manuscript. AS and NF participated in data collection and reviewed the manuscript. KO, BD, FT, and BV participated in the design and coordination of the study and helped draft the manuscript. IGG performed the genetic and statistical analysis. All authors read and approved the final manuscript.

Competing interests

The authors declare that they have no competing interests.

Author details

[1]German Center for Pediatric and Adolescent Rheumatology, Gehfeldstrasse 24, 82467 Garmisch-Partenkirchen, Germany. [2]Department of Pediatrics, Universitätsklinikum Aachen, Aachen, Germany. [3]IZKF Research Group Bioinformatics, RWTH Aachen Medical Faculty, Aachen, Germany. [4]University Medical Center Utrecht, Utrecht, Netherlands.

References

1. Singh-Grewal D, Schneider R, Bayer N, Feldman BM. Predictors of disease course and remission in systemic juvenile idiopathic arthritis: significance of early clinical and laboratory features. Arthritis Rheum. 2006;54:1595–601.
2. Mellins ED, Macaubas C, Grom AA. Pathogenesis of systemic juvenile idiopathic arthritis: some answers, more questions. Nat Rev Rheumatol. 2011;7:416–26.
3. Petty RE, Southwood TR, Manners P, Baum J, Glass DN, Goldenberg J, He X, Maldonado-Cocco J, Orozco-Alcala J, Prieur AM, et al. International League of Associations for Rheumatology classification of juvenile idiopathic arthritis: second revision, Edmonton, 2001. J Rheumatol. 2004;31:390–2.
4. Allantaz F, Chaussabel D, Stichweh D, Bennett L, Allman W, Mejias A, Ardura M, Chung W, Smith E, Wise C, et al. Blood leukocyte microarrays to diagnose systemic onset juvenile idiopathic arthritis and follow the response to IL-1 blockade. J Exp Med. 2007;204:2131–44.
5. Barnes MG, Grom AA, Thompson SD, Griffin TA, Pavlidis P, Itert L, Fall N, Sowders DP, Hinze CH, Aronow BJ, et al. Subtype-specific peripheral blood gene expression profiles in recent-onset juvenile idiopathic arthritis. Arthritis Rheum. 2009;60:2102–12.
6. Brachat AH, Grom AA, Wulffraat N, Brunner HI, Quartier P, Brik R, McCann L, Ozdogan H, Rutkowska-Sak L, Schneider R, et al. Early changes in gene expression and inflammatory proteins in systemic juvenile idiopathic arthritis patients on canakinumab therapy. Arthritis Res Ther. 2017;19:13.
7. Lainka E, Bielak M, Hilger V, Basu O, Neudorf U, Wittkowski H, Holzinger D, Roth J, Niehues T, Foell D. Translational research network and patient registry for auto-inflammatory diseases. Rheumatology (Oxford). 2011; 50:237–42.
8. Wallace CA, Giannini EH, Huang B, Itert L, Ruperto N, Childhood Arthritis Rheumatology Research A, Pediatric Rheumatology Collaborative Study G, Paediatric Rheumatology International Trials O. American College of Rheumatology provisional criteria for defining clinical inactive disease in select categories of juvenile idiopathic arthritis. Arthritis Care Res (Hoboken). 2011;63:929–36.
9. Irizarry RA, Hobbs B, Collin F, Beazer-Barclay YD, Antonellis KJ, Scherf U, Speed TP. Exploration, normalization, and summaries of high density oligonucleotide array probe level data. Biostatistics. 2003;4:249–64.
10. Wang J, Duncan D, Shi Z, Zhang B. WEB-based gene set analysis toolkit (WebGestalt): update 2013. Nucleic Acids Res. 2013;41:W77–83.
11. Ombrello MJ, Remmers EF, Tachmazidou I, Grom A, Foell D, Haas JP, Martini A, Gattorno M, Ozen S, Prahalad S, et al. HLA-DRB1*11 and variants of the MHC class II locus are strong risk factors for systemic juvenile idiopathic arthritis. Proc Natl Acad Sci U S A. 2015;112:15970–5.
12. Okada Y, Terao C, Ikari K, Kochi Y, Ohmura K, Suzuki A, Kawaguchi T, Stahl EA, Kurreeman FA, Nishida N, et al. Meta-analysis identifies nine new loci associated with rheumatoid arthritis in the Japanese population. Nat Genet. 2012;44:511–6.
13. Gerss J, Roth J, Holzinger D, Ruperto N, Wittkowski H, Frosch M, Wulffraat N, Wedderburn L, Stanevicha V, Mihaylova D, et al. Phagocyte-specific S100 proteins and high-sensitivity C reactive protein as biomarkers for a risk-adapted treatment to maintain remission in juvenile idiopathic arthritis: a comparative study. Ann Rheum Dis. 2012;71:1991–7.
14. Holzinger D, Frosch M, Kastrup A, Prince FH, Otten MH, Van Suijlekom-Smit LW, ten Cate R, Hoppenreijs EP, Hansmann S, Moncrieffe H, et al. The toll-like receptor 4 agonist MRP8/14 protein complex is a sensitive indicator for

disease activity and predicts relapses in systemic-onset juvenile idiopathic arthritis. Ann Rheum Dis. 2012;71:974–80.
15. Ombrello MJ, Arthur VL, Remmers EF, Hinks A, Tachmazidou I, Grom AA, Foell D, Martini A, Gattorno M, Ozen S, et al. Genetic architecture distinguishes systemic juvenile idiopathic arthritis from other forms of juvenile idiopathic arthritis: clinical and therapeutic implications. Ann Rheum Dis. 2017;76:906–13.
16. de Jager W, Hoppenreijs EP, Wulffraat NM, Wedderburn LR, Kuis W, Prakken BJ. Blood and synovial fluid cytokine signatures in patients with juvenile idiopathic arthritis: a cross-sectional study. Ann Rheum Dis. 2007;66:589–98.
17. Gohar F, Kessel C, Lavric M, Holzinger D, Foell D. Review of biomarkers in systemic juvenile idiopathic arthritis: helpful tools or just playing tricks? Arthritis Res Ther. 2016;18:163.
18. Yilmaz M, Kendirli SG, Altintas D, Bingol G, Antmen B. Cytokine levels in serum of patients with juvenile rheumatoid arthritis. Clin Rheumatol. 2001; 20:30–5.
19. Eberhardt CS, Haas JP, Girschick H, Schwarz T, Morbach H, Rosen-Wolff A, Foell D, Dannecker G, Schepp C, Ganser G, et al. No association of IL-12p40 pro1.1 polymorphism with juvenile idiopathic arthritis. Pediatr Rheumatol Online J. 2015;13:61.
20. Teng F, Klinger CN, Felix KM, Bradley CP, Wu E, Tran NL, Umesaki Y, Wu HJ. Gut microbiota drive autoimmune arthritis by promoting differentiation and migration of Peyer's patch T follicular helper cells. Immunity. 2016;44:875–88.
21. Chavele KM, Merry E, Ehrenstein MR. Cutting edge: circulating plasmablasts induce the differentiation of human T follicular helper cells via IL-6 production. J Immunol. 2015;194:2482–5.
22. Nigrovic PA, Mannion M, Prince FH, Zeft A, Rabinovich CE, van Rossum MA, Cortis E, Pardeo M, Miettunen PM, Janow G, et al. Anakinra as first-line disease-modifying therapy in systemic juvenile idiopathic arthritis: report of forty-six patients from an international multicenter series. Arthritis Rheum. 2011;63:545–55.
23. Hugle B, Hinze C, Lainka E, Fischer N, Haas JP. Development of positive antinuclear antibodies and rheumatoid factor in systemic juvenile idiopathic arthritis points toward an autoimmune phenotype later in the disease course. Pediatr Rheumatol Online J. 2014;12:28.
24. Heinrich PC, Behrmann I, Haan S, Hermanns HM, Muller-Newen G, Schaper F. Principles of interleukin (IL)-6-type cytokine signalling and its regulation. Biochem J. 2003;374:1–20.
25. Yokota S, Imagawa T, Mori M, Miyamae T, Aihara Y, Takei S, Iwata N, Umebayashi H, Murata T, Miyoshi M, et al. Efficacy and safety of tocilizumab in patients with systemic-onset juvenile idiopathic arthritis: a randomised, double-blind, placebo-controlled, withdrawal phase III trial. Lancet. 2008;371:998–1006.
26. Hinks A, Bowes J, Cobb J, Ainsworth HC, Marion MC, Comeau ME, Sudman M, Han B, Juvenile Arthritis Consortium for I, Becker ML, et al. Fine-mapping the MHC locus in juvenile idiopathic arthritis (JIA) reveals genetic heterogeneity corresponding to distinct adult inflammatory arthritic diseases. Ann Rheum Dis. 2017;76:765–72.
27. Kerlan-Candon S, Combe B, Vincent R, Clot J, Pinet V, Eliaou JF. HLA-DRB1 gene transcripts in rheumatoid arthritis. Clin Exp Immunol. 2001;124:142–9.
28. Holoshitz J. The rheumatoid arthritis HLA-DRB1 shared epitope. Curr Opin Rheumatol. 2010;22:293–8.
29. Prahalad S, Thompson SD, Conneely KN, Jiang Y, Leong T, Prozonic J, Brown MR, Ponder LA, Angeles-Han ST, Vogler LB, et al. Hierarchy of risk of childhood-onset rheumatoid arthritis conferred by HLA-DRB1 alleles encoding the shared epitope. Arthritis Rheum. 2012;64:925–30.
30. Awandare GA, Hittner JB, Kremsner PG, Ochiel DO, Keller CC, Weinberg JB, Clark IA, Perkins DJ. Decreased circulating macrophage migration inhibitory factor (MIF) protein and blood mononuclear cell MIF transcripts in children with Plasmodium falciparum malaria. Clin Immunol. 2006;119:219–25.
31. Terrazas CA, Huitron E, Vazquez A, Juarez I, Camacho GM, Calleja EA, Rodriguez-Sosa M. MIF synergizes with Trypanosoma cruzi antigens to promote efficient dendritic cell maturation and IL-12 production via p38 MAPK. Int J Biol Sci. 2011;7:1298–310.
32. Matsuda S, Matsuda Y, D'Adamio L. CD74 interacts with APP and suppresses the production of Abeta. Mol Neurodegener. 2009;4:41.
33. Stroncek DF, Caruccio L, Bettinotti M. CD177: a member of the Ly-6 gene superfamily involved with neutrophil proliferation and polycythemia vera. J Transl Med. 2004;2:8.
34. Matsuo K, Lin A, Procter JL, Clement L, Stroncek D. Variations in the expression of granulocyte antigen NB1. Transfusion. 2000;40:654–62.
35. Bayat B, Werth S, Sachs UJ, Newman DK, Newman PJ, Santoso S. Neutrophil transmigration mediated by the neutrophil-specific antigen CD177 is influenced by the endothelial S536N dimorphism of platelet endothelial cell adhesion molecule-1. J Immunol. 2010;184:3889–96.
36. Hu N, Mora-Jensen H, Theilgaard-Monch K, Doornbos-van der Meer B, Huitema MG, Stegeman CA, Heeringa P, Kallenberg CG, Westra J. Differential expression of granulopoiesis related genes in neutrophil subsets distinguished by membrane expression of CD177. PLoS One. 2014;9:e99671.

6

The majority of patients with newly diagnosed juvenile idiopathic arthritis achieve a health-related quality of life that is similar to that of healthy peers: results of the German multicenter inception cohort (ICON)

Miriam Listing[1*], Kirsten Mönkemöller[2], Ina Liedmann[1], Martina Niewerth[1], Claudia Sengler[1], Joachim Listing[1], Dirk Foell[3], Arnd Heiligenhaus[4], Ariane Klein[5], Gerd Horneff[5], Gerd Ganser[6], Johannes-Peter Haas[7], Jens Klotsche[1,8†] and Kirsten Minden[1,8†]

Abstract

Background: Achieving the best possible health-related quality of life (HRQoL) for a patient is an important treatment goal in juvenile idiopathic arthritis (JIA). We investigated the 36-month trajectories of HRQoL in children with JIA compared with healthy peers and identified the predictors of an unfavorable HRQoL.

Methods: Patients with a recent JIA diagnosis were enrolled in the German inception cohort study ICON. As a peer group, friends of patients of the same age and sex were asked to cooperate. Children were prospectively followed and regularly questioned about their HRQoL using the Pediatric Quality of Life Inventory 4.0 (PedsQL). Disease activity was assessed by the clinical Juvenile Arthritis Disease Activity Score (cJADAS-10), and the burden of the child's chronic illness on their family was assessed by the Family Burden Questionnaire (FaBel). Linear mixed models were used to compare the HRQoL of the patients and their peers. Associations between the health status of a patient at enrollment and an unfavorable HRQoL (PedsQL total < 79.3) at their 3-year follow-up (FU) were analyzed by logistic regression.

Results: Data from 953 patients (median symptom duration 6 months, mean age 7.9 years) and 491 healthy peers (aged 8.4 years) were analyzed. During 3 years of FU, the disease activity and HRQoL of the patients improved significantly (cJADAS-10 from 9.8 (6.2) to 2.7 (3.6) and PedsQL total score from 71.7 (18.2) to 87.3 (13.9)). While the HRQoL of the patients varied among the several JIA categories at the time of enrollment, no significant differences were found at the 3-year FU. After 36 months, the HRQoL of the patients had largely converged with that of their healthy peers. JIA patients had a psychosocial health status comparable with their healthy peers, whereas a small significant mean difference remained in physical health (5.8, 95% confidence interval (CI) 4.1–7.6). Up to the 36-month FU, three-quarters of JIA patients attained a favorable HRQoL (PedsQL ≥ 79.3) which was achieved by 90% of the peers. A higher family burden, higher pain level, and lower well-being at enrollment were associated with an unfavorable HRQoL.

(Continued on next page)

* Correspondence: mlisting@gmx.net
†Equal contributors
[1]Deutsches Rheuma-Forschungszentrum Berlin, Epidemiology Unit, Charitéplatz 1, 10117 Berlin, Germany
Full list of author information is available at the end of the article

(Continued from previous page)

Conclusions: Under current therapeutic conditions, an HRQoL corresponding with that of healthy children is a realistic treatment goal in JIA.

Keywords: Inception cohort, Juvenile idiopathic arthritis, Quality of life, Outcome

Background

Juvenile idiopathic arthritis (JIA) is the most common chronic inflammatory rheumatic illness in children, with an incidence of 2–20 cases per 100,000 at-risk children [1]. JIA encompasses a clinically heterogeneous group of disorders with unknown causes which begin before the age of 16 years. These diseases cause both temporary and permanent disability as well as an impaired quality of life [2–4]. The treatment of JIA currently aims at achieving an inactive disease state, preventing disability and damage, and ensuring the age-appropriate development of affected children and adolescents. As JIA influences virtually all aspects of the child's life and those of his or her family, achievement of an optimal health-related quality of life (HRQoL) is an important goal in clinical care. HRQoL is a complex, multidimensional concept that encompasses physical, emotional, social, and behavior-related well-being and functioning. A patient's individual perception of health is affected by his/her social and cultural background as well as his/her personal value system [5–7]. Several studies [4, 8–15] have shown that JIA patients have a lower HRQoL compared with healthy controls. Most prior studies were cross-sectional in their study design [8, 12–14], and the assessment of HRQoL was often conducted several years after diagnosis [4, 11]. Longitudinal studies of HRQoL in JIA patients are rare [4, 16–18], and some were performed to examine the effects of disease-modifying antirheumatic drugs (DMARDs) [16–18].

A large Canadian inception cohort [19] investigated changes in the HRQoL of patients with JIA. They found that the HRQoL of children with JIA improved gradually over time. Another inception cohort from Scandinavia [20] found reduced physical health in only 20% of JIA patients approximately 8 years after disease onset. Some indicators of a poor quality of life have been identified [9, 21–24] and include the persistence of a high level of disease activity, the presence of disabilities, chronic pain, and low social or emotional resources. However, some questions remain unanswered; for example, it has remained unclear why patients with clinically inactive disease nevertheless report a reduced quality of life [25]. Identifying the factors that predict a poor outcome with continued low HRQoL is a vital step toward providing appropriate interventions.

To the best of our knowledge, there are no published data that evaluate the course of HRQoL in newly diagnosed JIA patients compared with healthy peers. We therefore used data from the German Inception Cohort Of patients with Newly diagnosed JIA (ICON) to investigate the HRQoL of affected children during the first years of pediatric rheumatologic care in order to: 1) describe changes in HRQoL over time; 2) compare the HRQoL of patients with that of healthy peers; and 3) identify the predictors of a suboptimal HRQoL in the course of the disease.

Methods

Study design

ICON is an ongoing, prospective, observational cohort study into which patients with a recent onset of JIA and healthy controls were enrolled from May 2010 to December 2012 at 11 of the largest pediatric rheumatology sites in Germany. For the recruitment of the comparator group, patients and/or their parents were asked to recruit some of their friends of equal age and gender from kindergarten or school to participate as healthy peers. Informed consent was obtained from children (≥ 8 years) and their parents. The study protocol was approved by the ethics committee of the Charité – University Medicine Berlin. For more details on the ICON cohort study, see Sengler et al. [26].

Participants

Patients had to have a diagnosis of JIA (according to the International League of Associations for Rheumatology (ILAR) classification criteria [27]) for less than 12 months. A total of 953 consecutively observed patients with confirmed JIA and 491 healthy peers were included in the ICON study. Data available by 21 June 2017 were used for this analysis. After enrollment, JIA patients were assessed every 3 months in the first year and every 6 months thereafter, while healthy peers were questioned once a year. For this analysis, the 36-month follow-up (FU) was chosen as the study endpoint.

Measurements

Demographic data (age, sex, parent education, income, country of origin, and actual place of residence) were reported by the parents of the JIA patients and their healthy peers. At each study visit, the pediatric rheumatologist recorded treatment modalities and assessed the patient's disease state, for example the number of active (range 0–70) joints, and disease activity (physician's global assessment of disease activity (PGA)) on a 21-point numeric rating scale (NRS; 0–10). Parents of the JIA patients and their healthy peers assessed their child's overall well-being (parent's global assessment) and pain on a 21-point NRS (0–10) at each visit. Laboratory parameters such as the erythrocyte sedimentation rate (ESR), C-reactive protein (CRP), antinuclear antibodies (ANA), rheumatoid factor (RF), and human leukocyte antigen-B27 (HLA-B27) were also recorded. JIA categories according to ILAR criteria were reported by physicians at enrollment and 1-year and 3-year FU and were reviewed by two pediatric rheumatologists (KM and CS) [26, 27].

JIA disease activity was evaluated by the clinical Juvenile Arthritis Disease Activity Score (cJADAS-10). The cJADAS-10 (range 0–30) is calculated with the physician's global assessment, the parent's global assessment, and the number of actively involved joints (maximum 10). The cJADAS was found to be valid, feasible, and applicable in all JIA categories [28]. The cJADAS-10 thresholds proposed by Consolaro et al. [29, 30] were applied to define disease activity state (inactive disease, and minimal, moderate, or high disease activity). In patients with oligoarticular disease course (≤ 4 active joints), the cut-off points 1, 1.5, and 4 were used. The thresholds 1, 2.5, and 8.5 were used in those with polyarticular disease course (> 4 active joints).

The Childhood Health Assessment Questionnaire (CHAQ) [31] was used to measure the functional ability of the patients. To evaluate the HRQoL in JIA patients and healthy peers, the German version of the Pediatric Quality of Life Inventory generic core scales 4.0 (PedsQL) was used [32, 33]. The PedsQL consists of four subscales (physical functioning, emotional functioning, social functioning, and school functioning) which can be combined into physical health and psychosocial health composite scales, as well as the PedsQL total score. PedsQL scores range from 0 (being the worst) to 100 (being the best possible HRQoL). The parents of all participants completed the PedsQL at each visit.

The Strength and Difficulties Questionnaire (SDQ) [34, 35] was administered to the parents of all children aged 5 years or above at the time of enrollment. The total difficulties score ranges from 0 to 40. Higher scores are an indicator of more severe psychosocial problems, e.g., emotional and behavioral problems: scores ≤ 13 are classified as 'normal'; scores 14–16 as 'borderline'; and scores ≥ 17 as 'conspicuous'.

Parents of JIA patients also completed the German version of the Impact on Family Scale [36], the Family Burden Questionnaire (FaBel) 3 months after enrollment. The FaBel [37] measures the burden of a chronic illness on the family of the patient. The summary scale ranges from 0 to 4, and higher scores indicate a greater family burden.

Socioeconomic status

An established German multidimensional aggregated index was used to measure the socioeconomic status (SES) of the child. This index was evaluated and adapted from a representative German population sample of 17,641 study participants aged up to 17 years [38]. Since the parental work status was not ascertained in the ICON study, the calculation of this index was modified to be based only on parental education level (including schooling and vocational training) and household net income. According to Lampert et al. [38], the highest education level of the mother or father was used to assign the specific education score (ranging from low (1) to high (7)). The household equivalence net income score was calculated by dividing the net income by the square root of the number of family members (range from low (1) to high (7)) (http://www.oecd.org/els/soc/OECD-Note-EquivalenceScales.pdf). Based on the education level of the parents, missing net income data were imputed separately for parents of patients and parents of peers using the SAS® procedure MI. One imputation was used to calculate the household equivalence net income score since this is not a main outcome parameter. The lower and upper quartiles of the sum of the education and income scores (6.55, 12.1) were used as cut-points to define low, moderate, and high SES.

Study questions

The PedsQL total score and the PedsQL physical health as well as psychosocial health scales were used to compare the 36-month trajectories of HRQoL of JIA patients with that of healthy peers (aims 1 and 2, respectively). PedsQL scores of the peers were used to define optimal and suboptimal HRQoL states. Predictors of a suboptimal HRQoL status were identified in JIA patients (aim 3). In addition, as secondary outcomes, the disease activity measured by the cJADAS-10 and functional ability assessed by the CHAQ were investigated.

Statistical analysis

Marginal structural models were applied to achieve an approximation of age and gender distribution and social status characteristics between patients and peers. The following approach was applied. Logistic regression with the binary dependent variable patient or peer and the covariables age, sex, country of origin, parental education, and household equivalence net income was used to calculate weighted samples. For example, peers with a low social status underrepresented in the peer group were given a weight > 1, while the overrepresented group of peers with a high social status received a weight < 1. This weighting resulted in balanced samples which were used for the statistical analysis. Only columns 2 and 3 of Table 1 and Table 2 refer to unweighted samples; all

Table 1 Demographic data and proxy-reported health-related quality of life outcomes of patients and healthy peers at baseline

	Patients (*n* = 953)	Peer group (*n* = 491)	Weighted patients (*n* = 953)	Weighted peers (*n* = 491)
Female, *n* (%)	640 (67.2%)*	290 (59.1%)	613 (64.3%)	311 (64%)
Age at study enrollment (years), mean (SD)	7.9 (4.8)*	8.4 (4.6)	8.1 (4.9)	8.3 (4.5)
Country of origin Germany, *n* (%)	697 (76.9%)**	413 (84.5%)	726 (79.8%)	390 (80.6%)
Parent's education score, mean (SD)	4.7 (1.6)**	5.4 (1.5)	5.0 (1.6)	5.0 (1.5)
Equivalence household net income score, mean (SD)	4.0 (1.9)**	4.7 (1.8)	4.2 (1.9)	4.2 (1.9)
SES, mean (SD)	8.7 (3.0)**	10.1 (2.9)	9.2 (3.1)	9.3 (3.0)
Low (≤ 6.55), *n* (%)	288 (30.2%)	78 (15.9%)	241 (25.3%)	120 (24.7%)
Moderate, *n* (%)	486 (51.0%)	238 (48.5%)	485 (50.8%)	239 (49.3%)
High (≥ 12.1), *n* (%)	179 (18.8%)	175 (35.6%)	229 (24.0%)	126 (26.0%)
PedsQL total score, mean (SD)	71.5 (18.4)**	89.9 (7.7)	71.7 (18.2)**	89.6 (7.9)
PedsQL physical health, mean (SD)	66.0 (24.6)**	95.1 (7.1)	66.4 (24.4)**	94.9 (7.2)
PedsQL psychosocial health, mean (SD)	74.8 (17.4)**	87.1 (9.5)	74.9 (17.3)**	86.7 (9.7)
PedsQL emotional functioning, mean (SD)	68.9 (22.1)**	80.4 (13.8)	69.0 (21.9)**	80.1 (14.1)
PedsQL school functioning, mean (SD)	72.9 (20.9)**	88.1 (12.1)	73.1 (20.8)**	87.6 (12.3)
PedsQL social functioning, mean (SD)	82.0 (19.1)**	92.7 (10.0)	82.0 (19.0)**	92.5 (10.0)
SDQ, total scale (range 0–40), mean (SD)	9.4 (5.8)**	5.8 (4.8)	9.2 (5.9)**	6.1 (4.9)
Parent's global (NRS 0–10), mean (SD)	3.0 (2.3)**	0.7 (1.0)	3.0 (2.3)**	0.7 (1.0)
Pain (NRS 0–10), mean (SD)	3.0 (2.8)**	0.4 (0.8)	2.9 (2.8)**	0.4 (0.9)

*$p < 0.05$, **$p < 0.001$

NRS, numeric rating scale; PedsQL, Pediatric Quality of Life Inventory; SD, standard deviation; SDQ, Strength and Difficulties Questionnaire; SES, socioeconomic status

other analyses have been calculated on the basis of weighted samples.

Linear mixed models were applied to compare the primary outcome (PedsQL scores) between the groups. We applied this model to yield unbiased estimates in the presence of missing data. A characteristic of these models is that observations with partly missing data are not discarded from the analysis and will contribute to the estimate of the overall mean response.

To set thresholds for the suboptimal HRQoL we used the data from our German weighted peer sample. To facilitate a simple interpretation, the threshold in the PedsQL was defined as the point which was exceeded by 90% of the peers. Ninety percent of the peers had a PedsQL total score of 79.3 or above, a PedsQL physical health score of 84.4 or above, and a psychosocial health score of 73.3 or above. We used these values as thresholds to differentiate between a favorable or high quality of life, and suboptimal HRQoL. Univariable and multiple backward logistic regressions were used to identify the predictors of suboptimal HRQoL at 3-year FU. Age was included in the multiple analyses to adjust for the dropout of older children during the study course.

Linear regression analyses were applied to investigate associations between HRQoL and sociodemographic variables, parent-reported outcomes, and disease-specific clinical outcomes at the same point in time.

Patients with active disease at enrollment (cJADAS-10 > 1) were stratified into groups with minimal, moderate, high, and very high improvement. The quartiles and median changes in cJADAS-10 between enrollment and the 36-month visit were used to calculate the corresponding cut-off points (3, 6.5, and 11.5). Linear mixed models were used to investigate the PedsQL outcome in the JIA subgroups (JIA categories, groups of cJADAS-10 improvement). Means and frequencies of other secondary outcomes (e.g., disease activity, pain, and physical disability) were provided as observed.

Results

Baseline characteristics and comparisons between JIA patients and healthy peers

Data from 953 patients with newly diagnosed JIA and 491 healthy peers were included in the analysis. Dropout rates over the observation period were low and ranged between 2% and 6% per year (Fig. 1). Baseline characteristics of both groups differed significantly regarding health-related parameters, as well as for age, sex, and SES (Table 1). An adjustment was made (see the Statistical analysis section above) for this reason. Comparisons between both groups are based on the resulting

Table 2 Characteristics of JIA patients at baseline, and at the 1-year, 2-year, and 3-year follow-up (FU)

	Baseline	1-year FU	2-year FU	3-year-FU
n	953	850	805	761
JIA categories				
Oligoarthritis, *n* (%)	441 (46.3%)	–	–	–
Persistent oligoarthritis, *n* (%)		315 (37.1%)	–	253 (33.3%)
Extended oligoarthritis, *n* (%)		74 (8.7%)	–	98 (12.9%)
RF-negative polyarthritis, *n* (%)	250 (26.2%)	226 (26.6%)	–	205 (27.0%)
RF-positive polyarthritis, *n* (%)	16 (1.7%)	15 (1.8%)	–	15 (2.0%)
Enthesitis-related arthritis, *n* (%)	100 (10.5%)	92 (10.8%)	–	75 (9.9%)
Psoriatic arthritis, *n* (%)	40 (4.2%)	41 (4.8%)	–	35 (4.6%)
Systemic-onset JIA, *n* (%)	35 (3.7%)	29 (3.4%)	–	28 (3.7%)
Undifferentiated arthritis, *n* (%)	71 (7.5%)	58 (6.9%)	–	51 (6.7%)
Disease activity				
PGA (NRS 0–10), mean (SD)	3.8 (2.6)	1.0 (1.5)	0.8 (1.4)	0.8 (1.3)
cJADAS-10 (0–30), mean (SD)	9.8 (6.2)	3.4 (4.0)	2.8 (3.4)	2.7 (3.6)
Inactive disease, *n* (%)	56 (6.0%)	288 (39.8%)	309 (46.8%)	297 (52.0%)
Minimal disease activity, *n* (%)	24 (2.6%)	89 (12.3%)	85 (12.9%)	64 (11.2%)
Moderate disease activity, *n* (%)	159 (17.0%)	218 (30.2%)	175 (26.5%)	132 (23.1%)
High disease activity, *n* (%)	698 (74.5%)	128 (17.7%)	92 (13.9%)	78 (13.7%)
Parent's reported outcomes				
Functional status (CHAQ; range 0–3), mean (SD)	0.6 (0.7)	0.3 (0.5)	0.2 (0.5)	0.2 (0.5)
FaBel (total scale; range 0–4), mean (SD)[a]	1.7 (0.4)	–	–	–
Treatment				
NSAIDs, *n* (%)	800 (84.0%)	289 (37.8%)	191 (26.1%)	150 (22.4%)
Systemic glucocorticoids, *n* (%)	230 (24.1%)	83 (10.9%)	49 (6.7%)	32 (4.8%)
DMARDs, *n* (%)	394 (41.3%)	493 (64.5%)	427 (58.3%)	390 (58.2%)
csDMARDs, *n* (%)	387 (40.6%)	454 (59.4%)	350 (47.8%)	313 (46.7%)
MTX, *n* (%)	364 (38.2%)	422 (55.2%)	324 (44.2%)	285 (42.5%)
Sulfasalazine, *n* (%)	19 (2%)	22 (2.9%)	12 (1.6%)	11 (1.6%)
bDMARDs, *n* (%)	38 (4.0%)	156 (20.4%)	179 (24.4%)	163 (24.3%)
Etanercept, *n* (%)	21 (2.2%)	86 (11.3%)	105 (14.3%)	86 (12.8%)
Adalimumab, *n* (%)	7 (0.7%)	35 (4.6%)	37 (5.1%)	46 (6.9%)

bDMARD, biologic DMARD; CHAQ, Childhood Health Assessment Questionnaire; cJADAS-10, clinical Juvenile Arthritis Disease Activity Score; csDMARD, conventional synthetic DMARD; DMARD, disease-modifying antirheumatic drug; FaBel, Family Burden Questionnaire; JIA, juvenile idiopathic arthritis; MTX, methotrexate; NRS, numeric rating scale; NSAID, nonsteroidal anti-inflammatory drug; PGA, physician's global assessment of disease activity; RF, rheumatoid factor; SD, standard deviation
[a]Reported 3 months after baseline

weighted samples. Compared with the healthy peers, the HRQoL in JIA patients was impaired in both physical and psychosocial health (Table 1). Significantly higher SDQ total scores were found in JIA patients. JIA patients with borderline or conspicuous psychosocial problems at enrollment (SDQ total score ≥ 14) had a lower HRQoL (mean total score = 59, standard deviation (SD) 16). In multivariate linear regression analyses, the PedsQL total score was significantly associated with the SDQ total score and the parent's global score in both groups, and with pain in patients with JIA (all $p < 0.001$).

Characteristics of JIA patients, disease activity, and treatment from enrollment to 36 months

The mean age at JIA diagnosis was 7.7 years (SD 4.8). The median time from JIA diagnosis to enrollment was 2 months (interquartile range (IQR) 0–4). A history of uveitis or psoriasis was present in 5.9% and 3.5% of patients at enrollment, respectively. Nearly half of the patients had oligoarthritis (OA), and one-quarter had RF-negative polyarthritis (Table 2). At enrollment, categorization into persistent and extended OA was possible only in a minority of patients. Among these, 25 were diagnosed as having extended OA and, during follow-up, another 78 developed an

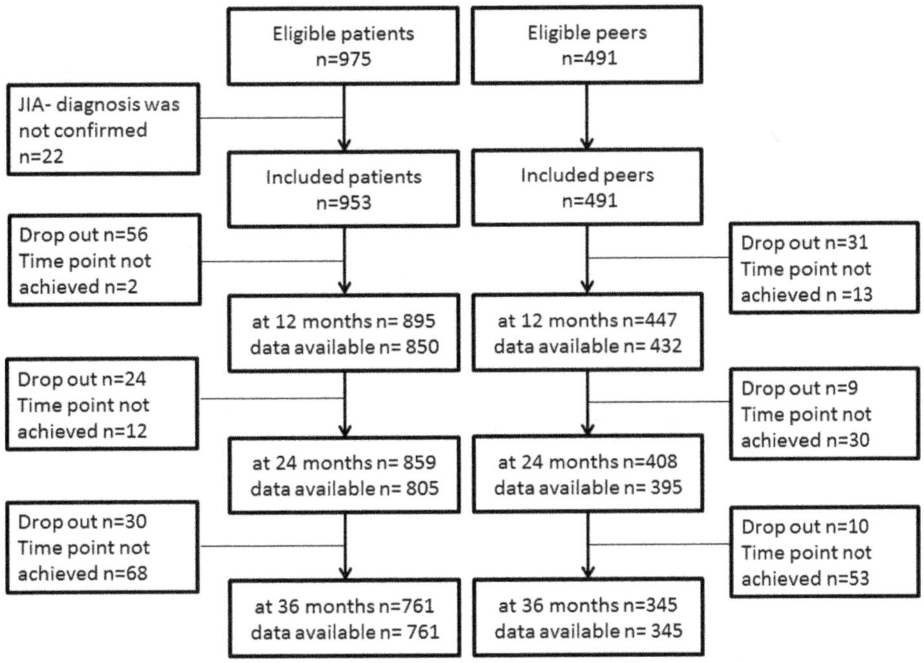

Fig. 1 Disposition of ICON participants included in the present analysis. JIA, juvenile idiopathic arthritis

extended disease course. Furthermore, in 16 children the JIA category was changed mainly due to the onset of psoriasis, enthesitis, sacroiliitis, or dactylitis, or new information on the onset of psoriasis in first-degree relatives.

Prior to, and at enrollment, almost all patients had received nonsteroidal anti-inflammatory drugs (NSAIDs), and 48% were treated with intra-articular glucocorticoids. Prior to their inclusion in the ICON study, treatment with conventional synthetic disease-modifying antirheumatic drugs (csDMARDs) was initiated in 44.2% of patients, whereas 55.5% were DMARD naive. This treatment pattern changed within the first 6 to 12 months after enrollment. About one-quarter were treated with tumor necrosis factor (TNF) inhibitors or other biologic DMARDs (bDMARDs) at the 2-year and 3-year FU. Intra-articular glucocorticoids were used in 11% of the patients within 6 months of the 2- and 3-year FU. Treatment was accompanied by a significant improvement in the HRQoL (PedsQL scores) of patients, disease activity, and functional ability (CHAQ). The mean cJADAS-10 reduced significantly within the first 6 months of standard care from 9.8 to 4.2 (SD 4.2). Half of the JIA patients were in a clinically inactive disease state at their 3-year FU (Table 2).

Course of HRQoL over 36 months, comparing children with JIA with healthy peers

Over the first 3 years of rheumatologic care, the HRQoL improvement in patients was statistically significant. On average, improvements of 11.2 (95% confidence interval (CI) 10.1–12.3), 21.7 (20.2–23.2), and 15.0 (13.9–16.1) units were observed in the psychosocial, physical health, and PedsQL total scores, respectively. There was a sharp increase in the PedsQL scores of the JIA patients within the first 6 months. The mean psychosocial health scores of patients with JIA were equivalent to those of their healthy peers (Fig. 2a). Mean significant differences between JIA patients and healthy peers for physical health and PedsQL total scores of 5.8 (95% CI 4.1–7.6) and 2.4 (0.9–4.0) remained (Fig. 2b, c).

Decreased disease activity was accompanied by an improvement in HRQoL. JIA patients with an inactive disease status at 3-year FU had a higher mean PedsQL total score of 92.8 (SD 8.8) than those with moderate (80.4 (16.0)) or high disease activity (73.6 (17.4)). A similar result was found by comparing the change in cJADAS with the change in PedsQL, which both depend on the baseline level. In patients with minimal improvement (see Statistical analysis section) in cJADAS-10 (32.7%), the PedsQL total score increased from 79.1 (95% CI 76.7–81.5) at enrollment to 83.1 (81.0–85.1) at 3-year FU; in those with moderate improvement (19.9%), it increased from 75.5 (72.5–78.5) to 87.7 (85.2–90.2); in patients with high improvement (24.2%), it increased from 68.6 (65.9–71.4) to 88.4 (86.1–90.8); and in those with very high improvement (23.1%), it increased from 59.8 (56.9–62.8) to 89.3 (86.9–91.8).

Changes in HRQoL in children with different JIA categories

At enrollment, the PedsQL total score differed significantly between JIA categories ($p < 0.001$). In particular,

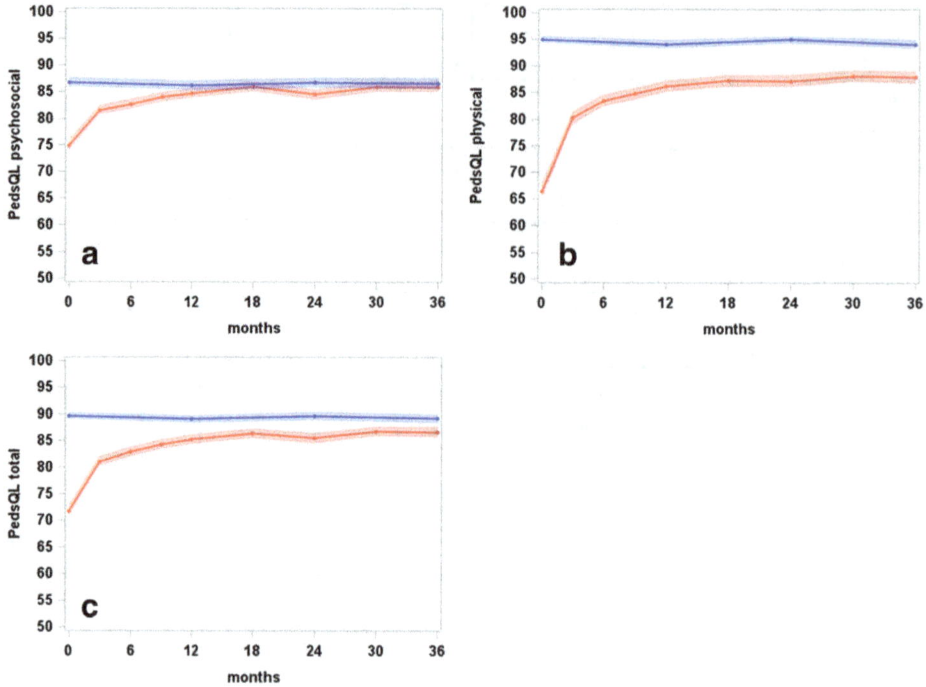

Fig. 2 Least square means of (**a**) Pediatric Quality of Life Inventory (PedsQL) psychosocial scores, **b** PedsQL physical scores, and (**c**) PedsQL total scores, and corresponding 95% confidence bands, of JIA patients (red) and healthy peers (blue) over 3 years of observation in ICON (results of linear mixed model analyses)

patients with RF-negative polyarthritis, psoriatic arthritis, and systemic arthritis reported a low HRQoL at baseline. An improvement in HRQoL was observed in all JIA categories, but to varying degrees (Fig. 3). The change in HRQoL was more distinct in patients with RF-negative polyarthritis and systemic JIA and was less pronounced in patients with psoriatic arthritis. At 12-month FU, differences between the JIA categories were still significant ($p = 0.03$), with ranges in PedsQL total score from 79.2 to 87.1. In particular, patients with psoriatic arthritis differed from others due to their low HRQoL. There was no statistically significant ($p = 0.44$) difference in HRQoL at the 3-year FU.

Predictors of suboptimal HRQoL at the 3-year FU

Lower HRQoL at the 36-month FU was strongly associated with higher pain, increased functional disability, and worse parent global score at baseline (all p values < 0.01, $R^2 = 0.54$) in a multivariable linear stepwise regression.

Using the PedsQL data of the peers to define a favorable HRQoL (score ≥ 79.3), we found that 76% of patients with JIA attained this HRQoL, with a mean PedsQL total value of 93.6 (SD 6.3). Those who did not achieve this threshold had a mean total score of 66.1 (11.4). With regard to physical and psychosocial health, 70% versus 82% of patients reached a favorable HRQoL (scores ≥ 84.4 and ≥ 73.3, respectively), with mean PedsQL physical health and psychosocial health values of 96.9 (4.3) and 91.9 (8.1). Mean levels of 68.2 (15.5) and 61.0 (10.4) were observed in children with suboptimal physical and psychosocial health, respectively. Associations between baseline parameters and the likelihood of a suboptimal HRQoL at the 36-month FU are shown in Table 3. The FaBel total score had a consistently large effect on poor HRQoL in multivariable regression analyses. In addition, subjectively perceived pain and the parent global score were significantly associated. Overall, a higher burden on the family, increased pain, and a worse parent global score at enrollment increased the likelihood of suboptimal HRQoL after 3 years of rheumatologic care.

Discussion

Our results confirm earlier findings using the ICON cohort of a noticeable reduction in disease activity in early JIA which can currently be achieved within the first 6 months of routine rheumatologic care [26]. Half of the JIA patients achieved an inactive disease status after 3 years of treatment if the cJADAS-10, which also includes the parent's perspective, is used for assessment. A greater decrease in cJADAS-10 was associated with a greater increase in HRQoL. Parent-reported functional disability, pain, and parent global scores were significantly associated with HRQoL. The level of psychosocial health of JIA patients was comparable with that of

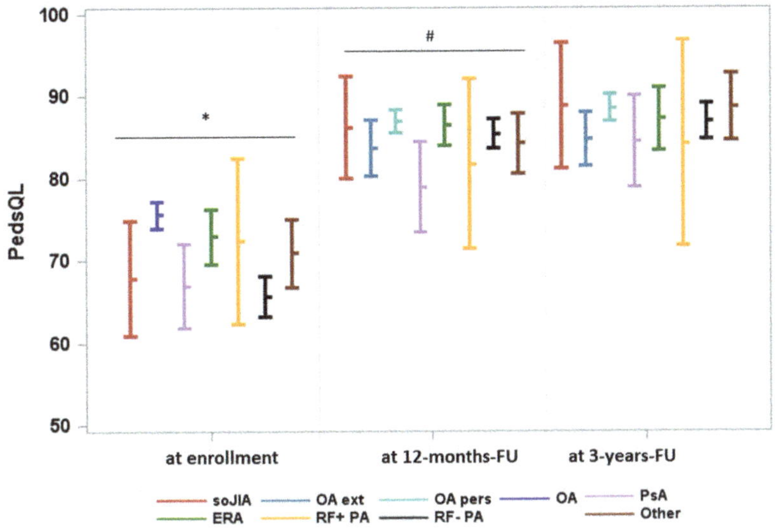

Fig. 3 HRQoL of patients with JIA differentiated by JIA category at baseline, at 12-month follow-up (FU), and at 3-year FU. Values are shown as least square means with corresponding 95% confidence intervals. Patients were assigned to the JIA category they refer to at the corresponding point in time. ERA, enthesitis-related arthritis; OA, oligoarthritis; OA ext, extended oligoarthritis; OA pers, persistent oligoarthritis; PedsQL, Pediatric Quality of Life Inventory; PsA, psoriatic arthritis; RF+ PA, rheumatoid factor-positive polyarthritis; RF- PA, rheumatoid factor-negative polyarthritis; soJIA, systemic-onset juvenile idiopathic arthritis. $^{*}p < 0.001$, $^{\#}p < 0.001$

healthy peers after 3 years of rheumatologic care, whereas a minor but significant difference remained in physical health. Different JIA categories showed unique HRQoL trajectories but, at 3-year FU, the PedsQL total scores had reached a comparable level in all categories. Three-quarters of patients with JIA reached a favorable HRQoL. Predictors of a suboptimal HRQoL (PedsQL total score < 79.3) were the parent global and pain scores at enrollment, as well as the burden borne by the family as a result of their child's illness.

Different methods are applied to measure disease activity in JIA. We used the cJADAS-10 because of its multidimensional concept. Our findings are consistent with those of others who also observed a clear decrease in disease activity and functional limitations following treatment for recent-onset JIA [20, 39, 40].

Many studies found a lower HRQoL in patients with JIA compared with healthy controls [4, 8–15, 41]. However, their results cannot simply be transferred to recent-onset JIA patients treated in pediatric rheumatologic care since patients were often sampled in the pre-biologic era of the 1980s or 1990s [8, 11, 41] or had a disease duration of more than 10 years [4, 8, 11, 41]. It should also be considered that most of these studies were cross-sectional in nature [8, 12–15, 41] and therefore did not permit conclusions about the HRQoL in JIA patients during the course of their disease.

After 36 months of rheumatologic care, we observed a clear approximation of the patients' PedsQL values to those of healthy peers. Regarding psychosocial health, our findings are in accordance with prior studies that found that psychosocial health was similar in patients with JIA and healthy peers [4, 10, 41, 42]. It is in line with other studies on the HRQoL of patients with JIA [4, 15] that physical health is more affected than psychosocial health, which was also shown in our analysis. Findings from the literature suggest that parents of children with health problems tend to underestimate their child's HRQoL, whereas parents from nonclinical samples tend to report a higher HRQoL than the children themselves [43]. Considering these findings, we suppose that the convergence of PedsQL values of JIA patients to levels of age-, sex-, and SES-comparable peers is more likely to be under- rather than overestimated in our cohort.

Until now, longitudinal studies on the HRQoL of children with JIA are rare [4, 16, 19]. Oen et al. [19] investigated the HRQoL of 1249 newly diagnosed patients with JIA using the Juvenile Arthritis QoL Questionnaire (JAQQ; range 1–7). They described an improvement in median JAQQ score from 2.7 at the first visit to 1.9 at 7 months and 1.5 at 37 months after diagnosis. Similar to our data, an improvement in HRQoL was most marked within the first 6 months. We identified mean HRQoL changes that were two- to three-times higher than the corresponding minimal clinically important different PedsQL scores calculated by Varni et al. [33]. This underlines the clear clinically relevant improvement in HRQoL that was already achieved during the first months of treatment and whose level could be maintained over time.

Table 3 Predictors at enrollment of a suboptimal HRQoL at the 36-month follow-up

Predictors	PedsQL score of suboptimal HRQoL at the 36-month follow up			
	Total < 79.3		Physical health < 84.4	Psychosocial health < 73.3
	Univariate	Multiple	Multiple	Multiple
Age[a]	1.01 (0.97–1.05)	1.02 (0.97–1.07)	1.06 (1.02–1.11)**	1.04 (0.99–1.09)
Sex[b]	1.01 (0.70–1.45)		0.57 (0.38–0.85)**	
SES score	0.97 (0.92–1.03)			
Time between symptom onset and diagnosis	1.01 (1.00–1.03)			
Uveitis	0.86 (0.41–1.66)			
JIA categories				
Persistent oligoarthritis	Referent			
Extended oligoarthritis	1.58 (0.91–2.71)			
RF-negative polyarthritis	1.10 (0.69–1.73)			
RF-positive polyarthritis	2.24 (0.63–7.22)			
Psoriatic arthritis	1.53 (0.66–3.36)			
Enthesitis-related arthritis	0.95 (0.48–1.80)			
Systemic-onset JIA	1.22 (0.42–3.12)			
Undifferentiated arthritis	0.80 (0.34–1.71)			
Disease activity				
cJADAS-10	1.03 (1.00–1.06)*			
PGA	1.02 (0.96–1.09)			
Parent's global	1.19 (1.10–1.29)***	1.15 (1.05–1.26)**		1.14 (1.03–1.26)**
Active joint count	1.00 (0.97–1.02)			
Pain				
Numeric rating scale	1.14 (1.07–1.22)***		1.21 (1.13–1.30)***	
Functional ability				
CHAQ	1.74 (1.36–2.23)***			
Psychosocial burden of families				
FaBel total	4.82 (2.96–7.98)***	3.88 (2.27– 6.72)***	2.97 (1.78–5.02)***	3.63 (2.04–6.53)***

*$p < 0.05$, **$p < 0.01$, ***$p < 0.0001$

CHAQ, Childhood Health Assessment Questionnaire; cJADAS-10, clinical Juvenile Arthritis Disease Activity Score; FaBel, Family Burden Questionnaire; HRQoL, health-related quality of life; JIA, juvenile idiopathic arthritis; PedsQL, Pediatric Quality of Life Inventory; PGA, physician's global assessment of disease activity; RF, rheumatoid factor; SES, socioeconomic status

[a] Admitted to multivariate analyses to adjust for missing data

[b] Female referent

In the ICON cohort, an improvement in HRQoL to the level measured in healthy peers was observed in each JIA category. At enrollment, each disease category differed significantly in their PedsQL total score, with particularly low scores in those patients with systemic JIA and RF-negative polyarthritis. At the onset of disease, systemic JIA is characterized by daily spiking fevers and is accompanied by a variety of other systemic signs [27] associated with a high disease burden and a decreased quality of life [8]. Patients with RF-negative polyarthritis may have low PedsQL scores at disease onset because of the restricted mobility caused by the inflammation in more than four joints. After 3 years, there were no relevant differences in HRQoL between the various JIA categories.

Our results are consistent with those reported by Oen et al. [19], who observed equivocal quality of life scores in the different JIA categories within 50 months of diagnosis. In our findings, this convergence was reached 12 months earlier. The almost equal quality of life of the different JIA categories was not found 10 years ago [8, 12, 14], which may be due to the improved effects of new treatment options. In the ICON cohort, patients with JIA were intensively treated (see [26]) according to current treatment recommendations [44–46]. Within the first year of observation, patients with systemic arthritis who received an interleukin (IL)-1 or IL-6 inhibitor most commonly achieved an inactive disease status [26] and had the highest mean PedsQL total score at the 1-year FU. In contrast, patients with psoriatic arthritis reached an inactive disease state less frequently [26] and had the lowest HRQoL scores at FU. Earlier findings [4, 41, 47] of a better HRQoL in JIA patients with inactive disease were confirmed in our study. The association between HRQoL and the clinical parameters of JIA have already been investigated in several studies [4, 9, 11, 12, 22, 48]. Significant associations between HRQoL and disease activity, physical disability, and pain have been described [4, 9, 22]. The impact of disability and pain was found to be stronger than that of disease activity in general, which is in line with our findings. Patient-reported (or, as in our study, parent-reported) outcomes were particularly associated with the patient's HRQoL, while clinical parameters such as the physician's global score or the number of actively involved joints played a minor role.

The proportion of JIA patients with a suboptimal HRQoL was investigated in other studies [9, 25, 49] which used a similar PedsQL cut-off to our work (< 78.6 versus < 79.3) to differentiate between optimal and suboptimal HRQOL. Lundberg et al. [49] and Haverman et al. [9] observed a suboptimal HRQoL in nearly half of their patients with JIA after a median of 2–5 and 3. 6 years of disease duration, respectively. In ICON, the outcome was more favorable. Only a quarter of the patients with JIA had a suboptimal HRQoL after 3 years of rheumatologic care. We identified pain and the parent's global assessment at enrollment as predictors of a suboptimal HRQoL status at FU. This is similar to the findings of others [4, 21, 50]. We further found that the burden caused by the disease on the child's family is another important predictor of a suboptimal quality of life. This is in accordance with other findings [24, 51] that described an association between HRQoL and the child's perception of social support and parental distress.

The strength of this study is the large sample size that accounts for differences in sociodemographic parameters such as age, sex, and social status between JIA patients and healthy peers. Only proxy-reported HRQoL was used to make conclusions for the whole cohort over the entire age range, rather than only in older patients and peers by self-reported HRQoL. It should be considered that proxy-reported HRQoL estimates may be biased compared with self-reports. However, the agreement between data reported by children and their parents is often high, especially in the case of sick children [47, 52]. In cases of discordance, the parents of sick patients described on average a lower HRQoL than the children themselves [43], resulting in an underestimation in HRQoL. There is another limitation that should not go unmentioned. We did not investigate the impact of individual treatment modalities on quality of life outcomes, as the ICON is an observational cohort study and treatment decisions prior to or after enrollment were confounded by their clinical indication.

Conclusion

With current treatment strategies, it is possible to achieve a favorable quality of life in most patients with JIA. After 3 years of pediatric rheumatology care, JIA patients have almost the same quality of life as healthy peers. This is a crucial finding for the counseling of patients and their parents. Among characteristics assessed at enrollment, family burden, pain, and functional impairment were more important than disease activity as predictors of a suboptimal quality of life over the course of this study. It is therefore important to look for these risk factors in clinical practice to be able to set the course at an early stage of the disease with targeted support measures.

Abbreviations

ANA: Antinuclear antibodies; bDMARD: Biologic disease-modifying antirheumatic drug; CHAQ: Childhood Health Assessment Questionnaire; CI: Confidence interval; cJADAS: Clinical Juvenile Arthritis Disease Activity Score; CRP: C-reactive protein; csDMARD: Conventional synthetic disease-modifying antirheumatic drug; DMARD: Disease-modifying antirheumatic drug; ESR: Erythrocyte sedimentation rate; FaBel: Family Burden Questionnaire; FU: Follow-up; HLA-B27: Human leukocyte antigen-B27; HRQoL: Health-related quality of life; ICON: Inception cohort of patients with newly diagnosed juvenile idiopathic arthritis; IL: Interleukin; ILAR: International League of Associations for Rheumatology; JAQQ: Juvenile Arthritis Quality of Life Questionnaire; JIA: Juvenile idiopathic arthritis; NRS: Numeric rating scale; NSAID: Nonsteroidal anti-inflammatory drug; OA: Oligoarthritis; PedsQL: Pediatric Quality of Life Inventory; PGA: Physician's global assessment of disease activity; RF: Rheumatoid factor; SD: Standard deviation; SDQ: Strength and Difficulties Questionnaire; SES: Socioeconomic status

Acknowledgements

We would like to thank all physicians engaged in the ICON cohort: Tilmann Kallinich, Berlin; Hans-Iko Huppertz, Bremen; Ivan Foeldvari, Hamburg; Angelika Thon, Hannover; Anton Hospach, Stuttgart; Jasmin Kümmerle-Deschner, Tübingen. We are especially grateful to all patients and their parents for their participation in ICON.

Funding

The ICON study is funded by the German Federal Ministry of Education and Research (BMBF, FKZ 01ER0812, 01ER0813, and 01ER0828).

Authors' contributions

ML performed data analysis and interpretation and drafted the paper. KM, IL, MN, CS, DF, AH, AK, GH, GG, and JPH participated in the design of the study and helped to draft the manuscript. JL and JK performed the data analysis and helped to draft the manuscript. KM was involved in the conception of the study, contributed to study design and performed interpretation. All authors read and approved the final manuscript.

Competing interests

The authors declare that they have no competing interests.

Author details

[1]Deutsches Rheuma-Forschungszentrum Berlin, Epidemiology Unit, Charitéplatz 1, 10117 Berlin, Germany. [2]Kinderkrankenhaus Amsterdamer Straße, Kliniken der Stadt Köln gGmbH, Köln, Germany. [3]Department of

Pediatric Rheumatology and Immunology, University of Münster, Münster, Germany. [4]Department of Ophthalmology at St. Franziskus Hospital Münster, University of Duisburg-Essen, Duisburg, Germany. [5]Asklepios Klinik Sankt Augustin, Sankt Augustin, Germany. [6]St. Josef-Stift Sendenhorst, Sendenhorst, Germany. [7]Deutsches Zentrum für Kinder- und Jugendrheumatologie, Garmisch-Partenkirchen, Germany. [8]Charité – Universitätsmedizin Berlin, Department of Rheumatology and Clinical Immunology, Berlin, Germany.

References

1. Prakken B, Albani S, Martini A. Juvenile idiopathic arthritis. Lancet. 2011; 377(9783):2138–49.
2. Magni-Manzoni S, Pistorio A, Labo E, Viola S, Garcia-Munitis P, Panigada S, Visconti C, Buoncompagni A, Martini A, Ravelli A. A longitudinal analysis of physical functional disability over the course of juvenile idiopathic arthritis. Ann Rheum Dis. 2008;67(8):1159–64.
3. Packham JC, Hall MA. Long-term follow-up of 246 adults with juvenile idiopathic arthritis: functional outcome. Rheumatology (Oxford). 2002;41(12): 1428–35.
4. Tollisen A, Selvaag AM, Aulie HA, Lilleby V, Aasland A, Lerdal A, Flato B. Physical functioning, pain and health-related quality of life in adults with juvenile idiopathic arthritis: a longitudinal 30-year follow-up study. Arthritis Care Res (Hoboken). 2017;. https://doi.org/10.1002/acr.23327. [Epub ahead of print]
5. Bullinger M, Hasford J. Evaluating quality-of-life measures for clinical trials in Germany. Control Clin Trials. 1991;12(4 Suppl):91S–105S.
6. The World Health Organization Quality of Life assessment (WHOQOL): position paper from the World Health Organization. Soc Sci Med. 1995; 41(10):1403–9.
7. Saxena S, Orley J, Group W. Quality of life assessment: The World Health Organization perspective. Eur Psychiatry. 1997;12(Suppl 3):263s–6s.
8. Foster HE, Marshall N, Myers A, Dunkley P, Griffiths ID. Outcome in adults with juvenile idiopathic arthritis: a quality of life study. Arthritis Rheum. 2003;48(3):767–75.
9. Haverman L, Grootenhuis MA, van den Berg JM, van Veenendaal M, Dolman KM, Swart JF, Kuijpers TW, van Rossum MA. Predictors of health-related quality of life in children and adolescents with juvenile idiopathic arthritis: results from a web-based survey. Arthritis Care Res (Hoboken). 2012;64(5): 694–703.
10. Manczak M, Rutkowska-Sak L, Raciborski F. Health-related quality of life in children with juvenile idiopathic arthritis—child's and parent's point of view. Reumatologia. 2016;54(5):243–50.
11. Bertilsson L, Andersson-Gare B, Fasth A, Petersson IF, Forsblad-D'elia H. Disease course, outcome, and predictors of outcome in a population-based juvenile chronic arthritis cohort followed for 17 years. J Rheumatol. 2013; 40(5):715–24.
12. Oliveira S, Ravelli A, Pistorio A, Castell E, Malattia C, Prieur AM, Saad-Magalhaes C, Murray KJ, Bae SC, Joos R, et al. Proxy-reported health-related quality of life of patients with juvenile idiopathic arthritis: the Pediatric Rheumatology International Trials Organization multinational quality of life cohort study. Arthritis Rheum. 2007;57(1):35–43.
13. Barth S, Haas JP, Schlichtiger J, Molz J, Bisdorff B, Michels H, Hugle B, Radon K. Long-term health-related quality of life in German patients with juvenile idiopathic arthritis in comparison to German general population. PLoS One. 2016;11(4):e0153267.
14. Gutierrez-Suarez R, Pistorio A, Cespedes Cruz A, Norambuena X, Flato B, Rumba I, Harjacek M, Nielsen S, Susic G, Mihaylova D, et al. Health-related quality of life of patients with juvenile idiopathic arthritis coming from 3 different geographic areas. The PRINTO multinational quality of life cohort study. Rheumatology (Oxford). 2007;46(2):314–20.
15. Solari N, Viola S, Pistorio A, Magni-Manzoni S, Vitale R, Ruperto N, Ullmann N, Filocamo G, Martini A, Ravelli A. Assessing current outcomes of juvenile idiopathic arthritis: a cross-sectional study in a tertiary center sample. Arthritis Rheum. 2008;59(11):1571–9.
16. Anink J, Prince FH, Dijkstra M, Otten MH, Twilt M, ten Cate R, Gorter SL, Koopman-Keemink Y, van Rossum MA, Hoppenreijs EP, et al. Long-term quality of life and functional outcome of patients with juvenile idiopathic arthritis in the biologic era: a longitudinal follow-up study in the Dutch Arthritis and Biologicals in Children Register. Rheumatology (Oxford). 2015; 54(11):1964–9.
17. Prince FH, Geerdink LM, Borsboom GJ, Twilt M, van Rossum MA, Hoppenreijs EP, Cate RT, Koopman-Keemink Y, van Santen-Hoeufft M, Raat H, et al. Major improvements in health-related quality of life during the use of etanercept in patients with previously refractory juvenile idiopathic arthritis. Ann Rheum Dis. 2010;69(1):138–42.
18. Ruperto N, Lovell DJ, Li T, Sztajnbok F, Goldenstein-Schainberg C, Scheinberg M, Penades IC, Fischbach M, Alcala JO, Hashkes PJ, et al. Abatacept improves health-related quality of life, pain, sleep quality, and daily participation in subjects with juvenile idiopathic arthritis. Arthritis Care Res (Hoboken). 2010;62(11):1542–51.
19. Oen K, Guzman J, Dufault B, Tucker LB, Shiff NJ, Watanabe Duffy K, Lee JJ, Feldman BM, Berard RA, Dancey P, et al. Health-related quality of life in an inception cohort of children with juvenile idiopathic arthritis: a longitudinal analysis. Arthritis Care Res (Hoboken). 2018;70(1):134-44. https://doi.org/10.1002/acr.23236. Epub 2017 Dec 6.
20. Nordal E, Zak M, Aalto K, Berntson L, Fasth A, Herlin T, Lahdenne P, Nielsen S, Straume B, Rygg M, et al. Ongoing disease activity and changing categories in a long-term nordic cohort study of juvenile idiopathic arthritis. Arthritis Rheum. 2011;63(9):2809–18.
21. Klotsche J, Minden K, Thon A, Ganser G, Urban A, Horneff G. Improvement in health-related quality of life for children with juvenile idiopathic arthritis after start of treatment with etanercept. Arthritis Care Res (Hoboken). 2014; 66(2):253–62.
22. Shaw KL, Southwood TR, Duffy CM, McDonagh JE. Health-related quality of life in adolescents with juvenile idiopathic arthritis. Arthritis Rheum. 2006; 55(2):199–207.
23. van Dijkhuizen EH, Wulffraat NM. Early predictors of prognosis in juvenile idiopathic arthritis: a systematic literature review. Ann Rheum Dis. 2015; 74(11):1996–2005.
24. Seid M, Huang B, Niehaus S, Brunner HI, Lovell DJ. Determinants of health-related quality of life in children newly diagnosed with juvenile idiopathic arthritis. Arthritis Care Res (Hoboken). 2014;66(2):263–9.
25. Seid M, Opipari L, Huang B, Brunner HI, Lovell DJ. Disease control and health-related quality of life in juvenile idiopathic arthritis. Arthritis Rheum. 2009;61(3):393–9.
26. Sengler C, Klotsche J, Niewerth M, Liedmann I, Foll D, Heiligenhaus A, Ganser G, Horneff G, Haas JP, Minden K. The majority of newly diagnosed patients with juvenile idiopathic arthritis reach an inactive disease state within the first year of specialised care: data from a German inception cohort. RMD Open. 2015;1(1):e000074.
27. Petty RE, Southwood TR, Manners P, Baum J, Glass DN, Goldenberg J, He X, Maldonado-Cocco J, Orozco-Alcala J, Prieur AM, et al. International League of Associations for Rheumatology classification of juvenile idiopathic arthritis: second revision, Edmonton, 2001. J Rheumatol. 2004;31(2):390–2.
28. McErlane F, Beresford MW, Baildam EM, Chieng SE, Davidson JE, Foster HE, Gardner-Medwin J, Lunt M, Wedderburn LR, Thomson W, et al. Validity of a three-variable juvenile arthritis disease activity score in children with new-onset juvenile idiopathic arthritis. Ann Rheum Dis. 2013;72(12):1983–8.
29. Consolaro A, Bracciolini G, Ruperto N, Pistorio A, Magni-Manzoni S, Malattia C, Pederzoli S, Davi S, Martini A, Ravelli A, et al. Remission, minimal disease activity, and acceptable symptom state in juvenile idiopathic arthritis: defining criteria based on the juvenile arthritis disease activity score. Arthritis Rheum. 2012;64(7):2366–74.
30. Consolaro A, Ravelli A. Defining criteria for disease activity states in juvenile idiopathic arthritis. Rheumatology (Oxford). 2016;55(4):595–6.
31. Singh G, Athreya BH, Fries JF, Goldsmith DP. Measurement of health status in children with juvenile rheumatoid arthritis. Arthritis Rheum. 1994;37(12): 1761–9.
32. Varni JW, Seid M, Smith Knight T, Burwinkle T, Brown J, Szer IS. The PedsQL in pediatric rheumatology: reliability, validity, and responsiveness of the Pediatric Quality of Life Inventory Generic Core Scales and Rheumatology Module. Arthritis Rheum. 2002;46(3):714–25.
33. Varni JW, Burwinkle TM, Seid M, Skarr D. The PedsQL 4.0 as a pediatric population health measure: feasibility, reliability, and validity. Ambul Pediatr. 2003;3(6):329–41.
34. Goodman R. The Strengths and Difficulties Questionnaire: a research note. J Child Psychol Psychiatry. 1997;38(5):581–6.
35. Stone LL, Janssens JM, Vermulst AA, Van Der Maten M, Engels RC, Otten R. The Strengths and Difficulties Questionnaire: psychometric properties of the parent and teacher version in children aged 4-7. BMC Psychol. 2015;3(1):4.

36. Stein RE, Riessman CK. The development of an impact-on-family scale: preliminary findings. Med Care. 1980;18(4):465–72.
37. Ravens-Sieberer U, Morfeld M, Stein RE, Jessop DJ, Bullinger M, Thyen U. The testing and validation of the German version of the impact on family scale in families with children with disabilities. Psychother Psychosom Med Psychol. 2001;51(9–10):384–93.
38. Lampert T, Muters S, Stolzenberg H, Kroll LE, Ki GGSSG. Measurement of socioeconomic status in the KiGGS study: first follow-up (KiGGS Wave 1). Bundesgesundheitsblatt Gesundheitsforschung Gesundheitsschutz. 2014; 57(7):762–70.
39. McErlane F, Foster HE, Carrasco R, Baildam EM, Chieng SE, Davidson JE, Ioannou Y, Wedderburn LR, Thomson W, Hyrich KL. Trends in paediatric rheumatology referral times and disease activity indices over a ten-year period among children and young people with juvenile idiopathic arthritis: results from the childhood arthritis prospective Study. Rheumatology (Oxford). 2016;55(7):1225–34.
40. Oen K, Duffy CM, Tse SM, Ramsey S, Ellsworth J, Chedeville G, Chetaille AL, Saint-Cyr C, Cabral DA, Spiegel LR, et al. Early outcomes and improvement of patients with juvenile idiopathic arthritis enrolled in a Canadian multicenter inception cohort. Arthritis Care Res (Hoboken). 2010;62(4):527–36.
41. Flato B, Lien G, Smerdel A, Vinje O, Dale K, Johnston V, Sorskaar D, Moum T, Ploski R, Forre O. Prognostic factors in juvenile rheumatoid arthritis: a case-control study revealing early predictors and outcome after 14.9 years. J Rheumatol. 2003;30(2):386–93.
42. Noll RB, Kozlowski K, Gerhardt C, Vannatta K, Taylor J, Passo M. Social, emotional, and behavioral functioning of children with juvenile rheumatoid arthritis. Arthritis Rheum. 2000;43(6):1387–96.
43. Upton P, Lawford J, Eiser C. Parent-child agreement across child health-related quality of life instruments: a review of the literature. Qual Life Res. 2008;17(6):895–913.
44. Ringold S, Weiss PF, Beukelman T, DeWitt EM, Ilowite NT, Kimura Y, Laxer RM, Lovell DJ, Nigrovic PA, Robinson AB, et al. 2013 update of the 2011 American College of Rheumatology recommendations for the treatment of juvenile idiopathic arthritis: recommendations for the medical therapy of children with systemic juvenile idiopathic arthritis and tuberculosis screening among children receiving biologic medications. Arthritis Rheum. 2013;65(10):2499–512.
45. Dueckers G, Guellac N, Arbogast M, Dannecker G, Foeldvari I, Frosch M, Ganser G, Heiligenhaus A, Horneff G, Illhardt A, et al. Evidence and consensus based GKJR guidelines for the treatment of juvenile idiopathic arthritis. Clin Immunol. 2012;142(2):176–93.
46. Beukelman T. Treatment advances in systemic juvenile idiopathic arthritis. F1000Prime Rep. 2014;6:21.
47. Ringold S, Wallace CA, Rivara FP. Health-related quality of life, physical function, fatigue, and disease activity in children with established polyarticular juvenile idiopathic arthritis. J Rheumatol. 2009;36(6):1330–6.
48. Mulligan K, Kassoumeri L, Etheridge A, Moncrieffe H, Wedderburn LR, Newman S. Mothers' reports of the difficulties that their children experience in taking methotrexate for juvenile idiopathic arthritis and how these impact on quality of life. Pediatr Rheumatol Online J. 2013;11(1):23.
49. Lundberg V, Lindh V, Eriksson C, Petersen S, Eurenius E. Health-related quality of life in girls and boys with juvenile idiopathic arthritis: self- and parental reports in a cross-sectional study. Pediatr Rheumatol Online J. 2012; 10(1):33.
50. Taxter AJ, Wileyto EP, Behrens EM, Weiss PF. Patient-reported outcomes across categories of juvenile idiopathic arthritis. J Rheumatol. 2015;42(10): 1914–21.
51. Aasland A, Flato B, Vandvik IH. Psychosocial outcome in juvenile chronic arthritis: a nine-year follow-up. Clin Exp Rheumatol. 1997;15(5):561–8.
52. April KT, Feldman DE, Platt RW, Duffy CM. Comparison between children with juvenile idiopathic arthritis (JIA) and their parents concerning perceived quality of life. Qual Life Res. 2006;15(4):655–61.

Predicting unfavorable long-term outcome in juvenile idiopathic arthritis: results from the Nordic cohort study

Veronika Rypdal[1,2*], Ellen Dalen Arnstad[3,4], Kristiina Aalto[5], Lillemor Berntson[6], Maria Ekelund[6,7], Anders Fasth[8], Mia Glerup[9], Troels Herlin[9], Susan Nielsen[10], Suvi Peltoniemi[5], Marek Zak[10], Marite Rygg[3,11], Martin Rypdal[12], Ellen Nordal[1,2] For the Nordic Study Group of Pediatric Rheumatology (NoSPeR)

Abstract

Background: The aim was to develop prediction rules that may guide early treatment decisions based on baseline clinical predictors of long-term unfavorable outcome in juvenile idiopathic arthritis (JIA).

Methods: In the Nordic JIA cohort, we assessed baseline disease characteristics as predictors of the following outcomes 8 years after disease onset. Non-achievement of remission off medication according to the preliminary Wallace criteria, functional disability assessed by Childhood Health Assessment Questionnaire (CHAQ) and Physical Summary Score (PhS) of the Child Health Questionnaire, and articular damage assessed by the Juvenile Arthritis Damage Index-Articular (JADI-A). Multivariable models were constructed, and cross-validations were performed by repeated partitioning of the cohort into training sets for developing prediction models and validation sets to test predictive ability.

Results: The total cohort constituted 423 children. Remission status was available in 410 children: 244 (59.5%) of these did not achieve remission off medication at the final study visit. Functional disability was present in 111/340 (32.7%) children assessed by CHAQ and 40/199 (20.1%) by PhS, and joint damage was found in 29/216 (13.4%). Model performance was acceptable for making predictions of long-term outcome. In validation sets, the area under the curves (AUCs) in the receiver operating characteristic (ROC) curves were 0.78 (IQR 0.72–0.82) for non-achievement of remission off medication, 0.73 (IQR 0.67–0.76) for functional disability assessed by CHAQ, 0.74 (IQR 0.65–0.80) for functional disability assessed by PhS, and 0.73 (IQR 0.63–0.76) for joint damage using JADI-A.

Conclusion: The feasibility of making long-term predictions of JIA outcome based on early clinical assessment is demonstrated. The prediction models have acceptable precision and require only readily available baseline variables. Further testing in other cohorts is warranted.

Keywords: Juvenile idiopathic arthritis, Disease activity, Prediction, Outcome research

Background

Juvenile idiopathic arthritis (JIA) is a heterogeneous childhood disease, with chronic joint inflammation as the common feature. The JIA categories differ by the number of joints affected, and the presence of extra-articular involvement [1]. Disease course and prognosis differ between JIA categories, but there is also large variability within each category [2, 3]. Therefore, efforts have been made to discern baseline clinical prognostic factors that can predict the severity, course, and long-term outcome of the disease [4, 5].

The primary goal of JIA treatment is to achieve remission [6]. Early prediction of the disease course for the individual child can facilitate tailored treatment. There is increasing evidence for the concept of "the window of therapeutic opportunity" in JIA, where early aggressive treatment with biologic agents and/or other disease-modifying anti-rheumatic drugs (DMARDs) may modify the disease course and improve long-term prognosis [7–9]. On the other hand, it is

* Correspondence: veronika.rypdal@unn.no
[1]Department of Pediatrics, University Hospital of North Norway, Tromsø, Norway
[2]Department of Clinical Medicine, UIT the Arctic University of Norway, Tromsø, Norway
Full list of author information is available at the end of the article

also essential to avoid unnecessary, costly, and potentially toxic treatment in children with a favorable prognosis.

Guzman et al. have recently presented a model for prediction of severe disease course, with outcomes developed specifically for their study [10]. In a systematic literature review, Dijkhuizen and Wulffraat state the need for prospective longitudinal studies of baseline clinical predictors using standardized validated outcome measures [4]. In the Nordic JIA cohort, we studied prediction of four established and validated outcomes, and aimed to construct prediction models that may aid decision on early aggressive treatment.

Methods

Study population

The initial prospective longitudinal multicenter Nordic JIA cohort consisted of consecutive children with incident JIA from 12 participating centers in defined geographical areas of Denmark, Finland, Norway and Sweden. All children in these areas with newly diagnosed JIA and disease onset in the study periods between 1 January 1997 and 30 June 2000 were included. The study was designed to be as close to population-based as possible, as previously reported [11].

In the current study, 440 children met the criteria of having a baseline study visit and a final study visit 8 years after disease onset. Out of these, 17 patients with systemic JIA were excluded, because systemic JIA is considered to have autoinflammatory rather than autoimmune disease mechanisms, and the clinical characteristics of predominantly fever, rash and serositis differs from other JIA-categories [12].

The baseline study visit was planned 6 months after disease onset. At this visit, disease activity variables, complete joint count, physician's global assessment of disease activity (physician's GA) on a 10-cm visual analogue scale (VAS), patient's/parent's global assessment (GA), medication and blood tests were registered [13]. Disease onset was defined as the time of presentation of symptoms of active arthritis, and the JIA categories were determined according to the International League of Associations for Rheumatology (ILAR) criteria [14].

Outcomes

At follow up, we evaluated 4 outcomes: (1) the main outcome was non-achievement of remission off medication, chosen as the best available validated measure of an adverse disease state over time. This included active disease, inactive disease of less than 12 months of duration, and clinical remission on medication (according to the preliminary Wallace criteria) [15, 16]. For the remainder of the paper, not in remission or non-achievement of remission refers to non-achievement of remission off medication unless otherwise specified; (2) and (3) functional disability was evaluated using the Childhood Health Assessment Questionnaire (CHAQ), and the Child Health Questionnaire Parent form (CHQ-PF50), aiming to achieve a broad evaluation of functional disability using both the JIA-specific CHAQ and the generic CHQ-PF50 instruments. CHAQ addresses functional ability in different activities of everyday life [17]. The CHAQ was completed by children of age >9 years, and otherwise by their parents, and the corresponding Health Assessment Questionnaire (HAQ) by participants > 18 years of age. From this point on in the text, CHAQ will refer to both the CHAQ and HAQ scores. The CHQ-PF50 consists of 50 items and 12 domains assessing health-related quality of life, yielding a physical summary score (PhS) and a psychological summary score (PsS) [17]. PhS ranges from 0 to 100, with a higher score indicating better functional ability; and (4) joint damage was assessed using the Juvenile Arthritis Damage Index of articular damage (JADI-A) ranging from 0 to a maximum of 72, where 36 joints, or joint groups, are scored 0 for no damage, 1 for partial damage, or 2 for severe damage [18]. All 4 outcomes were dichotomized; remission was dichotomized into clinical remission (those achieving remission without medication), and non-achievement of remission off medication (those not achieving remission or achieving remission on medication), CHAQ and JADI-A into score = 0, indicating no functional disability or no joint damage, and positive score >0, PhS into good functional ability, defined as score ≥40, and functional disability <40. This latter cut-off level is based on a reference score of 40 being one standard deviation below the mean score of healthy children in the USA [19].

Laboratory tests

Antinuclear antibodies (ANA) and rheumatoid factor (RF) were tested at least twice with a minimum of 3 months apart. ANA was analyzed by immunofluorescence on Hep-2 cells. Tests were interpreted according to cutoff values of the local immunological laboratories. HLA-B27 was analyzed using standardized methods [20]. C-reactive protein (CRP) was measured with immunoassays, with values <10 mg/L considered normal.

Statistics

Conventional descriptive statistics (absolute numbers, median, 1st and 3rd quartile, and percentage) were used to describe demographics and clinical characteristics. Univariate logistic regression was performed to assess baseline variables as predictors for each outcome. Variables that were significant at $p < 0.05$ in the univariate analysis were considered as candidates in a prediction model.

For each outcome, multivariable logistic regression models were constructed using a combination of predefined core variables, and additional variables selected using a forward stepwise selection method. Since the predictive ability of the models is assessed using cross-validation, the conventional limitations related to the screening of a large number of covariates in multivariable models are evaded [21]. Cross-validation controlled for overfitting of the data (internal validation), and the degree of overfitting is reflected in the performance in validation sets.

Clinical characteristics included in the Wallace provisional criteria for remission were a priori included in the prediction models; the cumulative active joint count, erythrocyte sedimentation rate (ESR), CRP, physician's GA, and morning stiffness [22]. Uveitis activity applies only to a minority of the cohort and was therefore not included. The additional baseline variables were included in a stepwise fashion if they contributed to the multivariable model with $p < 0.05$ when included. Symmetric joint involvement was not considered a candidate predictor as it correlates strongly with the specific joint involvement (Fig. 1). To ensure model simplicity the total number of variables was not allowed to exceed 10. Once the set of variables were selected, the model coefficients β_i for each predictor variable x_i were estimated using multivariable logistic regression, and the probability of unfavorable outcome was given as:

$$P = 1/\left(1 + e^{-A}\right), \text{where } A = \beta_0 + \beta_1 x_1 + \ldots + \beta_n x_n.$$

For each of the four outcomes, cross-validation of the method was performed by partitioning the cohort randomly in training sets consisting of three quarters of the patients ($N = 317$) and validation sets consisting of one quarter of the patients ($N = 106$). In each realization of the random partitioning we constructed prediction models using the algorithm described above, using *only* the training set to select variables and estimate coefficients. For each of the patients in the corresponding validation set the multivariable logistic model provides a probability of the unfavorable outcome. By comparing the predicted probability of unfavorable outcome with the actual outcome at the final study visit, the receiver operating characteristic (ROC) curve was computed, and the area under the curve (AUC) was estimated. The median AUC with interquartile range (IQR) was estimated from 100 realizations of the random partitioning of the cohort. For each step in the cross-validation we omitted any patients where the outcome or the required predictor variables were not available.

Finally, in our cohort we tested the prediction model for severe disease course developed by Guzman et al. [10]. We tested Guzman's model using the 4 outcome measures described above, i.e. not the outcomes for which their model was constructed. The analysis was performed using the software packages STATA version 14, and Wolfram Mathematica version 11.1.1.0.

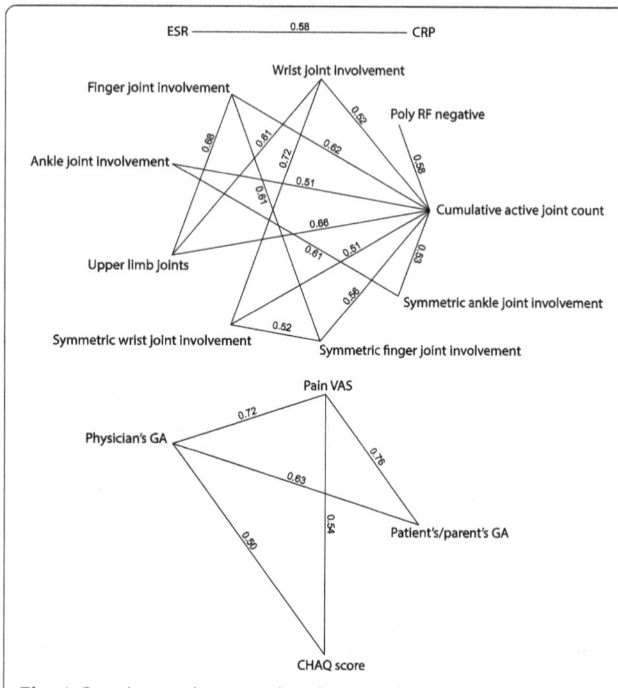

Fig. 1 Correlations between baseline variables. Lines are drawn only between pairs of baseline variables for which the sample Spearman correlation coefficient is ≥ 0.50. Baseline variables without correlation ≥0.50 are not included in the figure. RF, rheumatoid factor; VAS, visual analogue scale; GA, global assessment; CHAQ, Childhood Health Assessment Questionnaire

Ethical considerations

Approvals from medical research ethical committees and data protection authorities were granted according to the regulations of each participating country. Written informed consent was obtained from parents of children aged < 16 years, and from the children themselves if aged ≥ 16 years of age.

Results

The main finding is that in the Nordic cohort, long-term outcome in JIA can be predicted, with acceptable sensitivity and specificity, using only a handful of readily available clinical variables.

Study cohort

Characteristics of the 440 patients in the cohort have previously been published [11]. The study cohort constituted 423 children, after 17 patients with systemic JIA were excluded. The median time between disease onset and the baseline study visit was 7 (IQR 6–8) months,

Table 1 Baseline clinical characteristics as predictors of non-achievement of remission off medication in univariate logistic regression

Baseline characteristics	Total *N*	Remission off medication[a]	Not in remission[b]	OR (95% CI)	*p*
Gender female, *n* (%)	410	106 (38.8)	167 (61.2)	0.8 (0.5–1.2)	0.334
Age at disease onset, years	410	6.3 (2.5–10.0)	5.2 (2.5–9.6)	0.9 (0.9–1.0)	0.401
Time from onset to diagnosis, months	388	1.5 (0.5–2.9)	1.7 (0.5–3.6)	1.0 (1.0–1.1)	0.152
Cumulative active joint count	410	2 (1–4)	4 (2–7)	1.1 (1.1–1.2)	< 0.001
Physician's global assessment VAS	227	0.8 (0.0–1.3)	2.0 (1.0–3.8)	3.5 (1.9–6.2)	< 0.001
Polyarticular RF-positive, *n* (%)	410	1 (25.0)	3 (75.0)	2.1 (0.2–20.0)	0.535
Polyarticular RF-negative, *n* (%)	410	25 (26.9)	68 (73.1)	2.2 (1.3–3.6)	0.003
Oligoarticular, *n* (%)	410	107 (49.1)	111 (50.9)	0.5 (0.3–0.7)	< 0.001
Psoriatic arthritis, n (%)	410	3 (50.0)	3 (50.0)	0.7 (0.1–3.4)	0.635
Enthesitis-related arthritis (ERA), *n* (%)	410	11 (32.4)	23 (67.6)	1.5 (0.7–3.1)	0.315
Undifferentiated arthritis, *n* (%)	410	19 (34.5)	36 (65.5)	1.3 (0.7–2.4)	0.336
ANA-positive, ≤ 6 years, *n* (%)[c]	397	22 (31.4)	48 (68.6)	1.6 (0.9–2.7)	0.107
Specific joint involvement, *n* (%)					
Hip joint	409	18 (32.1)	38 (67.9)	1.5 (0.8–2.8)	0.168
Ankle joint	409	57 (31.0)	127 (69.0)	2.1 (1.4–3.1)	< 0.001
Tarsal joint	409	6 (16.7)	30 (83.3)	3.8 (1.5–9.2)	0.004
Subtalar joint	409	14 (26.9)	38 (73.1)	2.0 (1.1–3.8)	0.034
Wrist joint	409	33 (30.6)	75 (69.4)	1.8 (1.1–2.9)	0.014
Finger joint	409	36 (27.7)	94 (72.3)	2.3 (1.5–3.6)	< 0.001
Neck	409	9 (26.5)	25 (73.5)	2.0 (0.9–4.4)	0.085
Upper limb joints	410	67 (32.7)	138 (67.3)	1.9 (1.3–2.9)	0.001
Lower limb joints	410	144 (39.0)	225 (61.0)	1.8 (0.9–3.5)	0.073
Symmetric involvement, *n* (%)					
Hip joints	409	5 (21.7)	18 (78.3)	2.6 (0.9–7.1)	0.067
Ankle joints	409	27 (28.4)	68 (71.6)	2.0 (1.2–3.3)	0.006
Wrist joints	409	22 (34.4)	42 (65.6)	1.4 (0.8–2.4)	0.272
Finger joints	409	13 (22.0)	46 (78.0)	2.7 (1.4–5.3)	0.002
Patient-reported outcomes					
Patient's/parent's global assessment VAS	250	0.5 (0.0–2.2)	1.7 (0.5–3.5)	2.2 (1.4–3.4)	0.001
CHAQ score	257	0.1 (0.0–0.6)	0.5 (0.0–1.1)	2.0 (1.3–3.0)	0.002
Pain VAS	246	0.4 (0.0–3.0)	2.3 (0.5–4.2)	1.9 (1.3–2.8)	0.002
Morning stiffness for > 15 min, *n* (%)	314	25 (22.1)	88 (77.9)	3.6 (2.1–6.0)	< 0.001
Laboratory tests					
ESR mm/h	332	11.0 (6.0–18.0)	17.0 (9.5–34.0)	1.4 (1.2–1.7)	< 0.001
CRP >10 mg/L, *n* (%)	329	12 (16.7)	60 (83.3)	3.9 (2.0–7.5)	< 0.001
ANA-positive, *n* (%)	397	37 (33.0)	75 (67.0)	1.5 (1.0–2.4)	0.075
RF-positive, *n* (%)	221	5 (50.0)	5 (50.0)	0.6 (0.2–2.0)	0.376
HLA-B27 positive, *n* (%)	382	21 (25.9)	60 (74.1)	2.1 (1.2–3.6)	0.010

Values are the median (interquartile range, IQR), or number (percentage)

OR odds ratio, *CI* confidence interval, *VAS* visual analogue scale, *CHAQ* Childhood Health Assessment Questionnaire, *ESR* erythrocyte sedimentation rate for an increase in 10 mm/h, *CRP* C-reactive protein, *ANA* antinuclear antibody, *RF* rheumatoid factor, *HLA-B27* human leucocyte antigen

[a]Inactive disease off medication for 12 months according to the preliminary Wallace criteria

[b]Not in remission equals non-achievement of remission off medication

[c]ANA-positive patients ≤6 years at disease onset, with oligoarticular, polyarticular RF negative, psoriatic or undifferentiated arthritis

and between disease onset and the final study visit it was 98 (IQR 95–102) months. The median time from disease onset to diagnosis was 1.6 (IQR 0.5–3.3) months. A total of 280 patients (66.2%) were female, and the median age of disease onset in the cohort was 5.5 (IQR 2.5–9.7) years (Additional file 1: Table S1).

At the baseline study visit, 227/423 patients (53.7%) had oligoarthritis, 94/423 (22.2%) had rheumatoid factor (RF)-negative polyarthritis, and 4/423 (1.0%) had RF-positive polyarthritis (Additional file 1: Table S1). The median cumulative number of active joints within the first visit was 3 (IQR 1–6), and 381/423 patients (90.1%) had one or more affected lower limb joints at the baseline visit. Antinuclear antibodies (ANA) were present in 115/410 patients (28.1%), and HLA-B27 in 85/393 patients (21.6%) [23], presented in Additional file 1: Table S1. None of the children had started biologic agents before the baseline study visit, and early medications are shown in Additional file 2: Table S2. A total of 410/423 (96.9% of the total cohort) had baseline assessments and data on remission 8 years after disease onset. The corresponding numbers were 340/423 (80.4%) for CHAQ, 199/423 (47.0%) for PhS and 216/423 (51.1%) for JADI-A.

Correlation between baseline variables

The clinical predictor variables were analyzed with respect to correlation. There was significantly positive, moderate to strong correlation between several variables, especially between cumulative number of active joints, the joint-specific variables, and the polyarthritis RF-negative category. Physician's GA and the patient-reported outcomes also correlated positively with each other. The correlation structure between the predictor variables is illustrated in Fig. 1.

Prediction of non-achievement of remission off medication

Remission status at the final study visit was available for 410 patients. There were 166 (40.5%) children in remission without medication, while 38 (9.3%) were in remission on medication, and 206 (50.2%) were not in remission: 244/410 children (59.5%) did not achieve remission off medication. The baseline predictors of not achieving remission off medication were analyzed by univariate logistic regression and are presented in Table 1.

The following predictor variables were included in the multivariable prediction model for non-achievement of remission: Cumulative active joint count, ESR, CRP, morning stiffness, physician's GA, ANA, HLA-B27, and ankle joint arthritis. The first five variables were chosen a priori, and ANA, HLA-B27, and ankle joint arthritis were the variables included through the stepwise selection method (Table 2). The model has an AUC of 0.84 in the total cohort. Cross-validation yielded a median AUC = 0.78 (IQR 0.72–0.82) in the validation sets (Table 3). The corresponding ROC curves are shown in Figs. 2 and 3.

Table 2 Prediction of unfavorable outcome by multivariable modeling of baseline clinical characteristics

	Coef.	Std.Err
Not in remission[a] $N = 156$		
	β_0=-1.58	0.44
Cumulative active joint count	β_1=0.04	0.05
ESR mm/h	β_2=0.03	0.02
CRP >10 mg/L	β_3=-0.07	0.69
Morning stiffness > 15 min	β_4=1.16	0.45
Physician's global assessment VAS	β_5=0.16	0.46
ANA-positive	β_6=1.25	0.50
HLA-B27-positive	β_7=1.37	0.54
Ankle joint arthritis	β_8=1.10	0.49
Functional disability (CHAQ), $N = 141$		
	β_0=-1.68	0.35
Cumulative active joint count	β_1=-0.02	0.03
ESR mm/h	β_2=0.01	0.01
CRP > 10 mg/L	β_3=-0.20	0.63
Morning stiffness > 15 min	β_4=1.03	0.42
Physician's global assessment VAS	β_5=-0.40	0.56
Finger joint arthritis	β_6=1.21	0.54
Pain VAS	β_7 = 0.77	0.40
Functional disability (PhS), $N = 92$		
	β_0=-3.40	0.75
Cumulative active joint count	β_1=0.10	0.05
ESR mm/h	β_2=0.01	0.02
CRP > 10 mg/L	β_3=-2.06	1.28
Morning stiffness > 15 min	β_4=1.68	0.80
Physician's global assessment VAS	β_5=-0.71	0.88
Pain VAS	β_6=1.30	0.64
Joint damage (JADI-A), $N = 141$		
	β_0=-3.84	0.76
Cumulative active joint count	β_1=0.02	0.04
ESR mm/h	β_2=0.01	0.02
CRP > 10 mg/l	β_3= -0.11	0.83
Morning stiffness > 15 min	β_4=-0.59	0.61
Physician's global assessment VAS	β_5=0.28	0.52
Finger joint arthritis	β_6=1.84	0.68
Older age at disease onset (years)	β_7= 0.16	0.07

Coef. coefficients in the logistic regression, *Std.Err.* standard error in the coefficients, *VAS* visual analogue scale, *ESR* erythrocyte sedimentation rate for an increase in 10 mm/h, *CRP* C-reactive protein, *ANA* antinuclear antibody, *HLA-B27* human leucocyte antigen

[a]Not in remission equals non-achievement of remission off medication

We also developed a prediction model without the blood samples (ESR, CRP, ANA, and HLA-B27). This model yielded an AUC = 0.76 (IQR 0.72–0.80) for non-achievement of remission in the validation sets (Additional file 3: Figure S1).

Prediction of functional disability and joint damage

The CHAQ score at the final study visit was available in 340 children, and 111 (32.7%) had a CHAQ score >0. Three of the four patients with RF-positive polyarthritis reported functional disability. For univariate logistic regression results see Additional file 4: Table S3.

The prediction model for CHAQ score >0 uses cumulative active joint count, ESR, CRP, morning stiffness, physician's GA, finger joint arthritis, and pain VAS as variables (Table 2). The AUC of this model was 0.79 in the total cohort, and cross validation gave a median AUC of 0.73 (IQR 0.67–0.76) in the validation sets (Table 3). The ROC curve for the total cohort, and validation sets are shown in Figs. 2 and 3, respectively. The AUC for the model without blood samples was 0.72 (IQR 0.67–0.76) in the validation sets (Additional file 3: Figure S1).

Of the 199 patients with a physical summary score, 40 (20.1%) had a score <40. Results of the univariate analysis with PhS <40 as the outcome variable are shown in Additional file 5: Table S4. Variables included in the prediction model for PhS were cumulative active joint count, ESR, CRP, morning stiffness, Physician's GA, and pain VAS (Table 2). The AUC was 0.90 in the total cohort, and cross-validation gave a median AUC = 0.74 (IQR 0.65–0.80) in the validation sets (Table 3, Figs. 2 and 3). The AUC for the model without blood samples was 0.73 (0.66–0.79) in the validation sets (Additional file 3: Figure S1).

The JADI-A was collected for 216 patients at the final study visit, and 29 patients (13.4%) had joint damage registered 8 years after disease onset. The baseline predictors of joint damage are presented in Additional file 6: Table S5. In the prediction model, older age at disease onset and finger joint arthritis were included in addition to the five previously included variables (Table 2). The AUC was 0.84 in the cohort, and the median AUC was 0.73 (IQR 0.63–0.76) in the validation sets. The results are summarized in Table 3 and Figs. 2 and 3. Without blood tests the median AUC in the validation sets was 0.73 (IQR 0.63–0.80) (Additional file 3: Figure S1).

Other prediction models

The prediction model developed by Guzman et al. [10] was tested in our cohort by testing the ability of their model to predict the four outcomes described above. The model yielded an AUC = 0.69 for prediction of not achieving remission. For CHAQ >0, PhS <40, and JADI-A >0 the AUCs were 0.68, 0.69, and 0.71, respectively (Additional file 7: Figure S2).

Discussion

In the Nordic JIA cohort, we have developed and evaluated prediction models for long-term unfavorable outcome with acceptable sensitivity and specificity based on variables easily available at baseline, which may guide individually tailored treatment. Prediction of long-term unfavorable outcome early in the disease course may be useful in deciding when to start aggressive treatment in JIA.

To our knowledge, this is the first study on long-term prediction of well-established disease outcomes in a prospective population-based JIA cohort. Cross-validation analysis of model performance yielded AUCs of 0.78, 0.73, 0.74, and 0.73, for non-achievement of remission, CHAQ >0, PhS <40, and JADI-A >0, respectively.

An important step in developing applicable prediction models for JIA was carried out by Guzman et al. in a Canadian JIA cohort [10]. The authors recommended that their results should be tested in other JIA cohorts. We were not able to reproduce the predictive ability of their model in the Nordic JIA cohort (Additional file 7: Figure S2). One obvious reason for the discrepancy could be that Guzman's model is constructed to predict severe disease course, and not per se, any of the four pre-established, validated adverse outcomes that we assessed. Other reasons may be differences in the population-based approach, cohort composition, or ethnicity, or overfitting of models to the cohort.

The primary goal in the treatment of children with JIA is to achieve remission off medication, and the main implication of the current study is that prediction models may be useful in guiding decisions about treatment. Previous studies have indicated that the disease course may be modified by starting appropriate treatment early

Table 3 Cross-validation of the four prediction models of unfavorable long-term outcome in the Nordic JIA cohort

	Not in remission[a]	Functional disability (CHAQ)	Functional disability (PhS)	Joint damage (JADI-A)
AUC total cohort	0.84	0.79	0.90	0.84
AUC validation sets[b]	0.78 (0.72–0.82)	0.73 (0.67–0.76)	0.74 (0.65–0.80)	0.73 (0.63–0.76)

AUC area under the receiver operating characteristic curve, *CHAQ* Childhood Health Assessment Questionnaire, *PhS* Physical Summary Score, *JADI-A* Juvenile Arthritis Damage Index-Articular

[a]Not in remission equals non-achievement of remission off medication

[b]The AUCs in the validation sets are the median AUCs with the interquartile range of the 100 constructed models

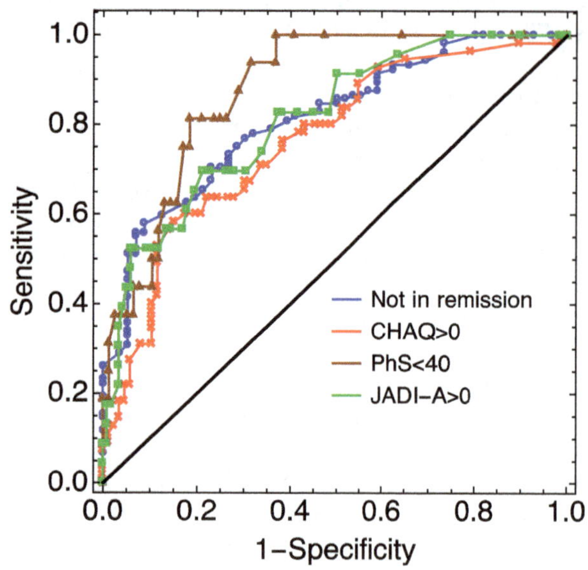

Fig. 2 Receiver operating characteristic (ROC) curves for the four unfavorable clinical outcomes in the total cohort. Non-achievement of remission off medication; CHAQ, Childhood Health Assessment Questionnaire; PhS, Physical Summary Score; JADI-A, Juvenile Arthritis Damage Index-Articular

[9, 24, 25]. To reach the goal of early inactive disease, a treat-to-target strategy including shared decision-making with well-informed children and parents is currently recommended [6, 9]. Even with promising advances in using gene expression profiles and biomarkers as predictors of treatment response and flare risk [26–29], the practical value of prediction based on a handful of readily available clinical variables cannot be understated.

The main strengths of our study are the use of validated outcome measures, the simplicity of the models, and the strict cross-validations. The use of validated outcomes is called for in reports on prognosis in JIA [3, 30, 31]. Model simplicity is ensured through the model construction method, where the main variables in the preliminary Wallace criteria of remission are included in the models a priori [15, 22]. The additional variables that were included in our models have independently been associated with adverse outcomes in previous studies [4, 23, 32–36].

The model performance was assessed using cross-validations, where predictions were performed on validation sets that were completely separate from the data used to construct the models. The 100 repeated model constructions and evaluations prevent overfitting the data. Despite

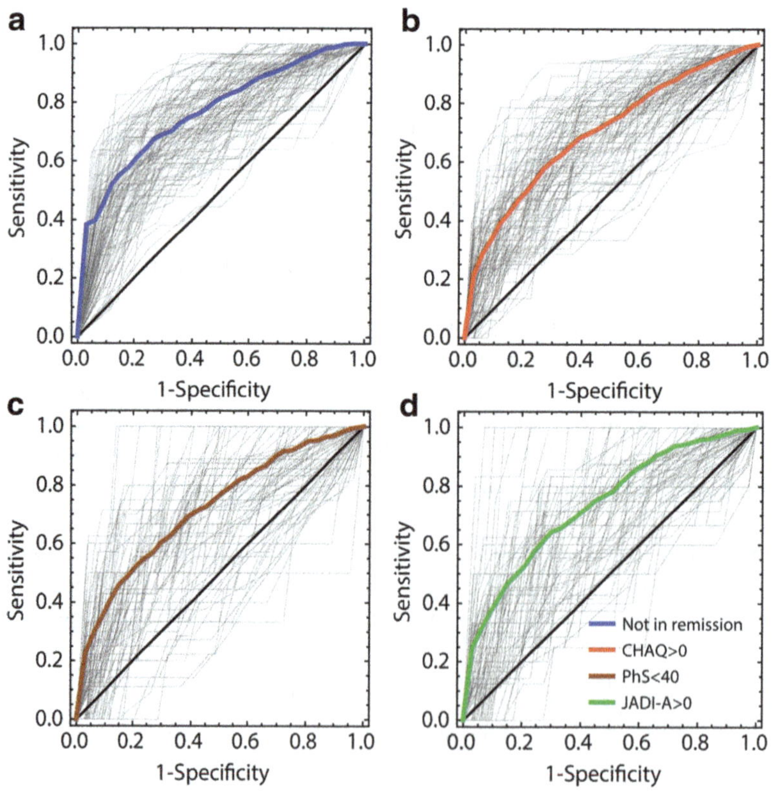

Fig. 3 Receiver operating characteristic (ROC) curves for the four unfavorable clinical outcomes in the validation sets. The colored lines are the mean ROC curves for the 100 different realizations of the partitioning of the cohort into training sets and validation sets (thin gray curves). **a** Not in remission. **b** Childhood Health Assessment Questionnaire (CHAQ) >0. **c** Physical Summary Score (PhS) <40. **d** Juvenile Arthritis Damage Index-Articular (JADI-A) >0

the strictness of the model-developing procedure, we still obtained acceptable predictive ability. The robustness and applicability of the prediction rules are emphasized by the fact that when the analyses were repeated without any blood tests, the performance was similar. An online calculator based on our models is available at the web-page http://predictions.no. An iOS app is also designed, and the test versions are available on request.

One of the limitations of our study is that for some of the patients, the baseline study visit scheduled 6 months after disease onset was not the first clinical visit. Some children had therefore already started treatment, mostly with nonsteroidal anti-inflammatory drugs (NSAIDs) or intraarticular corticosteroids, and were not treatment naïve when the predictor variables were assessed. This baseline time point, however, allowed use of the cumulative active joint count during the first 6 months of the disease, which is an important measure of early disease severity in line with the International League of Associations for Rheumatology (ILAR) criteria. A limitation is also that the primary outcome, non-achievement of remission off medication, is defined as inactive disease for more than 1 year, and this outcome does not necessarily reflect the disease course during the whole 8-year period. In addition, JADI-A is a rather crude measure of joint damage, and future predictive studies should therefore include imaging in joint damage assessment. Finally, the treatment given during the disease course may have altered the disease outcome, even though biologic medications were not generally available in the beginning of the study period in 1997. The natural history of JIA disease course without treatment is clearly impossible and unethical to study.

Conclusion

We have developed statistical models for predicting non-achievement of remission off medication, functional disability, and joint damage in children with JIA. The models are easy to use, and may provide a valuable tool to aid early treatment decisions on the need for DMARDs including biologic agents if validation in other JIA cohorts and across ethnicities can confirm our results [37]. We encourage further testing of our models before the applicability can be generalized and recommended.

Additional files

Additional file 1: Table S1. Characteristics of the 423 children in the Nordic juvenile idiopathic arthritis cohort at baseline. (PDF 134 kb)

Additional file 2: Table S2. Medications given before the baseline study visit. (PDF 108 kb)

Additional file 3: Figure S1. Receiver operating characteristic (ROC) curves for the four unfavorable clinical outcomes in the validation sets, but for models constructed without using blood samples as predictors. The colored lines are the mean ROC curves for the 100 different realizations of the partitioning of the cohort into training sets and validation sets (thin gray curves). (**a**) Not in remission. (**b**) Childhood Health Assessment Questionnaire (CHAQ) >0. (**c**) Physical Summary Score (PhS) <40. (**d**) Juvenile Arthritis Damage Index-Articular (JADI-A) >0. (PDF 435 kb)

Additional file 4: Table S3. Baseline clinical characteristics as predictors of functional disability (CHAQ) in univariate logistic regression. (PDF 125 kb)

Additional file 5: Table S4. Baseline clinical characteristics as predictors of functional disability (PhS) in univariate logistic regression. (PDF 163 kb)

Additional file 6: Table S5. Baseline clinical characteristics as predictors of joint damage (JADI-A) in univariate logistic regression. (PDF 161 kb)

Additional file 7: Figure S2. Receiver operating characteristic (ROC) curves for a test in the Nordic JIA cohort of the prediction model for severe disease course by Guzman et al. The area under the curve (AUC) values were 0.69 for non-achievement of remission off medication, 0.68 for Childhood Health Assessment Questionnaire (CHAQ) >0, 0.69 for Physical Summary Score (PhS) <40, and 0.71 for joint damage (JADI-A) >0. (PDF 287 kb)

Abbreviations

ANA: Antinuclear antibodies; AUC: Area under the receiver operating characteristic curve; CHAQ: Childhood Health Assessment Questionnaire; CRP: C-reactive protein; DMARD: Disease-modifying anti-rheumatic drug; ESR: Erythrocyte sedimentation rate; GA: Global assessment; ILAR: International League of Associations for Rheumatology; IQR: Interquartile range; JADI-A: Juvenile Arthritis Damage Index-Articular; JIA: Juvenile idiopathic arthritis; NSAIDs: Nonsteroidal anti-inflammatory drugs; PhS: Physical Summary Score; RF: Rheumatoid factor; ROC: Receiver operating characteristics; VAS: Visual analogue scale

Acknowledgements

We thank all the children and parents participating in the study. We also thank the other members of the Nordic Study group of Pediatric Rheumatology (NoSPeR), Gudmund Marhaug (Trondheim), Freddy Karup Pedersen (Copenhagen), Pekka Lahdenne (Helsinki), and Boel Anderson-Gäre (Jonköping), for their inspiring cooperation. We thank the following participating physicians who contributed by collecting data: Nils Thomas Songstad, Astri Lang and Anne Elisabeth Ross (Tromsø), Kjell Berntzen and Nina Moe (Trondheim), Mikael Damgaard and Nils Olof Jonsson (Jönköping), Anders Berner and Hans Ekström (Karlstad), Eric Ronge (Skövde), Agne Lind and Lars Hammarèn (Borås), Johan Robinsson (Trollhättan), and Anna-Lena Nilsson (Östersund). Finally, we thank Tom Willsgaard (Tromsø) for discussions regarding statistical methods.

Funding

The work was supported by grants from the Helse Nord Research Funds.

Authors' contributions

VR, EN, AF, TH, LB, SN, and MR were involved in the conception and design of the study, and/or basic analysis and interpretation of data, drafting of the manuscript, and revising it critically for important intellectual content. VR and MR performed the statistical analysis. VR, KA, MZ, EA, MG, SP, and ME were involved in the acquisition of data, and/or drafting of the manuscript and revising it critically for important intellectual content. All authors read and approved the final manuscript.

Consent for publication

Not applicable.

Competing interests

The authors declare that they have no competing interests.

Author details
[1]Department of Pediatrics, University Hospital of North Norway, Tromsø, Norway. [2]Department of Clinical Medicine, UIT the Arctic University of Norway, Tromsø, Norway. [3]Department of Clinical and Molecular Medicine, NTNU - Norwegian University of Science and Technology, Trondheim, Norway. [4]Department of Pediatrics, Levanger Hospital, Nord-Trøndelag Hospital Trust, Levanger, Norway. [5]Hospital for Children and Adolescents, University of Helsinki, Helsinki, Finland. [6]Department of Women's and Children's Health, Uppsala University, Uppsala, Sweden. [7]Department of Pediatrics, Ryhov County Hospital, Jonkoping, Sweden. [8]Department of Pediatrics, Institute of Clinical Sciences, Sahlgrenska Academy, University of Gothenburg, Gothenburg, Sweden. [9]Department of Pediatrics, Aarhus University Hospital, Aarhus, Denmark. [10]Department of Pediatrics, Rigshospitalet Copenhagen University Hospital, Copenhagen, Denmark. [11]Department of Pediatrics, St. Olavs Hospital, Trondheim, Norway. [12]Department of Mathematics and Statistics, UIT the Arctic University of Norway, Tromsø, Norway.

References

1. Prakken B, Albani S, Martini A. Juvenile idiopathic arthritis. Lancet. 2011; 377(9783):2138–49.
2. Adib N, Silman A, Thomson W. Outcome following onset of juvenile idiopathic inflammatory arthritis: I. frequency of different outcomes. Rheumatology (Oxford). 2005;44(8):995–1001.
3. Adib N, Silman A, Thomson W. Outcome following onset of juvenile idiopathic inflammatory arthritis: II. predictors of outcome in juvenile arthritis. Rheumatology (Oxford). 2005;44(8):1002–7.
4. van Dijkhuizen EH, Wulffraat NM. Early predictors of prognosis in juvenile idiopathic arthritis: a systematic literature review. Ann Rheum Dis. 2015; 74(11):1996–2005.
5. Flato B, Lien G, Smerdel A, Vinje O, Dale K, Johnston V, Sorskaar D, Moum T, Ploski R, Forre O. Prognostic factors in juvenile rheumatoid arthritis: a case-control study revealing early predictors and outcome after 14.9 years. J Rheumatol. 2003;30(2):386–93.
6. Consolaro A, Negro G, Lanni S, Solari N, Martini A, Ravelli A. Toward a treat-to-target approach in the management of juvenile idiopathic arthritis. Clin Exp Rheumatol. 2012;30(4 Suppl 73):S157–62.
7. Wallace CA, Giannini EH, Spalding SJ, Hashkes PJ, O'Neil KM, Zeft AS, Szer IS, Ringold S, Brunner HI, Schanberg LE, et al. Trial of early aggressive therapy in polyarticular juvenile idiopathic arthritis. Arthritis Rheum. 2012;64(6):2012–21.
8. Wallace CA, Giannini EH, Spalding SJ, Hashkes PJ, O'Neil KM, Zeft AS, Szer IS, Ringold S, Brunner HI, Schanberg LE, et al. Clinically inactive disease in a cohort of children with new-onset polyarticular juvenile idiopathic arthritis treated with early aggressive therapy: time to achievement, total duration, and predictors. J Rheumatol. 2014;41(6):1163–70.
9. Albers HM, Wessels JA, van der Straaten RJ, Brinkman DM, Suijlekom-Smit LW, Kamphuis SS, Girschick HJ, Wouters C, Schilham MW, le Cessie S, et al. Time to treatment as an important factor for the response to methotrexate in juvenile idiopathic arthritis. Arthritis Rheum. 2009;61(1):46–51.
10. Guzman J, Henrey A, Loughin T, Berard RA, Shiff NJ, Jurencak R, Benseler SM, Tucker LB, Re A-OI. Predicting which children with juvenile idiopathic arthritis will have a severe disease course: results from the ReACCh-Out Cohort. J Rheumatol. 2017;44(2):230–40.
11. Nordal E, Zak M, Aalto K, Berntson L, Fasth A, Herlin T, Lahdenne P, Nielsen S, Straume B, Rygg M, et al. Ongoing disease activity and changing categories in a long-term nordic cohort study of juvenile idiopathic arthritis. Arthritis Rheum. 2011;63(9):2809–18.
12. Vastert SJ, Kuis W, Grom AA. Systemic JIA: new developments in the understanding of the pathophysiology and therapy. Best Pract Res Clin Rheumatol. 2009;23(5):655–64.
13. Giannini EH, Ruperto N, Ravelli A, Lovell DJ, Felson DT, Martini A. Preliminary definition of improvement in juvenile arthritis. Arthritis Rheum. 1997;40(7):1202–9.
14. Petty RE, Southwood TR, Manners P, Baum J, Glass DN, Goldenberg J, He X, Maldonado-Cocco J, Orozco-Alcala J, Prieur AM, et al. International League of Associations for Rheumatology classification of juvenile idiopathic arthritis: second revision, Edmonton, 2001. J Rheumatol. 2004;31(2):390–2.
15. Wallace CA, Ravelli A, Huang B, Giannini EH. Preliminary validation of clinical remission criteria using the OMERACT filter for select categories of juvenile idiopathic arthritis. J Rheumatol. 2006;33(4):789–95.
16. Wallace CA, Ruperto N, Giannini E, Childhood A, Rheumatology Research A, Pediatric Rheumatology International Trials O, Pediatric Rheumatology Collaborative Study G. Preliminary criteria for clinical remission for select categories of juvenile idiopathic arthritis. J Rheumatol. 2004;31(11):2290–4.
17. Ruperto N, Ravelli A, Pistorio A, Malattia C, Cavuto S, Gado-West L, Tortorelli A, Landgraf JM, Singh G, Martini A. Cross-cultural adaptation and psychometric evaluation of the Childhood Health Assessment Questionnaire (CHAQ) and the Child Health Questionnaire (CHQ) in 32 countries. Review of the general methodology. Clin Exp Rheumatol. 2001;19(4 Suppl 23):S1–9.
18. Viola S, Felici E, Magni-Manzoni S, Pistorio A, Buoncompagni A, Ruperto N, Rossi F, Bartoli M, Martini A, Ravelli A. Development and validation of a clinical index for assessment of long-term damage in juvenile idiopathic arthritis. Arthritis Rheum. 2005;52(7):2092–102.
19. Landgraf JMAL, Ware JE. The CHQ user's manual. Boston: New England Medical Center; 1996.
20. Hulstaert FAJ, Hannet I, Lancaster P, Buchner L, Kunz J, et al. An optimized method for routine HLA-B27 screening using flow cytometry. Cytometry. 1994;18(1):21–9.
21. Lydersen S. Statistical review. Frequently given comments. Ann Rheum Dis. 2015;74(2):323–5. https://doi.org/10.1136/annrheumdis-2014-206186.
22. Wallace CA, Giannini EH, Huang B, Itert L, Ruperto N, Childhood Arthritis Rheumatology Research A, Pediatric Rheumatology Collaborative Study G, Paediatric Rheumatology International Trials O. American College of Rheumatology provisional criteria for defining clinical inactive disease in select categories of juvenile idiopathic arthritis. Arthritis Care Res (Hoboken). 2011;63(7):929–36.
23. Berntson L, Nordal E, Aalto K, Peltoniemi S, Herlin T, Zak M, Nielsen S, Rygg M, Nordic Study Group of Paediatric R. HLA-B27 predicts a more chronic disease course in an 8-year followup cohort of patients with juvenile idiopathic arthritis. J Rheumatol. 2013;40(5):725–31.
24. Bartoli M, Taro M, Magni-Manzoni S, Pistorio A, Traverso F, Viola S, Magnani A, Gasparini C, Martini A, Ravelli A. The magnitude of early response to methotrexate therapy predicts long-term outcome of patients with juvenile idiopathic arthritis. Ann Rheum Dis. 2008;67(3):370–4.
25. Tynjala P, Vahasalo P, Tarkiainen M, Kroger L, Aalto K, Malin M, Putto-Laurila A, Honkanen V, Lahdenne P. Aggressive combination drug therapy in very early polyarticular juvenile idiopathic arthritis (ACUTE-JIA): a multicentre randomised open-label clinical trial. Ann Rheum Dis. 2011;70(9):1605–12.
26. Gerss J, Roth J, Holzinger D, Ruperto N, Wittkowski H, Frosch M, Wulffraat N, Wedderburn L, Stanevicha V, Mihaylova D, et al. Phagocyte-specific S100 proteins and high-sensitivity C reactive protein as biomarkers for a risk-adapted treatment to maintain remission in juvenile idiopathic arthritis: a comparative study. Ann Rheum Dis. 2012;71(12):1991–7.
27. SA JK, Frank MB, Chen Y, Wallace CA, Jarvis JN. Whole blood gene expression profiling predicts therapeutic response at six months in patients with polyarticular juvenile idiopathic arthritis. Arthritis Rheumatol. 2014;66(5):1363–71.
28. Fall N, Barnes M, Thornton S, Luyrink L, Olson J, Ilowite NT, Gottlieb BS, Griffin T, Sherry DD, Thompson S, et al. Gene expression profiling of peripheral blood from patients with untreated new-onset systemic juvenile idiopathic arthritis reveals molecular heterogeneity that may predict macrophage activation syndrome. Arthritis Rheum. 2007;56(11):3793–804.
29. Anink J, Van Suijlekom-Smit LW, Otten MH, Prince FH, van Rossum MA, Dolman KM, Hoppenreijs EP, ten Cate R, Ursu S, Wedderburn LR, et al. MRP8/14 serum levels as a predictor of response to starting and stopping anti-TNF treatment in juvenile idiopathic arthritis. Arthritis Res Ther. 2015;17:200.
30. Ravelli A, Martini A. Early predictors of outcome in juvenile idiopathic arthritis. Clin Exp Rheumatol. 2003;21(5 Suppl 31):S89–93.
31. Wallace CA, Huang B, Bandeira M, Ravelli A, Giannini EH. Patterns of clinical remission in select categories of juvenile idiopathic arthritis. Arthritis Rheum. 2005;52(11):3554–62.
32. Ravelli A, Varnier GC, Oliveira S, Castell E, Arguedas O, Magnani A, Pistorio A, Ruperto N, Magni-Manzoni S, Galasso R, et al. Antinuclear antibody-positive patients should be grouped as a separate category in the classification of juvenile idiopathic arthritis. Arthritis Rheum. 2011;63(1):267–75.
33. Alberdi-Saugstrup M, Zak M, Nielsen S, Herlin T, Nordal E, Berntson L, Fasth A, Rygg M, Klaus M, Nordic Study Group of Pediatric R. High-sensitive CRP as a predictive marker of long-term outcome in juvenile idiopathic arthritis. Rheumatol Int. 2017;37(5):695–703.

8

Fluorescence optical imaging and musculoskeletal ultrasonography in juvenile idiopathic polyarticular disease before and during antirheumatic treatment - a multicenter non-interventional diagnostic evaluation

Ariane Klein[1*], Georg Werner Just[1], Stephanie Gabriele Werner[2], Prasad T. Oommen[3], Kirsten Minden[4], Ingrid Becker[5], Hans-Eckhard Langer[6], Dirk Klee[7] and Gerd Horneff[1]

Abstract

Background: Valid detection of inflamed joints is essential for correct classification, therapeutic decisions, prognosis and assessment of treatment efficacy in juvenile idiopathic arthritis (JIA). Fluorescence optical imaging (FOI) enables visualization of inflammation in arthritis of finger and hand joints and might be used for monitoring.

Methods: A 24-week observational study in polyarticular JIA patients newly starting treatment with methotrexate or an approved biologic was performed in three centers. Patients were evaluated clinically, by gray-scale ultrasonography (GSUS), power-Doppler ultrasonography (PDUS) and FOI at baseline, week 12 and week 24.

Results: Of 37 patients enrolled, 24 patients started methotrexate and 13 patients a biologic for the first time (etanercept $n = 11$, adalimumab and tocilizumab $n = 1$ each). Mean JADAS 10 decreased significantly from 17.7 at baseline to 12.2 and 7.2 at week 12 and 24 respectively. PedACR 30/50/70/100 response rates at week 24 were 85%/73%/50%/27%. The total number of clinically active joints in hand and fingers at baseline/week 12/week 24 was 262 (23.6%)/162 (16.4%)/162 (9.0%). By GSUS, at baseline/week 12/week 24, 192 (19.4%)/135 (16.1%)/83 (11.5%) joints showed effusions and 186 (18.8%)/107 (12.7%)/69 (9.6%) showed synovial thickening, and by PDUS 68 (6.9%)/15 (1.8%)/36 (5%) joints showed hyperperfusion. Any sign of arthritis was detected by US in a total of 243 joints (24.5%) at baseline, 161 joints (19.2%) at week 12 and 123 joints (17%) at week 24. By FOI at baseline/week 12/week 24, 430 (38.7%)/ 280 (29.2%)/215 (27.6%) showed a signal enhancement in at least one phase.

Summarizing all three points of time, the highest numbers of signals were detected by FOI with 32% of joints, especially in phase 2, while by US 20.7% and by clinical examination 17.5% of joints were active. A high number of joints (21.1%) had FOI signals but were inactive by clinical examination. A total 20.1% of joints with signals in FOI did not show effusion, synovial thickening or hyperperfusion by US.

Because of the high number of negative results, specificity of FOI compared with clinical examination/US/PD was high (84–95%), and sensitivity was only moderate.

(Continued on next page)

* Correspondence: ar.klein@asklepios.com
[1]Centre for Paediatric Rheumatology, Department of Paediatrics, Asklepios Clinic Sankt Augustin, Arnold-Janssen-Strasse 29, 53757 Sankt Augustin, Germany
Full list of author information is available at the end of the article

(Continued from previous page)

Conclusion: FOI and US could detect clinical but also subclinical inflammation. FOI detected subclinical inflammation to a higher extent than US. Improvement upon treatment with either methotrexate or a biologic can be visualized by FOI and US.

Keywords: Juvenile idiopathic arthritis, Imaging, Fluorescence optical imaging, Xiralite, Arthrosonography, Ultrasonography, Power Doppler

Background

Juvenile idiopathic arthritis (JIA) is the most common chronic inflammatory rheumatic disease in childhood and can lead to severe disability [1–3]. The validity of diagnosis, classification and prognosis as well as therapeutic decisions for each JIA patient depends on reliable detection of joint involvement. Careful clinical assessment is of great importance but may be difficult, especially in children. Subclinical inflammation could also be missed, for example in early stages of the disease or with minimal disease activity. Ultrasonography (US) in grayscale (GSUS) and power Doppler (PDUS) modes is often available for assessment of synovial thickening, joint effusions and hyperperfusion, thus helping to detect active joints. In clinical practice this procedure is usually used on a limited number of joints due to limitations of time. Fluorescence optical imaging (FOI) is a contrast-enhanced optical procedure for visualization of changes in microcirculation. It has been used for over 30 years for various indications [4]. In experimental models of arthritis, indocyanine green (ICG)-enhanced FOI findings corresponded to histologically proven synovitis [5, 6]. This approach was also tested in humans [7, 8]. FOI is time efficient and operator independent. The image interpretation, however, is dependent on visual perceptions and imaging experience of the examiner and is limited to wrist and finger joints. Increased focal optical signal intensities visualize areas of high perfusion, altered microcirculation and/or capillary leakage, which may not show in GSUS, especially in the small finger joints [9–11]. In adult RA patients, FOI has been shown to be a reliable technique to detect inflammation with good agreement with magnetic resonance imaging (MRI). The authors distinguished three different phases and a computer-generated composite image; their meaning still being unclear, they may give varying information such as changes in perfusion, microcirculation, capillary leakage or neovascularization. In the opinion of the authors, very early arthritis could be observed with FOI as well as subclinical inflammation [10, 11].

FOI might be a valuable tool to assess subclinical and very early arthritis, to differentiate between arthritis and pain syndrome and to assess treatment response.

This observational study intended to analyze improvement upon newly instituted treatment with a DMARD or with a biologic clinically, using commonly used tools (PedACR, JADAS, number of active, swollen and tender joints) and by imaging methods (GSUS and PDUS) as well as by FOI. We intended for the first time to compare clinical and imaging results with the new FOI method to explore the clinical utility. Of further interest is the presentation of residual inflammation which might not be detected clinically but by imaging and whether an early decrease of inflammation detected by FOI is predictive for remission later on.

The results of the first study using the FOI technique and US examination in children with JIA before and during antirheumatic treatment are reported here.

Methods

Patients

In three German centers a total number of 37 patients starting a new treatment with either a DMARD or a biologic approved for polyarticular JIA were recruited for this observational study. Inclusion criteria were: diagnosis of polyarticular JIA according to ILAR criteria (seropositive, seronegative polyarthritis JIA and extended oligoarthritis) [12], active disease with at least three clinically active joints in the hand region, age 6–18 years and agreement of patient and parents/legal guardian to participate in the study. Patients had to be either naïve to methotrexate in the cohort starting methotrexate or naïve to any biologic.

The study was performed in compliance with the Declaration of Helsinki. The study protocol was approved by the ethics committee Ärztekammer Nordrhein (Number: 2012026) and the ethics committee of the Charité university clinic Berlin (Number EA2/039/12). Written informed consent forms were obtained for all participants.

Clinical and laboratory assessment

All patients were evaluated by clinical examination (CE) at baseline, after 12 and 24 weeks. Swollen, tender joints and joints with limitation of motion (LOM) were scored for presence or absence (0–1). Joints with swelling not due to deformity or joints without swelling, LOM plus pain and/or tenderness were defined as active joints.

The ESR and C-reactive protein (CRP) test were recorded at each visit. Disease activity was also measured by patient/parent visual analog scale (0–100) of overall well-being, by physician visual analog scale of overall disease activity and by CHAQ scores (0–3) [13]. The JADAS 10 score was calculated for each visit [14].

Ultrasonography

Thirty joints were examined by ultrasonography for each patient (wrists, MCP 1–5, PIP 1–5, DIP 2–5) at three different time points (week 0, 12 and 24). Evaluation was done semiquantitatively (grades 0–3) for synovial thickening, joint effusions in GSUS and hyperperfusion in PDUS according to Manggi-Manzoni et al. [15]. Joints graded 1–3 were scored as active in the respective examination mode [10]. Ultrasonography examination was performed using LOGIQ e notebook with 12-MHz linear transducer by General Electrics Healthcare, Toshiba Aplio XG and MyLab70 XVG Esaote.

Fluorescence optical imaging

At each visit (week 0, 12 and 24) a standardized FOI examination was performed as described by Werner et al. [10, 11]. An ICG bolus (ICG-Pulsion®, 0.1 mg/kg BW; Pulsion Medical Systems AG, Munich, Germany) was injected into the cubital vein; thereafter one image/second over 6 minutes was obtained, resulting in 360 images. Three phases according to signal intensities in the fingertips and an electronically generated composite image (CI), automatically obtained by means of the integrated software XiraView (version 3.6), were analyzed. Phase 1 includes all images until clearly increased signal intensities are visible in the fingertips, phase 2 includes all images during increased intensities in the fingertips and phase 3 includes all images from the end of phase 2 until the end of the examination. For each phase and the composite image, each joint was scored semiquantitatively (0–3: 0 = no increased signal intensity; 1 = low increased signal intensity, <25% of affected joint area; 2 = moderate intensity, >25 and <50% of affected joint area; and 3 = strong increased signal intensity, >50% of affected joint area). Joints were counted as active if they reached at least a score of 1 [10, 11]. The commercially available Xiralite X4 device (Mivenion) was used for the examination. Reading was done by a single experienced observer, who had knowledge of the typical pitfalls of FOI interpretation.

Efficacy parameters

Clinical response was measured by the pediatric ACR (PedACR) criteria, JADAS reduction and reduction in the number of active joints. PedACR improvement was calculated as described previously in detail [16]. The categories contributing to the PedACR 30 Score are physician's global assessment of the subject's disease activity (numeric rating scale (NRS)), parents' global assessment of the subject's overall well-being (NRS), number of active joints (swelling not due to deformity or in joints without swelling, LOM plus pain and/or tenderness), number of joints with LOM, Childhood Health Assessment Questionnaire (CHAQ) and CRP. The JADAS minimal disease activity (defined as JADAS10 ≤ 3.8) and the JADAS remission activity (defined JADAS10 ≤ 1) according to the definition of Consolaro et al. [17] was calculated.

Safety parameters

Clinical and laboratory evidence of adverse events was investigated at each study visit. The investigator assessed and recorded any adverse event in detail on the adverse event form, including the date and time of onset, description, severity, time course, duration and outcome, relationship of the adverse event to the study drug and alternative etiology for events not considered 'probably related' to the study drug.

Statistical analysis

Analyses were conducted at patient and individual joint levels. Mean values and standard deviations were calculated for quantitative variables. Demographic and baseline characteristics were summarized by descriptive statistics. Efficacy and safety analyses were performed in the intention-to-treat population (ITT), and tests were two-sided. $p < 0.05$ was considered statistically significant. Frequencies were compared using the chi-square test or Fisher's exact test as appropriate. Agreement was reached when a joint was assessed as affected (>0) or not affected (0) with both modalities. Clinical examination and ultrasonography was used as the standard reference method for calculation of sensitivity and specificity. Receiver operating characteristic (ROC) curves were generated to assess sensitivity and specificity of FOI versus ultrasonography and clinical standards of care. The area under the curve (AUC) was calculated. Improvement of continuous disease activity parameters were compared using the t test. Data were entered into an Access 2010 database and analyzed with Excel 2010 (Microsoft, Redmond, WA, USA) or IBM SPSS Statistics version 23.

Results

Study population

Thirty-seven patients with active polyarticular JIA were enrolled in this study. Of these, 24 patients started treatment with methotrexate and 13 patients received therapy with a biologic for the first time (11 patients started etanercept, one patient adalimumab and one patient tocilizumab). Thirty-four patients (21 on methotrexate and 13 on biologic) could be evaluated at week 12, and 25 patients (17 on methotrexate, eight on biologic) completed the study through week 24. Mean age at enrollment was 13.9 years (range 9–18 years).

There were no significant differences regarding patient characteristics and disease activity parameters between the two cohorts at baseline, although patients in the biologics cohort tended to have higher disease activity parameters than patients in the methotrexate cohort (Table 1).

Of all patients, 35% received oral corticosteroids at baseline. Also the number of patients using oral corticosteroids at baseline was slightly but insignificantly higher in the biologics cohort (seven of 13 patients) than in the methotrexate cohort (six of 24 patients). No patient had active uveitis or history of uveitis and no patient had signs or history of systemic inflammation.

Efficacy

Response rates according to the PedACR 30/50/70/100 and the JADAS in this study were as expected. After 12 weeks of treatment, PedACR 30/50/70/100 scores were reached by 69%/45%/24%/10% in the methotrexate cohort and 82%/45%/19%/0% in the biologics cohort. Response rates improved further until week 24, with 85%/73%/50%/27% reaching PedACR 30/50/70/100 scores (83%/72%/44%/22% in the methotrexate cohort and 88%/75%/63%/38% in the biologics cohort).

All but eight patients showed decreased JADAS 10 scores at week 12, and four of these showed JADAS improvement at week 24. Mean JADAS 10 values decreased significantly during treatment for all patients. In the cohort completing week 24 of this study, the mean JADAS 10 values decreased from 17.7 at baseline to 12.2 at week 12 and 7.2 at week 24. Patients treated with DMARDs showed a decrease from 18.8 at baseline to 12.7 at week 12 and 7.6 at week 24. Patients treated with biologics started with a higher JADAS of 19.6 at baseline, but then decreased more rapidly to a JADAS 10 of 11 at week 12 and further to 6.1 at week 24.

Clinical examination

In total, 2970 separate joints of the hand region were evaluated by CE at three different points of time; of these, 2551 joints had complete data for US evaluation and 2910 had complete datasets for FOI analysis. Altogether, 519 of 2970 joints (17.5%) were clinically classified as active (434 (14.6%) swollen joints, 542 (18.2%) tender joints and 348 (11.7%) joints with limited range of motion). The joints PIP 2 and 3, followed by PIP 4 and 5, MCP 2 and 3 and the wrist were affected most frequently.

At baseline, 1110 joints were evaluated by CE and with FOI, and 990 joints were evaluated with US. In CE, 262 of the 1110 joints (23.6%) were classified as active joints (237 (21.4%) swollen joints, 267 (24.1%) tender joints and 181 (16.3%) joints with limited range of motion).

Upon treatment with either methotrexate or a biologic, a significant decrease of the mean number of active/swollen/tender or LOM joints at week 12 and week 24 compared with baseline was documented (Fig. 1a).

At week 12, 162 of 990 joints (16.4%) of the hand region evaluated by CE were assessed as clinically active. This decreased further in week 24 to 70 of 780 (9.0%).

Table 1 Patients' baseline characteristics

	All patients (*n* = 37)	DMARD cohort (*n* = 24)	Biologics cohort (*n* = 13)
Male/female	7/30	5/19	2/11
Age (years)	13.9 (2.2)	14.3 (2.1)	13.5 (2.4)
Disease duration (years)	3.6 (3.2)	3.2 (4.1)	4.1 (3.7)
CHAQ-DI	0.61 (0.7)	0.54 (0.58)	0.66 (0.84)
JADAS 10	16.9 (5.7)	15.5 (5.6)	19.0 (5.0)
ESR (mm/h)	17.6 (20.1)	18.9 (21.8)	14.4 (15)
CRP(mg/l)	5.0 (12.2)	2.7 (4.5)	8.7 (18.3)
Physician Global Assessment VAS (cm)	4.8 (2.1)	4.4 (1.8)	5.5 (2.3)
Parents Global Assessment VAS (cm)	4.5 (2.5)	4.5 (2.1)	4.5 (3.2)
Number of active joints	7.1 (5.2)	6.7 (5.2)	8.3 (5.0)
Number of tender joints	9.6 (8.9)	9.6 (8.0)	10.0 (11.4)
Number of swollen joints	7.2 (5.7)	6.8 (5.7)	8.1 (5.5)
Number of joints with LOM	6.5 (6.7)	5.4 (5.3)	8.4 (8.4)

Data presented as number or mean (standard deviation)

DMARD disease-modifying antirheumatic drug, *CHAQ* Childhood Health Assessment Questionnaire, *CRP* C-reactive protein, *ESR* erythrocyte sedimentation rate, *JADAS* Juvenile Diseases Activity Score, *LOM* limitation of motion, *VAS* visual analog scale

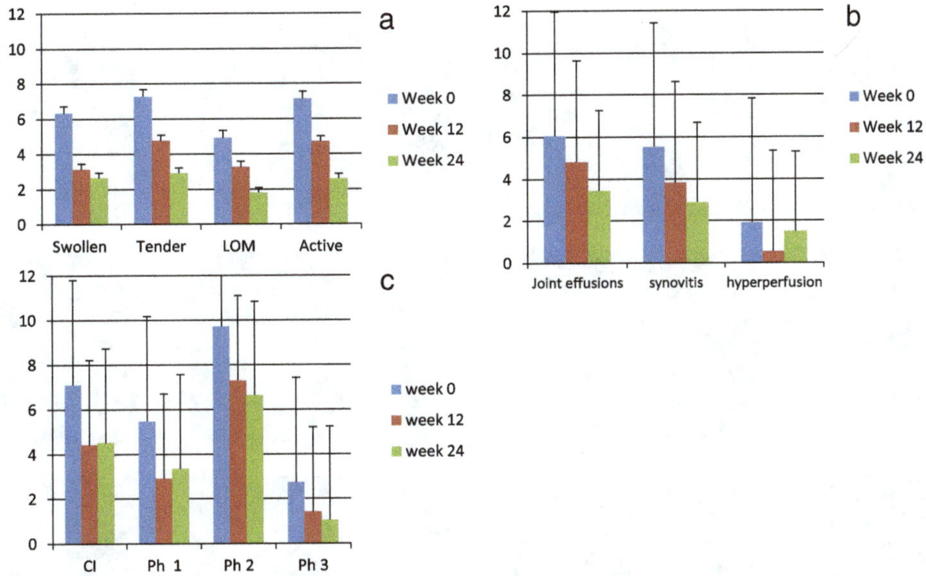

Fig. 1 Mean affected joints of the hand region for the three examination techniques before the start of treatment and after 12 and 24 weeks of treatment. **a** Clinical examination. **b** US/PD examination. **c** Signal intensity on FOI examination. Mean values and standard deviations are shown. *LOM* limitation of motion, *CI* composite image, *Ph* phase

Ultrasonography findings

At baseline, 990 joints of the hand region were evaluated by US examination. Here 192 joints (19.4%) showed joint effusions, 186 joints (18.8%) showed signs of synovial thickening on GSUS and 68 joints (6.9%) showed signs of hyperperfusion on PDUS. These numbers had decreased at week 12 to 135 joints (16.1%) with joint effusions, 107 joints (12.7%) with synovial thickening and 15 joints (1.8%) with hyperperfusion of 840 joints of the hand region evaluated by US. At week 24, 720 joints of the hand region were assessed by US. While the numbers of joints with joint effusions and synovial thickening improved further (83 and 69 joints (11.5% and 9.6%) respectively), more joints showed signs of hyperperfusion compared with week 12 (36 joints (5%)).

At baseline, in total 243 joints (24.5%) showed signs of inflammation for any of the three US parameters, 161 joints (19.2%) at week 12 and 123 joints (17%) at week 24. As outlined in Fig. 1b, a decrease of the mean number of joints with effusion, synovial thickening and hyperperfusion at week 12 and week 24 compared with baseline was documented.

Fluorescence optical findings

Overall, FOI revealed focal joint-related increased signal intensity as signs of synovitis/tenosynovitis in 947 joints. At baseline, 430 of 1110 evaluated joints (38.7%) showed increased signal intensity in one or more phases in FOI. This figure decreased to 280 of 960 evaluated joints (29.2%) at week 12 and 215 of 780 evaluated joints (27.6%) at week 24. With the phase1/phase 2/phase 3 and composite image, 215/369/108 and 266 joints were detected at baseline, 93/229/45 and 142 joints at week 12 and 84/166/26 and 115 joints at week 24 (Fig. 1c). Mean semiquantitative intensity of FOI signals in all examined joints decreased significantly between baseline and week 12 in all three phases and the composite image ($p < 0.0001$ for all), with only minimal changes between weeks 12 and 24.

Figure 2a shows FOI examinations of one patient at the three different time points. At baseline, high signals in FOI were noted, especially in PIP joints and in phase 2. These joints were also assessed active by clinical examination. All but one of the joints showed signs of effusions and most also synovial thickening on US, and PIP 3 of the right hand also showed hyperperfusion by PD. Upon treatment, the number of joints as well as the signal intensity decreased. At week 24, residual inflammation was visible by FOI and by clinical investigation especially in PIP 2–5 of the left hand.

Figure 2b shows FOI examinations of a second patient at four different time points. At baseline, both wrists and PIP 2–5 joints of both sides showed high signals in FOI, especially in phase 2 and in the composite image. In addition, signals over the DIP region indicate DIP joint involvement but cannot be clearly distinguished from fingertip hyperemia. Clinically DIP 2–5 of the left hand, MCP 1 of the left hand and PIP 2–5 of both hands were assessed as active, only PIP 2, 4 and 5 of the left hand showed sonographic effusions and PIP 5 of the left hand showed synovial thickening. Upon treatment, the number of joints as well as the signal intensity decreased. At week 24,

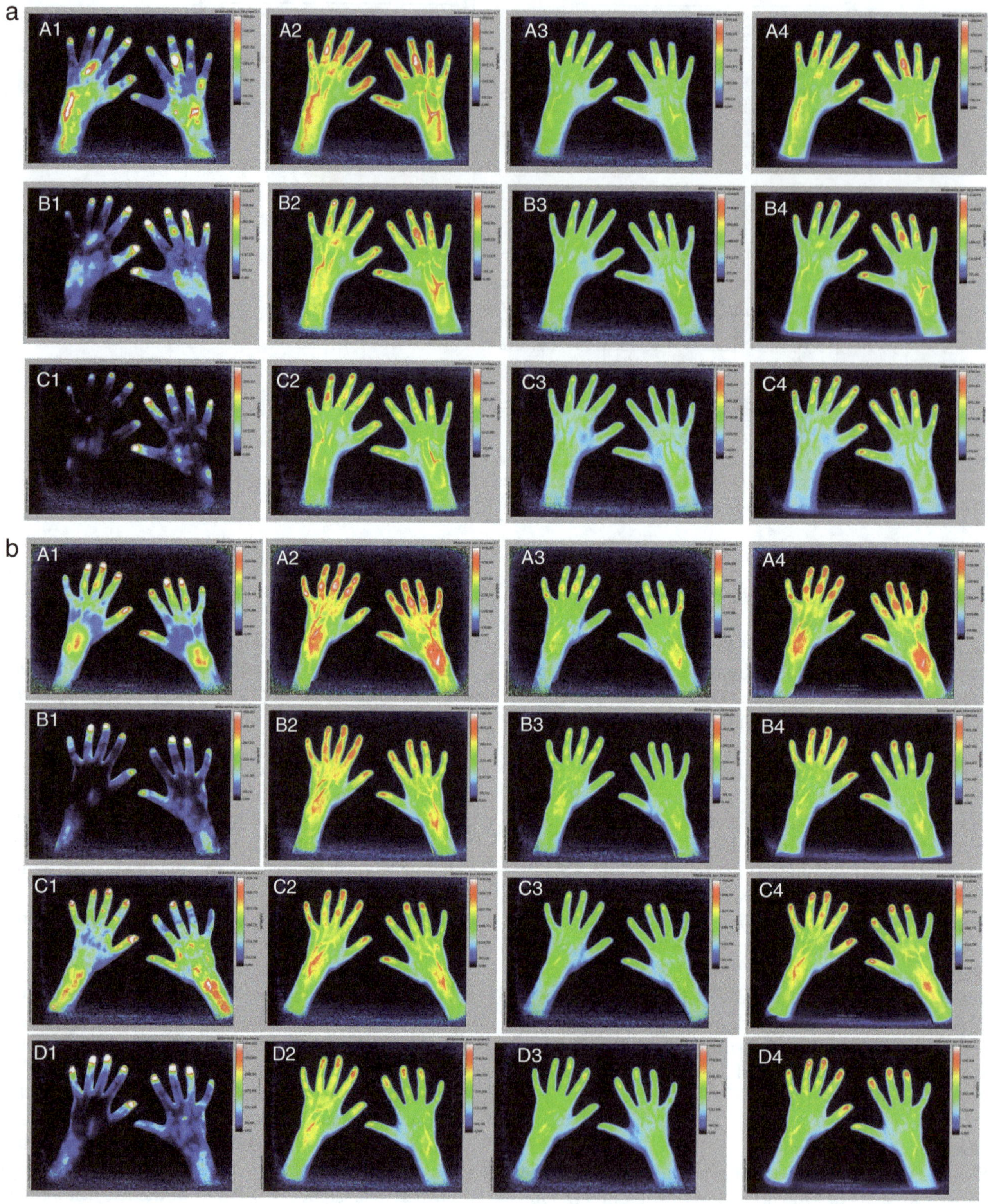

Fig. 2 (See legend on next page.)

(See figure on previous page.)
Fig. 2 a FOI of a patient treated with adalimumab. *Row A*, baseline; *row B*, week 12; *row C*, week 24; *column 1*, phase 1; *column 2*, phase 2; *column 3*, phase 3; *column 4*, composite image. At baseline, signals detected were grade 3 over PIP 3 of the right hand in phases 1 and 2 and composite image. Left-hand PIP 2–5 showed grade 2 signals in phase 2 and grade 1 signal in phase 3 and composite image. Left-hand PIP 1 showed grade 2 in phase 2, grade 0 in phase 3 and grade 1 in composite image. After 12 weeks of treatment, improvement of signal intensity was visible. Especially, right-hand PIP 3 still shows grade 3 signal in phase 2. Further reduction of signaling was noted at week 24. **b** FOI of a patient with polyarticular JIA who started etanercept treatment. *Row A*, baseline; *row B*, week 12; *row C*, week 24; *row D*, week 52; *column 1*, phase 1; *column 2*, phase 2; *column 3*, phase 3; *column 4*, composite image. At baseline, both wrists, both side PIP 2–5 and DIP 2–4 showed grade 3 signals in phase 2 but grade 1 in phase 3. Both DIP 5 showed weaker signals. Twenty-four-week imaging, especially in phase 2, demonstrates subclinical activity. At clinical examination the patient already had no active joints. Upon constant clinical remission on treatment, there is further improvement of FOI findings visible after 1 year

residual inflammation was visible in the region of PIP joints and wrist, while clinically and with US/PD no joint was assessed as active. Thus, clinically the patient was in remission, showing residual inflammation in FOI only. This patient had an FOI examination 1 year after baseline following completion of the study, while reporting pain in DIP and wrist joints. Clinically there were no abnormal findings in joint status and US/PD. FOI showed only minor signal enhancement.

Predictive value of FOI and clinical outcome

Joints showing improvement of FOI semiquantitative score at month 3 were more likely to improve clinically by month 6 than joints that stayed consistent or deteriorated with their FOI semiquantitative score (32–37% versus 18–20%). Logistic regression analysis, however, failed to produce reliable models. No positive correlation could be found between improvement of semiquantitative FOI score after 3 months and joint status after 6 months. Also no association between improvement in FOI scores of more than 30% at month 12 and JADAS minimal disease activity or JADAS remission could be shown.

Comparison of FOI, US and CE

The total number of joints evaluated for the hand region was 2970. Figure 3 summarizes CE, FOI and US results on the single joint level, showing the differences between the joints concerning frequency of detection of pathology by examination technique. FOI detected the highest number of joints (947 joints, 32%). Abnormal US findings were present in 527 of 2550 joints (20.7%) evaluated by US. A total 519 of the evaluated joints (17.5%) had active arthritis CE. A high number of joints (627 joints, 66.2%) showing increased signal intensity by FOI were rated clinically inactive by CE. Of the joints rated active in CE, 61.7% also showed FOI increased signal intensity. A total of 199 joints with clinical abnormalities did not show signaling by FOI (Table 2).

Also 513 (61.7%) joints that did not show sonographic signs of synovial thickening, effusions or hyperperfusion were detected by FOI. Especially, phase 2 showed increased signal intensity more often than the other phases and composite image.

On US examination, 211 of the 519 (40.6%) clinically active joints over all three time points showed effusion, 164 (31.6%) synovial thickening and 47 (9%) signs of hyperperfusion.

Ultrasonography did not detect signs of effusion, signs of synovial thickening or signs of hyperperfusion in numerous joints that were clinically classified as active. Effusions and synovial thickening were detected by US in 219 (8.9%) and 211 (8.6%) of 2451 clinically inactive joints and hyperperfusion was detected by power Doppler in 73 (3.0%) clinically inactive joints (Table 2).

Agreement of FOI with US was analyzed with obvious differences between different joints and in the different phases of FOI. Interestingly, agreement was 75–100% in DIP joints and MCP 1 (phase 2, CI), was 64–92% (CI) and 72–91% (phase 2) for MCP 2–5 and was 41–63% (CI) and 38–69% (phase 2) for PIP 2–4. A high variance between patients was also detected: mean agreement over patients (for all joints) ranged from 33 to 100% with a width of the confidence interval from 16 to 21%, depending on the compared pair of analysis methods.

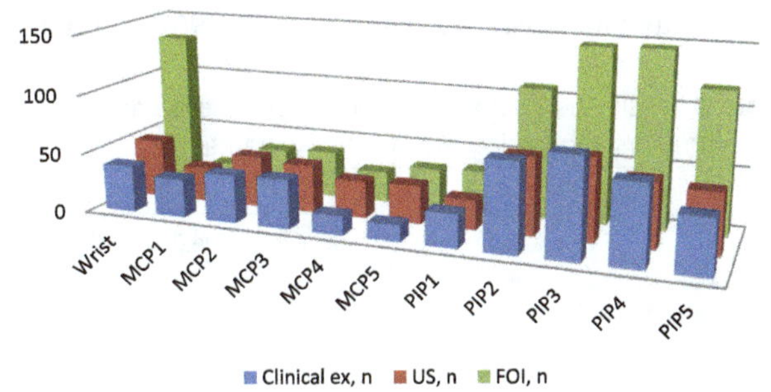

Fig. 3 Clinical, US and FOI results on the single joint level (all points of time summarized). Clinical examination considered active joint definition. US considered any sign of effusion, synovial thickening or PD positivity. FOI considered signal enhancement in any phase. *ex* examination, *FOI* fluorescence optical imaging, *PIP* proximal interphalangeal joint, *MCP* metacarpophalangeal joint, *US* ultrasonography

Table 2 Number of joints from a total of 2970 evaluated joints at three different points of time and comparison of number of joints with increased FOI signal and detection by US according to detection by clinical examination

	FOI					US/PD			
	Any signal (*n* = 947)	Composite image (*n* = 530)	Phase 1 (*n* = 396)	Phase 2 (*n* = 783)	Phase 3 (*n* = 180)	Any signal (*n* = 527)	Effusion (*n* = 430)	Synovitis (*n* = 375)	Hyperperfusion (*n* = 120)
Signal in clinically active joints (*n* = 519)	320 (33.8%/ 61.7%)[a]	205 (38.7%/ 39.5%)	161 (40.7%/ 31.0%)	277 (35.4%/ 53.4%)	81 (45.0%/ 15.6%)	239 (45.4%/ 46.0%)	211 (49.1%/ 40.7%)	164 (43.7%/ 31.6%)	47 (39.2%/ 9.0%)
Signal in clinically inactive joints (*n* = 2451)	627 (66.2%/ 25.6%)	325 (61.3%/ 13.3%)	235 (59.3%/ 9.6%9)	506 (64.6%/ 20.6%)	99 (55.0%/ 4.0%)	288 (54.6%/ 11.8%)	219 (51.0%/ 8.9%)	211 (56.2%/ 8.6%)	73 (60.8%/ 3.0%)

Data on US examination were available for 2550 joints in total
FOI fluorescence optical imaging, *PD* Power Doppler mode, *US* ultrasonography
[a]Percentages refer to columns/rows

FOI in phase 2 agreed best with detection of US effusions and synovial thickening, while the detection of PDUS hyperperfusion correlated best with FOI in phase 1 and to a slightly lesser extent phase 2.

Specificity of FOI compared with CE and US as the standard of reference showed high percentages for all parameters. Comparison of FOI phase 2 with clinical and US parameters showed specificity between 73 and 80%, composite image 82–87% and the other phases around or over 90%. Comparison of US parameters of inflammation and CE as standard of reference specificity was between 86 and 97% (Table 3).

Sensitivities comparing FOI and US with CE as the standard of reference as well as comparing FOI with US as the standard of reference were lower, with FOI phase 2 delivering the best values (45–56%) (Table 4).

ROC curves comparing FOI and US versus CE as the standard of care showed the highest values of the AUC for FOI phase 2 (AUC = 0.67 (95% CI 0.64–0.70)) and US B-mode joint effusions (AUC = 0.68 (95% CI 0.65–0.71)), followed by FOI composite image (AUC 0.63 (95% CI 0.60–0.66)) and US B-mode synovitis (AUC = 0.63 (95% CI 0.60–0.66)) (Fig. 4). Comparing FOI with US B-mode parameter joint effusions, phase 2 (AUC = 0.68 (95% CI 0.65–0.71)) followed by composite image (AUC = 0.63 (95% CI 0.60–0.66)) had the highest AUC values. Comparing FOI with US B-mode parameter synovitis, FOI phase 2 (AUC = 0.64 (95% CI 0.61–0.67)) and FOI phase 1 (AUC = 0.63 (95% CI 0.59–0.66)) had the highest AUC values. When calculating AUC with PDUS as the reference, FOI phase 1 had the highest values (AUC = 0.72 (95% CI 0.67–0.78)) (Figs. 5 a–c).

Safety

During the 24 weeks of this study, 15 adverse events (AE) were reported in 10 different patients. These included six infectious events, four events with gastrointestinal complaints, three patients with flare of JIA and two intraarticular injections. None of the events were serious. No events in correlation to FOI examination were noted.

Discussion

Musculoskeletal ultrasonography (in GSUS and PDUS) provides an imaging method which has a solid component in the clarification of inflammatory joint diseases. A disadvantage of the method is the relatively strong investigator dependency [18].

Table 3 Sensitivities: comparison of FOI parameters and parameters of clinical examination and US parameters, and comparison of US parameters and clinical examination parameters

Reference	FOI				US		
	Composite image	Phase 1	Phase 2	Phase 3	Joint effusion	Synovitis	Hyperperfusion power Doppler
Clinical active joints	0.395	0.314	0.543	0.160	0.471	0.360	0.103
Clinical swollen joints	0.394	0.323	0.534	0.169	0.474	0.365	0.103
Clinical tender joints	0.315	0.237	0.442	0.108	0.306	0.269	0.068
LOM	0.481	0.423	0.664	0.209	0.497	0.440	0.173
US joint effusion	0.393	0.316	0.565	0.191			
US synovitis	0.358	0.358	0.522	0.139			
Hyperperfusion by power Doppler	0.306	0.604	0.477	0.126			

FOI fluorescence optical imaging, *LOM* limitation of motion, *US* ultrasonography

Table 4 Specificities: comparison of FOI parameters and parameters of clinical examination and US parameters, and comparison of US parameters and clinical examination parameters

Reference	FOI				US		
	Composite image	Phase 1	Phase 2	Phase 3	Joint effusion	Synovitis	Hyperperfusion power Doppler
Clinical active joints	0.865	0.902	0.791	0.958	0.897	0.906	0.969
Clinical swollen joints	0.856	0.896	0.777	0.955	0.887	0.899	0.967
Clinical tender joints	0.848	0.884	0.767	0.947	0.862	0.888	0.962
LOM	0.859	0.903	0.785	0.957	0.874	0.899	0.974
US joint effusion	0.856	0.909	0.784	0.959			
US synovitis	0.841	0.904	0.762	0.945			
Hyperperfusion by power Doppler	0.818	0.888	0.730	0.935			

FOI fluorescence optical imaging, *LOM* limitation of motion, *US* ultrasonography

Morphological features of the inflammation are hypervascularization, increased blood perfusion and capillary permeability [19]. The (neo)angiogenesis is a very early event in the pathogenesis of chronic inflammation [20]. The angiogenesis of the synovial membrane leads to a dense capillary network in the inflamed joint membrane. Vasodilatation and increased capillary permeability maintain synovitis.

It has been shown in rheumatoid arthritis patients that the synovial vascularization correlates with the disease activity of an affected joint [21]. Arthrosonographic procedures, including power Doppler sonography, are limited in resolution, however, and are not capable of displaying an increased blood flow in the submillimeter region and thus on the capillary plane.

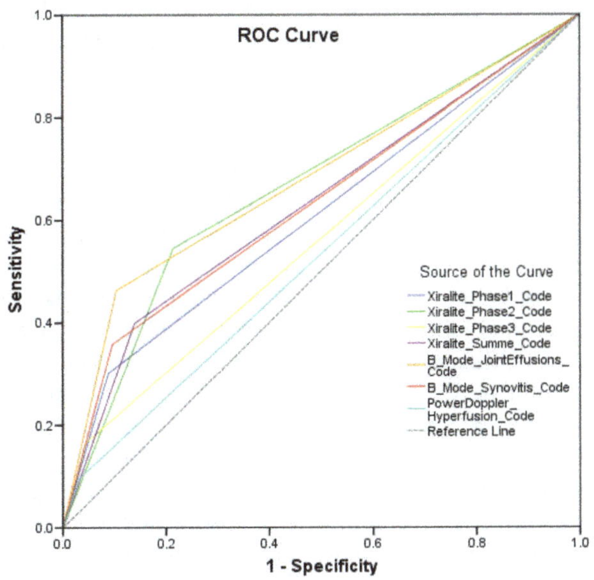

Fig. 4 ROC curves for FOI parameters in phases 1–3 and CI and US parameter B-mode joint effusion, B-mode synovitis and PDUS compared with clinical examination (active joint). Area under the curve (95% CI): FOI phase 1, 0.61 (0.58–0.64); FOI phase 2, 0.67 (0.64–0.70); FOI phase 3, 0.56 (0.53–0.59); FOI CI, 0.63 (0.60–0.66); US joint effusion, 0.68 (0.65–0.71); US synovitis, 0.63 (0.60–0.66); PDUS, 0.53 (0.50–0.56). *ROC* Receiver operating characteristic

Magnetic resonance imaging (MRI) is today regarded as the gold standard for the representation of synovitis. Furthermore, bone marrow edema detectable in MRI is the strongest independent predictor of the radiological progression of rheumatoid arthritis [22, 23]. The exact significance of MRI for the diagnosis and prognosis of an early arthritis has not yet been clarified conclusively [24]. Overall, MRI is used for early diagnosis in clinical routine and above all in clinical trials. For standardization, the OMERACT criteria for the use and evaluation of MRI were developed [25]. However, there are limitations to the use of MRI in everyday practice due to the high cost of an examination and the limited availability. The use of gadolinium and some contraindications also limit their use in clinical routine. Furthermore, there were several limitations especially in younger children, such as maintaining an immobile position or the necessity for sedation.

In human medicine, FOI methods have so far been used predominantly in ophthalmology as fluorescence angiography for the imaging diagnostics of retinal and choroidal diseases. Furthermore, FOI use is described in vascular surgery, in neurosurgery after clipping of a brain aneurysm in oncology to delineate tumor tissue and in plastic and reconstructive surgery [9, 26, 27].

FOI is a relatively new imaging technique for the detection of inflammation and arthritis in the joints of the hand by visualizing altered microcirculation and angiogenesis in adults with rheumatoid arthritis [9, 28]. FOI findings agreed well with US [10, 11] and MRI [11] findings in two studies with 252 and 32 RA patients and 46 and 6 patients respectively without signs of inflammatory disease as control groups. Early arthritis as well as subclinical inflammation could be detected by FOI.

There are almost no data concerning FOI use in pediatric patients with JIA. Werner et al. [29] described FOI use and results in three children. The aim of this study was to evaluate patients with JIA of hand and

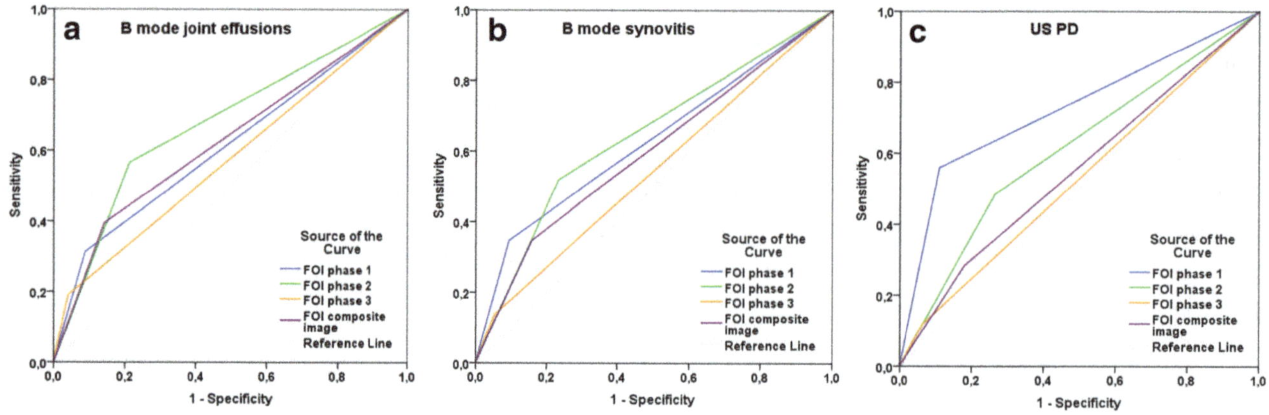

Fig. 5 ROC curves for FOI parameters in phases 1–3 and CI compared with US parameters B-mode joint effusion, B-mode synovitis and PD hyperperfusion. **a** US parameter B-mode joint effusion (area under the curve (95% CI)): FOI phase 1, 0.61 (0.58–0.64); FOI phase 2, 0.68 (0.65–0.71); FOI phase 3, 0.57 (0.54–0.61); FOI CI, 0.63 (0.60–0.66). **b** US parameter B-mode synovitis (area under the curve (95% CI)): FOI phase 1, 0.63 (0.59–0.66); FOI phase 2, 0.64 (0.61–0.67); FOI phase 3, 0.54 (0.51–0.57); FOI CI, 0.59 (0.56–0.63). **c** US parameter PD hyperperfusion (area under the curve (95% CI)): FOI phase 1, 0.72 (0.67–0.78); FOI phase 2, 0.61 (0.56–0.66); FOI phase 3, 0.53 (0.47–0.58); FOI CI, 0.55 (0.50-0.61). *ROC* Receiver operating characteristic

finger joints using the FOI technique along with US and CE, and to show its usefulness for demonstration of improvement upon treatment. Thus a follow-up analysis before and after 12 and 24 weeks of treatment (either methotrexate or a biologic antirheumatic drug) using the FOI technique in comparison with US and CE was performed in an open-label study. Clinical findings were all as expected. A high rate of treatment success on either a newly initiated therapy with methotrexate or a biologic was documented, similar to that observed in other trials, with earlier improvement in the biologics cohort.

As one result of our study, the number of joints with increased signal intensity in FOI was higher than the number of joints rated clinically active and even higher than the joints with signs of inflammation on US. These findings are consistent with the results of former studies using FOI in adults [10, 11]. In comparative studies of CE and GSUS, PDUS, and MRI, inflammatory changes were documented in clinically asymptomatic joints [30–32]. It can be assumed that FOI detected clinical and also subclinical activity.

There were differences in the specific phases of the analysis. The interpretation of the different phases is still not clear. Especially, phase 2 showed increased signal intensity in more joints than any other phase, including the composite image. Comparison of FOI with CE showed that phase 2 was best at detecting clinical active joints and also showed more activity in clinical inactive joints compared with the other FOI phases. FOI phase 2 also agreed best with US signs of synovial thickening and effusions. This may be the most sensitive phase and may be best suited to detect subclinical activity.

Phase 3 rarely showed increased FOI signals. In the former studies in adults, the authors considered phase 3 to show increased capillary permeability in which ICG is more persistent than normal [10, 11].

In joints with hyperperfusion detected by PDUS, FOI phase 1 most often showed increased signal intensity, followed by phase 2. This can also be shown in the ROC curves; when comparing the different FOI phases with PDUS, FOI phase 1 reached the best AUC values. As proposed by studies in adult patients, phase 1 may mirror increased vascularity as a sign of high disease activity [10, 11].

With CE as the standard of reference, FOI and US showed moderate sensitivities and high specificities, partly due to the high number of negative results. The findings for sensitivity and specificity for FOI with US as the standard of reference were comparable. This could also be shown in the ROC curves. Compared with CE, FOI phase 2 and US B-mode joint effusions were the most accurate parameters with similar values for the AUC. FOI phase 2 also had the highest AUC values when compared with the US mode parameters of joint effusion and synovitis. Because of the lack of an assured standard of reference, the interpretation of sensitivity and specificity is a delicate issue. Of course the majority of examined joints were expected to be inactive. Specificity was influenced by higher rates of positive findings in FOI compared with the other two methods. Because of the lack of a control group and an assured standard of reference like histopathological findings, sensitivity and specificity should be valued carefully. Results for agreement were added to complete the diagnostic description, but it should be considered that high numbers are partly based on the high amount of negative results.

In the detection of inflammatory changes, FOI was more sensitive than CE. The higher rate of positive findings compared with GDUS/PDUS suggests that the method is more sensitive than the other two procedures. It could be argued that only mild increases in FOI signal intensity might not be a sign of active arthritis and discreet findings in FOI should be interpreted carefully. Only FOI signals attributable to and limited to a specific joint were rated as FOI-positive joints. Also, Werner et al. [10, 11] state in their former studies that, because healthy subjects and controls with arthralgia but without signs of inflammatory disease had virtually no pathological increased signal intensity in FOI using the Xiralite method, the detected FOI signals appear to reflect actual inflammatory activity and are not all to be interpreted as false-positive findings.

Using MRI as a standard reference method, ICG-assisted fluorescence-optical diagnostics demonstrated high sensitivity (up to 85%) and high specificity (up to 95%) for the detection of MRI synovitis and tenosynovitis, as well as high consistency rates with MRI [10]. Unfortunately we were not able to also include MRI analyses in our study.

Improvement after 12 and 24 weeks of antirheumatic treatment could be shown with all three techniques, while the decrease in the number of joints with a FOI signal was slower than the clinical changes. To a lesser extent this was seen for the US as well. This indicates that joints becoming clinically inactive with treatment may show undetected subclinical activity, even after months of treatment. This is obvious in our patient shown in Fig. 3b who had residual inflammation at week 24 demonstrated by FOI although being in clinical remission. Hence, FOI can be useful to assess treatment response.

FOI improvement at month 3 did not show reliable predictive value for clinical improvement at month 6. Although more joints had changed from active at month 0 to inactive at month 6, when they had improved in FOI semiquantitative scores at month 3 (all FOI phases) the difference from 19 to about 35% is not huge. Logistic regression analysis could not produce reliable models either. One problem might be differences in sample size, because the vast majority of joints were inactive in the first place and did not show clinical or FOI changes during the investigation. But calculating only with initially active joints did not change the probability of outcome prediction.

There were some limitations to our study. The mean age of our patient cohort was relatively high, the youngest patient being 9 years old. This was due to reduced compliance in younger patients because the methodology is limited to older children able to comply with the procedure which takes 6 minutes and to the arm length of the children.

One further limitation of the FOI method is the lack of visualization of anatomical structures such as synovial proliferation or erosion, as well as the limited ability to assess the palmar inflammation, especially in the area of the hand and MCP joints. Furthermore, any inflammation of the hand region, for example lacerations of the skin, will result in increased signal intensity. In this study all patient hands were also examined for signs of inflammation and injury other than arthritis; this was documented and visible findings were documented and considered for FOI reading. Finally, FOI examination was tolerated well, with no report of AE correlated with the examination. We did not observe any serious adverse events in our cohort and in no patients did the analysis have to be stopped or interrupted.

Conclusion

ICG-supported FOI with the Xiralite method is a new imaging method for rheumatological questions. This technology allows sensitive detection of inflammatory changes. It is a useful technique to supplement clinical and ultrasonographic investigation in assessment of JIA activity in the joints of the hand. It can provide useful additional information for diagnosis and assessment of treatment response in JIA. Subclinical activity probably can be detected with this method. The procedure could be particularly important for the diagnosis of early arthritis as well as for follow-up under long-term anti-inflammatory therapy or for evaluation of remission.

Abbreviations

AUC: Area under the curve; CE: Clinical examination; CHAQ: Childhood Health Assessment Questionnaire; CI: Composite image; CRP: C-reactive protein; DIP: Distal interphalangeal joint; DMARD: Disease-modifying antirheumatic drug; ESR: Erythrocyte sedimentation rate; FOI: Fluorescence optical imaging; GS: Grey-scale mode; ILAR: International League of Rheumatology; ITT: Intention to treat; JADAS: Juvenile arthritis disease activity score; JIA: Juvenile idiopathic arthritis; LOM: Limitation of motion; MCP: Metacarpophalangeal joint; MRI: Magnetic resonance imaging; MTX: Methotrexate; NRS: Numeric rating scale; OMERACT: Outcome Measures in Rheumatology; PD: Power Doppler mode; PedACR: American College of Rheumatology pediatric criteria; PIP: Proximal interphalangeal joint; ROC: Receiver operating characteristic; US: Ultrasonography

Acknowledgements

Not applicable.

Funding

Unrestricted grant from Pfizer.

Authors' contributions

AK analyzed the data and wrote the manuscript. GH conceived the study, participated in its design and coordination, and was a major contributor to the manuscript. GWJ contributed to the manuscript and provided statistical analyses. IB analyzed the data and provided statistical support. DK, PTO, H-EL, and KM performed examination and data collection at the respective centers. SGW conceived the study, participated in its design and coordination, and read the fluorescence optical images, and was a contributor to the manuscript. H-EL conceived the study, and participated in its design and coordination. All authors read and approved the final manuscript.

Competing interests

AK, GWJ, SGW, IB, H-EL, and DK declare no competing interests. PTO is on the Advisory Board of Novartis. KM has received honoraria for lectures from Pfizer, Roche and Pharm-Allergan. GH has received grants and honorary fees from Abbvie, Pfizer, Novartis and Roche/Chugai.

Consent for publication

By signing informed consent the participations in this study (patients and parents) approved the use of their pseudonymized data for scientific analysis.

Author details

[1]Centre for Paediatric Rheumatology, Department of Paediatrics, Asklepios Clinic Sankt Augustin, Arnold-Janssen-Strasse 29, 53757 Sankt Augustin, Germany. [2]HELIOS Klinikum Duisburg, Klinik für Rheumatologie, Duisburg, Germany. [3]Department of Pediatric Oncology, Hematology and Clinical Immunology, University Children's Hospital, Medical Faculty, Heinrich-Heine-University, Düsseldorf, Germany. [4]Charité University Medicine and Epidemiology Unit, German Rheumatism Research Centre, Berlin, Germany. [5]Institute of Medical Statistics, University of Cologne, Cologne, Nordrhein-Westfalen, Germany. [6]RHIO (Rheumatologie, Immunologie, Osteologie) Düsseldorf, Düsseldorf, Germany. [7]Department of Diagnostic and Interventional Radiology, University Düsseldorf, Medical Faculty, Moorenstraße 5, 40225 Düsseldorf, Germany.

References

1. Petty RE. Prognosis in children with rheumatic diseases: justification for consideration of new therapies. Rheumatology (Oxford). 1999;38(8):739–42.
2. Woo P, Wedderburn LR. Juvenile chronic arthritis. Lancet. 1998;351(9107): 969–73.
3. Minden K, et al. Prognosis of patients with juvenile chronic arthritis and juvenile spondyloarthropathy. J Rheumatol. 2000;27(9):2256–63.
4. Gompels LL, Lim NH, Vincent T, Paleolog EM. In vivo optical imaging in arthritis—an enlightening future? Rheumatology (Oxford). 2010;49:1436–46.
5. Fischer T, Gemeinhardt I, Wagner S, et al. Assessment of unspecifi c near-infrared dyes in laser-induced fluorescence imaging of experimental arthritis. Acad Radiol. 2006;13:4–13.
6. Meier R, Krug C, Golovko D, et al. Indocyanine green-enhanced imaging of antigen induced arthritis with an integrated optical imaging/radiography system. ArthritisRheum. 2010;62:2322–7.
7. Ebert B, Berger J, Voigt J, et al. Early detection of rheumatoid arthritis in humans by fluorescence imaging. Optical Society of America meeting. Biomed. 2008; 2008 Mar 16-19; St. Petersburg, Florida. Biomedical Optics, OSA Technical Digest, 2008. BTuF19.
8. Fischer T, Ebert B, Voigt J, et al. Detection of rheumatoid arthritis using non-specific contrast enhanced fluorescence imaging. Acad Radiol. 2010;17:375–81.
9. Bremer C, Werner S, Langer HE. Assessing activity of rheumatic arthritis with fluorescence optical imaging. Eur Musculoskelet Rev. 2009;4:96–100.
10. Werner SG, Langer HE, Ohrndorf S, Bahner M, Schott P, Schwenke C, et al. Inflammation assessment in patients with arthritis using a novel in vivo fluorescence optical imaging technology [published erratum appears in Ann Rheum Dis 2012;71:1756 and Ann Rheum Dis 2013;72:156]. Ann Rheum Dis. 2012;71:504–10.
11. Werner SG, Langer HE, Schott P, Bahner M, Schwenke C, Lind-Albrecht G, et al. Indocyanine green-enhanced fluorescence optical imaging in patients with early and very early arthritis. A comparative study with magnetic resonance imaging. Arthritis Rheum. 2013;65:3036–44.
12. Petty RE, Southwood TR, Manners P, Baum J, Glass DN, Goldenberg J, et al. International League of Associations for Rheumatology. International League of Associations for Rheumatology classification of juvenile idiopathic arthritis: second revision, Edmonton, 2001. J Rheumatol. 2004;31:390–2.
13. Foeldvari I, Ruperto N, Dressler F, Häfner R, Küster RM, Michels H, et al. The German version of the Childhood Health Assessment Questionaire (CHAQ) and the Child Health Questionaire. Clin Exp Rheumatol. 2001;19(4 Suppl 23):71–4.
14. Consolaro A, et al. Development and validation of a composite disease activity score for juvenile idiopathic arthritis. Arthritis Rheum. 2009;61(5):658–66.
15. Magni-Manzoni S, Epis O, Ravelli A, Klersy C, Veisconti C, Lanni S, Muratore V, Sciré CA, Rossi S, Montecucco C. Comparison of clinical versus ultrasound-determined synovitis in juvenile idiopathic arthritis. Arthritis Rheum. 2009;61(11):1497–504.
16. Giannini EH, Ruperto N, Ravelli A, Lovell DJ, Felson DT, Martini A. Preliminary definition of improvement in juvenile arthritis. Arthritis Rheum. 1997;40:1202–9.
17. Consolaro A, et al. Remission, minimal disease activity, and acceptable symptom state in juvenile idiopathic arthritis: defining criteria based on the juvenile arthritis disease activity score. Arthritis Rheum. 2012;64(7):2366–74.
18. Lassere M, McQueen F, Østergaard M, et al. OMERACT Rheumatoid Arthritis Magnetic Resonance Imaging Studies. Exercise 3: an international multicenter reliability study using the RA-MRI Score. J Rheumatol. 2003;30(6):1366–75.
19. Scheel AK, Schmidt WA, Hermann K-G, et al. Interobserver reliabiltiy of rheumatologists performing musculoskeletal ultrasonography: results from a EULAR "Train the trainers" course. Ann Rheum Dis. 2005;64(7):1043–9.
20. Andersson SE, Johansson A, Lexmuller K, Ekstrom GM. Physiological characterization of mBSA antigen induced arthritis in the rat. II. Joint blood flow, glucose metabolism, and cell proliferation. J Rheumatol. 1998;25:1778–84.
21. Kennedy A, Ng CT, Biniecka M, et al. Angiogenesis and blood vessel stability in inflammatory arthritis. Arthritis Rheum. 2010;62:711–21.
22. McQueen FM, Benton N, Perry D, et al. Bone edema scored on magnetic resonance imaging scans of the dominant carpus at presentation predicts radiographic joint damage of the hands and feet six years later in patients with rheumatoid arthritis. Arthritis Rheum. 2003;48(7):1814–27.
23. Hetland ML, Ejbjerg B, Horslev-Petersen K, et al. MRI bone oedema is the strongest predictor of subsequent radiographic progression in early rheumatoid arthritis. Results from a 2-year randomised controlled trail (CIMESTRA). Ann Rheum Dis. 2009;68(3):384–90.
24. Suter LG, Fraenkel L, Braithwaite RS. Role of magnetic resonance imaging in the diagnosis and prognosis of rheumatoid arhtirits. Arthritis Care Res (Hoboken). 2011;63(5):675–88.
25. Lindblad S, Hedfors E. Intraarticular variation in synovitis: local macroscopic and microscopic signs of inflammatory activitiy are significantly correlated. Arthritis Rheum. 1985;28(9):977–86.
26. Ishizawa T, Fukushima N, Shibahara J, et al. Real-time identification of liver cancers by using indocyanin green fluorescent imaging. Cancer. 2009;115:2491–504.
27. Desmettre T, Devoisselle JM, Mordon S. Fluorescence properties and metabolic features of indocyanine green (ICG) as related to angiography. Surv Ophthalmol. 2000;45(1):15–27.
28. Fischer T, Ebert B, Voigt J, et al. Detection of rheumatoid arthritis using non-specific contrast enhanced fluorescence imaging. Acad Radiol. 2010:17;375–81.
29. Werner SG, Langer HE, Horneff G. Fluorescence optical imaging of juvenile arthritis. J Rheumatol. 2011;38(7):1447.
30. Brown AK, Conaghan PG, Karim Z, Quinn MA, Ikeda K, Peterfy CG, et al. An explanation for the apparent dissociation between clinical remission and continued structural deterioration in rheumatoid arthritis. Arthritis Rheum. 2008;58:2958–67.
31. Brown AK, Quinn MA, Karim Z, Conaghan PG, Peterfy CG, Hensor E, et al. Presence of significant synovitis in rheumatoid arthritis patients with disease-modifying antirheumatic drug-induced clinical remission: evidence from an imaging study may explain structural progression. Arthritis Rheum. 2006;54:3761–73.
32. Saleem B, Brown AK, Keen H, Nizam S, Freeston J, Wakefield R, et al. Should imaging be a component of rheumatoid arthritis remission criteria? A comparison between traditional and modified composite remission scores and imaging assessments. Ann Rheum Dis. 2011;70:792–8.

9

Early changes in gene expression and inflammatory proteins in systemic juvenile idiopathic arthritis patients on canakinumab therapy

Arndt H. Brachat[1], Alexei A. Grom[2], Nico Wulffraat[3], Hermine I. Brunner[2], Pierre Quartier[4], Riva Brik[5], Liza McCann[6], Huri Ozdogan[7], Lidia Rutkowska-Sak[8], Rayfel Schneider[9], Valeria Gerloni[10], Liora Harel[11], Maria Terreri[12], Kristin Houghton[13], Rik Joos[14], Daniel Kingsbury[15], Jorge M. Lopez-Benitez[16], Stephan Bek[1], Martin Schumacher[1], Marie-Anne Valentin[1], Hermann Gram[1], Ken Abrams[17], Alberto Martini[18], Daniel J. Lovell[2], Nanguneri R. Nirmala[19], Nicolino Ruperto[20*] and for the Pediatric Rheumatology International Trials Organization (PRINTO) and the Pediatric Rheumatology Collaborative Study Group (PRCSG)

Abstract

Background: Canakinumab is a human anti-interleukin-1β (IL-1β) monoclonal antibody neutralizing IL-1β-mediated pathways. We sought to characterize the molecular response to canakinumab and evaluate potential markers of response using samples from two pivotal trials in systemic juvenile idiopathic arthritis (SJIA).

Methods: Gene expression was measured in patients with febrile SJIA and in matched healthy controls by Affymetrix DNA microarrays. Transcriptional response was assessed by gene expression changes from baseline to day 3 using adapted JIA American College of Rheumatology (aACR) response criteria (50 aACR JIA). Changes in pro-inflammatory cytokines IL-6 and IL-18 were assessed up to day 197.

Results: Microarray analysis identified 984 probe sets differentially expressed (≥2-fold difference; $P < 0.05$) in patients versus controls. Over 50% of patients with ≥50 *a*ACR JIA were recognizable by baseline expression values. Analysis of gene expression profiles from patients achieving ≥50 *a*ACR JIA response at day 15 identified 102 probe sets differentially expressed upon treatment (≥2-fold difference; $P < 0.05$) on day 3 versus baseline, including IL-1β, IL-1 receptors (IL1-R1 and IL1-R2), IL-1 receptor accessory protein (IL1-RAP), and IL-6. The strongest clinical response was observed in patients with higher baseline expression of dysregulated genes and a strong transcriptional response on day 3. IL-6 declined by day 3 (≥8-fold decline; $P < 0.0001$) and remained suppressed. IL-18 declined on day 57 (≥1.5-fold decline, $P \leq 0.002$).

Conclusions: Treatment with canakinumab in SJIA patients resulted in downregulation of innate immune response genes and reductions in IL-6 and clinical symptoms. Additional research is needed to investigate potential differences in the disease mechanisms in patients with heterogeneous gene transcription profiles.

Keywords: Biomarkers, Canakinumab, Gene expression, Interleukin-1β, Juvenile idiopathic arthritis, SJIA

* Correspondence: nicolaruperto@gaslini.org
[20]Istituto Giannina Gaslini, Pediatria II-PRINTO, Genoa, Italy
Full list of author information is available at the end of the article

Background

Systemic juvenile idiopathic arthritis (SJIA) is a rare, multigenic, autoinflammatory disease of unknown etiology characterized by chronic arthritis; intermittent high-spiking fever, rash, and elevated levels of acute-phase reactants [1–3]. The clinical course is highly variable, ranging from a monocyclic course with a single episode of active disease to the more common persistent clinical course in which the disease remains clinically active. In a minority of patients, the disease follows a polycyclic course, with periods of quiescent disease interrupted by flares of systemic features and mild arthritis [3–5].

SJIA is currently recognized as a distinct subtype of juvenile idiopathic arthritis (JIA), although it is unique among the various forms of JIA in both its epidemiologic and immunopathologic features [1–3]. In contrast to the other JIA phenotypes, which are characterized by abnormalities in adaptive immune response, SJIA is driven by dysregulation of innate immune pathways, with monocytes and neutrophils—rather than lymphocytes—acting as the predominant effector cells [3]. The innate immune signature and clinical features of SJIA, also known as Still's disease, bear a striking resemblance to adult onset Still's disease, a rare autoinflammatory disorder characterized by daily spiking temperature, maculopapular rash, and arthritis [6]. Indeed, it has been suggested that these two clinical phenotypes are part of the same disease continuum with different ages of onset [6, 7].

A substantial and growing body of evidence suggests that the pro-inflammatory cytokines interleukins 1, 6, and 18 (IL-1, IL-6, IL-18), and tumor necrosis factor play central roles in the aberrant innate immune response observed in SJIA. In vitro exposure of healthy donor peripheral blood mononuclear cells (PBMCs) to sera from subjects with SJIA induces transcription of genes associated with the IL-1 signaling pathway and markedly increases IL-1β protein secretion [8]. Additionally, treatment of patients with SJIA with agents that block IL-1 signaling pathways resolves clinical symptoms with corresponding improvements in laboratory markers of inflammation [8–14]. Finally, it was recently reported that the proteomics signature associated with disease flares in patients with SJIA is characterized by the differential expression of a small group of proteins that are centrally mediated by IL-1 [15].

Canakinumab is a high-affinity human IL-1β monoclonal antibody that selectively binds to human IL-1β, thereby inactivating IL-1β signaling pathways and neutralizing its downstream effects [16, 17]. Clinical evidence of the efficacy and safety of canakinumab in patients with SJIA was demonstrated in two international phase-3 trials that served as the basis for the approval of canakinumab for the treatment of SJIA by United States and European regulatory authorities [13, 18, 19].

In the present analysis, we sought to characterize the molecular response to treatment with canakinumab and explore potential markers of disease activity and therapeutic response in patients with SJIA using blood-derived biomarker samples from the two phase-3 trials.

Methods

Patients

The source population for the biomarker analyses included all patients enrolled in the two phase-3 trials evaluating canakinumab for SJIA (ClinicalTrials.gov, NCT00886769 (trial 1) and NCT00889863 (trial 2)) conducted by the members of the Pediatric Rheumatology International Trials Organization (PRINTO) and the Pediatric Rheumatology Collaborative Study Group (PRCSG) [13]. All patients with available samples who received treatment with either canakinumab or placebo in trial 1 or who were treated with canakinumab in the open-label phase of trial 2 were selected for inclusion in the biomarker study. For selected biomarker analyses, donor samples from age-matched, race-matched, and gender-matched healthy subjects were used as a comparator.

Eligibility criteria and study designs for the original phase-3 trials have been previously described [13]. Briefly, eligible subjects were 2 to 19 years of age with a confirmed diagnosis of SJIA according to published criteria, and who had fever [20]. Concomitant therapy with a prednisone equivalent (up to 1.0 mg/kg/day) and stable doses of nonsteroidal anti-inflammatory drugs and methotrexate (≤20 mg/m^2 per week) were permitted.

The studies (trials 1 and 2) were conducted according to the ethical principles of the Declaration of Helsinki. The study was approved by the ethics committee of all participating centers according to the local regulations (see SJIA gene expression ethics approval.docx).

Study design

In trial 1, patients were randomly assigned to receive a single subcutaneous dose of canakinumab (4 mg/kg) or matched placebo. In trial 2, patients were treated with subcutaneous canakinumab (4 mg/kg) every 4 weeks for up to 32 weeks during an initial open-label phase. Patients who achieved a 30 aACR JIA response (defined as improvement of ≥30% in at least three of the six core criteria for JIA, worsening of >30% in no more than one of the criteria, and resolution of fever) and were not receiving glucocorticoids or who had undergone successful tapering and were receiving a stable dose of glucocorticoids, were included in a second withdrawal phase in which they were randomly assigned to continued treatment with canakinumab or placebo.

Blood samples for ribonucleic acid (RNA) isolation were collected at baseline and at day 3 in both trials. For quantification of IL-6 and IL-18, pharmacokinetic serum samples collected at baseline and on days 3, 29, 57, and 197 in trial 2 were used. The parent or guardian of each patient with SJIA and each healthy volunteer provided separate written informed consent (or assent for minors) for the collection and analysis of blood-derived biomarkers.

Biomarker analyses

SJIA gene transcription profile

Global gene transcription was measured in whole blood samples collected from patients with SJIA and age-matched healthy subjects. Microarray analyses were conducted by the Biomarker Development (BMD) group at the Novartis Institutes for Biomedical Research (Basel, Switzerland). Samples were stored at −80 °C and total RNA was subsequently isolated using the PAXgene Blood RNA Kit (Qiagen, Hilden, Germany). Complementary deoxyribonucleic acid (cDNA) was synthesized from total RNA using the Ovation® RNA Amplification System V2 and the Ribo-SPIA® amplification process according to the instructions of the manufacturer (NuGen Technologies Inc., San Carlos, CA, USA). Labeled cDNA was hybridized to GeneChip® U133plus 2.0 arrays as specified by the manufacturer (Affymetrix, Santa Clara, CA, USA). Integrity and purity of RNA and cDNA was confirmed using the Agilent 2100 Bioanalyzer system (Agilent Technologies Inc., Wilmington, DE, USA). Gene expression values were derived using Affymetrix MAS 5.0 software and scaled to a trimmed mean value of 150. Expression values were stored in CEL files and were analyzed using Bioconductor packages or customized R-scripts [21–23].

For group-wise comparison of transcript levels, robustly expressed transcripts were identified by filtering for probe sets with a median expression value of at least 64 in at least one of the groups (typically around 16,000 probe sets). The Wilcoxon test was applied with a threshold P value of ≤0.05 to identify genes that were significantly differentially expressed at baseline in patients with SJIA relative to healthy controls. An additional exploratory filtering step for effect size was performed using a 1.5-fold, 2-fold, and 3-fold difference in the median expression value as thresholds. The fold-change cutoffs are arbitrary and were selected before data analysis a priori, and were intended to either describe the more global changes in gene expression or to focus on the most strongly affected genes. Global changes in gene expression were evaluated using the more sensitive threshold of a 1.5-fold difference to facilitate identification of "hits" to signaling pathways (accepting a presumably elevated false positive rate), while the more rigorous threshold of a 3-fold difference was used to identify the most promising biomarker candidates. No correction for multiple comparisons was performed.

Differentially expressed transcripts were displayed using unsupervised two-dimensional hierarchical clustering to group baseline SJIA samples and healthy controls according to gene expression profiles. Expression values were median-centered per gene. Genes with a ≥1.5-fold median increase in baseline SJIA samples relative to normal controls were mapped to protein interaction networks using METACORE™ pathway maps (Thompson Reuters, New York, NY, USA).

Early transcriptional response to canakinumab

The early transcriptional response to canakinumab was evaluated by comparing gene expression values in patients with SJIA at day 3 with the values measured at baseline. The magnitude of effect was expressed as the median of the per-patient fold changes in transcription levels at day 3 compared with baseline. Differentially expressed transcripts were identified using the paired sample t test (P value ≤0.05, ≥1.5-fold differential expression). One-dimensional hierarchical clustering of transcripts was used to display gene expression values ordered according to the aACR JIA response at day 15 to visualize the relationship between baseline gene expression, day 3 transcriptional response, and day 15 clinical response (see Additional file 1: Table S1 for the criteria for each level of response).

The data discussed in this publication have been deposited in the NCBI Gene Expression Omnibus and are accessible through GEO [GEO:GSE80060] (http://www.ncbi.nlm.nih.gov/geo/query/acc.cgi?token=wdyteywqfbuzvgf&acc = GSE80060).

Protein biomarkers

A panel of peripheral blood protein markers was selected for analysis based on prior evidence of their association with disease status in patients with SJIA [24–26]. Selected protein markers included IL-6 and IL-18, both of which have been shown to be upregulated in SJIA.

Concentrations of IL-6 and IL-18 were quantified using commercial immunoassay (Quantikine HS Human IL-6 Immunoassay, Catalogue No. SS600B, R&D Systems; Human IL-18 ELISA Kit, Catalogue No. 7620, MBL) validated in human EDTA plasma; three levels of quality controls prepared in human EDTA plasma were used to validate the runs.

Sample preparation

Unknown samples (clinical study samples and the human EDTA plasma sample used to prepare quality controls) were stored at −80 °C. On the day of analysis, samples were thawed at room temperature. Once thawed, samples were stored at 2 – 8 °C or on ice if not immediately analyzed. A minimum dilution of 1:5 was applied for the analysis of IL-18.

Results

Patients with SJIA had a median age of 9 years, 52% were female, and 77% were white, whereas controls had a median age of 9 years, 50% were female, and 91% were white. Patients were characterized by high levels of disease activity at baseline, 99.4% of 177 patients had a juvenile arthritis disease activity score (JADAS)-27 > 8.5, indicating high disease activity [27].

SJIA gene transcription signature

Microarray analysis of whole blood samples collected from patients with SJIA at the baseline study visit identified a total of 984 probe sets with at differential expression at least twofold compared with aged-matched healthy controls. Of these, 704 probe sets were upregulated at least twofold and 280 downregulated at least twofold relative to controls. Unsupervised hierarchical clustering of upregulated genes perfectly discriminated baseline SJIA samples from healthy control samples (Fig. 1a). Clustering of downregulated genes had a more heterogeneous pattern; while the majority of patients with SJIA were grouped in a single cluster that was separated from controls, transcription patterns for downregulated genes in a minority of patients with SJIA were not distinguished from healthy controls (Fig. 1b).

On examination of which genes were more strongly expressed in patients with SJIA, the number of upregulated genes exceeded the number of downregulated genes by nearly 10-fold among the genes with the most marked differences. There were 111 probe sets indicating ≥3-fold upregulation compared with only 12 probe sets indicating ≥3-fold downregulation. Among the strongly upregulated genes were genes that encode neutrophil-expressed proteins like CD177, olfactomedin 4 (OLFM4) or defensin, alpha 4 (DEFA4) and several other regulators of immune function such as tumor necrosis factor, alpha-induced protein 6 (TNFAIP6), IL-1 receptor antagonist (IL1RN), C-type lectin domain family 4 (CLEC4D) or IL-1 receptor-associated kinase 3 (IRAK3); a complete list of strongly differentially expressed genes is available in Additional file 1: Table S2.

To further examine the functional pathways affected by genes that were differentially expressed in baseline SJIA samples, we mapped SJIA-induced genes (≥1.5-fold differential expression) to protein interaction networks as defined in the METACORE™ database/software. Network maps indicated a strong innate immune response, with widespread activation of inter-related pro-inflammatory signaling pathways. Figure 2 illustrates the interactions between key signaling pathways mediated by selected pro-inflammatory proteins, including IL-1β, IL-6, and the toll-like receptors TLR2 and TLR4.

Early transcriptional response to canakinumab

Microarray analysis of samples from patients with SJIA treated with canakinumab and achieving ≥50 aACR JIA response at day 15 identified a total of 1305 probe sets

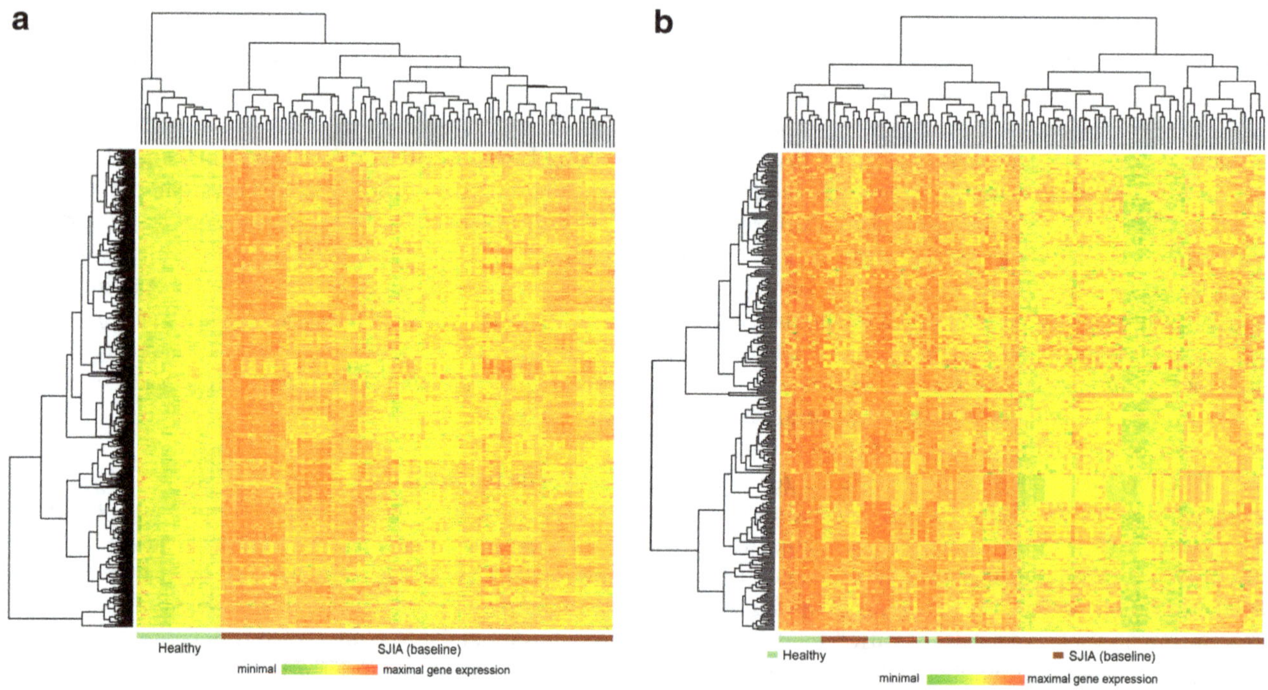

Fig. 1 Hierarchical clustering of genes that were upregulated (**a**) and downregulated (**b**) at least twofold in baseline systemic juvenile idiopathic arthritis (*SJIA*) samples compared with healthy control samples. Subjects are shown in *columns* and genes (probe sets) are shown in *rows*. Relative gene expression values are *color*-coded. With upregulated probe sets the hierarchical clustering of subjects perfectly segregated patients with SJIA from healthy controls. Using downregulated genes, the majority of patients with SJIA clustered together; however, a subset of patients with SJIA was indistinguishable from healthy controls

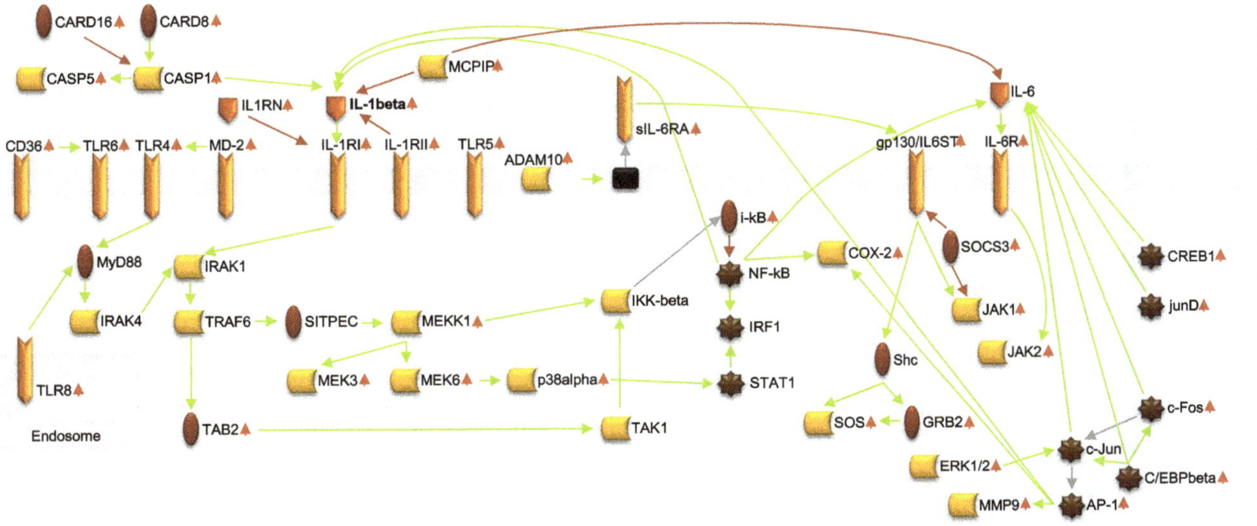

Fig. 2 Pathway map for selected proteins encoded by genes that were upregulated in baseline systemic juvenile idiopathic arthritis (*SJIA*) samples. Protein interaction networks for selected proteins that were upregulated in baseline SJIA samples compared with healthy control samples. Proteins were mapped using Metacore™ pathway maps (Thompson Reuters, New York, NY, USA). The network displayed here represents a combination of maps for the signaling pathways for IL-1β, IL-6, and the toll-like receptors TL2 and TL4. *Small red arrows* adjacent to gene/protein names indicate upregulation in SJIA. *ADAM10* disintegrin and metalloproteinase domain-containing protein 10, *AP-1* activator protein 1, *CARD* caspase recruitment domain, *CASP* caspase, *C/EBP CCAAT/* enhancer binding protein, *COX2* cyclooxlygenase-2, *CREB* cyclic AMP responsive element binding protein, *GRB* growth factor receptor-bound protein, *IL-1beta* interleukin-1 beta, *IL-R1* interleukin-1 receptor, *IL1RN* interleukin-1 receptor antagonist, *IL-6* interleukin-6, *IL-6R* interleukin-6 receptor, *sIL-6RA* soluble interleukin-6 receptor antagonist, *IL6ST* interleukin-6 signal transducer, *IRAK* interleukin receptor-associated kinase, *IRF* interferon regulatory factor, *JAK* Janus kinase, *MCPIP* monocyte chemotactic protein-induced protein, *MEK* mitogen activated kinase kinase, *MMP* matrix metalloproteinase, *NFκB* nuclear factor-κB, *SOS* son of sevenless protein, *STAT* signal transducer and activator of transduction, *TAB* TGFβ-activated kinase binding protein, *TAK* TGFβ-activated kinase, *TLR* toll-like receptor

indicating at least 1.5-fold differential expression between baseline and day 3 (no other post-treatment time points were available). These transcripts largely overlapped with those that were dysregulated (in the opposite direction) in baseline SJIA samples as compared with healthy donor samples. The response to canakinumab treatment of SJIA dysregulated genes is shown in Fig. 3, which displays samples ordered by time point (baseline or day 3) and by aACR JIA response score on day 15. These results indicated stronger dysregulation at baseline and also a stronger transcriptional response to canakinumab treatment in a majority of those patients who later (at day 15) reached higher aACR JIA response scores.

Patients who achieved a 100 aACR JIA response at day 15 had high expression of SJIA-induced genes at baseline and a large transcriptional response (downregulation) at day 3, with day-3 values resembling those of healthy controls. In contrast, patients who did not achieve a 30 aACR JIA response on day 15 had weak upregulation of SJIA-induced genes at baseline and essentially unaltered transcription levels on day 3.

Consistent with the observation described, the gene encoding IL-1β—the therapeutic target of canakinumab—also had a robust transcriptional response that was more pronounced in patients who achieved the strongest clinical outcomes. Among patients who did not achieve a 50 aACR, the relative mean gene expression (standard deviation (SD)) at baseline and at day 3 was 894 (501) and 657 (248), respectively. For patients who achieved ≥50 aACR, the relative mean gene expression (SD) at baseline and at day 3 was 1738 (780) and 735 (369), respectively. Transcription levels were also reduced for several IL-1β-related genes, including IL-1RN, IL-1R1, IL-1R2, and IL-1RAP, an essential component of the IL-1 receptor complex that is required for IL-1 signal transduction.

Protein biomarkers

Longitudinal analysis of soluble biomarkers in canakinumab-treated patients showed a marked reduction in serum IL-6 concentration that was evident by the first assessment at day 3 and persisted throughout the duration of observation (Fig. 4a). A more modest reduction was observed for IL-18 serum levels following canakinumab treatment. Additionally, in contrast to IL-6, which declined rapidly following treatment, the reduction in serum concentrations of IL-18 occurred later and was not statistically significant until day 57 (Fig. 4b).

To assess the potential utility of IL-6 and IL-18 as markers of SJIA disease activity status, we compared serum protein levels in patients who achieved a clinical response that was classified as "inactive disease" with those who had clinical evidence of active disease at the

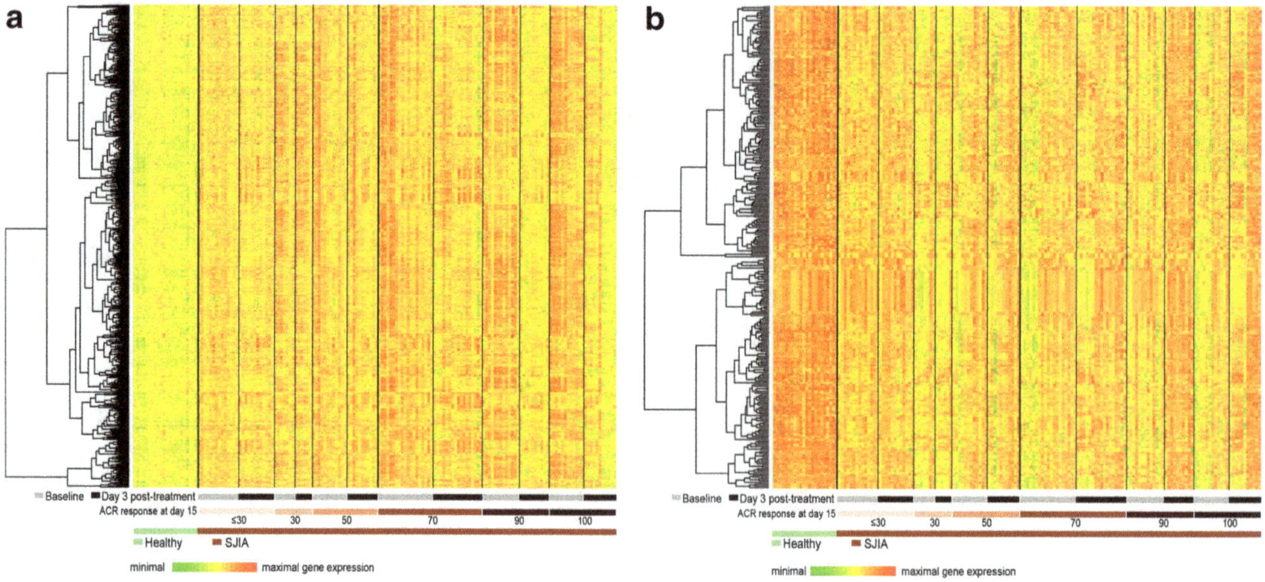

Fig. 3 Early transcriptional response to canakinumab treatment of dysregulated genes in systemic juvenile idiopathic arthritis (*SJIA*). Genes (probe sets) are shown in *rows* and subjects are shown in *columns*, ordered according to disease status (SJIA versus healthy), assessment time point (baseline versus day 3), and by response according to American College of Rheumatology (*ACR*) criteria at day 15. Relative gene expression values are *color*-coded. **a** Genes that were upregulated ≥2-fold in baseline SJIA samples compared with healthy control sample. **b** Genes that were downregulated ≥2-fold in baseline SJIA samples compared with healthy control samples

corresponding study visit. As per the modified Wallace criteria, inactive disease was defined as absence of active arthritis, fever, and signs or symptoms of SJIA; normal C-reactive protein level; and physician's global assessment of disease activity ≤10 mm) [28].

Statistically significant differences in serum IL-6 levels were observed at each time point in patients with inactive disease compared with the active disease group. At day 29 the mean IL-6 serum concentration in patients with active disease was 24.3 pg/mL (SD 41.2), whereas in patients with inactive disease the mean concentration was 1.4 pg/mL (SD 1.1) ($P = 0.0002$). Similarly at day 57 the mean IL-6 serum concentration in patients with active disease was 25.2 (SD 31.2), whereas in patients with inactive disease, the mean concentration was 1.5 pg/mL (SD 1.4) ($P = 8.9e^{-6}$). At day 197 the mean IL-6 serum concentration in patients with active disease was 45.0 (SD 85.7), whereas in patients with inactive disease, the mean concentration was 1.5 pg/mL (SD 0.5) ($P = 0.01$). Additionally, serum IL-6 levels were normal in all patients classified as having inactive disease; however, normal levels were also observed in patients with active disease. Analysis of serum IL-18 concentrations showed no statistically significant differences between patients with active and inactive disease. At day 29 the mean serum IL-18 concentration in patients with active disease was 14080 pg/mL (SD 26733), whereas in patients with inactive disease, the mean concentration was 21090 pg/mL (SD 30291) ($P = 0.3$). At day 57 the mean IL-18 concentration in the patients with active disease was 10830 pg/mL (SD 16875), whereas in patients with inactive disease the mean concentration was 16790 pg/mL (SD 21661) ($P = 0.2$). At day 197 the mean IL-18 concentration in patients with active disease was 6218 pg/mL (SD 8784), whereas in patients with inactive disease the mean concentration was 7970 pg/mL (SD 12140) ($P = 0.7$).

Discussion

The current study of blood-derived biomarkers in patients with SJIA treated with canakinumab in a phase-3 clinical trial program yielded several observations with potential implications for patient management and subsequent research. First, analysis of global gene expression in whole blood samples from patients with SJIA and age-matched healthy controls identified robust disease-related alterations of the transcriptome involving key mediators of innate immune response. Consistent with prior research [29–31], differentially expressed genes were typically upregulated relative to healthy controls, supporting the hypothesis that the immune-pathologic process in SJIA is characterized by transcriptional activation of "disease genes" rather than suppression of "health-associated" genes.

Second, we identified a canakinumab response signature in many patients with SJIA that was characterized by the rapid normalization of transcript levels for SJIA overexpressed genes, including those associated with IL-1 and IL-6 signaling pathways. For example, we observed a marked decline in transcription levels of the gene encoding the therapeutic target of canakinumab, IL-1β, suggesting that

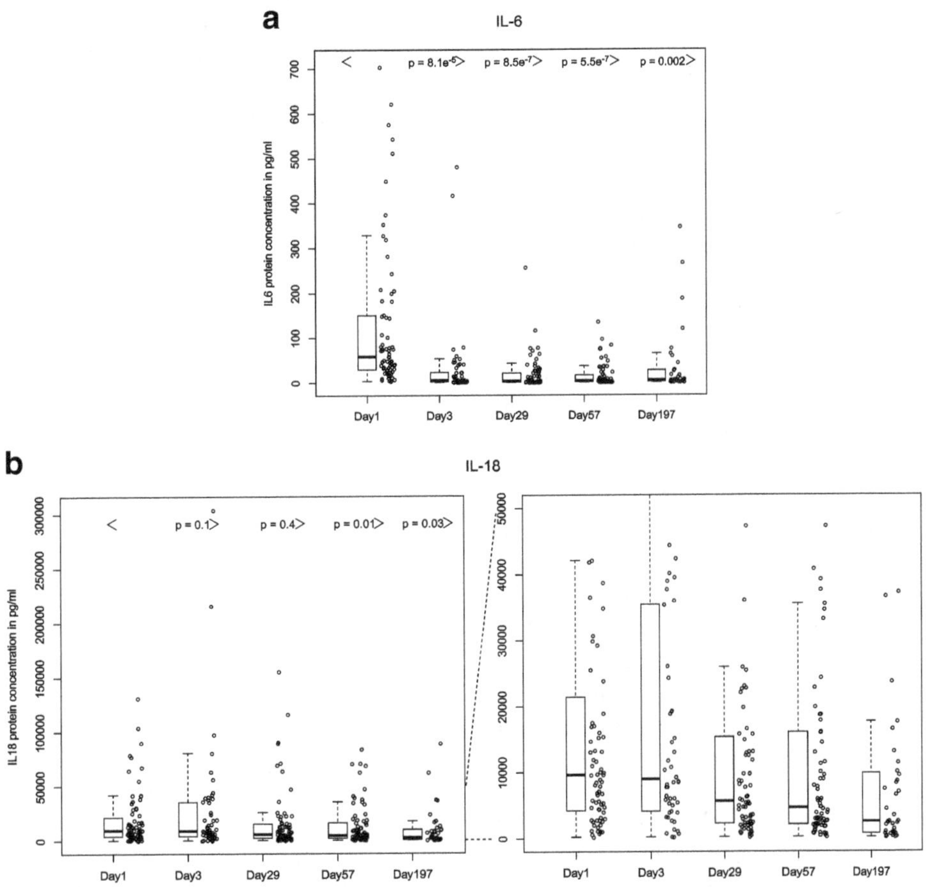

Fig. 4 Longitudinal change in serum concentrations of IL-6 (**a**) and IL-18 (**b**) after treatment with canakinumab. Data are shown for trial 2. Similar results were observed for plasma samples in trial 1 (data available until day 29; not shown). The *left panel* (**b**) shows all data; the *right panel* represents a magnification of the lower portion of the *y-axis*. *IL-6* interleukin-6, *IL-18* interleukin 18

canakinumab disrupts a positive feedback loop between IL-1β signaling and IL-1β production. The strongest clinical response to canakinumab was observed in patients with higher baseline expression of SJIA-induced genes and a larger transcriptional reduction at day 3; poor clinical response was typically associated with low differential expression of dysregulated genes at baseline and a negligible transcriptional response at day 3.

It is noteworthy that the group of genes comprising the canakinumab response signature in this study closely corresponds with the group of genes that define the transcription signature of adult-onset Still's disease (AOSD). Indeed, comparison of baseline gene transcription data from patients with AOSD enrolled in a recent trial evaluating canakinumab in healthy adult subjects showed that the mean expression of all of the genes that were downregulated following canakinumab treatment in the current study were upregulated prior to treatment in patients with AOSD relative to healthy controls ($P < 0.00002$) [32, 33]. Similarly, most of the genes that were upregulated following canakinumab treatment in patients with SJIA were downregulated prior to treatment in patients with AOSD compared with healthy controls ($P < 0.00002$). Collectively, these findings support the concept of a Still's disease continuum that includes both a juvenile-onset and an adult-onset form.

Third, consistent with the early transcriptional effects of canakinumab on genes encoding proteins involved in innate immunity, serum concentrations of the pro-inflammatory cytokines IL-6 and IL-18 declined following treatment with canakinumab. While IL-6 levels declined markedly by day 3 and remained suppressed throughout the duration of treatment, the decline in IL-18 was less robust and occurred much later than the observed declines in IL-6. This might be explained by slow-acting regulatory mechanisms controlling peripheral IL-18 secretion or by residual ongoing pro-inflammatory stimulation of unknown origin. It is important to note that circulating levels of IL-18 have been shown to be markedly elevated in patients with SJIA with macrophage activation syndrome (MAS) [34–36]. While high IL-18 was observed in the three patients who developed MAS during the phase-3 trial of canakinumab, there were quite a few patients with equally high or higher IL-18 who did not develop MAS during the course of the study. Evidence from recent studies suggests a complex interaction between IL-18 and other cytokines in the development of MAS and provides intriguing clues on the potential contribution of free IL-18 levels, the IL-18/IFN-γ ratio, and the IL-18/IL-6 ratio to the prediction of MAS in patients with SJIA [35, 36]. Each of these clues warrants further investigation; however, the limited number of patients with MAS in this cohort precludes meaningful interpretation of the available data.

Fourth, the presence of a number of SJIA-induced genes at baseline, e.g., CD177, OLFM4, and the gene encoding IL-1β, among others, appeared to lead to a stronger transcriptional response to canakinumab treatment and higher ACR responses at day 15. However, in a significant proportion of canakinumab responders, these transcriptional effects were not observed, and therefore, baseline gene expression would not correctly predict good canakinumab responders. The predictive performance of baseline gene expression, with respect to other previously identified markers of response to IL-1 inhibition, will be the subject of future investigation.

The findings of the present study should be interpreted in the context of certain limitations. First, while the observed changes in gene expression were presumably influenced by changes in the cellular composition of the samples, the precise contribution of changes in blood cell populations to the observed transcriptional response cannot be reliably ascertained. Additionally, the degree to which the findings might have been influenced by factors such as disease duration and severity, prior treatment with other biologic therapies, and concomitant exposure to corticosteroids during the study is unknown. Second, baseline gene transcription was evaluated using the single pre-treatment blood sample that was available for each patient. Given the dynamic nature of the disease with frequent spikes in fever, it is possible that the differences between patients with SJIA and healthy controls were attenuated or obscured and that the contrast in gene transcription profiles might be enhanced by integrating data from multiple pre-treatment measurements. This might also reduce the apparent heterogeneity observed in subgroups of patients who achieved a comparable clinical response to canakinumab. Finally, patients without fever and with a more prominent polyarticular disease course were excluded from enrollment in the original phase-3 clinical trials from which blood samples for the current study were obtained. Accordingly, the effect of canakinumab on gene expression in patients with SJIA with a polyarticular disease course is unknown.

Conclusions

Our findings demonstrate that canakinumab treatment in patients with SJIA results in rapid reductions in the expression of genes related to inflammation, with corresponding reductions in circulating levels of pro-inflammatory cytokines and clinical symptoms, suggesting that canakinumab can, at least in part, reverse molecular disease patterns.

Abbreviations

aACR: adapted American college of rheumatology; ACR: American College of Rheumatology; BMD: biomarker development; cDNA: complimentary deoxyribonucleic acid; CLEC4D: C-type lectin domain family 4; DEFA4: defensin, alpha 4; IL: interleukin; IL1-R: interleukin-1 receptor; IL1-RAP: interleukin-1 receptor accessory protein; IL1RN: interleukin-1 receptor antagonist; IRAK3: interleukin-1 receptor-associated kinase 3; JADAS: juvenile arthritis disease activity score; JIA: juvenile idiopathic arthritis; OLFM4: olfactomedin 4; PBMCs: peripheral blood mononuclear cells; PRCSG: Pediatric Rheumatology Collaborative Study Group; PRINTO: Pediatric Rheumatology International Trials Organization; RNA: ribonucleic acid; SJIA: systemic juvenile idiopathic arthritis; TNFAIP6: tumor necrosis factor, alpha-induced protein 6

Acknowledgments

We thank all remaining PRINTO and PRCSG participating centers that participated in the trial. Argentina: Ruben Cuttica, MD; Austria: Wolfgang Emminger, MD; Belgium: Bernard Lauwerys, MD, Carine Wouters, MD, Laurence Goffin, MD; Brazil: Flavio Sztajnbok, MD, Sebastiao Radominski, MD, Sheila Oliveira, MD; Canada: Elie Haddad, MD; France: Isabelle Kone-Paut, MD, Marine Desjonqueres, MD, Michel Fischbach, MD; Germany: Angelika Thon, MD, Dirk Foell, MD, Elisabeth Weibarth-Riedel, MD, Gerd Horneff, MD, Ralph Trauzeddel, MD, Reinhard Berner, MD, Tilmann Kallinich, MD; Greece: Maria Trachana, MD; Hungary: Tamás Constantin, MD; Israel: Judith Barash, MD, Yackov Berkun, MD, Yosef Uziel, MD; Italy: Fabrizia Corona, MD, Maria Alessio, MD, Rolando Cimaz, MD, Stefania Viola, MD; Norway: Berit Flato, MD; Peru: Manuel Ferrandiz, MD; Spain: Inmaculada Calvo, MD, Jordi Anton, MD, Juan Carlos Robledillos, MD, Maria Luz Gamir, MD; Sweden: Bo Magnusson, MD; Switzerland: Michael Hofer, MD; Turkey: Erbil Unsal, MD, Muferet Erguven, MD, Seza Ozen, MD; United Kingdom: Nick Wilkinson, MD, Alice Chieng, MD, Athimalaipet Ramanan, MD, Helen Foster, MD, Kiran Nistala, MD; USA: Gloria Higgins, MD, Katherine Marzan, MD, Kenneth Schikler, MD, Paula Morris, MD. We also thank Elise Hellinger and BioScience Communications for providing editorial support on behalf of Novartis Pharma AG.

Funding

This study was sponsored and funded by Novartis Pharma.

Authors' contributions

AHB and NRN carried out the gene expression analysis. AHB carried out the statistical analysis. NRN, HG, KA, HIB, DJL, AM, and NR were involved in protocol writing, manuscript drafting, and manuscript revision. NW, PQ, RB, LM, HO, LRS, RS, VG, LH, MT, KH, RJ, DK, JMLB, HIB, DJL, AM, and NR were involved in the clinical trials, provided the patient samples for this analysis, and were involved in the writing and revision of the manuscript. AHB, AAG, MAV, HG, KA, SB, and MS were involved in the writing and revision of the manuscript. All authors read and approved the final manuscript.

Competing interests

K. Abrams is an employee of Novartis Pharmaceuticals Corporation. S. Bek was an employee of Novartis Institutes for Biomedical Research. A. Brachat is an employee of Novartis Institutes for Biomedical Research and a shareholder of Novartis Pharma AG. R. Brik receives consulting fees from Novartis. H. Brunner is on the speakers' bureau and serves as a consultant for Novartis, and is involved in unrelated research with Novartis. V. Gerloni has nothing to declare. H. Gram is an employee of Novartis Institutes for Biomedical Research. A. Grom receives speaker/consulting fees from Novartis, and collaborates on research with NovImmune. L. Harel receives fees for recruiting patients for clinical trials. K. Houghton has nothing to declare. R. Joos receives consultant fees from Pfizer, BMS, AbbVie, Roche, Cellgene, and UCB. D. Kingsbury has nothing to declare. J.M. Lopez-Benitez has nothing to declare. D.J. Lovell is on the speakers' bureau and serves as a consultant for Novartis, and is involved in unrelated research with Novartis. A. Martini is on the speakers' bureau and serves as a consultant for Novartis, and is involved in unrelated research with Novartis. L. McCann has nothing to declare. N. Nirmala was an employee of Novartis Institutes for Biomedical Research. H. Özdoğan receives speaker fees and collaborates on research with Novartis. P. Quartier receives speaker/consulting fees from Novartis, Swedish Orphan Biovitrum (SOBI), and Roche, and collaborates on research with Novartis, Swedish Orphan Biovitrum (SOBI), and Roche. N. Ruperto is on the speakers' bureau and serves as a consultant for Novartis, and is involved in unrelated research with Novartis. L. Rutkowska-Sak has nothing to declare. R. Schneider receives consultant fees from Novartis. M. Schumacher was an employee of Novartis Pharma AG. M. Terreri collaborates on research with Novartis. M.A. Valentin is an employee of Novartis Pharma AG. N. Wulffraat has nothing to declare. No other nonfinancial conflicts of interest exist for any of the authors other than those listed above.

Ethics approval and consent to participate

Independent ethics committee or institutional review board

The study protocol and all amendments were reviewed by the Independent Ethics Committee or Institutional Review Board for each center (see Additional file 1: Table S3 (trial 1) and Table S4 (trial 2) for a list of independent ethics committees or institutional review boards.

Ethical conduct of the studies

The studies were conducted according to the ethical principles of the Declaration of Helsinki (trials 1 and 2).

Patient information and consent

Informed consent was obtained from each patient in writing before randomization. The studies were described by a nurse/study coordinator/the investigator, who answered any questions, and written information was also provided (trials 1 and 2).

Author details

[1]Novartis Institutes for Biomedical Research, Basel, Switzerland. [2]Cincinnati Children's Hospital Medical Center, PRCSG, Cincinnati, OH, USA. [3]Wilhelmina Kinderziekenhuis, Department of Pediatric Immunology and Rheumatology, Utrecht, Netherlands. [4]Université Paris-Descartes, IMAGINE Institute, Hôpital Necker-Enfants Malades. Centre de référence national pour les Arthrites Juveniles, Unité d'Immunologie, Hématologie et Rhumatologie Pediatrique, Paris, France. [5]Rambam Medical Center, Department of Pediatrics B, Haifa, Israel. [6]Alder Hey Children's NHS Foundation Trust, Liverpool, UK. [7]Cerrahpasa Tip Fakultesi, Ic Hastaliklari ABD, Romatoloji BD, Istanbul, Turkey. [8]Institute of Rheumatology, Paediatric Clinic, Warsaw, Poland. [9]Hospital for Sick Children, Division of Rheumatology, Toronto, ON, Canada. [10]Istituto Gaetano Pini, Divisione di Reumatologia, Milano, Italy. [11]Schneider Childrens Medical Center, Pediatric Rheumatology Unit, Petach-Tikvah, Israel. [12]Universidade Federal de São Paulo, Pediatrics, São Paulo, Brazil. [13]British Columbia Children's Hospital, Vancouver, BC, Canada. [14]Universitair Ziekenhuis Gent, Centrum Voor Kinderreumatologie, Gent, Belgium. [15]Randall Children's Hospital at Legacy Emanuel, Portland, OR, USA. [16]Floating Hospital for Children, Rheumatology NEMC 286, Boston, MA, USA. [17]Novartis Pharmaceuticals Corporation, East Hanover, NJ, USA. [18]University of Genova and Istituto Giannina Gaslini, Pediatria II-PRINTO, Genoa, Italy. [19]Novartis Institutes for Biomedical Research, Cambridge, MA, USA. [20]Istituto Giannina Gaslini, Pediatria II-PRINTO, Genoa, Italy.

References

1. Prakken B, Albani S, Martini A. Juvenile idiopathic arthritis. Lancet. 2011;377: 2138–49.
2. Ravelli A, Martini A. Juvenile idiopathic arthritis. Lancet. 2007;369:767–78.
3. Mellins ED, Macaubas C, Grom AA. Pathogenesis of systemic juvenile idiopathic arthritis: some answers, more questions. Nat Rev Rheumatol. 2011;7:416–26.
4. Woo P. Systemic juvenile idiopathic arthritis: diagnosis, management, and outcome. Nat Clin Pract Rheumatol. 2006;2:28–34.
5. Singh-Grewal D, Schneider R, Bayer N, Feldman BM. Predictors of disease course and remission in systemic juvenile idiopathic arthritis: significance of early clinical and laboratory features. Arthritis Rheum. 2006;54:1595–601.
6. Jamilloux Y, Gerfaud-Ventin M, Martinon F, et al. Pathogenesis of adult-onset Still's disease: new insights from the juvenile counterpart. Immunol Res. 2015;61:53–62.
7. Martini A. It is time to rethink juvenile idiopathic arthritis classification and nomenclature. Ann Rheum Dis. 2012;71:1437–9.
8. Pascual V, Allantaz F, Arce E, et al. Role of interleukin-1 (IL-1) in the pathogenesis of systemic onset juvenile idiopathic arthritis and clinical response to IL-1 blockade. J Exp Med. 2005;201:1479–86.
9. Verbsky JW, White AJ. Effective use of the recombinant interleukin 1 receptor antagonist anakinra in therapy resistant systemic onset juvenile rheumatoid arthritis. J Rheumatol. 2004;31:2071–5.
10. Gattorno M, Piccini A, Lasigliè D, et al. The pattern of response to anti IL-1 treatment distinguishes two subset of patients with systemic onset juvenile idiopathic arthritis. Arthritis Rheum. 2008;58:1505–15.
11. Quartier P, Allantaz F, Cimaz R, et al. A multicenter, randomized, double-blind, placebo-controlled trial with the interleukin-1 receptor antagonist anakinra in patients with systemic-inset juvenile idiopathic arthritis (ANAJIS trial). Ann Rheum Dis. 2011;70:747–54.
12. Ruperto N, Quartier P, Wulffraat N, et al. A phase II, multicenter, open-label study evaluating dosing and preliminary safety and efficacy of canakinumab in systemic juvenile idiopathic arthritis with active systemic features. Arthritis Rheum. 2012;64:557–67.
13. Ruperto N, Brunner HI, Quartier P, et al. Two randomized trials of canakinumab in systemic juvenile idiopathic arthritis. N Engl J Med. 2012;367:2396–406.
14. Lovell DJ, Giannini EH, Reiff AO, et al. Long-term safety and efficacy of rilonacept in patients with systemic juvenile idiopathic arthritis. Arthritis Rheum. 2013;65:2486–96.
15. Ling XB, Park JL, Carroll T, et al. Plasma profiles in active systemic juvenile idiopathic arthritis: biomarkers and biological implications. Proteomics. 2010; 10:4415–30.
16. Lachmann HJ, Kone-Paut I, Kuemmerle-Deschner JB, et al. Use of canakinumab in the cryopyrin-associated periodic syndrome. N Engl J Med. 2009;360:2416–25.
17. Kuemmerle-Deschner JB, Ramos E, Blank N, et al. Canakinumab (ACZ885, a fully human IgG1 anti-IL-1beta mAb) induces sustained remission in pediatric patients with cryopyrin-associated periodic syndrome (CAPS). Arthritis Res Ther. 2011;13:R34.
18. Ilaris [package insert]. East Hanover, NJ: Novartis Pharmaceuticals Corporation; 2016.
19. Ilaris [summary of product characteristics]. Camberley, UK: Novartis Europharm Limited; 2014.
20. Petty RE, Southwood TR, Manners P, et al. International League of Associations for Rheumatology classification of juvenile idiopathic arthritis: second revision, Edmonton, 2001. J Rheumatol. 2004;31:390–2.
21. R development core team. R: A language and environment for statistical computing. R foundation for statistical computing. 2004, Vienna, Austria. http://www.r-project.org.
22. Ihaka R, Gentleman R. R: a language for data analysis and graphics. J Comput Graph Stat. 1996;3:299–314.
23. Irizarry RA, Bolstad BM, Collin F, Cope LM, Hobbs B, Speed TP. Summaries of Affymetrix GeneChip probe level data. Nucleic Acids Res. 2003;31:e15.
24. Lotito AP, Campa A, Silva CA, et al. Interleukin 18 as a marker of disease activity and severity in patients with juvenile idiopathic arthritis. J Rheumatol. 2007;34:823–30.
25. Frosch M, Ahlmann M, Vogl T, et al. The myeloid-related proteins 8 and 14 complex, a novel ligand of toll-like receptor 4, and interleukin-1beta form a positive feedback mechanism in systemic-onset juvenile idiopathic arthritis. Arthritis Rheum. 2009;60:883–91.
26. Wittkowski H, Frosch M, Wulffraat N, et al. S100A12 is a novel molecular marker differentiating systemic-onset juvenile idiopathic arthritis from other causes of fever of unknown origin. Arthritis Rheum. 2008;58:3924–31.
27. Ravelli A, Brunner HI, Ruperto N, et al. Use of the JADAS criteria to assess efficacy of canakinumab in patients with SJIA – an analysis of 12-week pooled data. Pediatr Rheumatol Online J. 2014;12 suppl 1:63.

28. Wallace CA, Ruperto N, Giannini EH, et al. Preliinary criteria for clinical remission for select categories of juvenile idiopathic arthritis. J Rheumatol. 2004;31:2290–4.
29. Allantaz F, Chaussabel D, Stichweh D, et al. Blood leukocyte microarrays to diagnose systemic onset juvenile arthritis and follow the response to IL-1 blockade. J Exp Med. 2007;204:2131–44.
30. Ogilve EM, Hkan A, Hubank M, et al. Specific gene expression profiles in systemic juvenile idiopathic arthritis. Arthritis Rheum. 2007;66:1954–65.
31. Fall N, Barnes M, Thornton S, et al. Gene expression profiling of peripheral blood from patients with new-onset systemic juvenile idiopathic arthritis reveals molecular heterogeneity that may predict macrophage activation syndrome. Arthritis Rheum. 2007;56:3793–804.
32. ClinicalTrials.gov. NCT02204293. https://clinicaltrials.gov/ct2/show/NCT02204293. Accessed 14 Aug 2015.
33. Nirmala N, Arndt Brachat A, Feist E, et al. Gene-expression analysis of adult-onset Still's disease and systemic juvenile idiopathic arthritis is consistent with a continuum of a single disease entity. Pediatr Rheumatol Online J. 2015;13:50.
34. de Jager W, Vastert SJ, Beekman JM, et al. Defective phosphorylation of interleukin-18 receptor beta causes impaired natural killer cell function in systemic-onset juvenile idiopathic arthritis. Arthritis Rheum. 2009;60:2782–93.
35. Shimizu M, Nakagishi Y, Inoue N, et al. Interleukin-18 for predicting the development of macrophage activation syndrome in systemic juvenile idiopathic arthritis. Clin Immunol. 2015;160:277–81.
36. Put K, Avau A, Brisse E, et al. Cytokines in systemic juvenile idiopathic arthritis and haemophagocytic lymphohistiocytosis: tipping the balance between interleukin-18 and interferon-γ. Rheumatology. 2015;54:1507–17.

10

Pharmacovigilance in juvenile idiopathic arthritis patients treated with biologic or synthetic drugs: combined data of more than 15,000 patients from Pharmachild and national registries

Joost Swart[1†], Gabriella Giancane[2†], Gerd Horneff[3,4], Bo Magnusson[5], Michael Hofer[6,7], Ekaterina Alexeeva[8,9], Violeta Panaviene[10], Brigitte Bader-Meunier[11], Jordi Anton[12], Susan Nielsen[13], Fabrizio De Benedetti[14], Sylvia Kamphuis[15,16], Valda Staņēviča[17], Maria Tracahana[18], Laura Marinela Ailioaie[19], Elena Tsitsami[20], Ariane Klein[3], Kirsten Minden[21,22], Ivan Foeldvari[23], Johannes Peter Haas[24], Jens Klotsche[21,22], Anna Carin Horne[5], Alessandro Consolaro[25,26], Francesca Bovis[2], Francesca Bagnasco[2], Angela Pistorio[27], Alberto Martini[28], Nico Wulffraat[1], Nicolino Ruperto[2*] and for the Paediatric Rheumatology International Trials Organisation (PRINTO), BiKeR and the board of the Swedish Registry

Abstract

Background: The availability of methotrexate and the introduction of multiple biological agents have revolutionized the treatment of juvenile idiopathic arthritis (JIA). Several international and national drug registries have been implemented to accurately monitor the long-term safety/efficacy of these agents. This report aims to present the combined data coming from Pharmachild/PRINTO registry and the national registries from Germany (BiKeR) and Sweden.

Methods: Descriptive statistics was used for demographic, clinical data, drug exposure, adverse events (AEs) and events of special interest (ESIs). For the Swedish register, AE data were not available.

Results: Data from a total of 15,284 patients were reported: 8274 (54%) from the Pharmachild registry and 3990 (26%) and 3020 (20%) from the German and the Swedish registries, respectively. Pharmachild children showed a younger age (median of 5.4 versus 7.6 years) at JIA onset and shorter disease duration at last available visit (5.3 versus 6.1–6.8) when compared with the other registries. The most frequent JIA category was the rheumatoid factor–negative polyarthritis (range of 24.6–29.9%). Methotrexate (61–84%) and etanercept (24%–61.8%) were the most frequently used synthetic and biologic disease-modifying anti-rheumatic drugs (DMARDs), respectively. There was a wide variability in glucocorticoid use (16.7–42.1%). Serious AEs were present in 572 (6.9%) patients in Pharmachild versus 297 (7.4%) in BiKeR. Infection and infestations were the most frequent AEs (29.4–30.1%) followed by gastrointestinal disorders (11.5–19.6%). The most frequent ESIs were infections (75.3–89%).

(Continued on next page)

* Correspondence: nicolaruperto@gaslini.org; http://www.printo.it; http://www.pediatric-rheumatology.printo.it
[†]Joost Swart and Gabriella Giancane contributed equally to this work.
[2]IRCCS Istituto Giannina Gaslini, Clinica Pediatrica e Reumatologia, PRINTO, Via Gaslini, 5, 16147 Genoa, Italy
Full list of author information is available at the end of the article

(Continued from previous page)
Conclusions: This article is the first attempt to present a very large sample of data on JIA patients from different national and international registries and represents the first proposal for data merging as the most powerful tool for future analysis of safety and effectiveness of immunosuppressive therapies in JIA.

Keywords: Juvenile idiopathic arthritis, Registry, Safety, Adverse events, Methotrexate, Biologics

Background

Juvenile idiopathic arthritis (JIA) [1] is the most common chronic pediatric rheumatic disease and an important cause of short- and long-term disability and quality-of-life impairment [2–8]. Although none of the available drugs for JIA has curative potential, prognosis has greatly improved as the result of substantial progress in disease management with the introduction of biologics. Despite the good efficacy results of all phase III trials on biologic agents, the long-term safety profile needs to be further characterized. For example, spontaneous reporting from countries with a low incidence of tuberculosis suggested that tuberculosis might be problematic in patients treated with biologics [9]. In August 2009, the US Food and Drug Administration (FDA) announced through a boxed warning that an increased risk of certain cancers in children might occur, and labeling for the tumor necrosis factor (TNF) blocker products was updated [10–14]. A Cochrane review from February 2011 compared the adverse events (AEs) of biologics and concluded that there is an urgent need for more research regarding their long-term safety of different biologics [15]. The availability of a large observational international and national registry could enable clinicians and regulatory agencies to properly monitor the long-term or rare safety events and effectiveness of these agents in the relatively low prevalent JIA.

The aim of this project is to present the combined data of the "Pharmacovigilance in JIA patients treated with biologic agents and/or MTX" (Pharmachild) international registry and two consenting JIA national registries: the "Biologics in Pediatric Rheumatology Registry" (BiKeR) from Germany and the JIA registry from Sweden. The secondary goal was to test a sharing system for future merging of data to address specific JIA scientific and clinical questions.

Methods

Description of registries

The Pharmachild registry

Pharmachild is an observational international registry that started in 2011 with European Union initial funding support and that enrolled children from member centers of the Paediatric Rheumatology International Trials Organisation (PRINTO) [16].

Inclusion criteria were children with JIA as per International League of Associations for Rheumatology (ILAR) criteria [17] receiving biologics or other synthetic disease-modifying anti-rheumatic drugs (DMARDs) as per physician decision. The registry contains two specific populations. The first is a retrospective cohort of all patients under treatment or previously treated with DMARDs by one-time clinical chart revision of safety events and complete drug exposure since disease onset to last available follow-up. The second is a prospective cohort including all cases newly treated with DMARDs since enrollment in the registry and cases still under treatment with any drug. To avoid selection bias, each center performed a census for all patients previously treated with DMARDs at that specific center, used as the reference to evaluate the enrollment capability. In a second step, the center entered retrospective data, considered successful if they retrieved at least 70% of the patients listed in the census. Finally, in a third step, the prospective data collection started.

Data collection included full and complete details for ILAR classification criteria; demographic, clinical, and laboratory information; and efficacy (only for the prospective cohort) and safety data on a long-term basis. Centers reported the whole drug exposure of the patient along with dates of start and discontinuation of the drug, dosages, route of administration, reasons for discontinuation, and possible correlation with the AEs. All the AEs of at least moderate/severe/very severe intensity and serious AEs, using the latest release of the Medical Dictionary for Regulatory Activities (MedDRA) dictionary, were reported; mild intensity was reported only for those AEs which did not resolve and require a follow-up report. Some AEs were classified as by consensus of PRINTO members as events of special interest (ESIs).

Efficacy data were collected in the prospective cohort through the JIA core set measures with whole joint count [18], the disease activity status measured through the Juvenile Arthritis Disease Activity Score (JADAS), and the annual evaluation of damage through the Juvenile Arthritis Damage Index (JADI) [19] and of growth and pubertal development and key information on imaging and bio-specimen local collection. As patient-reported outcome (PRO), families completed online the Juvenile Arthritis Multidimensional Assessment Report (JAMAR) [20] before the scheduled clinic visit or in the hospital (on tablets or paper) in order to provide key notes to the treating physician before the clinical examination.

The system also provided data on drug exposure and occurrence of AEs (Fig. 1) as a tool to discuss the health status of a patient with the family.

Data collection was performed online via the secured PRINTO website on a dedicated server with a username and timely password on an https-encrypted platform. English was the official language used for all forms completed by the physicians, and the PROs were available in the appropriate language spoken by parents/patients. The web system was designed to be user-friendly, modular, and upgradable. During data entry, several hundred automatic checks were in place to ensure data quality and consistency. In particular, safety events were checked for accuracy by PRINTO-certified MedDRA coders, which could go back to the center with electronic query tickets in case of missing or unclear information (Additional file 1). A designated pediatric rheumatologist acted as medical monitor (JS) by performing an electronic check and revision of the AEs and ESIs; in addition, for some ESIs (for example, infection), adjudicating committees were in place.

The BiKeR registry

The BiKeR registry in Germany focused, from 2001, on AEs and efficacy data in patients treated with etanercept (ETN), the first biologic licensed in Germany [21]. From that time, surveillance was extended to all biologics approved for JIA [22–24]. Information on biologics not approved for JIA was also collected for such patients who have been admitted for an approved biologic if patients were switched. The BiKeR registry was founded by pharmaceutical companies with independent bilateral contracts. BiKeR was approved by the ethics committee of the physician board of Aerztekammer Nordrhein, Düsseldorf. The BiKeR registry includes about 80 study sites and since its inception has followed more than 4000 patients in Germany and Austria who were 2 to 18 years old and who meet the ILAR criteria for JIA. Written consent was obtained from patients and parents and repeated if the patient became an adult. Only pseudonymized data were collected.

Patient demographic characteristics, disease history, and previous treatments are documented at the time of patient enrollment. Details about relevant treatment and reasons for discontinuation, concomitant therapy, disease activity, and AEs are prospectively collected by using standard case report forms (CRFs) at the start of treatment, at months 3 and 6, and every 6 months thereafter. Safety was analyzed on the basis of AE reporting. All reported AEs defined as any untoward medical occurrence in a subject administered a pharmaceutical product, even without a causal relationship with the treatment, were analyzed. Serious AEs and ESIs were defined as in Pharmachild. Onsite monitoring is performed in selected larger centers covering about 80% of admitted patients. In 2005, the registry was extended to include a control group of 1500 biologic-naïve JIA patients who started with the synthetic DMARD such as MTX to enable comparison of patients exposed to biologics with unexposed JIA cohorts [25, 26]. The "Juvenile arthritis MTX/Biologics long-term Observation" (JUMBO) was launched in 2007 to include data on long-term safety after transition to adulthood [27]. At present, 3990 patients are included in the JUMBO registry.

The Swedish registry

In 2009, the Swedish JIA registry began to follow all children on biologics and later expanded to all patients treated with or without DMARDs. Reports from care givers, patients, and medical records using JADAS, quality-of-life questionnaires, and arthritis-specific questions were included in the registry, which after 5 years includes 1700 children (60% of the total JIA population and above 90% of patients on cytokine modulators). Data on treatment as well as disease course and efficacy were included, while data on safety were not available [28].

Statistics

All registries and participating centers obtained approval from their respective ethics committee and obtained consent/assent based on existing national regulations.

Pharmachild, BiKeR, and the Swedish registries reported cumulative summary data into predefined spreadsheets in order to provide baseline descriptive statistics of demographic and clinical data. Safety data were available only for Pharmachild and BiKeR. ESIs common to the two registries are reported.

For qualitative data, frequencies (percentage) were reported, while quantitative data were expressed in terms of medians with first and third quartiles. No formal statistical comparisons were performed.

Results

Demographic characteristics and drug exposure

In Pharmachild, 11,796 patients in total were registered in the census registry as of January 2017 from 98 PRINTO centers in 32 countries. Clinical and safety data were provided for 8274 (70.1%) out of 11,796 patients

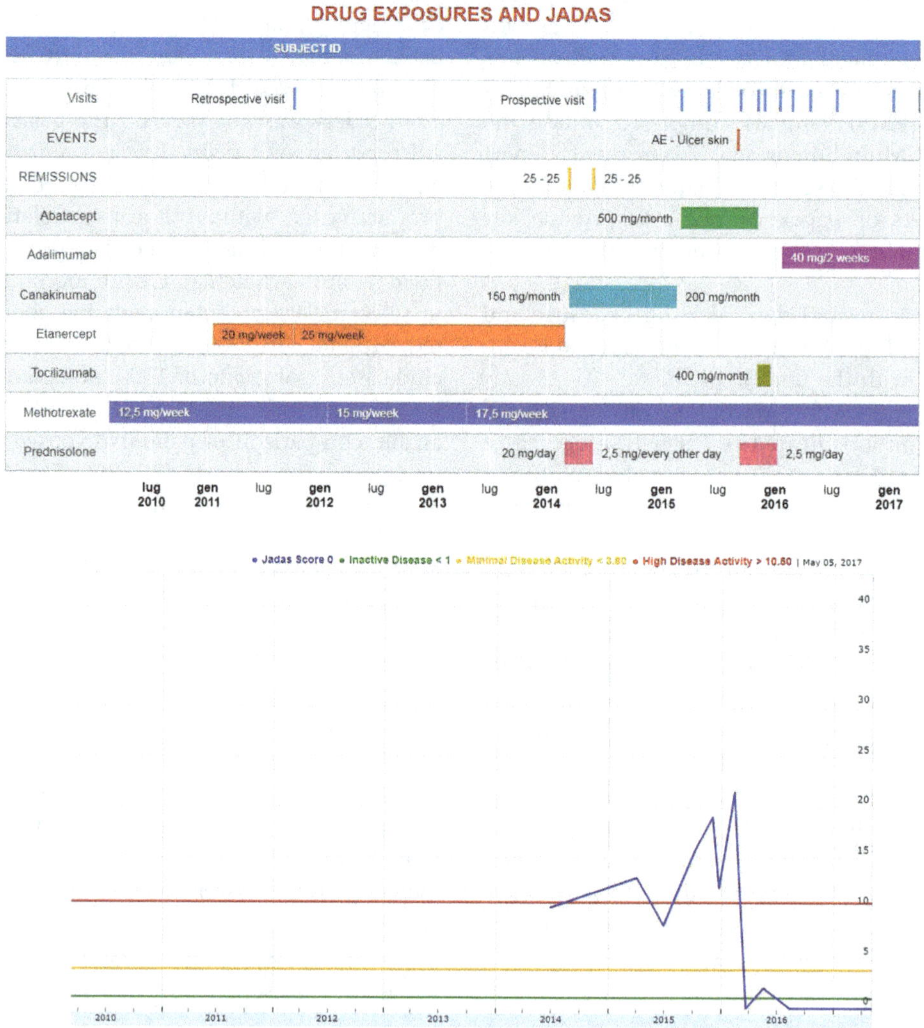

Visit date	29/05/2014	05/11/2015	26/11/2015	14/01/2016	05/04/2017
Physician global evaluation of disease activity (21 circle VAS)	1	4	2	5	0
Parents evaluation of child overall well-being (21 circle VAS)	8	9	8	9,5	0
ESR	20	30	7		10
CRP standardised	5	41	0,58	0,53	0,168
No. of joints with active arthritis	1	5	2	7	0
No. of joints with limitation of motion	1	5	2	7	0
JIA ACR inactive Disease	Active	Active	Active	Active	Inactive
JADAS10	10	19	12	21,5	0
JADAS inactive disease (<1)	N	N	N	N	Y
JADAS Minimal disease activity (< 3.80)	Y	N	Y	N	N
JADAS High disease activity (> 10.50)	N	Y	N	Y	N

Fig. 1 Pharmachild graphical depiction over time of the key efficacy and safety data. Drug exposure and adverse events are represented in parallel to Juvenile Arthritis Disease Activity Score (JADAS) pattern. The Excel spreadsheet with all the data could be downloaded automatically by all participating centers. In the figure, an example of a patient from an Italian center is presented

belonging to 86 participating centers. Sixty out (61.2%) of eighty-six centers provided at least 70% safety data of their local JIA patients, and the median was 55 patients per center. Prospective data were collected for a total of 3070 patients.

Table 1 reports the demographic and clinical data for a total of 15,284 patients: 8274 (54.1%) from the Pharmachild registry and 3990 (26.1%) from the German BiKeR and 3020 (19.8%) from the Swedish registry. The patients included in the German and Swedish registries were not overlapping with those in Pharmachild since the registries were created in different periods and included data from different patients with the same disease.

Patients coming from the Pharmachild database showed a younger age (median of 5.4 years versus

Table 1 Demographic and clinical characteristics of the juvenile idiopathic arthritis patients from different registries

	Pharmachild *N* = 8274	BiKeR *N* = 3990	Sweden *N* = 3020
Number of countries	32	2#	1
Number of centers	86	72	33
Number of patients per center	55.5 (17–124)	10.5 (3–39.8)	52 (31–78)
Age at onset	5.4 (2.4–10.0)	7.6 (3.2–11.7)	7.6 (2.9–11.7)[1]
Age at JIA diagnosis	6.2 (2.8–10.9)	–	8.3 (3.5–12.8)[2]
Disease duration at last visit	5.3 (2.7–8.8)	6.1 (3.5–9.5)	6.8 (4.3–10.1)[3]
Female	5584 (67.5%)	2670 (66.9%)	1989 (65.9%)
Antinuclear antibodies (ANA)*	1767 (21.4%)	1900 (47.6%)	–
ILAR JIA category		4	5
Systemic	911 (11.0%)	267 (6.7%)	109 (4.7%)
Oligo	3071 (37.1%)	1215 (30.5%)	1148 (49.6%)
Oligo persistent	2011 (24.3%)	494 (12.4%)	–
Oligo extended	1060 (12.8%)	721 (18.1%)	–
Polyarticular RF^-	2183 (26.4%)	1192 (29.9%)	568 (24.6%)
Polyarticular RF^+	322 (3.9%)	243 (6.1%)	85 (3.7%)
Psoriatic arthritis	285 (3.4%)	296 (7.4%)	160 (6.9%)
Enthesitis-related arthritis	924 (11.2%)	649 (16.3%)	185 (8.0%)
Undifferentiated arthritis	578 (7.0%)	127 (3.2%)	58 (2.5%)

Data are medians (1st–3rd quartiles) or frequencies (percentages)
*ANA at least two consecutively positive determinations according to local standards
Germany and Austria
[1]data available for 2477 subjects
[2]data available for 2197 subjects
[3]data available for 2479 subjects
[4]data available for 3989 subjects
[5]data available for 2313 subjects
Abbreviations: *BiKeR* Biologics in Pediatric Rheumatology Registry, *ILAR* International League of Associations for Rheumatology, *JIA* juvenile idiopathic arthritis, *RF* rheumatoid factor

7.6) at onset and shorter disease duration (5.3 versus 6.1–6.8) at the last available follow-up visit in comparison with the other registries. BiKeR reported a lower median number of children per center (10.5 versus 52–55.5). Antinuclear antibody (ANA) positivity was higher in BiKeR and missing in the Swedish registry.

The JIA category distribution differed among registries, but the most frequent JIA category was rheumatoid factor (RF)–negative polyarthritis (range of 24.6%–29.9%). The frequency of oligoarticular JIA was higher in the Swedish registry (49.6% versus about 30.5%–37.1% in the other two registries), while in BiKeR the frequencies of oligo- and poly-articular JIA RF-negative were similar (about 30%); Pharmachild depicted a higher frequency of systemic JIA (11% versus 4.7–6.7% in the German and Swedish registries, respectively).

Table 2 reports the number of patients who ever received a drug from onset to last available follow-up visit, with the corresponding days of drug exposure per medication from the first day of drug administration to the last available follow-up visit, excluding the days off therapy for any reason.

There was a global trend to use MTX as a first-choice synthetic DMARD and ETN as a first-line biologic, but the Swedish registry used these drugs in a lower percentage of patients (MTX 61% versus about 84% in Pharmachild and BiKeR; ETN 24% versus 43.5% in Pharmachild and 61.8% in BiKeR). Despite the similar percentage of patients using these medications, children from BiKeR were exposed for a shorter period to the drugs compared with Pharmachild children, whereas the Swedish registry demonstrated a much longer drug exposure, with a wide range of variability among patients. Adalimumab, among the most frequently used biologics, was administered in similar percentages of patients among all three databases (about 21% of patients). Systemic steroids were used in similar percentages of patients and with the same drug exposure in BiKeR and Pharmachild, whereas the Swedish registry administered shorter cycles of steroids in a smaller number of

Table 2 Number of patients who ever received a drug from onset to last available follow-up visit, with the corresponding days of drug exposure per medication from the first day of drug administration to the last available follow-up visit

		Pharmachild N = 8274 Days of drug exposure	BiKeR N = 3990 Days of drug exposure	Sweden N = 3020 Days of drug exposure
DMARDs	Methotrexate	6963 (84.2%); 924 (449–1747)	3344 (83.8%); 494 (173–957)	1842 (61%); 1198 (555–2127)
	Sulfasalazine	861 (10.4%); 360 (143–730)	274 (6.9%); 174 (32–470)	95 (3%) 443 (132–1042)
	Cyclosporine	518 (6.3%); 616 (235–1358)	113 (2.8%); 186 (62–580)	16 (0.5%); 584 (250–1452)
	Leflunomide	372 (4.5%); 434 (182–888)	219 (5.5%); 267 (68–701)	2 (0.1%); 840 (511–1169)
	Hydroxychloroquine	279 (3.4%); 486 (202–1022)	106 (2.7%); 182 (1–535)	32 (1.1%); 957 (311–1612)
	Azathioprine	108 (1.3%); 439 (187–973)	155 (3.9%); 186 (26–494)	31 (1%); 1171 (340–2179)
	Thalidomide	35 (0.4%); 290 (85–665)	0	0
Systemic glucocorticoids		3299 (39.9%) 206 (67–648)	1680 (42.1%) 196 (81–449)	503 (16.7%) 91 (35–437)
Biologics	Etanercept	3600 (43.5%); 719 (300–1338)	2467 (61.8%); 489 (184–934)	726 (24%); 827 (341–1666)
	Adalimumab	1778 (21.5%); 442 (174–927)	810 (20.3%); 350 (117–755)	657 (21.8%); 701 (292–1604)
	Infliximab	705 (8.5%); 425 (160–951)	68 (1.7%); 213 (129–717)	189 (6.3%); 825 (328–1738)
	Tocilizumab	633 (7.7%); 351 (126–742)	281 (7%); 377 (127–730)	122 (4%); 660 (193–1353)
	Abatacept	420 (5.1%); 342 (156–715)	101 (2.5%); 190 (83–582)	80 (2.6%); 378 (164–1125
	Anakinra	339 (4.1%); 299 (94–837)	50 (1.3%); 304 (9–806)	48 (1.6%); 422 (144–836)
	Golimumab	161 (1.9%); 270 (106–623)	63 (1.6%); 344 (88–783)	93 (3.1%); 796 (370–1743)
	Canakinumab	145 (1.8%); 351 (133–1032)	39 (1%); 364 (214–733)	7 (0.2%); 654 (604–1654)
	Rituximab	103 (1.2%); 42 (24–87)	4 (0.1%); 15 (0–108)	20 (0.7%); 129 (15–1550)
	Certolizumab	33 (0.4%); 166 (106–309)	4 (0.1%); 49 (0–110)	8 (0.3%); 984 (714–1538)
	Other biologic agents	14 (0.2%); 217 (54–432)	4 (0.1%); 77 (25–149)	2 (0.1%); 325 (223–426)

Data are numbers of patients with frequencies (percentage), and medians and 1st–3rd quartiles of days of drug exposure
Abbreviations: *BiKeR* Biologics in Pediatric Rheumatology Registry, *DMARD* disease-modifying anti-rheumatic drug

patients (about 40% of patients in Pharmachild and BiKeR versus 16.7% in the Swedish registry).

Safety data

Overall, the German registry showed a higher incidence of AEs but with lower intensity. In Pharmachild, 1599 (19.3%) of 8274 patients reported at least one moderate AE compared with 1747 (43.8%) of 3999 AEs of any intensity patients in BiKeR. Indeed, when the AEs of at least moderate intensity were compared between the two registries, the differences were less pronounced (18.5% for Pharmachild versus 10.2% in BiKeR). Serious AEs were present in 572 patients (6.9%) in Pharmachild versus 297 (7.4%) in BiKeR. Among them, 13 deaths were reported in Pharmachild and 3 in BiKeR mainly due to severe infections or malignancies or both.

Table 3 reports a total of 5173 AEs in Pharmachild and 5013 in BiKeR, according to the MedDRA dictionary divided by system organ class (SOC). Infection and infestations resulted as the most frequent SOC in

Table 3 Total number of adverse events by MedDRA system organ class ordered by decreasing frequencies

	Pharmachild *N* = 5173	BiKeR *N* = 5013
Infections and infestations	1523 (29.4%)	1509 (30.1%)
Gastrointestinal disorders	595 (11.5%)	984 (19.6%)
Injury, poisoning and procedural complications	325 (6.3%)	152 (3.1%)
Blood and lymphatic system disorders	291 (5.6%)	99 (2%)
Investigations	285 (5.5%)	377 (7.5%)
Eye disorders	270 (5.2%)	309 (6.2%)
Skin and subcutaneous tissue disorders	256 (4.9%)	217 (4.3%)
General disorders and administration site conditions	245 (4.7%)	410 (8.2%)
Hepatobiliary disorders	233 (4.5%)	24 (0.5%)
Surgical and medical procedures	209 (4.1%)	98 (2%)
Nervous system disorders	151 (2.9%)	227 (4.5%)
Musculoskeletal and connective tissue disorders	147 (2.8%)	138 (2.7%)
Respiratory, thoracic, and mediastinal disorders	112 (2.2%)	50 (1%)
Psychiatric disorders	105 (2.1%)	157 (3.1%)
Endocrine disorders	104 (2.0%)	6 (0.1%)
Metabolism and nutrition disorders	77 (1.5%)	34 (0.7%)
Renal and urinary disorders	66 (1.3%)	21 (0.4%)
Immune system disorders	33 (0.6%)	77 (1.5%)
Vascular disorders	30 (0.6%)	46 (0.9%)
Reproductive system and breast disorders	26 (0.5%)	13 (0.3%)
Congenital, familial, and genetic disorders	22 (0.4%)	9 (0.2%)
Cardiac disorders	19 (0.4%)	13 (0.3%)
Neoplasms benign, malignant, and unspecified (including cysts and polyps)	16 (0.3%)	29 (0.6%)
Ear and labyrinth disorders	13 (0.3%)	7 (0.1%)
Social circumstances	11 (0.2%)	0
Pregnancy, puerperium and perinatal conditions	9 (0.2%)	7 (0.1%)

Data are absolute numbers and frequencies (percentage)
Abbreviation: *BiKeR* Biologics in Pediatric Rheumatology Registry, *MedDRA* Medical Dictionary for Regulatory Activities

Pharmachild and BiKeR (29.4% versus 30.1%, respectively) followed by gastrointestinal disorders (11.5% versus 19.6%) whereas all remaining SOCs occurred in less than 10% of the AEs. In Pharmachild, more injuries, poisoning, and complications and hematological and hepatobiliary disorders were reported compared with BiKeR, which showed more investigations, general disorders and administration site conditions, and neurological and immune system disorders. The numbers of uveitis, included in "Eye disorders" category, were comparable in the two registries (5.2% versus 6.2% in Pharmachild and BiKeR, respectively).

These results were confirmed by analyzing the distribution of AEs separately for the retrospective and the prospective visits. We identified a total of 1050 AEs extracted from the prospective visits, and 4123 events by the retrospective data, divided by SOC. In general, the hierarchy and frequency of AEs were similar, and infections and infestations were the most frequent events (Additional file 2).

Table 4 reports details for the 2022 and 1697 common ESIs in Pharmachild and BiKeR, respectively. The most frequent ESIs were infections, which were the most prevalent in both registries (75.3% versus 89% in Pharmachild and BiKeR, respectively), followed by blood cell–related ESIs. In Pharmachild, infusion/injection-related reactions were more frequent than in BiKeR (10.8% versus 1.4%).

There were 27 cases of tuberculosis reported in Pharmachild (52% from Asia, 37% from Europe, and 11% from the US) and none in BiKeR, whereas all serious/targeted infections were 674 (33.3%) and 171 (10.1%), respectively; 17 cases of tuberculosis were during biologic therapy, namely TNF inhibitors in 14 patients.

There were few cases of malignancies reported in either registry. Besides the reported cases of hematological malignancies in Table 4, in Pharmachild we could observe 10 additional cases (neoplasm others), represented for one third by hemangioma, and with the remaining patients suffering from thyroid cancer, cervix neoplasm, skin tumors, breast fibroadenoma, colon adenoma, and osteochondroma. The German registry reported in the same group similar malignancies, in particular of the genital apparatus (thyroid carcinoma, germ cell tumor, anaplastic ependymoma, and cervix dysplasia).

Discussion

Since the 1990s, when the first immunomodulatory products for rheumatic diseases were introduced, the benefits of synthetic and biologic DMARDs became clear in the management of JIA. Currently, however, safety information for JIA is derived mainly from phase III clinical trials and more recent registries and administrative claims. Therefore, little information exists on the long-term safety of these agents. In 2009, a great scientific debate regarding the safety of TNF blockers started, prompting the FDA to issue a warning regarding a possible association between the use of TNF blockers and the development of lymphoma and other cancers in children and young adults with JIA [29]. Until now, owing to confounding factors such as the use of concomitant immunosuppressants, the effect of biological therapies on the risk to develop cancer or other risks such as infections in JIA is still controversial [30]. Literature has provided evidence that an increased risk of malignancy exists among children with JIA when compared with the

Table 4 Total number of events of special interest ordered by decreasing frequencies

	Pharmachild N = 2022	BiKeR N = 1697
Infections:	1523 (75.3%)	1509 (89%)
Serious/targeted infections (Epstein–Barr virus, cytomegalovirus, papilloma virus, herpes zoster primary and reactivation, and opportunistic infections)	674 (33.3%)	171 (10.1%)
Tuberculosis	27 (1,3%)	0
Other infections	822 (40.6%)	1338 (78.8%)
Infusion/injection related reactions:	218 (10.8%)	24 (1.4%)
Infusion related reaction	144 (7.1%)	11 (0.6%)
Injection related reaction	74 (3.7%)	13 (0.8%)
Blood cell–related events of special interest (ESI):	188 (9.3%)	90 (5.3%)
Pancytopenia	6 (0.3%)	65 (3.8%)
Neutropenia	107 (5.3%)	14 (0.8%)
Macrophage activation syndrome	75 (3.7%)	11 (0.6%)
Aplastic anemia	0	0
Autoimmune ESI:	50 (2.5%)	50 (2.9%)
Inflammatory bowel disease (IBD)	21 (1.1%)	23 (1.3)
Other autoimmune diseases excluding IBD, uveitis, and demyelinisation disorders	18 (0.9%)	24 (1.4%)
Lupus erythematosus systemic/lupus-like syndrome	4 (0.2%)	1 (0.1%)
Optic neuritis	4 (0.2%)	0
Multiple sclerosis	2 (0.1%)	0
Demyelination	1 (0.05%)	2 (0.2%)
Malignancies:	16 (0.8%)	13 (0.8%)
Leukemias	3 (0.1%)	2 (0.2%)
Lymphomas	2 (0.1%)	5 (0.3%)
Hematopoietic neoplasms (excluding leukemias and lymphomas)	1 (0.05%)	2 (0.2%)
Neoplasm (other)	10 (0.5%)	4 (0.2%)
Others ESI:	27 (1.3%)	11 (0.6%)
Gastrointestinal (GI) ulcer/GI bleed/GI perforation	17 (0.8%)	4 (0.2%)
Pregnancy	9 (0.4%)	7 (0.4%)
Congestive heart failure	1 (0.05%)	0

Data are absolute numbers and frequencies (percentage)

general population, irrespective of medication use. Conversely, other studies have not confirmed these findings, highlighting the need of further studies to estimate this risk more accurately [11, 13, 31, 32]. In order to address this and other safety concerns more reliably, several methods for pharmacovigilance could be implemented, spanning from the results of phase II and III clinical trials to post-marketing passive reporting or from registries (not-for-profit or sponsored by pharmaceutical companies) [10, 33]. For this purpose, several registries have been created in the last decade; in particular, the national pediatric rheumatology societies in European countries and in North America initiated independent registries or registries in collaboration with pharmaceutical companies for the long-term evaluation of the safety and effectiveness mainly of biologic DMARDs [26, 28, 33–37]. Other research groups have concentrated their efforts on the analysis of insurance claims [30, 38]. PRINTO implemented Pharmachild in order to guarantee a critical mass of patients' data and to provide systematically obtained evidence for provision of reliable scientific data for health professionals and health authorities. Aiming to avoid overlapping of data collection and to find an agreement on the proper way to share common data, a considerable number of European pediatric rheumatology societies (for example, in France, the Netherlands, Spain, and the Czech Republic primarily) agreed to use Pharmachild as their primary resource for data collection.

This article is the first attempt to present a very large sample of data on JIA patients from different registries, providing an overview on the baseline characteristics from international and national registries. This analysis highlights some differences but also similarities. An important difference that was observed was the higher frequency of AEs in the German BiKeR registry, even though associated with a lower intensity, which may reflect the different inclusion criteria of the two registries. Indeed, in Pharmachild, events of mild intensity, defined as transient or mild discomfort (<48 h) and no medical intervention/therapy required, are excluded. This difference is the trade-off implemented in Pharmachild in order to concentrate on more important safety events and facilitate data collection in everyday busy clinical practice.

Similarities among registries regarding therapies and AEs could be identified. MTX was the most used synthetic DMARD. ETN was the most frequently used biologic agent in all registries considered, followed by adalimumab. Drug exposure differed the three databases; in BiKeR, it was lower for almost all the medications; in the Swedish registry, it was much longer and had a wider range of exposure variability despite the similar disease duration. The relatively high rate of ETN use in the BiKeR registry might be explained by the fact that this registry originally started as a registry for this specific drug, when ETN was the only approved biological drug in pediatric rheumatology and then extended to other medications after their approval. However, in more recent years in BiKeR, ETN is the first biologic in about two thirds of patients with non-systemic JIA. Systemic steroids were used much less in Sweden and for shorter periods and this was maybe due to the lower incidence of systemic JIA. In regard to ESIs, infections were the most common event in both Pharmachild and BiKeR registries whereas malignancies were reported in a limited number of patients. The overall frequencies of the different AEs and ESIs were similar between Pharmachild and BiKeR. The major differences when comparing Pharmachild with BiKeR were higher frequencies of tuberculosis infection and infusion/injection-related reactions in the first for a possible interviewer bias elicited by the Pharmachild CRFs, which explicitly focus the attention of the clinicians to these AEs. The difference in the rate of tuberculosis infections may also reflect a different risk among European countries and the need for higher awareness of this problem in some regions.

Next to reporting baseline data from a large sample of patients with JIA , this study could not merge individual patient data because of the lack of homogeneous information. Therefore, it can be seen as a practical proposal for future studies that involve data merging. We propose a three-step procedure for future studies. In step 1, the CRFs of the different registries should be compared highlighting the similarities and differences. Step 2 will verify the database technical characteristic (for example, Sql server version 2005 and Access 2010) and the field coding (for example, gender, int, 1 = male; 2 = female). The third step related to the individual patient's data merging. An Excel spreadsheet with the data specifications related to a specific article will be shared with the participating registries. Each registry will have to add its own data related to the project. The coordinator of the project will merge the individual patients' data after proper coding transformation. A census (for example, few demographic data of all patients in the registry) will be provided by each registry as a preliminary step to check for a potential selection bias. The coordinator will then prepare an additional spreadsheet to highlight the important missing information (query log) to be resolved in a timely manner in order to proceed with the final analysis and drafting of the article. The entire procedure may meet some obstacles due to the lack of homogeneous information among registries and ethical and data protection regulations that often inhibit the exchange of patient data. Nevertheless, the methodological approach proposed to merge the data appears to be a successful tool for increasing the number of patients and data for future studies.

A possible limitation to our study is that a relevant part of clinical information comes from retrospective data with no efficacy results available. Nevertheless, as pointed out in Additional file 2, retrospective data in Pharmachild were mostly overlapping with prospective data, thus supporting the validity of these safety findings. This limitation becomes crucial when we consider efficacy data, which can be provided only by the prospective analysis. For this reason, further work in the future will be focused on these patients in order to advance the use of JIA drugs through the study of the Pharmachild population. Future analytical work will also have to report accumulated patient years of treatment for each of the registries.

Conclusions

This article is the first attempt to present a very large sample of data on JIA patients from different national and international registries and represents the first proposal for sharing of data from national and international registries as the most powerful tool for future analysis of safety and effectiveness, with the aim to address important questions on current daily practice in pediatric rheumatology.

Abbreviations

AE: Adverse event; BiKeR: Biologics in Pediatric Rheumatology Registry; CRF: Case report form; DMARD: Disease-modifying anti-rheumatic drug; ESI: Events of special interest; ETN: Etanercept; FDA: US Food and Drug Administration; ILAR: International League of Associations for Rheumatology; JADAS: Juvenile Arthritis Disease Activity Score; JIA: Juvenile idiopathic arthritis; JUMBO: Juvenile arthritis MTX/Biologics long-term Observation; MedDRA: Medical Dictionary for Regulatory Activities; MTX: Methotrexate; Pharmachild: Pharmacovigilance in JIA patients treated with biologic agents and/or MTX; PRINTO: Paediatric Rheumatology International Trials Organisation; PRO: Patient-reported outcome; RF: Rheumatoid factor; SOC: System organ class; TNF: Tumor necrosis factor

Acknowledgments

We thank all PRINTO centers which contributed to data collection.
The German registry is supported by an unrestricted grant from Pfizer, Germany; AbbVie, Germany; and Roche, Germany; Chugai; Pfizer; and Roche had no role in the study design or in the collection, analysis, or interpretation of the data; the writing of the manuscript; or the decision to submit the manuscript for publication. Publication of this article was not contingent upon approval by the study sponsors.
This study would not have been possible without the collaboration of numerous German and Austrian pediatric rheumatologists, patients, and their parents.
Collaborators: Berger, T; Böschow, G; Borte, M; Feddersen, I; Föll, D; Ganser, G; Geikowski, T; Girschick, H; Haller, M, H; Hedrich, C; Heubner, G; Hospach, T; Hufnagel, M; Keck, B; Kössel, H; Kümmerle-Deschner, J; Küster, M; Lilienthal, E; Maier, J; Mrusek, S; Müller, T; Oommen, P; Prelog, M; Quietzsch, J; Rietschel, C; Rogalski, B; Rühlmann, M; Rühner, P; Sailer-Höck, M; Schatz, R; Schmalbach, T; Seibert, W; Thon, A; Trauzeddel, R, Urban, A; Weller-Heinemann, F; Windschall, D; Florence Uettwiller, Richard Mouy, Ngoc-Phoi DUONG, and Thit-Thao TRUONG.

Funding

Pharmachild has been supported by a grant from the European Union (grant 260353) and by funding from the Italian public hospital IRCCS Istituto Giannina Gaslini.

Authors' contributions

JS, GG, FB, and NR drafted the first and subsequent version of the manuscript. JS, GG, FB, NR, GH, BM, and NW contributed to the planning of the study. All authors critically revised and approved the content of the final manuscript.

Consent for publication
Not applicable.

Competing interests
JS has received a research a grant from Pfizer. GH has received research funds from, has acted as a consultant for, and has participated in speaker bureaus for AbbVie, Chugai, Novartis, Pfizer Inc., and Roche. BM has acted as a principal investigator for Novartis and Enzyvant. MH has received a grant from AbbVie and a grant and personal fees from Novartis. EA has received research grants from Roche, Abbott, Pfizer, Bristol-Myers Squibb, Centocor, and Novartis and has received honoraria as a speaker for Roche, Novartis, and Pfizer. BB-M has participated as co-investigator to clinical trials from Pfizer, Abbott, Novartis, and Roche. JA has received grants and personal fees (consulting lecturers and speakers' bureau) and has been member of advisory groups for Pfizer, AbbVie, Roche, Sobi, Novartis, and Gebro. FDB receives consultancy/unrestricted research grants from AbbVie, Gilead, Novartis, Novimmune, Pfizer, Roche, Sanofi, Sobi, and UCB. VS has research collaborations with Pfizer and has received consulting fees from AbbVie and Roche. KM is funded by the German Rheumastiftung and has received research grants from Pfizer, AbbVie, and Roche and honoraria from AbbVie, Genzyme, Medac, and Pharm-Allergan. IF has received personal fees from AbbVie, Chugai, and Novartis and has acted as a consultant for Genentech, Bayer, Medac, and Lilly. AM does not have any conflict of interest to declare since March 2016, when he became the Scientific Director of the public hospital IRCCS Istituto Giannina Gaslini because this role does not allow him to render private consultancy resulting in personal income. He performed consultancy activities on behalf of the public hospital IRCCS Istituto Giannina Gaslini for AbbVie, Boehringer, Novartis, and R-Pharm and is the Scientific Director of the public hospital IRCCS Istituto Giannina Gaslini, which has received funds from Bristol-Myers Squibb, Hoffman-La Roche, Janssen, Novartis, Pfizer Inc., and Sobi for the coordination activity of the PRINTO network. NW has received research grants from Pfizer and AbbVie and personal fees from Novartis. NR has acted as a consultant and has participated in speaker bureaus for AbbVie, Ablynx, Amgen, AstraZeneca, Baxalta Biosimilars, Biogen Idec, Boehringer, Bristol-Myers Squibb, Celgene, Eli-Lilly, EMD Serono, Gilead Sciences, Janssen, Medimmune, Novartis, Pfizer Inc., R-Pharm, Roche, Sanofi, Servier, and Takeda and works as a full-time public employee of the public hospital IRCCS Istituto Giannina Gaslini, which has received funds from Bristol-Myers Squibb, Hoffman-La Roche, Janssen, Novartis, Pfizer Inc., and Sobi for the coordination activity of the PRINTO network. The other authors declare that they have no competing interests.

Author details
[1]Department of Pediatric Immunology and Rheumatology, Wilhelmina Children's Hospital, Lundlaan, 6 PO box 85090, Utrecht, The Netherlands. [2]IRCCS Istituto Giannina Gaslini, Clinica Pediatrica e Reumatologia, PRINTO, Via Gaslini, 5, 16147 Genoa, Italy. [3]Asklepios Clinic Sankt Augustin, Arnold-Janssen strasse 29, Sankt Augustin, Germany. [4]Department of Pediatric and Adolescents medicine, Medical faculty, University Hospital of Cologne, Kerpener Str. 62, Cologne, Germany. [5]Karolinska University Hospital, Pediatric Rheumatology Unit, Stockholm, Sweden. [6]Unité Romande d'Immuno-Rhumatologie Pediatrique/Centre Hospitalier Universitaire Vaudois (CHUV), Pediatrie, University of Lausanne, Av Bugnon 46, Lausanne, Switzerland. [7]University Hospital of Geneva, Geneva, Switzerland. [8]Federal State Autonomous Institution "National Medical Research Center of Children's Health" of the Ministry of Health of the Russian Federation, LOMONOSOVSKIJ PR-T,2/62, Moscow, Russia. [9]Federal State Autonomous Educational Institution of Higher Education I.M. Sechenov First Moscow State Medical University of the Ministry of Health of the Russian Federation, Moscow, Russia. [10]Vilnius University, Clinic of Children's Diseases, Vilnius, Lithuania and Children's Hospital, Affiliate of Vilnius University Hospital Santariskiu Klinikos, Santariskiu, 4, Vilnius, Lithuania. [11]Université Paris-Descartes, Institut IMAGINE, Centre de référence national pour les Rhumatismes inflammatoires et les maladies Auto-Immunes Systémiques rares de l'Enfant (RAISE), Unité d'Immunologie, Hématologie et Rhumatologie Pediatrique, Hôpital Necker-Enfants Malades, Assistance Publique Hôpitaux de Paris, 149 Rue De Sevres, Paris, France. [12]Hospital Sant Joan de Déu, Universitat de Barcelona, Unidad de Reumatología Pediátrica, Esplugues de Llobregat, Passeig Sant Joan de Deu 2, Barcelona, Spain. [13]Juliane Marie Centret, Rigshospitalet, Paediatric Rheumatology Unit, Blegdamsvej 9, Copenhagen, Denmark. [14]Division of Rheumatology, IRCCS Ospedale Pediatrico Bambino Gesù, Piazza S. Onofrio, 4, Rome, Italy. [15]Sophia Children's Hospital, Department of Paediatric Rheumatology, Erasmus University Medical Centre, Dr Molewaterplein 60, Rotterdam, The Netherlands. [16]Department of Rheumatology, Erasmus University Medical Centre, Rotterdam, The Netherlands. [17]Riga Stradins University, Department of Pediatrics, Children University Hospital, Vienibas gatve 45, Riga, LV, Latvia. [18]Hippokration General Hospital, First Department of pediatrics, Thessaloniki University School of Medicine, Konstantinoupoleos 49, Thessaloniki, Greece. [19]Alexandru Ioan Cuza University of Iasi, V. Lupu str.nr. 62, Iasi, Romania. [20]Aghia Sophia Childrens Hospital, First Department of Pediatrics, University of Athens Medical School, Thivon 1, Athens, Greece. [21]German Rheumatism Research Centre, Berlin, Germany. [22]Charité University Medicine, Charitéplatz 1, Berlin, Germany. [23]Hamburg Centre for Pediatric and Adolescent Rheumatology, Dehnhaide 120, Hamburg, Germany. [24]German Center for Pediatric and Adolescent Rheumatology, Deutsches Zentrum für Kinder- und Jugendrheumatologie, Zentrum für Schmerztherapie junger Menschen, Gehfeldstrasse 24, Garmisch-Partenkirchen, Germany. [25]IRCCS Istituto Giannina Gaslini, Clinica Pediatrica e Reumatologia, via Gaslini 5, Genoa, Italy. [26]Dipartimento di Neuroscienze, Riabilitazione, Oftalmologia, Genetica e Scienze Materno-Infantili (DiNOGMI), Università degli Studi di Genova, Genoa, Italy. [27]IRCCS Istituto Giannina Gaslini, Servizio di Epidemiologia e Biostatistica, via Gaslini 5, Genoa, Italy. [28]IRCCS Istituto Giannina Gaslini, Direzione Scientifica, via Gaslini 5, Genoa, Italy.

References

1. Ravelli A, Martini A. Juvenile idiopathic arthritis. Lancet. 2007;369:767–78.
2. Ruperto N, Levinson JE, Ravelli A, Shear ES, Tague BL, Murray K, et al. Longterm health outcomes and quality of life in American and Italian inception cohorts of patients with juvenile rheumatoid arthritis. I Outcome status. J Rheumatol. 1997;24:945–51.
3. Ruperto N, Ravelli A, Levinson JE, Shear ES, Murray K, Tague BL, et al. Longterm health outcomes and quality of life in American and Italian inception cohorts of patients with juvenile rheumatoid arthritis. II Early predictors of outcome. J Rheumatol. 1997;24:952–8.
4. Oliveira S, Ravelli A, Pistorio A, Castell E, Malattia C, Prieur AM, et al. Proxy-reported health-related quality of life of patients with juvenile idiopathic arthritis: the Pediatric Rheumatology International Trials Organization multinational quality of life cohort study. Arthritis Rheum. 2007;57:35–43.
5. Gutierrez-Suarez R, Pistorio A, Cespedes CA, Norambuena X, Flato B, Rumba I, et al. Health-related quality of life of patients with juvenile idiopathic arthritis coming from 3 different geographic areas. The PRINTO multinational quality of life cohort study. Rheumatology. 2007; 46:314–20.
6. Vanoni F, Suris JC, von Scheven-Gete A, Fonjallaz B, Hofer M. The difference of disease perception by juvenile idiopathic arthritis patients and their parents: analysis of the JAMAR questionnaire. Pediatr Rheumatol Online J. 2016;14:2.
7. Kuhlmann A, Schmidt T, Treskova M, Lopez-Bastida J, Linertova R, Oliva-Moreno J, et al. Social/economic costs and health-related quality of life in patients with juvenile idiopathic arthritis in Europe. Eur J Health Econ. 2016; 17(Suppl 1):79–87.
8. Oen K, Guzman J, Dufault B, Tucker LB, Shiff NJ, Duffy KW, et al. Health-Related Quality of Life in an Inception Cohort of Children With Juvenile Idiopathic Arthritis: A Longitudinal Analysis. Arthritis Care Res (Hoboken). 2018;70:134–44.
9. Keane J, Gershon S, Wise RP. Tuberculosis associated with infliximab, a tumor necrosis factor alpha-neutralizing agent. N Engl J Med. 2017;345: 1098–104.
10. Ruperto N, Vesely R, Saint-Raymond A, Martini A. Impact of the European paediatric legislation in paediatric rheumatology: past, present and future. Ann Rheum Dis. 2013;72:1893–6.
11. Horneff G, Klein A, Oommen PT. Update on malignancies in children with juvenile idiopathic arthritis in the German BIKER Registry. Clin Exp Rheumatol. 2016;34:1113–20.

12. Zahedi Niaki O, Clarke A, Ramsey-Goldman R. Malignancy incidence in 5294 patients with juvenile idiopathic arthritis. RMD Open. 2017;2:e000212.
13. Mannion ML, Beukelman T. What is the background incidence of malignancy in children with rheumatic disease? Curr Rheumatol Rep. 2013;15:310.
14. Beukelman T, Haynes K, Curtis JR, Xie F, Chen L, Bemrich-Stolz CJ, et al. Rates of malignancy associated with juvenile idiopathic arthritis and its treatment. Arthritis Rheum. 2012;64:1263–71.
15. Singh J, Wells GA, Christensen R. Adverse effects of biologics: a network meta-analysis and Cochrane overview. Cochrane Database Syst Rev. 2011;16: CD008794.
16. Ruperto N, Martini A. Networking in paediatrics: the example of the Paediatric Rheumatology International Trials Organisation (PRINTO). Arch Dis Child. 2011;96:596–601.
17. Petty RE, Southwood TR, Manners P, Baum J, Glass DN, Goldenberg J, et al. International League of Associations for Rheumatology classification of juvenile idiopathic arthritis: second revision, Edmonton, 2001. J Rheumatol. 2004;31:390–2.
18. Giannini EH, Ruperto N, Ravelli A, Lovell DJ, Felson DT, Martini A. Preliminary definition of improvement in juvenile arthritis. Arthritis Rheum. 1997;40: 1202–9.
19. Viola S, Felici E, Magni-Manzoni S, Pistorio A, Buoncompagni A, Ruperto N, et al. Development and validation of a clinical index for assessment of long-term damage in juvenile idiopathic arthritis. Arthritis Rheum. 2005;52: 2092–102.
20. Filocamo G, Schiappapietra B, Bertamino M, Pistorio A, Ruperto N, Magni-Manzoni S, et al. A new short and simple health-related quality of life measurement for paediatric rheumatic diseases: initial validation in juvenile idiopathic arthritis. Rheumatology (Oxford). 2010;49:1272–80.
21. Horneff G, De Bock F, Foeldvari I, Girschick HJ, Michels H, Moebius D, et al. Safety and efficacy of combination of etanercept and methotrexate compared to treatment with etanercept only in patients with juvenile idiopathic arthritis (JIA): preliminary data from the German JIA Registry. Ann Rheum Dis. 2009;68:519–25.
22. Schmeling H, Minden K, Foeldvari I, Ganser G, Hospach T, Horneff G. Efficacy and safety of adalimumab as the first and second biologic agent in juvenile idiopathic arthritis: the German Biologics JIA Registry. Arthritis Rheumatol. 2014;66:2580–9.
23. Horneff G, Klein A, Klotsche J, Minden K, Huppertz HI, Weller-Heinemann F, et al. Comparison of treatment response, remission rate and drug adherence in polyarticular juvenile idiopathic arthritis patients treated with etanercept, adalimumab or tocilizumab. Arthritis Res Ther. 2016;18:272.
24. Horneff G, Schulz AC, Klotsche J, Hospach A, Minden K, Foeldvari I, et al. Experience with etanercept, tocilizumab and interleukin-1 inhibitors in systemic onset juvenile idiopathic arthritis patients from the BIKER registry. Arthritis Res Ther. 2017;19:256.
25. Albarouni M, Becker I, Horneff G. Predictors of response to methotrexate in juvenile idiopathic arthritis. Pediatr Rheumatol Online J. 2014;12:35.
26. Becker I, Horneff G. Risk of Serious Infection in Juvenile Idiopathic Arthritis Patients Associated With Tumor Necrosis Factor Inhibitors and Disease Activity in the German Biologics in Pediatric Rheumatology Registry. Arthritis Care Res (Hoboken). 2017;69:552–60.
27. Minden K, Niewerth M, Zink A, Seipelt E, Foeldvari I, Girschick H, et al. Long-term outcome of patients with JIA treated with etanercept, results of the biologic register JuMBO. Rheumatology (Oxford). 2012;51:1407–15.
28. Magnusson B, Board of Registry. The Swedish paediatric JIA-registry. Pediatr Rheumatol. 2014;12:P5.
29. Diak P, Siegel J, La GL, Choi L, Lemery S, McMahon A. Tumor necrosis factor alpha blockers and malignancy in children: forty-eight cases reported to the Food and Drug Administration. Arthritis Rheum. 2010;62:2517–24.
30. Beukelman T, Xie F, Chen L, Baddley JW, Delzell E, Grijalva CG, et al. Rates of hospitalized bacterial infection associated with juvenile idiopathic arthritis and its treatment. Arthritis Rheum. 2012;64:2773–80.
31. Nordstrom BL, Mines D, Gu Y, Mercaldi C, Aquino P, Harrison MJ. Risk of malignancy in children with juvenile idiopathic arthritis not treated with biologic agents. Arthritis Care Res (Hoboken). 2012;64:1357–64.
32. Bernatsky S, Rosenberg AM, Oen KG, Duffy CM, Ramsey-Goldman R, Labrecque J, et al. Malignancies in juvenile idiopathic arthritis: a preliminary report. J Rheumatol. 2011;38:760–3.
33. Lionetti G, Kimura Y, Schanberg L. Using Registries to Identify Adverse Events in Rheumatic Diseases. Pediatrics. 2013;132:1384–94.
34. Davies R, Southwood TR, Kearsley-Fleet L, Lunt M, Hyrich KL. Medically Significant Infections Are Increased in Patients With Juvenile Idiopathic Arthritis Treated With Etanercept: Results From the British Society for Paediatric and Adolescent Rheumatology Etanercept Cohort Study. Arthritis Rheumatol. 2015;67:2487–94.
35. Kearsley-Fleet L, Davies R, Baildam E. Factors associated with choice of biologic among children with Juvenile Idiopathic Arthritis: results from two UK paediatric biologic registers. Rheumatology (Oxford). 2016;55:1556–65.
36. Mourao AF, Santos M, Melo-Gomes JA. Effectiveness and long-term retention of anti-tumour necrosis factor treatment in juvenile and adult patients with juvenile idiopathic arthritis: data from Reuma.pt. Rheumatology (Oxford). 2016;55:697–703.
37. Sauvain MJ, Schalm SB, Berthet G. Swiss registry for TNF-alpha blockers in children and adolescents with rheumatological diseases. Praxis (Bern 1994). 2010;99:649–54.
38. Hurd A, Beukelman T. Infectious complications in juvenile idiopathic arthritis. Curr Rheumatol Rep. 2013;15:327.

11

Comparison of treatment response, remission rate and drug adherence in polyarticular juvenile idiopathic arthritis patients treated with etanercept, adalimumab or tocilizumab

Gerd Horneff[1*], Ariane Klein[1], Jens Klotsche[2], Kirsten Minden[2], Hans-Iko Huppertz[3], Frank Weller-Heinemann[3], Jasmin Kuemmerle-Deschner[4], Johannes-Peter Haas[5] and Anton Hospach[6]

Abstract

Background: Treatment response, remission rates and compliance in patients with polyarticular juvenile idiopathic arthritis (polyJIA) treated with adalimumab, etanercept, or tocilizumab were analyzed in clinical practice.

Methods: Data collected in the German BIKER registry were analyzed in patients with polyJIA who started treatment with approved biologics, adalimumab, etanercept or tocilizumab, from 2011 to 2015. Baseline patient characteristics, treatment response, safety and drug survival were compared.

Results: Two hundred thirty-six patient started adalimumab, 419 etanercept and 74 tocilizumab, with differences in baseline patient characteristics. Baseline Juvenile Disease Activity Score (JADAS)10 (mean ± SD) in the adalimumab/etanercept/tocilizumab cohorts was 12.1+/−7.6, 13.8 ± 7.1 and 15.1 ± 7.4, respectively (adalimumab vs etanercept, $p = 0.01$), and Childhood Health Assessment Questionnaire (CHAQ)-disability index scores was 0.43 ± 0.58, 0.59 ± 0.6 and 0.63 ± 0.55, respectively (adalimumab vs etanercept, $p < 0.001$). Uveitis history was more frequent in the adalimumab cohort (OR 5.73; $p < 0.001$). Balanced patients' samples were obtained by a generalized propensity score to adjust for baseline differences. Pediatric ACR30/50/70/90 criterion improvement after 3 months treatment was achieved by 68%/60%/42%/24% in the etanercept cohort, 67%/59%/43%/27% in the adalimumab cohort and 61%/52%/35%/26% in the tocilizumab cohort. At 24 months, JADAS minimal disease activity was achieved in 52.4%/61.3%/52.4% and JADAS remission in 27.9%/34.8%/27.9% patients in the adalimumab/etanercept/tocilizumab cohorts, respectively. Etanercept was used in 95.5% of patients as a first biologic, adalimumab in 50.8% and tocilizumab in 20.2%. There were no important differences in efficacy between first-line and second-line use of biologics. In total 60.4%/49.4%/31.1% patients discontinued adalimumab/etanercept/tocilizumab, respectively (HR for adalimumab 1.67; $p < 0.001$; HR for tocilizumab 0.35; $p = 0.001$). Drug survival rates did not differ significantly in patients on biologic monotherapy compared with combination therapy with methotrexate. Over 4 years observation under etanercept/adalimumab/tocilizumab, 996/386/103 adverse events, and 148/119/26 serious adverse events, respectively, were reported.

(Continued on next page)

* Correspondence: g.horneff@asklepios.com
[1]Department of Pediatrics, Centre of General Pediatrics and Neonatology, Asklepios Clinic Sankt Augustin, 53757 Sankt Augustin, Germany
Full list of author information is available at the end of the article

(Continued from previous page)

Conclusions: In clinical practice, etanercept is most frequently used as first-line biologic. Adalimumab/etanercept/tocilizumab showed comparable efficacy toward polyJIA. Overall, tolerance was acceptable. Interestingly, compliance was highest with tocilizumab and lowest with adalimumab. This study provides the first indication for the comparison of different biologic agents in polyarticular JIA based on observational study data with all their weaknesses and demonstrates the need for well-controlled head-to-head studies for confirmation.

Keywords: Adalimumab, Etanercept, Tocilizumab, Juvenile idiopathic arthritis, Drug surveillance, JADAS

Background

Juvenile idiopathic arthritis (JIA) is a collective term for arthritides that are diagnosed before the age of 16 years. Diagnosis requires disease duration of at least 6 weeks and the exclusion of other causes of arthritis [1]. JIA is the most common chronic rheumatic inflammatory disease of childhood. If not successfully treated, it can lead to severe disability [2].

Pharmacologic treatment consists of nonsteroidal antirheumatic drugs, mainly for symptomatic relief, and disease-modifying antirheumatic drugs (DMARDs). Of the latter group, methotrexate (MTX) is the most common first-line DMARD and is a cornerstone drug in the treatment of patients with JIA. Its efficacy was first demonstrated two decades ago in a randomized controlled trial [3]. According to national and international guidelines and recommendations, patients with JIA who are refractory to MTX treatment are eligible for treatment with biologic agents [4, 5].

Etanercept, an anti-TNF-α receptor immunoglobulin Fc fragment fusion protein, was the first biologic agent approved by the US Food and Drug Administration for the treatment of polyarticular JIA (pJIA) in 1999 and by the European Medicines Evaluating Agency in 2000. Its efficacy and safety were demonstrated in a randomized controlled withdrawal trial and several long-term observational studies from national registries, including the German Biologics in Pediatric Rheumatology (BIKER) Registry [6–9]. In 2008, adalimumab, a monoclonal anti-TNF-α antibody, was approved for the treatment of polyarticular JIA, as monotherapy or in combination with MTX, after its efficacy was established in a placebo-controlled withdrawal trial [10]. Adalimumab was preferred over etanercept for the treatment of uveitis for years until a recent randomized placebo controlled trial demonstrated its efficacy for treatment of uveitis [11]. Observational data on the use of adalimumab for JIA are more limited than those on the use of etanercept [12]. Tocilizumab, a monoclonal interleukin-6 receptor antibody, was first approved for systemic onset JIA in 2011 and was found to be effective in a randomized controlled withdrawal trial [13]. Since 2013, Tocilizumab has been the third first-line biologic agent approved for treatment of polyarticular JIA.

The efficacy of these three agents for the treatment of JIA is considered to be equivalent [14]. However, no head-to-head trials have been conducted to compare etanercept, adalimumab or tocilizumab. All three biologic agents are approved for treatment of polyarticular JIA in children older than 2 years who do not respond to MTX. Therefore, the initial decision of which biologic agent to use must be determined based on limited evidence. The aim of this analysis was to compare baseline characteristics, efficacy, tolerability and drug survival in patients with polyarticular JIA initiating adalimumab, etanercept or tocilizumab.

Methods

The German BIKER Registry was approved by the local ethics committee. Written consent was obtained and pseudonymized data were collected. This registry has been extensively described in previous reports [9, 15]. Patients in the German BIKER registry initiating treatment with adalimumab, etanercept or tocilizumab between 1 January 2011 and 31 December 2015 were included in the study. The study population was restricted to patients who were classified in the following JIA categories: rheumatoid factor-positive polyarthritis, rheumatoid factor-negative polyarthritis and extended oligoarthritis. Patients with other JIA categories (systemic onset JIA, persistent oligoarthritis, psoriatic arthritis (PsA), enthesitis-related arthritis (ERA) and unclassified JIA) were excluded because of differences in the approval of the three biologics studied and to homogenize the study population.

For the efficacy analyses, assessments were performed at baseline and at follow up after 3 and 6 months and every 6 months thereafter. Due to the character of the registry study, the number of patients observed decreased with treatment duration. For this reason, efficacy was analyzed until month 24. Juvenile Disease Activity Score (JADAS) scores and improvement in the Pediatric American College of Rheumatology Criteria (PedACR) were calculated as previously described in detail [16, 17]. The JADAS minimal disease activity (MDA) (defined as JADAS10 ≤ 3.8) and JADAS remission rates (defined as JADAS10 ≤ 1) according to the definition of Consolaro et al. [18] were calculated. The JADAS10 was chosen because all four domains, number of active joints (truncated at 10), patient's/parent's global assessment of disease activity, physician's global assessment of disease activity, and erythrocyte sedimentation rate, ranged from 0 to 10 points. Functional status was determined using the Childhood Health Assessment Questionnaire (CHAQ) disability index [19].

Safety was analyzed based on adverse event reporting. An adverse event was defined as any untoward medical occurrence in a subject administered a pharmaceutical product, even without a causal relationship with the treatment. Serious adverse events included death, a life-threatening event or an event leading to or prolonging hospitalization, persistent or significant disability/incapacity or an important medical event requiring medical or surgical intervention to prevent a serious outcome or congenital anomaly or birth defect. For this analysis, reasons for discontinuation were classified as inefficacy, intolerance, remission or other reasons.

Statistical analysis

The adalimumab, etanercept and tocilizumab cohorts differed in their clinical characteristics and treatment history at baseline. A generalized propensity score was estimated to obtain balanced samples of patients in respect to baseline characteristics. The likelihood of being allocated to a cohort was estimated by a multinomial logistic regression model, including the predictors, sex, age at JIA onset, JIA category, disease duration, JADAS10, concomitant MTX use and the number of previously used biologic agents. Balanced samples of patients were obtained using an inverse probability of treatment weight. Generalised estimation equations (GEE) were applied to the weighted sample of patients to analyze the drug adherence and treatment response. Drug survival was analyzed by Kaplan-Meier plots and Cox proportional hazard model.

Results

Study population

The German BIKER registry database of 3547 patients with JIA was used to identify eligible patients. Patients diagnosed with rheumatoid factor-positive polyarthritis, rheumatoid factor-negative polyarthritis or extended oligoarthritis, who had initiated treatment with a biologic agent from 1 January 2011 to 31 December 2015, were considered. Up to December 2015, 236 patients started on adalimumab, 419 started on etanercept and 74 started on tocilizumab.

Clinical characteristics at treatment initiation significantly differed between the three groups (Additional file 1: Table S1). The propensity-score-weighted analyses of baseline characteristics resulted in balanced samples as reported in Table 1 except for sex and uveitis. Female predominance was more pronounced in the etanercept and adalimumab cohorts than in the tocilizumab cohort (Table 1). Compared with the etanercept cohort, patients in the adalimumab or tocilizumab cohort were slightly older. The distribution of the three analyzed JIA categories was comparable among medications despite a lower rate of patients diagnosed with extended oligoarthritis in the tocilizumab cohort compared with the other two cohorts combined.

Etanercept was used as a first biologic agent in 583 patients (79.9%), adalimumab in 174 patients (23.9%) and tocilizumab in 17 patients (2.3%). Thus, etanercept was preferred as a first-line biologic agent. Only 17 patients (4.1%) received etanercept as a second-line biologic agent. In the adalimumab cohort, approximately half (46.6%) of the patients received adalimumab as the first biologic agent, while only 18.9% in the tocilizumab cohort received tocilizumab as the first biologic agent.

Compared with the etanercept cohort, the baseline JADAS10 and CHAQ-disability index were lower in the adalimumab cohort. Concomitant uveitis was present in 23 (5.5%) of the etanercept cohort, in 58 (25%) of the adalimumab cohort and in no patients in the tocilizumab cohort. Thus, uveitis demonstrated the highest frequency in patients treated with adalimumab (odds ratio 3.41 (95% CI 3.21; 4.45); $p = 0.03$).

At baseline, 302 patients (72%) in the etanercept cohort but only 127 (54%) in the adalimumab and 34 (46%) in the tocilizumab cohort received concomitant therapy with MTX. The differences described were not statistically significant after weighting the analyses with the propensity score weight (Table 1).

Treatment response

The mean treatment duration was comparable among all cohorts (1.25 ± 1.05 years in the etanercept cohort, 1.0 ± 0.86 in the adalimumab cohort and 0.98 ± 0.59 in the tocilizumab cohort). Improvement according to PedACR30/50/70/90 criteria was reached after 3 months by 68%/60%/42 %/24 % in the etanercept cohort, 67%/59%/43%/27% in the adalimumab cohort and 61%/52%/35%/26% in the tocilizumab cohort, respectively. The response rates further increased or were stable with continuing treatment (Fig. 1). There were no statistically significant differences between the three groups in the PedACR response rates. PedACR response rates to etanercept/adalimumab/tocilizumab, either as first-line or second-line biologic agents, were comparable (Additional file 2: Figure S1).

At baseline, the mean observed JADAS10 was highest in the tocilizumab (15.1 ± 7.4) and etanercept (13.8 ± 7.1) cohorts ($p > 0.05$) and significantly lower in the adalimumab cohort (12.1 ± 7.6; $p = 0.003$ compared to etanercept; $p = 0.011$ compared to tocilizumab). The significant differences in baseline JADAS10 disappeared after weighting the analyses (Table 1, Fig. 2).

Table 1 Patients' characteristics (absolute number of patients, percentages, descriptive statistics as reported in BIKER; comparison between the three cohorts weighted by an inverse probability of treatment)

	Etanercept cohort *n* = 419	Adalimumab cohort *n* = 236	Tocilizumab cohort *n* = 74	Etanercept versus adalimumab[a] OR (95% CI); *p* value	Tocilizumab versus etanercept[a] OR (95% CI); *p* value	Tocilizumab versus adalimumab[a] OR (95% CI); *p* value
Female, *n* (%)	332 (79.2%)	192 (81.4%)	51 (68.8%)	0.96 (0.57; 1.62); 0.88	0.63 (0.45; 0.89); 0.03	0.58 (0.48; 0.98); 0.04
Age at baseline, years, mean ± SD	10.5 ± 4.4	11.8 ± 4.0	12.9 ± 3.6	0.63 (−0.31; 1.57); 0.19	1.65 (−0.67; 3.96); 0.16	1.02 (−1.31; 3.34); 0.39
Median (IQR)	11.1 (7.1–13.9)	12.7 (8.7– 15.0)	13.5 (11.2– 15.9)			
Disease duration at treatment start, mean ± SD	3.6 ± 3.3	5.8 ± 4.0	6.1 ± 3.5	0.40 (−0.17; 0.98); 0.17	1.13 (−0.05; 2.02); 0.07	0.73 (−0.21; 1.66); 0.13
Median (IQR)	2.6 (1.1–5.1)	4.9 (2.4–8.4)	5.8 (2.9–8.8)			
JIA category *n* (%)						
RF+ PA	37 (8.8%)	23 (9.7%)	9 (12.2%)	1.45 (0.74; 2.83); 0.28	0.95 (0.60; 1.49); 0.81	2.18 (0.48; 9.85); 0.31
RF- PA	224 (53.5%)	128 (54.2%)	47 (63.5%)	(ref)	(ref)	(ref)
ExOA	158 (37.7%)	85 (36.0%)	18 (24.3%)	3.17 (0.74; 13.60); 0.12	0.71 (0.22; 2.27); 0.57	0.75 (0.24; 2.41); 0.63
First biologic used	400 (95.5%)	110 (46.6%)	14 (18.9%)	0.54 (0.28; 1.03); 0.06	0.44 (0.16; 1.18); 0.10	0.81 (0.34; 1.96); 0.65
Co-med corticosteroids, *n* (%)	134 (32.0)	60 (25.4)	26 (35.1)	1.38 (0.96; 1.97)	1.15 (0.69; 1.94)	1.59 (091; 2.78)
Co-med MTX, *n* (%)	302 (72.1)	127 (53.8)	34 (45.9)	1.20 (0.76; 1.88); 0.44	0.76 (0.28; 2.06); 0.59	0.64 (0.24; 1.70); 0.37
JADAS10 (0–40), mean ± SD	13.8 ± 7.1	12.1 ± 7.6	15.1 ± 7.4	−0.41 (−2.30; 1.48); 0.67	−0.53 (−4.22; 3.17); 0.78	−0.12 (−3.84; 3.60); 0.95
Median (IQR)	13.6 (8.8–19.0)	11.7 (6.1–17.5)	14.8 (9.2–20.1)			
CHAQ-DI (0–3), mean ± SD	0.59 ± 0.60	0.43 ± 0.58	0.63 ± 0.55	−0.04 (−0.19; 0.12); 0.64	−0.10 (−0.30; 0.11); 0.35	−0.06 (−0.29; 0.17); 0.60
Median (IQR)	0.38 (0.13–0.88)	0.13 (0–0.623)	0.63 (0.19-1.0)			
Uveitis before start of biologic	23 (5.5%)	59 (25%)	0	3.41 (3.21; 4.45); 0.03	-	-

[a]Analyses weighted by an inverse probability of treatment estimated by a generalized propensity score. *beta* regression coefficient for continuous variables, *CI* confidence interval, *OR* odds ratio for categorical variable, *(ref)* reference group, *JIA* juvenile idiopathic arthritis, *RF* rheumatoid factor, PA, polyarthritis, ExOA extended oligoarthritis, *JADAS* Juvenile Disease Activity Score, *CHAQ-DI* Childhood Health Assessment Questionnaire disability index

A significant decrease in the adjusted JADAS10 was observed in all three cohorts (Fig. 2). From baseline to the last observation on treatment, the JADAS10 decreased by 8.6 (95% CI 7.6; 9.5) points in the etanercept cohort, by 7.3 (95% CI 5.8; 8.6) in the adalimumab cohort and by 5.1 (95% CI 1.5; 8.4) in the tocilizumab cohort. The decrease in JADAS10 did not significantly differ among the three cohorts. The mean decrease in JADAS10 was −7.7 (95% CI −8.47; −6.99) in patients with rheumatoid factor-negative polyarthritis or extended

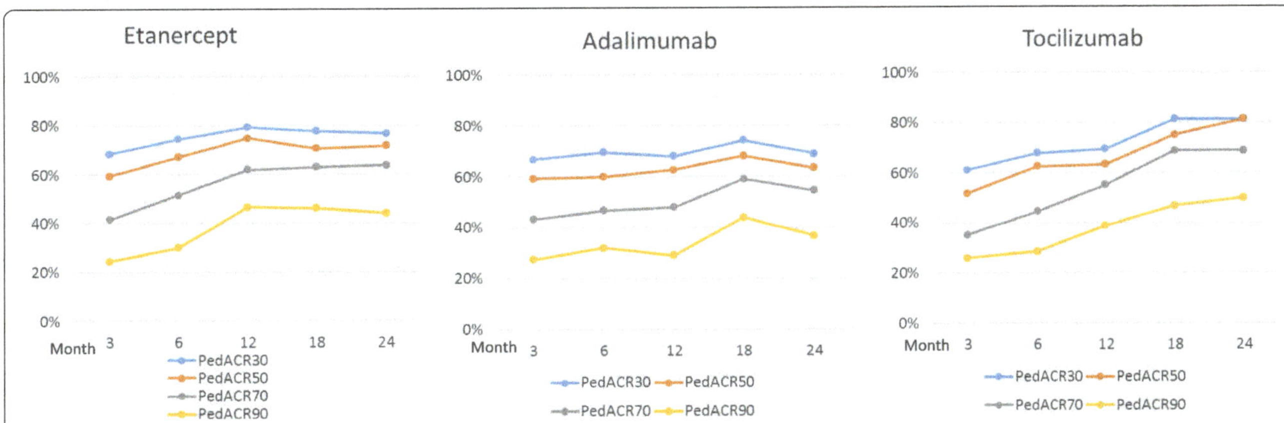

Fig. 1 Improvement in patients using etanercept, adalimumab or tocilizumab according to the Pediatric American College of Rheumatology (*PedACR*)30/50/70 and 90 criteria

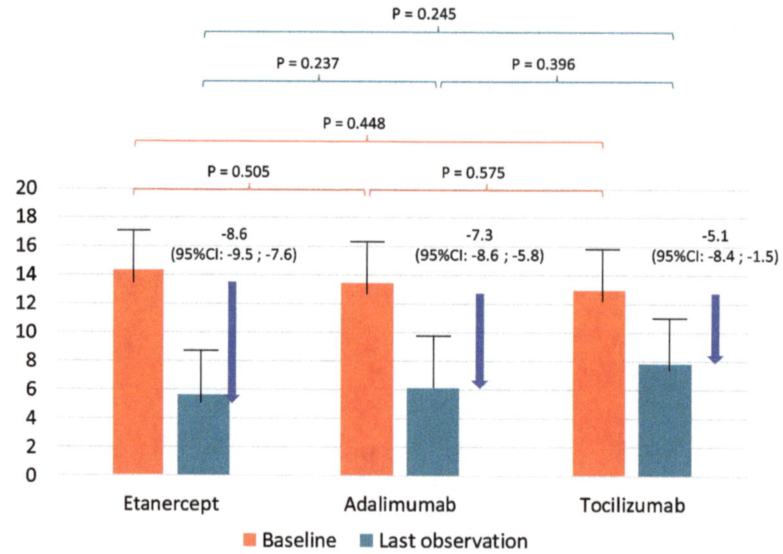

Fig. 2 Improvement in patients following etanercept, adalimumab or tocilizumab treatment according to Juvenile Disease Activity Score (*JADAS*)10 at baseline compared with the last observation on a study drug

oligoarthritis, and −9.4 (95% CI −12.13; −6.63) for rheumatoid factor-positive polyarthritis. The difference between the JIA categories in the JADAS10 response was not statistically significant (delta = 1.51; 95% CI −0.54; 3.56; $p = 0.149$).

JADAS remission and JADAS-MDA were used as further treatment response indicators. In the etanercept, adalimumab and tocilizumab cohorts, 131 patients (34.8%), 71 patients (27.9%) and 16 patients (23.5%), respectively, achieved JADAS remission (defined as JADAS10 ≤ 1.0) at the last observation. The three cohorts did not significantly differ in JADAS remission at the last observation adjusting for baseline differences between the three cohorts. The rates of achieving JADAS-MDA were comparable among all three cohorts (Fig. 3): 231 patients (61.3%), 133 patients (52.4%) and 32 patients (47.1%) in the etanercept, adalimumab and tocilizumab cohorts, respectively, achieved JADAS-MDA (defined as JADAS10 ≤ 3.8) at the last observation.

Patients who were first exposed to biologic agents were compared to those who switched from a first to a second biologic agent. The mean (± SD) JADAS10 in the cohort previously exposed to a biologic agent (14.8 ± 7.3) was not significantly lower than that in the biologic-agent-naïve cohort (16.5 ± 7.2). The decline in JADAS10 at 3, 6, 12, 18 and 24 months, respectively, was 3.9 ± 3.3, 6.2 ± 7.4, 9.6 ± 7.7, 6.6 ± 5.9 and 2.9 ± 2.4 in the biologic-naïve group, and 8.9 ± 6.5, 7.6 ± 8.2, 4.6 ± 5.6, 3.2 ± 4.5 and 7.7 ± 8.8 in the cohort switching from a first to a second biologic. The decline in JADAS and the rates of achieving JADAS remission and JADAS- MDA were again comparable among the cohorts.

Functional disability was analyzed using the CHAQ-DI. The observed baseline CHAQ-DI was highest in the

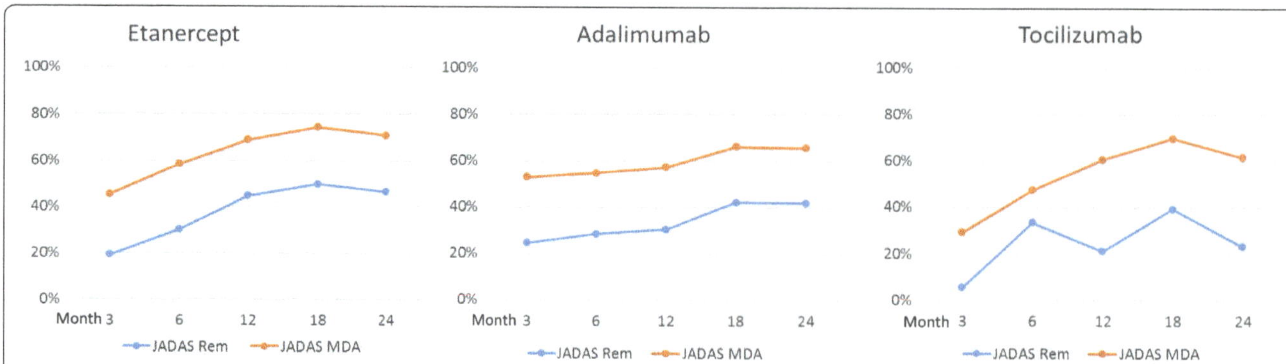

Fig. 3 Rates of Juvenile Disease Activity Score (*JADAS*)10 remission and minimal disease activity in patients taking etanercept, adalimumab or tocilizumab

tocilizumab cohort (0.63 ± 0.55), followed by the etanercept cohort (0.59 ± 0.60) and the adalimumab cohort (0.43 ± 0.58). However, the baseline CHAQ-DI did not differ among the three cohorts in the propensity-score-weighted analyses. Reductions in CHAQ-DI from baseline to the last observation in the tocilizumab, etanercept and adalimumab cohorts were (−0.31 ± 0.46), (−0.22 ± 0.54) and (−0.12 ± 0.47), respectively. Reduction in the CHAQ-DI was significantly greater in the etanercept cohort than in the adalimumab cohort ($p = 0.032$). There was no significant difference in the reduction in the CHAQ-DI between the tocilizumab and the etanercept cohort ($p = 0.261$). However, the residual CHAQ-DI at the last observation was comparable among all three cohorts (etanercept 0.31 ± 0.44, adalimumab 0.29 ± 0.48 and tocilizumab 0.36 ± 0.46).

Drug adherence and discontinuations

Drugs were discontinued by 142 patients (60.2%) in the adalimumab cohort versus 207 patients (49.4%) in the etanercept cohort and 23 patients (31.1%) in the tocilizumab cohort. The median drug survival before discontinuation due to inefficacy or intolerance was 2.85 years for adalimumab and 4.29 years for etanercept; this was not calculated for tocilizumab because more than 50% of the patients were still receiving treatment (Fig. 4). Survival analyses using Cox proportional hazard regression revealed significant differences between adalimumab and etanercept survival (hazard ratio 2.82, 95% CI 1.55; 5.14; $p < 0.001$), between adalimumab and tocilizumab survival (hazard ratio 4.71, 95% CI 2.58; 8.61; $p < 0.001$), and between etanercept and tocilizumab survival (hazard ratio 2.82, 95% CI 1.55; 5.14; $p = 0.001$).

Drug survival with adalimumab (hazard ratio 1.36, 95% CI 1.03; 1.78; $p = 0.029$) was improved but was significant lower compared to etanercept when restricting the analyses to patients who took etanercept and adalimumab as their first biologic agents. Interestingly, the survival rates of patients on monotherapy with a biologic agent compared with combination therapy with MTX were not significantly different ($p = 0.836$) regardless of whether they were calculated separately in the etanercept, adalimumab or tocilizumab cohort (data not shown) or for the combined analysis (Additional file 3: Figure S2). Patients with rheumatoid factor-negative polyarthritis or extended oligoarthritis had a comparable drug survival to patients with rheumatoid factor-positive polyarthritis (hazard ratio = 0.995, 95% CI 0.67; 1.47; $p = 0.98$). Drug survival also did not statistically significantly differ between the JIA categories in the adalimumab (hazard ratio = 1.15, 95% CI 0.62; 2.12; $p = 0.653$) and etanercept (hazard ratio = 0.83, 95% CI 0.48; 1.43; $p = 0.502$) cohorts.

The reasons for discontinuation are provided in Table 2. The most common reason for discontinuation was poor efficacy or unsatisfactory response. Significantly more patients discontinued adalimumab (odds ratio 4.89, 95% CI 1.65; 14.48; $p = 0.004$) for reasons of inefficacy ($n = 52$ (22%)) than tocilizumab ($n = 9$ (12.2%)). Remission was the second leading reason for discontinuation of a biologic

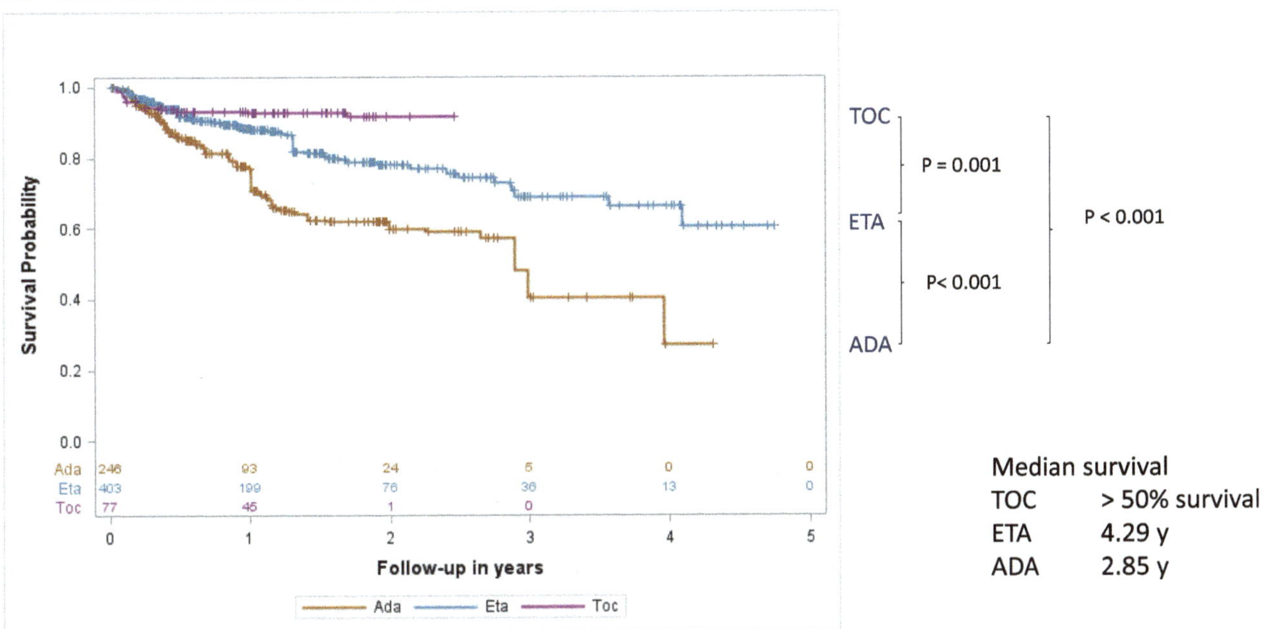

Fig. 4 Drug survival during treatment with etanercept (ETA), adalimumab (*ADA*) or tocilizumab (*TOC*); weighted Kaplan-Meier analyses weighted by an inverse probability of treatment estimated by a generalized propensity score. Significant differences were noted, using the Cox proportional hazard model, between the cohorts treated with adalimumab versus etanercept ($p < 0.001$, hazard ratio 0.60 (0.48–0.75)), adalimumab versus tocilizumab ($p = 0.001$, hazard ratio 0.21 (0.12 – 0.39)) and tocilizumab versus etanercept ($p < 0.001$, hazard ratio 2.82 (1.55 – 5.14))

Table 2 Rates and reasons for discontinuation

	Etanercept cohort	Adalimumab cohort	Tocilizumab cohort	Adalimumab versus etanercept[a]	Tocilizumab versus etanercept[a]	Tocilizumab versus adalimumab[a]
	$n = 419$	$n = 236$	$n = 74$	OR (95% CI); *p* value	OR (95% CI); *p* value	OR (95% CI); *p* value
Discontinuations, *n* (%)	207 (49.4)	142 (60.4)	23 (31.1)	1.57 (1.03; 2.41); 0.037	0.20 (0.09; 0.45); <0.001	0.13 (0.06; 0.29); <0.001
Inefficacy, *n* (%)	50 (11.9)	52 (22.0)	9 (12.2)	1.65 (0.88; 3.08); 0.118	0.34 (0.11; 1.00); 0.050	0.20 (0.07; 0.60); 0.004
Remission, *n* (%)	54 (12.9)	22 (9.3)	2 (2.7)	0.78 (0.43; 1.40); 0.404	0.12 (0.02; 0.79); 0.027	0.16 (0.02; 1.05); 0.056
Intolerance, *n* (%)	15 (3.6)	15 (6.4)	2 (2.7)	2.28 (1.03; 5.04); 0.042	0.84 (0.18; 4.01); 0.826	0.37 (0.08; 1.79); 0.216
Details	Hypersensitivity (5), uveitis (3), vasculitis (1),	Infections (4)[b]	Impetigo (1)			
	Lymphoma (1)	Hypersensitivity (3)	Neutropenia (1)			
	Elevated transaminases (1), neuro-psychiatric (4)[b]	Pustulosis (1), neuro-psychiatric (5)[b]		0.2	5	
Others*, *n* (%)	88 (16.0)	53 (22.4)	10 (13.4)	1.21 (0.74; 1.96); 0.443	0.27 (0.10; 0.72); 0.009	0.22 (0.08; 0.60); 0.003

[a]Analyses weighted by an inverse probability of treatment estimated by a generalized propensity score. [b]Infections included pneumonia and soft tissue infections; Neuropsychiatric included headache, nausea, aggressiveness, anxiety, and vertigo. *beta* regression coefficient for continuous variables, *CI* confidence interval, *OR* odds ratio for categorical variable

agent. Significantly more patients discontinued etanercept due to remission ($n = 54$ (12.9%; odds ratio 8.24 (95% CI 1.27; 53.53); $p = 0.027$) than tocilizumab ($n = 2$ (2.7%)). In general, few patients discontinued due to intolerance (etanercept, $n = 15$ (3.6%); adalimumab, $n = 15$ (6.4%); tocilizumab, $n = 2$ (2.7%)). Patients treated with adalimumab had a higher odds for discontinuation due to intolerance (odds ratio 2.28, 95% CI 1.03; 5.04; $p = 0.042$) than etanercept. The reasons for discontinuation included infections, hypersensitivity, neuropsychiatric events, vasculitis, lymphoma (one patient) and others (Table 2).

Safety

A total of 1484 adverse events (AE) were reported, of which there were 996 in patients receiving etanercept, 386 in patients receiving adalimumab and 102 in patients receiving tocilizumab. Of the adverse events, 148 were classified as serious adverse events (SAE), comprising 119 patients on etanercept, 26 patients on adalimumab and 3 patients on tocilizumab. Thus, the rates of AE and SAE were significantly higher with etanercept than with the other biologic agents (Table 3).

The AE and SAE were classified as adverse events of special interest (AESI) if they represented new onset or aggravation of uveitis ($n = 88$), serious or medically important infections ($n = 66$), neutropenia ($n = 26$), hepatitis/elevated transaminases ($n = 19$), chronic inflammatory bowel disease (CED, $n = 14$), intolerance ($n = 7$), new onset of autoimmunity ($n = 6$), pregnancy ($n = 6$), bleeding disorders ($n = 5$), hyperlipidemia ($n = 4$), stroke ($n = 2$), malignancy ($n = 1$), thrombosis ($n = 1$), or demyelination ($n = 1$). There were no deaths.

Serious or medically important infections observed in the etanercept cohort included pneumonia ($n = 9$), primary

Table 3 Safety

	ADA	ETA	TOC	ETA vs ADA	ADA vs TOC	ETA vs TOC
Patients, *n*	236; 236.4	419	74			
Patient years, *n*	236.4	524,096	72,47364819			
Exposure, years mean ± SD	1.00 ± 0.86	1.25 ± 1.05	0.98 ± 0.60			
Adverse events, *n*; *n*/patient	386; 1.63	996; 2.37	102: 1.38	$p = 0.011$		$p = 0.004$
Rate/100 PY (95% CI)	163.3 (148.8; 180.4)	190.0 (178.6; 202.2)	140,7 (113.5; 167.4)	RR 1.16 (1.03–1.31)	ns	RR 1.35 (1.1–1.66)
Serious adverse events, *n*; *n*/patient	26; 0.11	119; 0.28	3; 0.04	$p = 0.0008$		$p = 0.004$
Rate/100 PY (95% CI)	11.0 (7.5; 16.2)	22.07 (19.0; 27.2)	4.1 (1.3; 12.8)	RR 2.06 (1.35–3.16)	ns	RR 5.48 (1.74–17.25)
Autoimmunopathy, *n*; *n*/patient	3; 0.012	2; 0.004	1; 0.014			
Rate/100 PY (95% CI)	1.27 (0.41; 3.39)	0.38 (0.09; 1.53)	1.38 (0.19; 9.59)	ns	ns	ns
Bleeding disorder, n; *n*/patient	2; 0.008	3; 0.007	0			
Rate/100 PY (95% CI)	0.85 (0.21; 3.38)	0.57 (0.18; 1.17)		ns	ns	ns
CED, n; *n*/patient	1; 0.004	13; 0.031	0	$p = 0.09$		
Rate/100 PY (95% CI)	0.42 (0.06; 3.0)	2.48 (1.44; 4.27)		RR 5.86 (0.77–44.83)	ns	ns
Demyelinisation	0	1; 0.002	0			
Rate/100 PY (95% CI)		0.19 (0.03-1.35)		ns	ns	ns
Hepatitis	6; 0.025	10; 0.024	3; 0.041			
Rate/100 PY (95% CI)	2.54 (1.14; 5.65)	1.91 (1.03; 3.55)	4.14 (1.31; 12.57)	ns	ns	ns
Hyperlipidemia	0	3; 0.007	1; 0.014			
Rate/100 PY (95% CI)		0.57 (0.18; 1.17)	1.38 (0.19; 9.59)	ns	ns	ns
Infection. serious or medically important; *n*; *n*/patient	13; 0.055	50; 0.119	3; 0.041	$p = 0.076$		
Rate/100 PY (95% CI)	5.5 (3.19; 9.47)	9.54 (7.23; 12.59)	4.14 (1.31; 12.57)	RR 1.73 (0.94–3.19)	ns	ns
Intolerance, n; *n*/patient	2; 0.008	3; 0.007	2; 0.027			
Rate/100 PY (95% CI)	0.85 (0.21; 3.38)	0.57 (0.18; 1.17)	2.76 (0.68; 10.81)	ns	ns	ns
Malignancy, n; *n*/patient	0	1; 0.002	0			
Rate/100 PY (95% CI)		0.19 (0.03; 1.35)		ns	ns	ns

ADA adalimumab, *ETA* etanercept, *TOC* tocilimuzab, *PY* person years, *ns* not significant, *RR* relative risk varicella ($n = 7$, none were vaccinated), zoster ($n = 14$), pyelonephritis ($n = 5$), peritonitis ($n = 2$), appendicitis ($n = 2$) and cellulitis ($n = 2$). The events observed with adalimumab were pneumonia ($n = 2$), primary varicella ($n = 4$, none were vaccinated), zoster ($n = 3$), osteomyelitis ($n = 1$), septic arthritis [1] appendicitis ($n = 1$) and influenza ($n = 1$). For tocilizumab, one case each of pneumonia, appendicitis and influenza was reported. No cases of tuberculosis occurred, and apart from herpes zoster, no opportunistic infections were observed.

Some differences in the occurrence of specific AESI were noted among the three treatment cohorts. Neutropenia and serious or medically important infections occurred with significantly greater frequency in the etanercept cohort compared with the adalimumab cohort. Aggravation of uveitis occurred more frequently in the adalimumab cohort than in the tocilizumab cohort, whereas neutropenia occurred significantly less frequently. Compared with the tocilizumab cohort, aggravation and new onset of uveitis occurred more frequently in the etanercept cohort.

Notably, serious or medically important infections and events of chronic inflammatory bowel disease occurred more frequently in the etanercept cohort than in the adalimumab cohort. However, this difference was not significant ($p < 0.05$, Table 3).

Discussion

To our knowledge, this is the first study to directly compare adalimumab, etanercept, and tocilizumab as therapy for polyarticular JIA. Data analysis was restricted to patients initiating treatment after 2011, when tocilizumab became available for the treatment of JIA. The patient population was further restricted to patients with rheumatoid factor-positive or rheumatoid factor-negative polyarthritis and extended oligoarthritis. Patients with systemic JIA (sJIA), enthesitis-related arthritis (ERA) and psoriatic arthritis (PsA) were excluded to acquire a more homogenous patient population and to avoid the effect of differences in approval among the respective drugs; etanercept is approved for ERA and PsA, adalimumab for ERA and tocilizumab for sJIA.

Etanercept was approved for polyarticular JIA in 2000, and adalimumab was approved in 2008. Therefore, considerably more experience has been gained with etanercept than with adalimumab or tocilizumab. Accordingly, etanercept was used much more frequently than either adalimumab or tocilizumab. In the Dutch ABC registry, etanercept was also the most frequently prescribed biologic agent for non-systemic JIA [20]. In that study, greater drug experience was the most important factor driving the decision to use etanercept rather than adalimumab. Adalimumab was favored by Dutch pediatric rheumatologists for patients who had preceding uveitis. Similar findings were obtained in the current BIKER population.

For German pediatric rheumatologists, we may speculate that the number of patients starting on etanercept as their first biologic agent is higher because there is prolonged experience with etanercept compared to the other biologic agents. Adalimumab was predominantly chosen as the first biologic agent in patients with concomitant uveitis. Finally, the relative rarity of using tocilizumab can either be attributed to the fact that first, it is the biologic agent with the least experience of use and second, that currently only the intravenous infusion is approved, which means it can only be used in centers with an infusion facility. The decision as to which biologic agent is used is not influenced by a protocol, algorithm, national recommendation or guideline, or by the registry itself. Adalimumab was used more frequently than etanercept as a second-line biologic agent but had comparable efficacy in both second-line and first-line users [12].

There were few other differences among the studied cohorts. Patients in the adalimumab or tocilizumab cohorts were older than those in the etanercept cohort, and there were fewer patients with extended oligoarthritis in the tocilizumab cohort. A striking difference was observed in use of concomitant MTX, which was much more common in the etanercept cohort, followed by the adalimumab cohort. Fewer than 50% of the patients in the tocilizumab cohort received concomitant MTX therapy. This observation was surprising because etanercept is approved only for monotherapy, whereas both of the other biologic agents are also approved for combination therapy.

Despite these differences, PedACR treatment response rates were comparable for all three biologic agents. The majority of patients demonstrated marked improvement after 3 months of treatment. The response rates thereafter remained stable or increased further. No apparent differences among the three treatment cohorts were noted, in accordance with the response rates observed in open-label phases of the pivotal randomized controlled withdrawal studies of each of the drugs [6, 13, 21]. However, in the most recent clinical trial investigating etanercept, patients with extended oligoarticular JIA experienced a much higher rate of clinical improvement [9].

There was a small but significant difference in reported absolute disease activity at baseline, as measured by the JADAS10, which was highest in the tocilizumab cohort and lowest in the adalimumab cohort. This difference was balanced by the inverse probability of treatment allocation estimated by a generalized propensity score. The JADAS score fell significantly in all cohorts after treatment. The residual JADAS at the last observation (mean observation time in all cohorts of approximately 1 year) was highest in the etanercept cohort. The greatest adjusted mean reduction in the JADAS was observed in the etanercept cohort; in contrast, the greatest observed mean reduction was in the tocilizumab cohort.

As tocilizumab may have had a higher influence on the acute phase response via its inhibitory capability on the IL-6 axis, the JADAS10 and the clinical JADAS (cJADAS), which considers only three clinical parameters were compared. Interestingly, at baseline 144 of 407 patients (35.4%) in the etanercept cohort and 26 of 74 patients (35.1%) in the tocilizumab cohort had higher classic JADAS than cJADAS. Upon treatment (month 3 to 24), 91 of 856 patients (10.6%) in the etanercept cohort and 22 of 187 patients (12.4%) from the tocilizumab cohort had higher classic JADAS than cJADAS. Thus, both at baseline and after treatment the results were very much comparable, and direct inhibition of IL-6 seems not to influence the laboratory parameters of the JADAS10 more than TNF inhibition. As we used definitions for MDA and remission based on the complete JADAS, the original JADAS10 was preferred over the cJADAS, which considers only three clinical parameters. Comparable numbers of patients achieved JADAS remission and JADAS minimal disease activity in a large database study [16, 18]. No differences were identified among the cohorts in terms of either speed to remission/MDA or absolute remission/MDA rates.

Interestingly, the drug survival rates for the three biologic agents were different in this study. Whereas etanercept and tocilizumab showed comparable drug survival, significantly more patients discontinued adalimumab. The main reason for adalimumab discontinuation was lack of therapeutic response or inefficacy, which differed significantly compared with the discontinuation frequency with etanercept due to inefficacy/lack of therapeutic effect. This could have been influenced by the higher proportion of patients on MTX in the etanercept cohort. It is possible that Adalimumab in monotherapy could lead to more immunogenicity and secondary loss of efficacy.

Remission was the second leading reason for drug discontinuation. Significantly fewer patients discontinued tocilizumab than etanercept for reasons of remission. This finding is remarkable because the rates of JADAS remission were not different. The mean/median duration of treatment with both etanercept and tocilizumab were comparable. There were also no differences in the number of patients on prolonged treatment: a quarter of the patients had been treated with etanercept for more than 1.7 years, which was comparable to more than 1.5 years in a quarter of the patients using tocilizumab. It is likely that tocilizumab adherence was affected by its more frequent use as a second-line biologic agent compared with etanercept and thus an earlier biologic treatment had failed. It can be speculated that in this situation, successful drug treatment likely will not be discontinued.

Very few patients discontinued their biologic agent due to intolerance, which suggests that they are not only very effective but also very well-tolerated. The pattern of AE observed in this study of patients with pJIA is consistent with the known safety profile of adalimumab, etanercept and tocilizumab [6, 10, 13]. Interestingly, there were no cases of tuberculosis. Apart from herpes zoster, which has been regarded as an opportunistic infection by some authors, no other opportunistic infections were reported. Furthermore, only one case of malignancy was reported, in which an Epstein-Barr virus (EBV)-associated lymphoma developed in a child who had been treated with MTX and etanercept. This observation is preliminary due to the short observation period of this analysis to compare biologic agents used contemporaneously, thus restricting the analysis to patients treated after 2011. Notably, a significant number of malignancies have been observed in the BIKER registry since 2001 [22, 23].

The observed discontinuation rate was comparable to that reported in an Italian cohort, in which 165 of 301 patients with various categories of JIA discontinued biologic treatment [24]. The majority (135 patients) discontinued for reasons of treatment failure, including a lack or loss of efficacy, and AE. Most patients discontinued due to intolerance (34.6%), which was very different compared with our cohort. This discrepancy can be explained, in part, by the frequent use of infliximab in the Italian cohort. Among this cohort, 39% of patients discontinued biologic treatment due to adverse events. Because infliximab is not approved for JIA in Germany, it cannot by studied systematically in BIKER.

In the present analysis, the overall safety of the biologic agents was acceptable. The rate of serious or medically important infections (4.1–9.5/100 patient-years) was comparable to that observed in other registry cohorts. In a British cohort, medically important infections occurred more frequently among users of TNF inhibitors than in a non-biologic control cohort, but the rate of serious infections was not significantly different [25]. Interestingly, new onset Crohn's disease or ulcerative colitis mostly occurred in the etanercept cohort, which is consistent with previous findings [26]. Etanercept has been shown to lack efficacy toward CED [27]. However, the rate of uveitis was highest in the adalimumab cohort, which could be attributed to a selection bias, as described previously [28]. Patients with uveitis as a comorbidity had a four times higher chance of receiving adalimumab rather than etanercept [28]. Other AESI were reported infrequently. It is interesting to note that the rates of reported neutropenia, hyperlipidemia or elevated liver enzymes were not higher in the tocilizumab cohort, as might be expected based on analyses conducted in adult patients with rheumatoid arthritis [27].

The results from randomized controlled trials (RCT) cannot easily be extrapolated to routine care. Several specific features of the RCT must be considered. The inclusion and exclusion criteria may be responsible for a more homogenous study population; for example, comorbidities and concomitant drugs are usually exclusion criteria. Clinical control is tighter, prescribing practices are more stringent in a trial over time, and drug adherence may be influenced by the desire to retain a patient in the study. Thus, the RCT population may not reflect routine clinical care. By comparison, registry analyses reflect routine care and may, in part, be superior to RCTs despite having other limitations.

Observational studies of cohorts of unselected patients receiving routine care may allow better comparisons of the drugs used, although the lack of randomization must be considered when interpreting the results. In a smaller Dutch observational study of 214 patients with JIA [29], the use of etanercept and adalimumab was evaluated in routine care; however, neither the efficacy nor the survival rates were compared.

Our results reflect clinical practice and do not include the very early introduction of biologic agents, which has been evaluated in the TREAT and ACUTE-JIA studies [30, 31]. Furthermore, the observations obtained from a registry are not a substitute for clinical trials. Comparative head-to-head studies with biologic agents in juvenile idiopathic arthritis as performed in adult patients with rheumatoid arthritis would be an ideal approach, but the lower prevalence of JIA may render this an unrealistic target.

Conclusions

So far, in clinical practice etanercept remains the most frequently used first-line biologic agent for the treatment of polyarticular JIA. The three biologic agents adalimumab, etanercept and tocilizumab had comparable efficacy. Overall, tolerance was acceptable. Interestingly, compliance was highest with tocilizumab and lowest with adalimumab. This study provides the first indication for the comparison of different biologic agents in polyarticular JIA based on observational study data, with all their weaknesses, and demonstrates the need for well-controlled head-to-head studies for confirmation.

Additional files

Additional file 1: Table S1. Patient characteristics (unweighted as reported in BIKER). (DOCX 17 kb)

Additional file 2: Figure S1. Pediatric ACR30/50/70/90 improvement in patients receiving etanercept, adalimumab or tocilizumab as a first-line or second-line biologic agent. (PPT 172 kb)

Additional file 3: Figure S2. Drug survival during treatment with etanercept, adalimumab or tocilizumab (combined cohorts) depending on the concomitant use of methotrexate, weighted Kaplan-Meier analyses weighted by an inverse probability of treatment estimated by a generalized propensity score. No significant differences were found between the two groups. (PPT 74 kb)

Abbreviations

AE: adverse event; AESI: adverse events of special interest; BIKER: Biologics in Pediatric Rheumatology Registry; CHAQ: Childhood Health Assessment Questionnaire; DMARD: disease-modifying antirheumatic drug; ERA: enthesitis-related arthritis; GEE: generalised estimation equations; HR: hazard ratio; IL: interleukin; JADAS: Juvenile Disease Activity Score; JIA: juvenile idiopathic arthritis; MDA: minimal disease activity; MTX: methotrexate; PedACR: Pediatric ACR criteria; PsA: psoriatic arthritis; RCT: randomized controlled trials; SAE: serious adverse event; SD: standard deviation; sJIA: systemic juvenile idiopathic arthritis; TNF: tumor necrosis factor

Acknowledgements

The BIKER study group included the pediatric rheumatology departments at the following universities and hospitals in Austria and Germany: Aachen, Berlin-Charité, Berlin-Buch, Bremen, Celle, Duesseldorf, Hamburg, Innsbruck, Neunkirchen, Sankt Augustin, Stuttgart, Tuebingen, Ulm and Vienna. This study would not have been possible without the collaboration of numerous German and Austrian pediatric rheumatologists, patients and their parents. Collaborators: Angelika Thon, Gerd Ganser, Markus Hufnagel, Christian Hedrich, Andreas Urban, Ralf Trauzeddel, Daniel Windschall, Frank Dressler, Prasaad Oommen, Rolf Kuester, Doris Meyer, Gundula Böschow, Michael Rühlmann, Dirk Föll, Rietschel, Bernd-Ulrich, Keck, Michael Borte, Thomas Berger, Maria Haller, Betina Rogalski, Wolfgang Emminger, Ina Feddersen, Michaela Sailer-Hoeck, Catarina Schuetz, Hermann Girschick, Thilo Schmalbach, Sonja Mrusek

Funding

The study sponsor according to law is GH. The BIKER registry is supported by an unrestricted grant from Pfizer, Germany, Abbvie, Germany and Roche, Germany. The companies had no influence on study design or on the collection, analysis, or interpretation of the data, the writing of the manuscript or the decision to submit the manuscript for publication. Publication of this article was not contingent upon approval by the study sponsors, the German Registry.

Authors' contributions

GH conceived the study, contributed to study design, performed data analysis and interpretation and drafted the paper. AK performed data analysis and interpretation and drafted the paper. JK performed the statistical analysis. KM was involved in the conception of the study, contributed to study design and performed data analysis and interpretation. HIH, FWH, JKD, JPH and HA participated in the design of the study and helped to draft the manuscript. All authors read and approved the final manuscript.

Competing interests

Gerd Horneff has received research funds, advisory board membership and honorary fees from Abbvie, Pfizer and Roche. Kirsten Minden has received research grants from Abbvie, Pfizer and Roche and honorary fees from Abbvie, Pfizer, Genzyme and Pharm-Allergan. Toni Hospach has received advisory board membership and honoraria from Pfizer, Abbvie and Roche.

Consent for publication

Not applicable.

Ethics approval and consent to participate

The study was conducted in accordance with the protocol, ICH GCP, FDA regulations governing clinical study conduct, ethical principles that have their origin in the Declaration of Helsinki, 1996 revision and 2000 revision with subsequent clarifications, and all applicable local regulations. Before the study was initiated, the study protocol, the informed consent form and subject information were submitted to the responsible independent ethics committee of the Aerztekammer Nordrhein, Duesseldorf, Germany for review. Parents/legal guardian signed the informed consent form before any study-related procedures occurred.

Author details

[1]Department of Pediatrics, Centre of General Pediatrics and Neonatology, Asklepios Clinic Sankt Augustin, 53757 Sankt Augustin, Germany. [2]German Rheumatism Research Centre Berlin, and Children's University Hospital Charité, Berlin, Germany. [3]Prof Hess Children's Hospital, Bremen, Germany. [4]Department of Pediatrics, University of Tuebingen, 72076 Tuebingen, Germany. [5]German Centre for Pediatric and Adolescent Rheumatology, Garmisch-Partenkirchen, Germany. [6]Department of Pediatrics, Section of Rheumatology, Olgahospital, Klinikum, Stuttgart, Germany.

References

1. Petty RE, Southwood TR, Manners P, Baum J, Glass DN, Goldenberg J, et al. International league of associations for rheumatology classification of juvenile idiopathic arthritis: second revision, Edmonton, 2001. J Rheumatol. 2004;31:390–2.
2. Danner S, Sordet C, Terzic J, Donato L, Velten M, Fischbach M, et al. Epidemiology of juvenile idiopathic arthritis in Alsace, France. J Rheumatol. 2006;33:1377–81.
3. Giannini EH, Brewer EJ, Kuzmina N, Shaikov A, Maximov A, Vorontsov I, et al. Methotrexate in resistant juvenile rheumatoid arthritis. Results of the U.S.A.-U.S.S.R. double-blind, placebo-controlled trial. the Pediatric Rheumatology Collaborative Study Group and The Cooperative Children's Study Group. N Engl J Med. 1992;326:1043–9. doi:10.1056/NEJM199204163261602.
4. Dueckers G, Guellac N, Arbogast M, Dannecker G, Foeldvari I, Frosch M, et al. Evidence and consensus based treatment guidelines 2010 for juvenile idiopathic arthritis by the German Society of Paediatric Rheumatology. Klin Padiatr. 2011;223:386–94. doi:10.1055/s-0031-1287837.
5. Beukelman T, Patkar NM, Saag KG, Tolleson-Rinehart S, Cron RQ, DeWitt EM, et al. 2011 American College of Rheumatology recommendations for the treatment of juvenile idiopathic arthritis: Initiation and safety monitoring of therapeutic agents for the treatment of arthritis and systemic features. Arthritis Care Res. 2011;63:465–82. doi:10.1002/acr.20460.
6. Lovell DJ, Giannini EH, Reiff A, Cawkwell GD, Silverman ED, Nocton JJ, et al. Etanercept in children with polyarticular juvenile rheumatoid arthritis. Pediatric Rheumatology Collaborative Study Group. N Engl J Med. 2000;342:763–9. doi:10.1056/NEJM200003163421103.
7. Prince FH, Twilt M, ten Cate R, et al. Long-term follow-up on effectiveness and safety of etanercept in juvenile idiopathic arthritis: the Dutch national register. Ann Rheum Dis. 2009;68:635–41.
8. Horneff G, Schmeling H, Biedermann T, Foeldvari I, Ganser G, Girschick HJ, et al. The German etanercept registry for treatment of juvenile idiopathic arthritis. Ann Rheum Dis. 2004;63:1638–44. doi:10.1136/ard.2003.014886.
9. Horneff G, De Bock F, Foeldvari I, Girschick HJ, Michels H, Moebius D, et al. Safety and efficacy of combination of etanercept and methotrexate compared to treatment with etanercept only in patients with juvenile idiopathic arthritis (JIA): preliminary data from the German JIA Registry. Ann Rheum Dis. 2009;68:519–25. doi:10.1136/ard.2007.087593.
10. Ruperto N, Giannini EH, Pistorio A, Brunner HI, Martini A, Lovell DJ. Is it time to move to active comparator trials in juvenile idiopathic arthritis?: a review of current study designs. Arthritis Rheum. 2010;62:3131–9. doi:10.1002/art.27670.
11. Ramanan AV, Dick AD, McKay A, Jones A, Williamson P, Compeyrot-Lacassagne S, Hardwick B, Hickey H, Hughes D, Woo P, Benton D, Edelsten C, Beresford MW. A Randomised Controlled Trial of the Clinical Effectiveness, Safety and Cost-Effectiveness of Adalimumab in Combination with Methotrexate for the Treatment of Juvenile Idiopathic Arthritis Associated Uveitis [abstract]. Arthritis Rheumatol. 2015; 67(suppl 10). http://acrabstracts.org/abstract/a-randomised-controlled-trial-of-the-clinical-effectiveness-safety-and-cost-effectiveness-of-adalimumab-in-combination-with-methotrexate-for-the-treatment-of-juvenile-idiopathic-arthritis-associated/.
12. Schmeling H, Minden K, Foeldvari I, Ganser G, Hospach T, Horneff G. Efficacy and safety of adalimumab as the first and second biologic agent in juvenile idiopathic arthritis: the German Biologics JIA Registry. Arthritis Rheumatol. 2014;66:2580–9. doi:10.1002/art.38741.
13. Brunner HI, Ruperto N, Zuber Z, Keane C, Harari O, Kenwright A, et al. Efficacy and safety of tocilizumab in patients with polyarticular-course juvenile idiopathic arthritis: results from a phase 3, randomised, double-blind withdrawal trial. Ann Rheum Dis. 2015;74:1110–7. doi:10.1136/annrheumdis-2014-205351. annrheumdis-2014-205351.
14. Klein A, Horneff G. Treatment strategies for juvenile idiopathic arthritis. Expert Opin Pharmacother. 2009;10:3049–60. doi:10.1517/14656560903386300.
15. Horneff G, Schmeling H. Biedermann et al. The German Etanercept Registry for treatment of juvenile idiopathic arthritis (JIA). Ann Rheum Dis. 2004;63:1638–44.
16. Consolaro A, Ruperto N, Bazso A, Pistorio A, Magni-Manzoni S, Filocamo G, et al. Development and validation of a composite disease activity score for juvenile idiopathic arthritis. Arthritis Rheum. 2009;61:658–66. doi:10.1002/art.24516.
17. Giannini EH, Ruperto N, Ravelli A, Lovell DJ, Felson DT, Martini A. Preliminary definition of improvement in juvenile arthritis. Arthritis Rheum. 1997;40:1202–9. doi:10.1002/1529-0131(199707)40:7<1202::AID-ART3>3.0.CO;2-R.
18. Consolaro A, Bracciolini G, Ruperto N, Pistorio A, Magni-Manzoni S, Malattia C, et al. Remission, minimal disease activity, and acceptable symptom state in juvenile idiopathic arthritis: defining criteria based on the juvenile arthritis disease activity score. Arthritis Rheum. 2012;64:2366–74. doi:10.1002/art.34373.
19. Singh G, Athreya BH, Fries JF, Goldsmith DP. Measurement of health status in children with juvenile rheumatoid arthritis. Arthritis Rheum. 1994;37:1761–9. doi:10.1002/art.1780371209.
20. Otten MH, Anink J, Prince FH, Twilt M, Vastert SJ, Ten Cate R, et al. Trends in prescription of biological agents and outcomes of juvenile idiopathic arthritis: results of the Dutch national Arthritis and Biologics in Children Register. Ann Rheum Dis. 2015;74:1379–86. doi:10.1136/annrheumdis-2013-204641.
21. Lovell DJ, Ruperto N, Goodman S, Reiff A, Jung L, Jarosova K, et al. Adalimumab with or without methotrexate in juvenile rheumatoid arthritis. N Engl J Med. 2008;359:810–20. doi:10.1056/NEJMoa0706290.
22. Horneff G, Foeldvari I, Minden K, Moebius D, Hospach T. Report on malignancies in the German juvenile idiopathic arthritis registry. Rheumatology (Oxford). 2011;50:230–6.
23. Horneff G, Klein A, Oommen PT, Hospach A, Foeldvari I, Feddersen I, Minden K. Update on malignancies in children with juvenile idiopathic arthritis in the German BIKER Registry.Clin Exp Rheumatol. 2016 Sep 8. [Epub ahead of print]
24. Romano M, Pontikaki I, Gattinara M, Ardoino I, Donati C, Boracchi P, et al. Drug survival and reasons for discontinuation of the first course of biological therapy in 301 juvenile idiopathic arthritis patients. Reumatismo. 2013;65:278–85. doi:10.4081/reumatismo.2013.682.
25. Davies R, Southwood TR, Kearsley-Fleet L, Lunt M, Hyrich KL, British Society for Paediatric, Adolescent Rheumatology Etanercept Cohort Study. Medically significant infections are increased in patients with juvenile idiopathic arthritis treated with etanercept: results from the British Society for Paediatric and Adolescent Rheumatology Etanercept Cohort Study. Arthritis Rheumatol. 2015;67:2487–94. doi:10.1002/art.39197.
26. Barthel D, Ganser G, Kuester RM, Onken N, Minden K, Girschick HJ, et al. Inflammatory bowel disease in juvenile idiopathic arthritis patients treated with biologics. J Rheumatol. 2015;42:2160–5. doi:10.3899/jrheum.140472.
27. Sandborn WJ, Hanauer SB, Katz S, Safdi M, Wolf DG, Baerg RD, et al. Etanercept for active Crohn's disease: a randomised, double-blind, placebo-controlled trial. Gastroenterology. 2001;121:1088–94.
28. Foeldvari I, Becker I, Horneff G. Uveitis events during Adalimumab, Etanercept, and methotrexate therapy in juvenile idiopathic arthritis: data from the biologics in Pediatric Rheumatology Registry. Arthritis Care Res (Hoboken). 2015;67:1529–35.
29. Anink J, Otten MH, Gorter SL, Prince FHM, van Rossum MAJ, van den Berg JM, et al. Treatment choices of paediatric rheumatologists for juvenile idiopathic arthritis: etanercept or adalimumab? Rheumatology (Oxford). 2013;52:1674–9. doi:10.1093/rheumatology/ket170.
30. Wallace CA, Giannini EH, Spalding SJ, Hashkes PJ, O'Neil KM, Zeft AS, et al. Trial of early aggressive therapy in polyarticular juvenile idiopathic arthritis. Arthritis Rheum. 2012;64:2012–21. doi:10.1002/art.34343.
31. Tynjälä P, Vähäsalo P, Tarkiainen M, Kröger L, Aalto K, Malin M, et al. Aggressive combination drug therapy in very early polyarticular juvenile idiopathic arthritis (ACUTE-JIA): a multicentre randomised open-label clinical trial. Ann Rheum Dis. 2011;70:1605–12. doi:10.1136/ard.2010.143347.

12

The risk of hospitalized infection following initiation of biologic agents versus methotrexate in the treatment of juvenile idiopathic arthritis

Timothy Beukelman*, Fenglong Xie, John W. Baddley, Lang Chen, Melissa L. Mannion, Kenneth G. Saag, Jie Zhang and Jeffrey R. Curtis

Abstract

Background: In the present study, we compared the incidence of hospitalized infection among children with juvenile idiopathic arthritis (JIA) following initiation of treatment with biologic agents versus methotrexate (MTX).

Methods: We used national Medicaid claims data from 2000 through 2010 to create cohorts of children with JIA who were new users of tumor necrosis factor inhibitors (TNFi), anakinra, and MTX (without concurrent biologic agent use) as defined by a 6-month baseline period of nonuse. Because most anakinra users have systemic juvenile idiopathic arthritis (SJIA), we used claims to identify MTX users who likely had SJIA. Among TNFi users, concurrent MTX use was a time-varying covariate. The study outcome was a primary hospital discharge diagnosis of infection. We calculated adjusted hazard ratios (aHRs) to compare infection rates between biologic agents and MTX.

Results: We identified 3075 new MTX users (160 with SJIA), 2713 new TNFi users, and 247 new anakinra users. There was no increased risk of infection associated with TNFi monotherapy versus MTX (aHR 1.19, 95 % CI 0.72–1.94) or with TNFi + MTX combination therapy versus MTX (aHR 1.23, 95 % CI 0.69–2.17). Baseline high-dose oral glucocorticoid use (≥10 mg/day of prednisone) was associated with infection (aHR 2.03 [95 % CI 1.21–3.39] versus no oral glucocorticoid). Anakinra was associated with infection versus MTX (aHR 3.53 95 % CI 1.83–6.82), but less so compared with MTX users with SJIA (aHR 2.69, 95 % CI 0.82–8.82).

Conclusions: Neither TNFi monotherapy nor TNFi + MTX combination therapy was significantly associated with hospitalized infection compared with MTX. Anakinra was significantly associated with infection, but there was likely residual confounding by disease phenotype.

Background

Biologic agents, especially tumor necrosis factor inhibitors (TNFi), are widely used in the treatment of juvenile idiopathic arthritis (JIA), and the frequency of their use continues to increase [1–3]. All therapeutic agents are associated with risks, and serious infections are the most commonly occurring serious adverse events in JIA that are possibly caused by biologic agents. Assessing and contextualizing the risk of infection due to use of biologic agents is complicated by the facts that the disease process of JIA itself likely increases the rate of infection [4] and that active JIA must be treated with other systemic immunosuppression, if not with biologic agents, to prevent permanent disability [1]. Thus, there is a clear need for comparative studies of the relative safety of biologic agents in JIA. Despite the frequent use of biologic agents and the need for comparative studies, only a few such studies have been published to date [5, 6].

Among published comparative studies, some do not suggest a significant difference between infection rates

* Correspondence: tbeukelman@peds.uab.edu
The University of Alabama at Birmingham, 1720 2nd Ave S, Birmingham, AL, 35233, USA

associated with TNFi versus methotrexate (MTX) [4, 7], while others do suggest an increased rate associated with TNFi [8, 9]. Similar to the situation with studies of adults with rheumatoid arthritis in which investigators have reported discrepant results, these differences are likely attributable to variations in study populations and study designs [10]. For example, in our previously published study in which we reported no increased risk of infection with TNFi versus MTX, we used a prevalent-user design rather than a methodologically superior new-user design that was not feasible, owing to limited available data at the time [4, 11].

Current JIA treatment recommendations call for the addition of TNFi to MTX (rather than TNFi monotherapy) owing to the demonstrated increased effectiveness of this approach [1]. Nevertheless, many children with JIA are treated with TNFi monotherapy [2]. Importantly, the relative safety of combination therapy versus monotherapy is unclear. The rate of infection associated with TNFi + MTX combination therapy was not increased versus TNFi monotherapy in two published observational studies conducted outside the United States [8, 12], but this issue has not been fully assessed in other studies.

There are several non-TNFi biologic agents currently used for the treatment of JIA, including abatacept, anakinra, canakinumab, and tocilizumab [1, 13]. The relative risk of infection with these biologic agents in JIA is not known [5, 6]. The interleukin (IL)-1 inhibitors anakinra and canakinumab are currently used almost exclusively to treat systemic juvenile idiopathic arthritis (SJIA) [1, 3, 13, 14]. Limited reports of infections associated with anakinra suggest a possible increased risk of infection, but there are no published comparative studies [5]. Importantly, SJIA has a pathogenesis and treatment approach different from those for the other categories of JIA, including the more frequent use of systemic glucocorticoids (GCs) at higher doses [13, 15, 16]. Very little is known about the risks of infection associated with SJIA and its treatment in clinical practice.

In an attempt to address these knowledge gaps, we used national U.S. Medicaid administrative claims data to compare rates of hospitalized infection among children with JIA who were newly starting biologic agents versus those newly starting MTX without concurrent biologic agent use.

Methods

Data source

We obtained local institutional review board approval. We conducted this study using Medicaid Analytic eXtract (MAX) files from all 50 U.S. states and the District of Columbia from 2000 through 2010, inclusive. These were the most recent data available to us at the time of the study. MAX files contain medical and pharmacy administrative claims records for low-income children enrolled in Medicaid (U.S. government medical assistance). We have previously published studies of JIA using this data source [4, 17].

Study cohorts

Using pharmacy and infusion claims, we identified patients who were new users of MTX or biologic agents, including TNFi (etanercept, adalimumab, infliximab, golimumab, and certolizumab), abatacept, anakinra, canakinumab, and tocilizumab. New use was defined by a 6-month baseline clean period of nonuse during which the patient had full medical and pharmacy benefits. Additionally, new users of any TNFi had no use of any TNFi or any other biologic agent during the baseline period (i.e., those switching biologic agents were excluded). Only the first observed use of each medication was considered for new use. Individual patients could have more than one episode of new use during the study period (e.g., MTX and then TNFi). New users who had at least one physician diagnosis code consistent with JIA (International Classification of Diseases, Ninth Revision [ICD-9], codes 714, 696.0, 720) before age 16 years and prior to the new-use prescription fill date (index date) were included. We excluded patients who had any of the following at any time prior to the index date: (1) a physician diagnosis code for JIA when less than 6 months of age; (2) any physician diagnosis code or hospital discharge diagnosis code for inflammatory bowel disease (ICD-9 codes 555, 556); (3) any physician diagnosis code or hospital discharge diagnosis code for malignancy, organ transplant, or HIV infection; and (4) two or more physician diagnosis codes or hospital discharge diagnosis codes for other rheumatologic diseases (systemic lupus erythematosus and other diffuse connective tissue diseases, vasculitis, sarcoidosis) that were at least 7 days but more than 183 days apart. New MTX users were excluded if they used biologic agents at any time prior to the index date.

In order to better evaluate relative infection rates associated with the biologic agents used to treat SJIA, we attempted to identify patients within the MTX new-user cohort who were very likely to have SJIA. However, within ICD-9 there is no specific, reliable physician diagnosis code for SJIA. Therefore, we considered new users of MTX who met any of the following at any time in the data to have SJIA: (1) any physician diagnosis code or hospital discharge diagnosis code for macrophage activation syndrome (ICD-9 code 288.4); (2) any receipt of anakinra, canakinumab, or rilonacept following receipt of MTX; (3) any receipt of cyclosporine in the absence of any physician diagnosis code for uveitis; and (4) any receipt of thalidomide or lenalidomide. Among children with JIA, the development of macrophage activation syndrome [18] and use of the selected medications mentioned above [1, 13] occur nearly exclusively in children with SJIA.

Medication exposures

The baseline mean daily GC dose was determined by summing the total cumulative oral GC dose dispensed during the 6-month baseline period in milligrams of prednisone equivalents and dividing by 183 days. Baseline mean daily GC dose was categorized as none, low dose (<10 mg of prednisone equivalents per day), and high dose (≥10 mg of prednisone equivalents per day). Among new TNFi users, concurrent MTX use was determined on a time-varying basis during study follow-up. The resultant medication exposure categories were TNFi monotherapy and TNFi + MTX combination therapy, and patients changed exposure categories during follow-up on the basis of their treatment received. Owing to the small number of observed outcomes, we did not adjust or restrict for concurrent MTX use among new anakinra users. The concurrent use of cyclosporine was determined on a time-varying basis during follow-up.

Study follow-up

Follow-up began on the index date. Follow-up was censored at the first date that any of the following occurred: (1) prescription for corresponding medication cohort (MTX or specific biologic agent) not filled within 90 days of the days supplied by the previous filled prescription or typical infusion interval (e.g., 56 days for infliximab), (2) meeting any of the study cohort exclusion criteria, (3) experiencing the primary study outcome of hospitalized infection, or (4) end of the study period. Patients in the new MTX user cohort were immediately censored if they received a biologic agent.

Covariates

Sex, race, and age at index date were determined. The presence of physician diagnosis codes or hospital discharge diagnosis codes for the comorbid conditions of psoriasis, diabetes mellitus, and asthma during the 6-month baseline period was assessed. The occurrence of infection during the 6-month baseline period was assessed and assigned to one of three hierarchical levels: none, nonprimary hospital discharge diagnosis or outpatient physician diagnosis code, primary hospital discharge diagnosis (i.e., a nonprimary discharge or outpatient diagnosis was not considered in the presence of a primary hospital discharge diagnosis). Baseline GC use and time-varying concurrent cyclosporine use during follow-up were modeled as covariates.

Study outcome

The study outcome was a primary hospital discharge diagnosis of infection. The outcome included ICD-9 codes reflecting infections by all organisms (e.g., bacteria, viruses, fungi). As part of sensitivity analyses, we included any hospital discharge diagnosis of infection (i.e., primary and nonprimary hospital discharge diagnoses). The list of infection ICD-9 codes was adapted from previously validated lists [19–21].

Analyses

We determined the baseline characteristics of the patients in each new medication use cohort. We did not perform statistical tests of the differences between the cohorts, because individual patients could contribute to multiple cohorts and the MTX with SJIA cohort was a subset of the MTX cohort.

We determined crude infection rates for each new medication user cohort if there were at least ten observed infection outcomes. We considered all TNFi inhibitors together as a group compared with MTX in further analyses.

We used Cox proportional hazards regression models to compare the incidence of infections between new biologic agent users and new MTX users. For new users of TNFi, we compared TNFi monotherapy and TNFi + MTX combination therapy versus MTX within the same model. For the new users of anakinra, we separately compared ANA versus MTX and ANA versus MTX with SJIA. We calculated adjusted hazard ratios (aHRs) by using multivariable models to adjust for covariates that were potential confounders of the association between the medication exposures and the outcome. Because individual patients could contribute to more than one new-user cohort, a sandwich variance estimator was applied to account for additional correlations in the data [22]. To evaluate the possibility of statistical interaction between oral GC and biologic agent use and the association with hospitalized infection, we evaluated separate multivariable hazard models for children with and without use of oral GCs during the 6-month baseline period.

We analyzed infection rates among individual TNFi with etanercept as the referent when there were at least ten infection outcomes present. We compared patients' characteristics among the individual TNFi using chi-square tests. In the multivariable Cox regression models for the comparison of individual TNFi, we additionally adjusted for the number of prior biologic agents used (more than 6 months prior to the index date), and we ignored the concurrent use of MTX.

To evaluate the robustness of our primary results, we performed the following sensitivity analyses: expanded the outcome definition to include hospital discharge diagnosis for infection in any position (i.e., included nonprimary discharge diagnoses), decreased the infection risk window following the days supplied by the last prescription from 90 days to 30 days, decreased the time period used to calculate the baseline mean daily oral GC dose from 183 days to 60 days, and censored all follow-up at 6 months following the index date.

Results

The patients' characteristics at the time of newly starting MTX, TNFi, or anakinra are shown in Table 1. There was an insufficient number of infection outcomes to report on new users of abatacept, canakinumab, or tocilizumab. The characteristics of new MTX users with SJIA are also shown. Patients in the MTX with SJIA subcohort met our definition because of any use of cyclosporine without uveitis (55 %), future use of IL-1 inhibitor (51 %), diagnosis of macrophage activation syndrome (10 %), or any use of thalidomide or lenalidomide (8 %).

There were clear differences between the cohorts. Specifically, the TNFi users were older, and the anakinra users had higher baseline GC use and more frequent primary hospitalized infections during the baseline period. The MTX users with SJIA were more similar to the anakinra new users with respect to GC use and baseline infections than were all MTX users.

Table 2 shows the crude infection rates for each of the medication cohorts. The crude infection rates for all MTX users, TNFi monotherapy, and TNFi + MTX combination therapy were similar, and ranged from 1.46 to 1.74 infections per 100 person-years. The infection rate for anakinra users was markedly higher at 8.41 infections per 100 person-years. The infection rate for MTX with SJIA was higher than for all MTX users at 2.64 per 100 person-years.

The most commonly observed types of hospitalized infection overall were pneumonia (19 %), bladder and kidney (13 %), and cellulitis and abscess (10 %). The frequency distribution of the types of infection was not significantly different among new users of MTX, TNFi, and anakinra (data not shown). We observed two hospitalized infections that could be considered opportunistic infections: one case of herpes zoster in a patient receiving TNFi and one case of coccidioidal meningitis in a patient receiving MTX (without prior observed TNFi use).

Table 3 shows the relative hazards of infection in the analysis of TNFi versus MTX. There was not a significantly increased risk of infection associated with TNFi monotherapy or TNFi + MTX combination therapy compared with new use of MTX without concurrent or prior biologic agent use (aHR 1.19 [95 % CI 0.72–1.94] and aHR 1.23 [95 % CI 0.69–2.17], respectively). In the hazard models, adjustment for potential confounders slightly increased the relative hazard associated with TNFi. This is owing to confounding by patient age; older

Table 1 Characteristics of patients at the time of medication initiation

	MTX	All TNFi	Anakinra	MTX with SJIA
Number of patients	3075	2713	247	160
Mean age, years (SD)	9.0 (4.7)	10.9 (4.7)	9.4 (4.8)	7.4 (4.6)
Median age (IQR)	9.0 (5.0–13.0)	11.0 (7.0–15.0)	9.0 (6.0–13.0)	6.5 (3.0–11.0)
Female sex, %	66.0	68.3	64.4	56.9
Asthma, %	8.2	6.1	6.5	7.5
Diabetes mellitus, %	1.1	1.2	1.6	0.6
Psoriasis, %	2.7	3.9	0	8.8
Baseline oral GC dose, %				
None	67.1	57.5	22.3	40.0
Low (<10 mg/day)	24.1	29.7	33.6	26.3
High (≥10 mg/day)	8.8	12.9	44.1	33.8
MTX use on index date, %	N/A	47.8	37.3	N/A
Cyclosporine use on index date, %	0.4	1.0	3.6	6.9
Baseline infection, %				
None	47.7	55.8	45.3	35.0
Nonprimary hospitalized or outpatient	49.6	42.1	47.4	54.4
Primary hospitalized	2.7	2.1	7.3	10.6

Abbreviations: MTX Methotrexate, *TNFi* Tumor necrosis factor inhibitor, *SJIA* Systemic juvenile idiopathic arthritis, *GC* glucocorticoid, *mg* Milligrams of prednisone equivalent, *N/A* Not applicable

Table 2 Crude infection rates for each medication initiation cohort

Medication exposure	Person-years of follow-up	Number of infections	Infection rate per 100 person-years (95 % CI)
MTX	2668.5	39	1.46 (1.07–2.00)
TNFi monotherapy	2144.0	33	1.54 (1.09–2.17)
TNFi + MTX combination	1094.5	19	1.74 (1.11–2.72)
Anakinra with or without MTX	225.9	19	8.41 (5.36–13.2)
MTX with SJIA	113.7	3	2.64 (0.85–8.18)
Etanercept	2594.0	37	1.43 (1.03–1.97)
Adalimumab	413.2	12	2.90 (1.65–5.11)
Infliximab	227.1	3	1.32 (0.43–4.10)

MTX Methotrexate, *TNFi* Tumor necrosis factor inhibitor, *SJIA* Systemic juvenile idiopathic arthritis

age was associated both with TNFi use and with a lower baseline risk of infection. A primary hospital discharge diagnosis of infection during the baseline was strongly associated with subsequent infection after the index date compared with no infection during baseline (aHR 3.28 [95 % CI 1.44–7.48]), and this association was less strong for nonprimary hospital discharge and outpatient diagnoses (aHR 1.72 [95 % CI 1.12–2.63]). High-dose oral GC use during the baseline period was associated with infection compared with no GC use (aHR 2.03 [95 % CI 1.21–3.39]), whereas low-dose GC use was not (aHR 0.86 [95 % CI 0.50–1.46]). Sensitivity analyses that varied the outcome definition, medication risk window, duration of the baseline period to assess GC use, and duration of follow-up did not significantly change these results (data not shown). Stratified analyses of baseline GC users and nonusers did not suggest an interaction between TNFi and GCs with respect to infection (data not shown).

Table 2 also shows the infection rates observed with the individual TNFi. There were no infections observed among new users of certolizumab (0.7 person-years of observation) or golimumab (3.5 person-years of observation). Compared with etanercept, adalimumab use was associated with an increased risk of infection (unadjusted HR 1.99 [95 % CI 1.03–3.87]) that persisted after adjustment for potential confounders (aHR 2.39 [95 % CI 1.21–4.72]). The characteristics of patients newly initiating etanercept and adalimumab were different: 1.0 % of etanercept new users had prior biologic agent use, compared with 28.2 % of new adalimumab users ($p < 0.0001$). Physician diagnosis codes for uveitis were observed during the 6-month baseline period in 14.0 % of new adalimumab users versus 3.1 % for etanercept ($p < 0.0001$). Further restricting the analysis to patients with no prior use of any biologic agent in the available data did not change the result (aHR 2.36 [95 % CI 1.18–4.72]). Because adalimumab received its U.S. Food and Drug Administration (FDA)-approved label for the treatment of JIA in 2008, we also restricted the comparison with etanercept to new medication initiations in 2008 and later. The resulting infection rate associated with adalimumab appeared more similar to the infection rate associated with etanercept over the same period (aHR 1.39 [95 % CI 0.62–3.19]).

Table 4 shows the relative hazards of infection for the comparison of anakinra and MTX. Anakinra was significantly associated with an increased risk of infection

Table 3 Relative hazards of infection for tumor necrosis factor inhibitors versus methotrexate

Exposure	Comparator	Unadjusted relative hazard (95 % CI)	Adjusted[a] relative hazard (95 % CI)
TNFi monotherapy	MTX	1.12 (0.70–1.78)	1.19 (0.72–1.94)
TNFi + MTX combination	MTX	1.21 (0.69–2.10)	1.23 (0.69–2.17)
Hospitalized infection during baseline	No infection during baseline		3.28 (1.44–7.48)
Nonprimary hospitalized or outpatient infection during baseline	No infection during baseline		1.72 (1.12–2.63)
High-dose oral GC (≥10 mg/day)	No oral GC use during baseline		2.03 (1.21–3.39)
Low-dose oral GC (<10 mg/day)	No oral GC use during baseline		0.86 (0.50–1.46)

TNFi Tumor necrosis factor inhibitor, *MTX* Methotrexate, *GC* Glucocorticoid
[a]Multivariable model included the following variables: new TNFi use, age, sex, asthma, baseline oral GC dose, infection during baseline period

compared with all MTX users (aHR 3.53 [95 % CI 1.83–6.82]). High-dose oral GC use was associated with an increased risk of infection compared with no use of GCs (aHR 2.79 [95 % CI 1.35–5.78]). The increased risk of infection associated with anakinra was somewhat attenuated when the comparator cohort was restricted to MTX with SJIA (aHR 2.69 [95 % CI 0.82–8.82]).

Discussion

In an analysis of pooled TNFi exposure, we did not observe a significant increase in hospitalized infection rates following initiation of TNFi monotherapy or TNFi + MTX combination therapy compared with initiation of MTX without prior or concurrent biologic agent use among children with JIA. These results are consistent with those of several previously published studies, while other studies have shown an increased risk of infection associated with TNFi use. One of the earliest published studies about comparative rates of serious infections in clinical practice was a prospective cohort study in which investigators found no difference in infection rates between children with JIA receiving etanercept ($n = 103$), etanercept plus MTX ($n = 294$), or MTX alone ($n = 197$) [7]. Likewise, we previously published a study using U.S. Medicaid data reporting no difference in infection rates between TNFi regardless of MTX use versus MTX use alone [4], although this study was limited by its prevalent user design necessitated by limited available data [10, 11].

More recently, reports of serious infections based on data derived from large, drug-based JIA registries have been published. Davies et al. analyzed data derived from the British Society for Paediatric and Adolescent Rheumatology Etanercept Cohort Study (BSPAR-ETN) and reported an observed increased rate of "medically significant" infections among children receiving etanercept versus MTX (aHR 2.13 [95 % CI 1.22–3.74]) [8]. However, the definition of "medically significant" was based upon the judgment of the treating physician and potentially biased the results; when the outcome was limited to infections requiring hospitalization or intravenous antibiotics, there was no increased risk of infection associated with etanercept versus MTX (aHR 1.36 [95 % CI 0.60–3.07]) [8]. Of note, the crude rate of infections requiring hospitalization or intravenous antibiotics among children receiving etanercept in that study (2.2 per 100 person-years) was similar to our observed rate of hospitalized infection (1.4 per 100 person-years), whereas the rate of medically significant infections determined by the treating physician was much higher (5.5 per 100 person-years) [8]. Additionally, the authors reported no significant increased risk of infection with etanercept plus MTX versus etanercept monotherapy, regardless of the infection outcome definition [8]. Klotsche et al. analyzed data from the German Biologics in Paediatric Rheumatology (BiKeR) registry and its follow-up registry, Juvenile arthritis Methotrexate/Biologics long-term Observation (JuMBO), and reported an

Table 4 Relative hazards of infection for anakinra versus methotrexate and anakinra versus methotrexate with systemic juvenile idiopathic arthritis

Exposure	Comparator	Unadjusted relative hazard (95 % CI)	Adjusted[a] relative hazard (95 % CI)
Anakinra	MTX	5.69 (3.30–9.81)	3.53 (1.83–6.82)
Hospitalized infection during baseline	No infection during baseline		4.81 (1.94–11.9)
Nonprimary hospitalized or outpatient infection during baseline	No infection during baseline		1.76 (0.99–3.16)
High-dose oral GC (≥10 mg/day)	No oral GC use during baseline		2.79 (1.35–5.78)
Low-dose oral GC (<10 mg/day)	No oral GC use during baseline		1.06 (0.54–2.08)
Anakinra	MTX with SJIA	3.07 (0.93–10.2)	2.69 (0.82–8.82)
Hospitalized infection during baseline	No infection during baseline		3.10 (0.74–12.9)
Nonprimary hospitalized or outpatient infection during baseline	No infection during baseline		1.76 (0.66–4.72)
High-dose oral GC (≥10 mg/day)	No oral GC use during baseline		2.05 (0.57–7.30)
Low-dose oral GC (<10 mg/day)	No oral GC use during baseline		1.59 (0.41–6.09)

Abbreviations: MTX Methotrexate, *SJIA* Systemic juvenile idiopathic arthritis, *mg* Milligrams of prednisone equivalents, *GC* Glucocorticoid

[a]Multivariable model included the following variables: new anakinra use, age, sex, asthma, baseline oral GC dose, infection during baseline period, cyclosporine use (time-varying).

increased rate of infection with etanercept versus MTX (adjusted relative risk [aRR] 2.12 [95 % CI 1.08–4.17]) but no increased rate with adalimumab versus MTX (aRR 0.88 [95 % CI 0.18–4.28]) [9]. Importantly, this study was not able to adjust for systemic GC use. Also of note, the crude infection rates for MTX (0.52 per 100 person-years) and etanercept (0.92 per 100 person-years) in this study were lower than in other published studies of serious infection in JIA [9], suggesting the possibility of underreporting of infections by physicians.

We observed that high-dose GC use during the baseline period was a significant risk factor for subsequent hospitalized infection. The results of this study showed a somewhat less extreme risk association with high-dose GCs (aHR 2.03 [95 % CI 1.21–3.39]) than did our previously published study (aHR 3.1 [95 % CI 2.0–4.7]) [4]. This different result may be due to the new-user design employed in the present analysis. In the prior prevalent-user design, the estimate for GCs may have represented both the risks attributable to GCs and those attributable to high disease activity that is frequently associated with GC use. In the present analysis, some of the confounding by high disease activity was likely diminished by the new-user design, thus attenuating the risk estimate associated with GCs [10, 11]. The authors of the BSPAR-ETN analyses reported a univariate risk associated with any baseline GC use that was similar to our study's result (HR 2.13 [95 % CI 1.29–3.51]).

We observed a significantly increased risk of infection with adalimumab compared with etanercept. Although we restricted this analysis to patients without any use of biologic agents in the 6-month baseline period, we could not adequately adjust for the number of prior biologic agents ever used, because only 20 new users of etanercept (1 %) had any prior use of biologic agents, compared with 28 % of adalimumab users. Therefore, new users of adalimumab likely had more refractory disease and a potentially resultant increased baseline risk of infection. When we restricted the analysis to patients without any observed prior use of biologic agents, we obtained the same result, but the identification of any prior biologic agent use may have been limited by left censoring. Additionally, we observed only 12 infections among the adalimumab users, and therefore our results may be susceptible to random chance. Another consideration is that etanercept was available for several years prior to the availability of adalimumab, likely influencing prescribing patterns for both medications. When we restricted our analysis to the period after adalimumab received its FDA-approved label for JIA, the infection rates appeared more similar, but the estimate was imprecise because few infection outcomes were observed.

Interestingly, the authors of the BiKeR/JuMBO analyses reported the opposite observation. In that study, adalimumab was associated with fewer infections than etanercept (aRR 0.88 [95 % CI 0.18–4.28]), although there were only two infection outcomes in the adalimumab cohort with a resultant wide 95 % CI. Another important consideration when comparing these TNFi is the fact that adalimumab is frequently prescribed for the treatment of anterior uveitis associated with JIA and etanercept is not [14, 23]. There may be differential baseline infection risks based upon the presence of active uveitis versus synovitis. In our study, we were not able to reliably determine whether patients received TNFi for the treatment of active uveitis versus synovitis, but compared with etanercept users, the new users of adalimumab were much more likely to have diagnosis codes for uveitis during the baseline period.

In analyzing the largest published cohort, to our knowledge, of children with JIA initiating anakinra, we observed a significantly increased risk of infection compared with MTX, even with adjustment for GC dose during the baseline period. It can be assumed that most children receiving anakinra had SJIA [1, 3, 13, 14], but this could not be determined with certainty on the basis of our data, as we did not have access to medical records. When we restricted the new MTX user comparators to those very likely to have SJIA, the relative risk associated with anakinra was partially attenuated but still elevated. It must be noted that our definition of SJIA was limited by the lack of clinical data. Our definition could not be validated with the data available, and the sensitivity and specificity of the definition are unknown. For example, it is possible that a small minority of MTX users with SJIA received oral cyclosporine for treatment of skin psoriasis rather than SJIA, as suggested by the increased proportion of children with psoriasis in this subcohort compared with MTX (2.7 % versus 8.8 %). Additionally, we observed only three infections among the MTX users with SJIA; therefore, our results may be susceptible to random chance.

Previously reported rates of infection associated with anakinra are highly variable. On one hand, in one case series of 33 patients receiving anakinra [24] and one prospective cohort study of 20 newly diagnosed patients receiving anakinra without concurrent GCs [25], researchers reported no observed serious infections. On the other hand, investigators in a different published case series of 46 patients receiving anakinra as part of their initial treatment regimen reported 3 serious infections (approximate rate of 6 serious infections per 100 person-years) [26]. In addition, researchers in a clinical trial with an open-label extension period in which 22 total patients received anakinra reported 4 serious infections (approximate rate of 25 serious infections per 100 person-years) [27]. A different clinical trial of anakinra for polyarticular course JIA reported 2 serious infections among 86 total patients, but an approximate infection rate cannot be determined on the basis of the data published [28]. Similarly, published clinical trial data derived from studies of the other commercially available IL-1 inhibitors (canakinumab and rilonacept) do not allow for calculation of approximate serious infection rates for comparison [29, 30]. Looking beyond evidence in JIA, the authors of a published meta-analysis of randomized clinical trials of anakinra for adults with rheumatoid arthritis demonstrated a significantly increased risk of infection compared with placebo (odds ratio 3.40 [95 % CI 1.11–10.46]) [31].

Very little is known about background infection rates among children with SJIA compared with other categories of JIA, but it is plausible that the infection risk may be much greater. We controlled for baseline GC use to the extent possible in our study and still observed an increased risk associated with anakinra. One potential source of published evidence about the possibility of a differential baseline infection risk is a comparison of the infection rates in the two recently published clinical trials for tocilizumab, one for polyarticular JIA and the other for SJIA. In the polyarticular JIA trial, the serious infection rate was approximately 6.7 per 100 person-years during the open-label run-in portion of the trial and 3.1 per 100 person-years during the remainder of the study [32]. In the SJIA trial, the rate of serious infection was approximately 17 per 100 person-years [33], suggesting an increased risk of infection in children with SJIA that is independent of biologic agent use. Of course, these studies are not directly comparable, because the patients in the SJIA study received higher doses of tocilizumab and GCs. We attempted to control for the effects of SJIA by restricting the MTX comparator group to children with likely SJIA, but residual confounding by disease severity and disease activity was likely present, as we could not reliably assess these factors using administrative claims data.

It is notable that our study was limited by the data source. We used a new-user design to control for arthritis disease activity at the time of newly starting a medication [11] because disease activity is known to be associated with an increased risk of infection in adults with rheumatoid arthritis [34]. Nevertheless, administrative claims do not contain clinical data, and residual confounding by disease activity was possible in our results and could not be further evaluated in this study.

Conclusions

We did not observe an increased risk of infection with TNFi monotherapy or TNFi + MTX combination therapy compared with MTX alone. Recent infection and high-dose oral GC use were important risk factors for hospitalized infection. Adalimumab was associated with an increased risk of infection compared with etanercept, but this result may be confounded by disease severity. Anakinra was associated with increased risk of infection compared with MTX. More studies are needed to elucidate the risks of infection associated with SJIA and its treatment.

Abbreviations

aHR: Adjusted hazard ratio; aRR: Adjusted relative risk; BiKeR: Biologics in Paediatric Rheumatology; BSPAR-ETN: British Society for Paediatric and Adolescent Rheumatology Etanercept Cohort Study; FDA: U.S. Food and Drug Administration; GC: Glucocorticoid; ICD-9: International Classification of Diseases, Ninth Revision; IL: Interleukin; JIA: Juvenile idiopathic arthritis; JuMBO: Juvenile arthritis Methotrexate/Biologics long-term Observation; MAX: Medicaid Analytic eXtract; MTX: Methotrexate; N/A: Not applicable; SJIA: Systemic juvenile idiopathic arthritis; TNFi: Tumor necrosis factor inhibitor

Acknowledgements

Not applicable.

Funding

This work was supported by the Agency for Healthcare Research and Quality (AHRQ) as part of a grant (U19HS021110) administered through the AHRQ Center for Education and Research on Therapeutics Program. The AHRQ was not involved in the design of the study; the collection, analysis, and interpretation of data; or in the writing of the manuscript.

Authors' contributions

TB, FX, JWB, LC, MLM, KGS, JZ, and JRC were responsible for study conception and design. TB, KGS, and JRC acquired data. Analysis and interpretation of data: TB, FX, LC, and JRC analyzed and interpreted the data. TB wrote the manuscript. All authors critically revised the manuscript, and all authors read and approved the final manuscript.

Competing interests

The authors declare the following financial competing interests. TB has received consulting fees from UCB, Genentech/Roche, and Novartis. JWB has received consulting fees from Pfizer, Astellas Pharma, Merck, and Bristol-Myers Squibb as well as research funding from Bristol-Myers Squibb. KGS has received consulting fees from Abbot, Amgen, Ardea/AstraZeneca, Bristol-Myers Squibb, Crealta Pharmaceuticals, Eli Lilly and Co., Merck, Pfizer, and Genentech/Roche, as well as research funding from Amgen, Ardea/AstraZeneca, Crealta Pharmaceuticals, Eli Lilly and Co., Merck, and Takeda Pharmaceutical Co. JRC has received consulting fees from Genentech/Roche, UCB, Janssen, Corrona, Amgen, Pfizer, Bristol-Myers Squibb, Crescendo Bioscience, and AbbVie, as well as research funding from Genentech/Roche, UCB, Janssen, Corrona, Amgen, Pfizer, Bristol-Myers Squibb, Crescendo Bioscience, and AbbVie. The other authors declare that they have no competing interests.

Consent for publication

Not applicable.

References

1. Beukelman T, Patkar NM, Saag KG, Tolleson-Rinehart S, Cron RQ, DeWitt EM, et al. 2011 American College of Rheumatology recommendations for the treatment of juvenile idiopathic arthritis: initiation and safety monitoring of therapeutic agents for the treatment of arthritis and systemic features. Arthritis Care Res (Hoboken). 2011;63(4):465–82.

2. Mannion ML, Xie F, Curtis JR, Beukelman T. Recent trends in medication usage for the treatment of juvenile idiopathic arthritis and the influence of tumor necrosis factor inhibitors. J Rheumatol. 2014;41(10):2078–84.
3. Beukelman T, Ringold S, Davis TE, DeWitt EM, Pelajo CF, Weiss PF, et al. Disease-modifying antirheumatic drug use in the treatment of juvenile idiopathic arthritis: a cross-sectional analysis of the CARRA Registry. J Rheumatol. 2012;39(9):1867–74.
4. Beukelman T, Xie F, Chen L, Baddley JW, Delzell E, Grijalva CG, et al. Rates of hospitalized bacterial infection associated with juvenile idiopathic arthritis and its treatment. Arthritis Rheum. 2012;64(8):2773–80.
5. Swart JF, de Roock S, Wulffraat NM. What are the immunological consequences of long-term use of biological therapies for juvenile idiopathic arthritis? Arthritis Res Ther. 2013;15(3):213.
6. Hurd A, Beukelman T. Infectious complications in juvenile idiopathic arthritis. Curr Rheumatol Rep. 2013;15(5):327.
7. Giannini EH, Ilowite NT, Lovell DJ, Wallace CA, Rabinovich CE, Reiff A, et al. Long-term safety and effectiveness of etanercept in children with selected categories of juvenile idiopathic arthritis. Arthritis Rheum. 2009;60(9):2794–804.
8. Davies R, Southwood TR, Kearsley-Fleet L, Lunt M, Hyrich KL, British Society for Paediatric and Adolescent Rheumatology Etanercept Cohort Study. Medically significant infections are increased in patients with juvenile idiopathic arthritis treated with etanercept: results from the British Society for Paediatric and Adolescent Rheumatology Etanercept Cohort Study. Arthritis Rheumatol. 2015;67(9):2487–94.
9. Klotsche J, Niewerth M, Haas JP, Huppertz HI, Zink A, Horneff G, et al. Long-term safety of etanercept and adalimumab compared to methotrexate in patients with juvenile idiopathic arthritis (JIA). Ann Rheum Dis. 2016;75(5):855–61.
10. Solomon DH, Lunt M, Schneeweiss S. The risk of infection associated with tumor necrosis factor α antagonists: making sense of epidemiologic evidence. Arthritis Rheum. 2008;58(4):919–28.
11. Ray WA. Evaluating medication effects outside of clinical trials: new-user designs. Am J Epidemiol. 2003;158(9):915–20.
12. Horneff G, De Bock F, Foeldvari I, Girschick HJ, Michels H, Moebius D, et al. Safety and efficacy of combination of etanercept and methotrexate compared to treatment with etanercept only in patients with juvenile idiopathic arthritis (JIA): preliminary data from the German JIA Registry. Ann Rheum Dis. 2009;68(4):519–25.
13. Ringold S, Weiss PF, Beukelman T, Dewitt EM, Ilowite NT, Kimura Y, et al. 2013 update of the 2011 American College of Rheumatology recommendations for the treatment of juvenile idiopathic arthritis: recommendations for the medical therapy of children with systemic juvenile idiopathic arthritis and tuberculosis screening among children receiving biologic medications. Arthritis Care Res (Hoboken). 2013;65(10): 1551–63.
14. Kearsley-Fleet L, Davies R, Baildam E, Beresford MW, Foster HE, Southwood TR, et al. Factors associated with choice of biologic among children with juvenile idiopathic arthritis: results from two UK paediatric biologic registers. Rheumatology (Oxford). 2016;55(9):1556–65.
15. Beukelman T. Treatment advances in systemic juvenile idiopathic arthritis. F1000Prime Rep. 2014;6:21.
16. Bruck N, Schnabel A, Hedrich CM. Current understanding of the pathophysiology of systemic juvenile idiopathic arthritis (sJIA) and target-directed therapeutic approaches. Clin Immunol. 2015;159(1):72–83.
17. Beukelman T, Haynes K, Curtis JR, Xie F, Chen L, Bemrich-Stolz CJ, et al. Rates of malignancy associated with juvenile idiopathic arthritis and its treatment. Arthritis Rheum. 2012;64(4):1263–71.
18. Ravelli A, Davì S, Minoia F, Martini A, Cron RQ. Macrophage activation syndrome. Hematol Oncol Clin North Am. 2015;29(5):927–41.
19. Patkar NM, Curtis JR, Teng GG, Allison JJ, Saag M, Martin C, et al. Administrative codes combined with medical records based criteria accurately identified bacterial infections among rheumatoid arthritis patients. J Clin Epidemiol. 2009;62(3):321–7.
20. Grijalva CG, Chen L, Delzell E, Baddley JW, Beukelman T, Winthrop KL, et al. Initiation of tumor necrosis factor-α antagonists and the risk of hospitalization for infection in patients with autoimmune diseases. JAMA. 2011;306(21):2331–9.
21. Yun H, Xie F, Delzell E, Levitan EB, Chen L, Lewis JD, et al. Comparative risk of hospitalized infection associated with biologic agents in rheumatoid arthritis patients enrolled in Medicare. Arthritis Rheumatol. 2016;68(1):56–66.
22. Lin DY, Wei LJ. The robust inference for the Cox proportional hazards model. J Am Stat Assoc. 1989;84:1074–8.
23. Heiligenhaus A, Michels H, Schumacher C, Kopp I, Neudorf U, Niehues T, et al. Evidence-based, interdisciplinary guidelines for anti-inflammatory treatment of uveitis associated with juvenile idiopathic arthritis. Rheumatol Int. 2012;32(5):1121–33.
24. Zeft A, Hollister R, LaFleur B, Sampath P, Soep J, McNally B, et al. Anakinra for systemic juvenile arthritis: the Rocky Mountain experience. J Clin Rheumatol. 2009;15(4):161–4.
25. Vastert SJ, de Jager W, Noordman BJ, Holzinger D, Kuis W, Prakken BJ, et al. Effectiveness of first-line treatment with recombinant interleukin-1 receptor antagonist in steroid-naive patients with new-onset systemic juvenile idiopathic arthritis: results of a prospective cohort study. Arthritis Rheumatol. 2014;66(4):1034–43.
26. Nigrovic PA, Mannion M, Prince FH, Zeft A, Rabinovich CE, van Rossum MA, et al. Anakinra as first-line disease-modifying therapy in systemic juvenile idiopathic arthritis: report of forty-six patients from an international multicenter series. Arthritis Rheum. 2011;63(2):545–55.
27. Quartier P, Allantaz F, Cimaz R, Pillet P, Messiaen C, Bardin C, et al. A multicentre, randomised, double-blind, placebo-controlled trial with the interleukin-1 receptor antagonist anakinra in patients with systemic-onset juvenile idiopathic arthritis (ANAJIS trial). Ann Rheum Dis. 2011;70(5):747–54.
28. Ilowite N, Porras O, Reiff A, Rudge S, Punaro M, Martin A, et al. Anakinra in the treatment of polyarticular-course juvenile rheumatoid arthritis: safety and preliminary efficacy results of a randomized multicenter study. Clin Rheumatol. 2009;28(2):129–37.
29. Ruperto N, Brunner HI, Quartier P, Constantin T, Wulffraat N, Horneff G, et al. Two randomized trials of canakinumab in systemic juvenile idiopathic arthritis. N Engl J Med. 2012;367(25):2396–406.
30. Ilowite NT, Prather K, Lokhnygina Y, Schanberg LE, Elder M, Milojevic D, et al. Randomized, double-blind, placebo-controlled trial of the efficacy and safety of rilonacept in the treatment of systemic juvenile idiopathic arthritis. Arthritis Rheumatol. 2014;66(9):2570–9.
31. Salliot C, Dougados M, Gossec L. Risk of serious infections during rituximab, abatacept and anakinra treatments for rheumatoid arthritis: meta-analyses of randomised placebo-controlled trials. Ann Rheum Dis. 2009;68(1):25–32.
32. Brunner HI, Ruperto N, Zuber Z, Keane C, Harari O, Kenwright A, et al. Efficacy and safety of tocilizumab in patients with polyarticular-course juvenile idiopathic arthritis: results from a phase 3, randomised, double-blind withdrawal trial. Ann Rheum Dis. 2015;74(6):1110–7.
33. De Benedetti F, Brunner HI, Ruperto N, Kenwright A, Wright S, Calvo I, et al. Randomized trial of tocilizumab in systemic juvenile idiopathic arthritis. N Engl J Med. 2012;367(25):2385–95.
34. Au K, Reed G, Curtis JR, Kremer JM, Greenberg JD, Strand V, et al. High disease activity is associated with an increased risk of infection in patients with rheumatoid arthritis. Ann Rheum Dis. 2011;70(5):785–91.

13

Review of biomarkers in systemic juvenile idiopathic arthritis: helpful tools or just playing tricks?

Faekah Gohar, Christoph Kessel, Miha Lavric, Dirk Holzinger and Dirk Foell*

Abstract

Background: Diagnosing systemic juvenile idiopathic arthritis (SJIA) can be extremely challenging if typical arthritis is lacking. A variety of biomarkers have been described for the diagnosis and management of SJIA. However, very few markers have been well-validated. In addition, increasing numbers of biomarkers are identified by high throughput or multi-marker panels.

Method: We identified diagnostic or prognostic biomarkers by systematic literature review, evaluating each according to a predefined level of verification, validation or clinical utility. Diagnostic biomarkers were those identifying SJIA versus (1) non-SJIA conditions or healthy controls (HC) or (2) other non-systemic JIA subtypes. Prognostic biomarkers were those specifically tested for the prediction of (1) disease flare, (2) increased disease activity +/- discrimination of active versus inactive disease, or (3) macrophage activation syndrome (MAS).

Results: Fifty-five studies fulfilled the inclusion criteria identifying 68 unique biomarkers, of which 50/68 (74 %) were investigated by only a single research group. Candidate marker verification and clinical utility was evaluated according to whether markers were readily and reliably measurable, investigated by independent study groups, discovered by more than one method (i.e. verified markers) and validated in independent cohorts. This evaluation revealed diagnostic biomarkers of high interest for further evaluation in the diagnostic approach to SJIA that included heme oxygenase-1, interleukin-6 (IL-6), IL-12, IL-18, osteoprotegerin, S100 calcium-binding protein A12 (S100A12) and S100A8/A9.

Conclusion: In summary, a number of biomarkers were identified, though most had limited evidence for their use. However, our findings combined with the identified studies could inform validation studies, whether in single or multi-marker assays, which are urgently needed.

Background

Systemic juvenile idiopathic arthritis (SJIA), or Still's disease/syndrome, is a childhood rheumatic condition that is typically characterized by spiking fever in a quotidian pattern, transient rash and arthritis. Patients may alternate between periods of disease activity (flare) and inactive disease. SJIA accounts for around 10–20 % of juvenile idiopathic arthritis (JIA), which has an incidence of around 6.6–15 per 100,000 children [1]. Although defined as a subtype of JIA, patients often present with rather unspecific signs and symptoms initially, with the hallmark fever of unknown origin, but without chronic arthritis. Diagnosing SJIA is challenging in these cases as the disease is recognized as an autoinflammatory syndrome rather than classical autoimmune arthritis [2, 3]. Accordingly, most clinical symptoms can be attributed to dysregulated innate immune mechanisms with only minor involvement of adaptive immunity. Gene expression studies of circulating cells show increased levels of transcripts, reflecting monocyte/macrophage-associated activation in SJIA [4–6]. The innate immune cells such as monocytes and macrophages are thought to be drivers of SJIA, producing several mediators implicated in the pathogenesis of SJIA, including interleukin-1 (IL-1), IL-6 and IL-18 and phagocyte-specific S100 proteins [7]. IL-1 in particular seems to have a prominent role in SJIA. Serum from patients with SJIA induces the transcription of genes of the innate immune system including IL-1 in peripheral blood mononuclear cells (PBMC). Furthermore,

* Correspondence: dfoell@uni-muenster.de
Department of Paediatric Rheumatology and Immunology, University of Münster, Domagkstraße 3, D-48149 Münster, Germany

activated monocytes from patients with SJIA secrete significantly more IL-1β in comparison with monocytes from healthy controls [6].

Significant challenges to improving the clinical care of patients with SJIA include the discrimination of SJIA from other causes of fever, evidence-based evaluation of response to treatment, detection and limitation of subclinical inflammation and discrimination of SJIA without macrophage activation syndrome (MAS) from SJIA with MAS [8]. MAS is a serious complication of SJIA with a 10 % mortality risk, defined as an acute episode of overwhelming inflammation and characterized by activation and expansion of T lymphocytes and hemophagocytic macrophages. In the early stages, development of MAS is difficult to predict and diagnostic and prognostic biomarkers might enable early intervention.

These challenges could be addressed by the identification and validation of clinically relevant biomarkers, of which those circulating in serum and plasma are useful and easily obtainable from peripheral blood [9–13]. Mechanistic markers are those that are elevated or decreased in response to underlying pathological processes, whereas proxy markers, such as C-reactive protein (CRP), do not have a definite role in the pathology of the disease, and are non-specific markers of inflammation [14]. Therefore, measurement of a mechanistic biomarker can quantify a pathologic process. With such quantification, a level of severity can be defined, and cutoffs determined, allowing the use of such biomarkers as treatment targets (Fig. 1) [8, 15]. Diagnostic biomarkers, proxy or mechanistic, can aid detection of a disease or confirm it in uncertain cases e.g., evolving SJIA versus sepsis [15, 16].

Although a number of publications describe potential biomarkers, none have been recently validated or used in clinical studies aside from the IL-1 family cytokines and the S100-proteins, S100A12 and S100A8/A9 [17]. To date, discovery studies vastly outnumber validation studies, which are more challenging to perform given their requirement for independent cohorts and statistically valid sample sizes. Additionally, the number of identified candidates is usually large and the cost of validation high, leading to a need for unbiased prioritization of candidates for validation [18].

In conclusion, a combination of sensitive biomarkers could allow targeted and personalized treatment and improve treatment outcomes [8]. We therefore identified current candidate diagnostic and prognostic biomarkers from the literature, additionally evaluating their potential for validation/clinical use, function and association with other identified biomarkers. We also discuss the current and future potential of biomarkers for SJIA.

Method

Search criteria

A PubMed search was performed using the search terms as follows: "Arthritis, Juvenile"[Mesh] AND (("2000/11/01"[PDAT]: "2015/11/01"[PDAT]) AND "humans"[MeSH

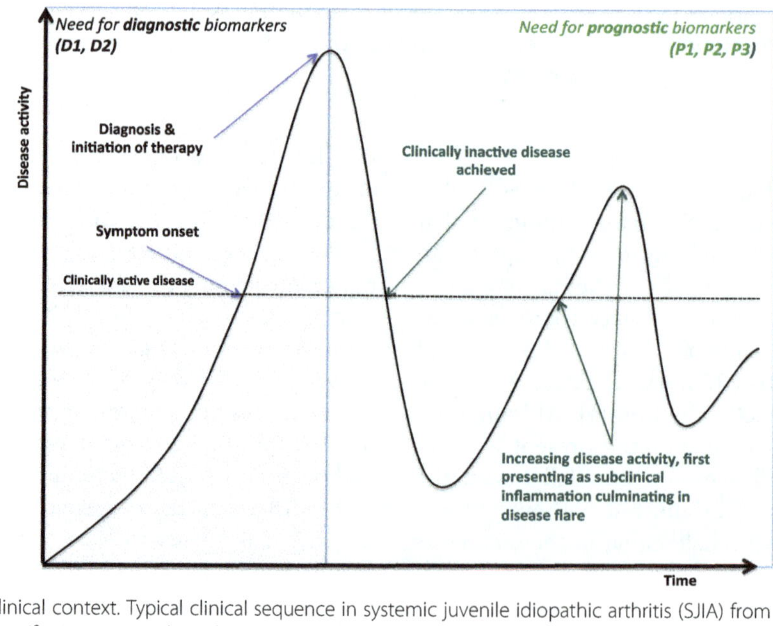

Fig. 1 Biomarker need in clinical context. Typical clinical sequence in systemic juvenile idiopathic arthritis (SJIA) from disease onset, diagnosis to clinical resolution and flare. Specific time points where there is a need for diagnostic and prognostic biomarkers are indicated. Diagnostic markers are indicated as follows: *D1* SJIA versus other non-JIA conditions, *D2* SJIA versus other JIA subtypes. Prognostic markers are indicated as follows: *P1* prognostic for flare, *P2* prognostic for increased disease activity, *P3* prognostic for macrophage activation syndrome (MAS) or differentiating MAS from SJIA flare. Adapted from Hinze et al. 2015 [8]

Terms] AND English [lang]) along with the additional keywords: 1) cytokine ("cytokines"[MeSH Terms] OR "cytokines"[All Fields] OR "cytokine"[All Fields]) ($n = 544$ individual studies identified), OR 2) biomarker ("biological markers"[MeSH Terms] OR ("biological"[All Fields] AND "markers"[All Fields]) OR "biological markers"[All Fields] OR "biomarker"[All Fields]) ($n = 307$), OR 3) validation ($n = 114$). Abstracts of identified studies were reviewed and any fulfilling exclusion criteria at the outset were excluded, and the full text scrutinized for those remaining.

Inclusion and exclusion criteria

Inclusion criteria were as follows: studies in which serum or plasma markers were analysed; original research studies; studies that specifically addressed the biomarkers with the diagnostic or prognostic functions as indicated in Table 1 and studies that also included SJIA-specific analyses. Exclusion criteria were: case studies or review articles; studies that included fewer than three patients with SJIA; studies with only negative findings reported (i.e. no statistically significant finding for the candidate marker for the use evaluated) and studies describing functional/cell-based assays or enzyme activity assays. We also excluded studies on adult-onset Still's disease (AOSD) [19] and genetic array/genotype or phenotype studies that described individual patients rather than disease signatures, without evaluation of individual biomarkers, even if performed as unbiased discovery studies. Genetic markers and gene expression profiles in SJIA have been previously discussed in a review by Nirmala et al. [20].

Data analysis and categorisation of biomarkers

Details recorded from identified studies included the aims, numbers of included patients and methods of biomarker assessment (Additional file 1). Biomarkers from each study were categorised as diagnostic (discriminating SJIA from non-JIA disorders or healthy controls (HC) termed "D1 biomarkers" or differentiating SJIA from other JIA subtypes, "D2 biomarkers") or prognostic (for flare, "P1 biomarkers", increased disease activity or discriminating active versus inactive disease, "P2 biomarkers", or prognostic for MAS or differentiating SJIA with and without MAS, "P3 biomarkers"), as defined in Table 1, according to the study objectives, and indicated in Fig. 1.

Evaluation of identified markers

Identified candidate biomarkers were scored and ranked by their potential to reach validation or clinical use, with potentially spurious or unreproducible candidate findings ranked the lowest. The biomarker scoring system (BMS) used (Table 2) was developed to identify whether identified candidates (1) were readily measurable, i.e. in standard collected biological samples and without special equipment, (2) had been measured by independent study groups, as confirmation that the biomarker is detectable, (3) had been discovered by more than one method, e.g., proteomic and enzyme-linked immunosorbent assay (ELISA) methods, (4) had been measured by an established assay, i.e. an assay that is well-described, with normal cutoff values available, as this would allow easier translation to clinical practice and finally (5) had been validated for the stated clinical question. Each evaluation question making up the BMS (Table 2) was answered using only the information collected during the review process, and each of the included five questions was scored 0 or 1.

Results and discussion

Identified candidate biomarkers

A total of 57 studies describing 68 unique biomarkers were identified (Table 3). All reported biomarkers were identified in serum unless otherwise indicated (Additional file 1: Table S1). The mean number of patients with SJIA included in studies was 21 (range 4–60). There were 50 biomarkers (74 %) investigated in studies performed by a single research group and 29/57 studies evaluated a single biomarker. Biomarkers included cytokines, soluble receptors, antibodies, alarmins and other functional molecules (Table 3). The most studied biomarkers were IL-18 ($n = 7$ individual studies), IL-6 ($n = 5$), S100A8/A9 ($n = 5$), S100A12 ($n = 4$) and soluble CD25

Table 1 Diagnostic and prognostic criteria for inclusion

Biomarker function	Description	Biomarkers identified (*n*)	Number of studies in which biomarkers were identified (*n*)
Diagnostic	D1: SJIA versus other non-arthritis conditions or HC	36	48
	D2: SJIA versus other JIA subtypes	25	25
Prognostic	P1: for flare (or relapse)	14	16
	P2: for increased disease activity and/or the discrimination of active and inactive disease	15	21
	P3: for MAS or discriminating MAS from SJIA flare	7	12

Table 2 Scoring system used to perform an unbiased evaluation of identified biomarkers

Q1	Readily measurable (e.g. in serum)	Yes = 1	No = 0
Q2	Measured by more than one independent study group	Yes = 1	No = 0
Q3	Discovered by more than one single method	Yes = 1	No = 0
Q4	Measured by a reproducible assay	Yes = 1	No = 0
Q5	Validated in a validation cohort	Yes = 1	No = 0
	Maximum score = 5, minimum score = 0		

(IL-2 receptor) ($n = 4$) (Table 3). Only two identified biomarkers, namely S100A8/A9 and S100A12, were described in JIA (but not SJIA) validation studies [21]. Hepcidin, also included as a diagnostic marker, was validated for differentiating SJIA-associated anaemia from anaemia of other causes, but not specifically for SJIA diagnosis [22].

Current clinical uses of identified biomarkers

This study identified some well-established markers of inflammation and/or SJIA, such as the S100-proteins (S100A12 and S100A8/A9 complex), IL-18 and IL-6, autoantibodies, non-specific inflammatory markers and some markers not classically associated with SJIA, such as B cell markers. S100A8/A9 is a predictive biomarker for subclinical disease activity and a predictor of JIA relapse after stopping medication [17, 21, 23]. IL-18 concentration is a known marker of disease activity in SJIA, while IL-18 and IL-6 can define subsets of SJIA [24–26]. While IL-6 and IL-1 are targets of the biological therapies tocilizumab, canakinumab, rilonacept and anakinra, respectively, neither cytokine is routinely measured in patients [27–30]. IL-1b, as already discussed, is usually undetectable in serum and IL-18 is not regularly measured due to technical limitations in performing bioassays [31]; however the reason for IL-6 not being used in routine care is unclear [32, 33].

A number of autoantibodies were identified as candidate biomarkers, including rheumatoid factor (RF), antinuclear antibodies (ANA) and anti-citrullinated protein antibodies (ACPA). RF has long been recognised as distinguishing RF-positive and RF-negative forms of polyarthritis (JIA subtypes) [34]. ANA are routinely evaluated in JIA as a screening factor for JIA-associated uveitis [35]. However, Shin et al. showed that ANA levels can change over time in patients with SJIA, which is a finding replicated by Huegle et al. [36, 37] ACPA are associated with joint damage, and are included in the classification criteria for rheumatoid arthritis, though they do not have an established use in SJIA [38–40].

CRP and ferritin, which are routinely measured, non-specific, acute phase reactants used as surrogate markers, were described as baseline parameters in most of the identified studies, but were not the subject of investigation in the studies, so were therefore excluded from Tables 1 and 3 and from further analyses. Other non-specific identified biomarkers of inflammation were serum amyloid (SAA), fibrin D-dimer and complement 4 (C4). While previously important in detecting long-term complications of inflammation such as amyloidosis, SAA measurement has become less important since the introduction of biological treatments, which have reduced complications in SJIA.

Candidate biomarkers categorised as diagnostic or prognostic

Some biomarkers were identified in more than one study as described above and evaluated for more than one clinical question (Tables 1 and 3). There were 51 markers characterised as diagnostic, 33 as prognostic and 16 were both diagnostic and prognostic (Table 3): these were ACPA, A proliferation-inducing ligand (APRIL), B-cell activating factor (BAFF), cartilage oligomeric matrix protein (COMP), follistatin-like protein 1 (FSTL-1), heme oxygenase-1 (HO-1), interferon gamma (IFNg), IL-10, IL-18, IL-18 binding protein (IL-18BP), IL-6, S100A12, S100A8/A9, SAA, soluble ST2/IL-1 receptor-like 1 (sST2) and transthyretin (TTr).

Evaluation of identified markers by clinical question

There were 36 biomarkers that differentiated SJIA from HC or other non-JIA disease (D1 biomarkers) and 25 markers differentiated SJIA from other JIA subtypes (D2 biomarkers). Of the prognostic markers, 14 P1 (flare), 15 P2 (disease activity) and seven P3 (MAS) biomarkers were identified (Table 1). Ten biomarkers were common to D1 and D2 (Fig. 2a); however, few markers overlapped between the prognostic groups (Fig. 2b). This analysis suggests that some biomarkers could have broad use as diagnostic or prognostics markers, rather than being useful only for specific questions. These markers might therefore be more useful than others in a clinical setting, and might therefore be prioritised for validation.

Evaluation of candidate markers

For unbiased and valid results, biomarker evaluation should be performed according to a predefined hypothesis [41] in order to identify candidates more likely to be specific, rather than a high number of unspecific candidates. High throughput methods are increasingly sensitive and producing ever larger numbers of candidate biomarkers; however, they can still be impeded by methodological limitations, such as in LC-MS/MS, by the presence of high abundant proteins [42, 43]. Therefore, careful and evidence-based hypothesis-driven evaluation and prioritisation of candidates for validation studies is vital. While discovery studies are usually unbiased, the

Table 3 Identified serum and plasma biomarkers

Biomarker		Detection method	Intended use (P/D) + Reference		BMS score[a] Q1 + Q2 + Q3 + Q4 + Q5 = total
Abbreviation/gene name	Full/alternative name		D	P	
A2M	Alpha-2-macroglobulin	Commercial ELISA		[45]	1 + 0 + 0 + 1 + 0 = 2
AB-oxLDL	Antibodies to oxidized low-density lipoprotein	Commercial ELISA	[68]		1 + 0 + 0 + 1 + 0 = 2
ACAN	Aggrecan core protein, cartilage-specific core protein	Immunoassay	[69]		1 + 0 + 0 + 1 + 0 = 2
ACPA	Anti-citrullinated protein antibodies	Commercial ELISA	[39]	[39]	1 + 0 + 0 + 1 + 0 = 2
ACT	Alpha-1-antichymotrypsin	Commercial ELISA		[45]	1 + 0 + 0 + 1 + 0 = 2
AECA	Anti-endothelial cell antibodies	In-house ELISA	[70]		1 + 0 + 0 + 1 + 0 = 2
AGP1	Alpha-1-acid-glycoprotein	Commercial ELISA		[45]	1 + 0 + 0 + 1 + 0 = 2
ANA	Antinuclear antibody	Fluorescence assay		[36]	1 + 1 + 0 + 1 + 0 = 3
		Commercial ELISA		[37]	
Anti-BiP	Anti-immunoglobulin binding protein/glucose regulated protein 78 (GRP78)	In-house ELISA	[71]		1 + 0 + 0 + 1 + 0 = 2
Anti-CCP	Anti-cyclic citrullinated peptide	Commercial ELISA	[72]		1 + 0 + 0 + 1 + 0 = 2
APO A1	Apolioprotein A1	Commercial ELISA		[45]	1 + 0 + 0 + 1 + 0 = 2
APO VI	Apolipoprotein VI	Commercial ELISA		[45]	1 + 0 + 0 + 1 + 0 = 2
APRIL	A proliferation-inducing ligand	Commercial ELISA	[73]	[73]	1 + 0 + 0 + 1 + 0 = 2
B2M	Beta -2-microglobulin	Not indicated		[74]	1 + 0 + 0 + 1 + 0 = 2
BAFF	B-cell activating factor	Commercial ELISA	[73]	[73]	1 + 0 + 0 + 1 + 0 = 2
C4	Complement C4	Commercial ELISA		[45]	1 + 0 + 0 + 1 + 0 = 2
CCL3	Chemokine (C-C motif) ligand 3	Luminex assay	[57]		1 + 0 + 0 + 1 + 0 = 2
CD10	Cluster of differentiation antigen 10, also called neprilysin	Fluorimetric assay	[75]		1 + 0 + 0 + 1 + 0 = 2
CFH	Complement factor H	Commercial ELISA		[45]	1 + 0 + 0 + 1 + 0 = 2
COMP	Cartilage oligomeric matrix protein	Commercial ELISA	[39]	[39]	1 + 1 + 0 + 1 + 0 = 3
			[76]	[77]	
				[78]	
CXCL9	Chemokine (C-X-C Motif) ligand 9	Luminex assay	[57]		1 + 0 + 0 + 1 + 0 = 2
Fibrin D-dimer		Commercial assay		[79]	1 + 0 + 0 + 1 + 0 = 2
FSTL-1	Follistatin-like protein 1	Commercial ELISA	[80]	[80]	1 + 1 + 0 + 1 + 0 = 3
				[81]	
GHRL	Ghrelin, appetite regulating hormone	Commercial ELISA	[82]		1 + 0 + 0 + 1 + 0 = 2
GSN	Gelsolin	Commercial ELISA		[45]	1 + 0 + 0 + 1 + 0 = 2
Hepcidin	Peptide hormone, released by hepatocytes	Commercial assay	[22]		1 + 0 + 0 + 1 + 0 = 2
HMGB1	High mobility group box protein 1	Commercial assay	[83]		1 + 0 + 0 + 1 + 0 = 2
HO-1	Heme oxygenase-1	Commercial ELISA	[84]	[85]	1 + 1 + 0 + 1 + 1 = 4
HP	Haptoglobin	Commercial ELISA		[45]	1 + 0 + 0 + 1 + 0 = 2
IFNg	Interferon gamma	Commercial ELISA	[86]	[86]	1 + 0 + 0 + 1 + 0 = 2
IgA RF	Ig A rheumatoid factor isotype	In-house ELISA	[87]		1 + 0 + 0 + 1 + 0 = 2
IgM RF	Ig M rheumatoid factor isotype	In-house ELISA	[87]		1 + 0 + 0 + 1 + 0 = 2
IL-10	Interleukin-10	Commercial ELISA	[88]	[85]	1 + 0 + 0 + 1 + 0 = 2
IL-12	Interleukin-12	Luminex assay	[57]		1 + 1 + 1 + 1 + 0 = 4
		Commercial ELISA	[89]		
IL-18	Interleukin-18	Commercial assay	[25]		1 + 1 + 1 + 1 + 0 = 4
		Luminex assay	[57]	[24]	

Table 3 Identified serum and plasma biomarkers *(Continued)*

			[86]	[90]	
			[90]	[91]	
			[92]		
IL-18BP	Interleukin-18 binding protein	Commercial assay	[86]		1 + 1 + 0 + 1 + 0 = 3
			[90]	[90]	
IL-1b	Interleukin-1beta	Commercial ELISA	[89]		1 + 0 + 0 + 1 + 0 = 2
IL-6	Interleukin-6	Luminex assay Commercial ELISA	[57]	[24]	1 + 1 + 1 + 1 + 0 = 4
			[86]		
			[89]		
			[76]		
IP-10/CXCL10	IFNg-induced protein 10, or C-X-C motif chemokine 10	Commercial ELISA Luminex assay	[57]		1 + 1 + 0 + 1 + 0 = 3
			[86]		
			[93]		
LGALS3	Galectin-3	Commercial ELISA	[94]		1 + 0 + 0 + 1 + 0 = 2
MIF	Macrophage migration inhibitory factor	Luminex assay	[57]		1 + 0 + 0 + 1 + 0 = 2
MMP-3	Matrix metalloprotinease-3/stromelysin-1 (SL-1)	Commercial ELISA	[72]		1 + 0 + 0 + 1 + 0 = 2
Neopterin		Commercial ELISA		[85]	1 + 0 + 0 + 1 + 0 = 2
NO	Nitric oxide	Spectrophotometry		[95]	1 + 0 + 0 + 1 + 0 = 2
OPG	Osteoprotegerin/TNF 11B	Luminex assay Commercial ELISA	[57]		1 + 1 + 1 + 1 + 0 = 4
			[96]		
OPN	Osteopontin, phosphoglycoprotein	Commercial ELISA	[97]		1 + 0 + 0 + 1 + 0 = 2
RA33	Anti-heterogeneous nuclear ribonucleoprotein A2 antibodies	Commercial ELISA	[98]		1 + 0 + 0 + 1 + 0 = 2
RANKL	TNF ligand superfamily member 11/receptor activator of nuclear factor kappa B ligand	Commercial ELISA	[96]		1 + 0 + 0 + 1 + 0 = 2
Resistin	Protein adipokine	Commercial ELISA	[99]		1 + 0 + 0 + 1 + 0 = 2
S100A12	S100 calcium-binding protein A12	In-house ELISA Commercial ELISA	[45]	[45]	1 + 1 + 1 + 1 + 0 = 4
			[100]	[100]	
			[101]	[102]	
S100A8/A9	MRP8/14 (myeloid regulatory protein 8/14) complex, complex of S100A8 (Calgranulin A) and S100A9 (Calgranulin B)	In-house ELISA Commercial ELISA	[23]		1 + 1 + 1 + 1 + 0 = 4
			[45]	[23]	
			[101]	[17]	
			[103]	[45]	
SAA	Serum amyloid A	Commercial ELISA	[45]	[45]	1 + 1 + 0 + 1 + 0 = 3
			[76]		
SAP	Serum amyloid P	Commercial ELISA		[45]	1 + 0 + 0 + 1 + 0 = 2
sCD163	Soluble cluster of differentiation 163/haemoglobin scavenging receptor	Commercial ELISA		[85]	1 + 1 + 0 + 1 + 0 = 3
				[104]	
sCD21	Soluble cluster of differentiation 21	Commercial ELISA	[105]		1 + 0 + 0 + 1 + 0 = 2
sCD23	Soluble cluster of differentiation 23/soluble low affinity immunoglobulin epsilon Fc receptor)	Commercial ELISA	[105]		1 + 0 + 0 + 1 + 0 = 2
sCD25	Soluble cluster of differentiation 25/soluble interleukin-2 receptor alpha	Commercial ELISA		[74]	1 + 1 + 0 + 1 + 0 = 3
				[104]	
				[106]	
				[107]	

Table 3 Identified serum and plasma biomarkers *(Continued)*

sE-selectin	Soluble E-selectin adhesion molecule	Commercial ELISA	[108] [109] [110]		1 + 1 + 0 + 1 + 0 = 3
sICAM-1	Soluble intracellular adhesion molecule-1	Commercial ELISA	[108] [109] [110]		1 + 1 + 0 + 1 + 0 = 3
sRAGE	Soluble receptor for advanced glycation end products	Commercial assay	[83]		1 + 0 + 0 + 1 + 0 = 2
sST2	Soluble ST2, also called interleukin 1 receptor-like 1 (IL-1RL1)	Commercial ELISA	[111]	[111]	1 + 0 + 0 + 1 + 0 = 2
sTM	Soluble thrombomodulin/CD141	Commercial ELISA	[112]		1 + 0 + 0 + 1 + 0 = 2
sTNFR55	Soluble tumour necrosis factor receptor 55	Commercial ELISA	[113]		1 + 0 + 0 + 1 + 0 = 2
sTNFR75	Soluble tumour necrosis factor receptor 75	Commercial ELISA	[113]		1 + 0 + 0 + 1 + 0 = 2
Survivin		Commercial ELISA	[76]		1 + 0 + 0 + 1 + 0 = 2
TIMP	Tissue inhibitors of metalloproteinases	Commercial ELISA	[96]		1 + 0 + 0 + 1 + 0 = 2
TNF-alpha	Tumour necrosis factor-alpha	Commercial ELISA	[88]		1 + 0 + 0 + 1 + 0 = 2
TTR	Transthyretin	Commercial ELISA	[45]	[45]	1 + 0 + 0 + 1 + 0 = 2

[a]Biomarker scoring system (BMS) biomarker score: each answer is scored as follows: yes = 1, no = 0. *D* diagnostic, *P* prognostic, *Q1* readily measurable (e.g. in serum), *Q2* measured by more than one independent study group, *Q3* discovered by more than one single method, *Q4* measured by a reproducible assay, *Q5* validated in a validation cohort, *IFN* interferon, *TNF* tumour necrosis factor

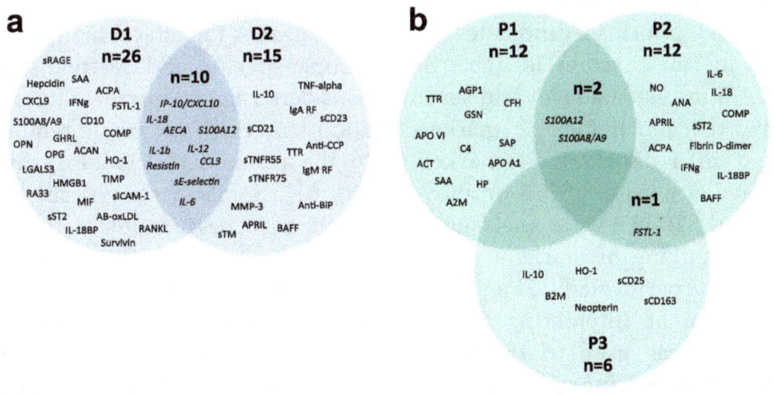

Fig. 2 Identified biomarkers grouped by clinical question. **a** Diagnostic biomarkers are shown that differentiated systemic juvenile idiopathic arthritis (SJIA) from healthy controls (HC) or other non-JIA disease (*D1*), SJIA vs other JIA subtypes (*D2*) or both (*D1* and *D2*). **b** Prognostic biomarkers for flare (*P1*), increased disease activity or discriminating active disease from inactive (*P2*), for macrophage activation syndrome (MAS) or discriminating MAS from SJIA flare (*P3*), or a combination of these are shown. The specific clinical question is very important in interpreting the results of biomarker studies. Little overlap between different diagnostic questions suggests a predominance of different pathways during different stages of disease and therefore a specific hypothesis and clinical question is more useful in studies to understand mechanisms. Biomarkers that are broad enough to cover more than one diagnostic or prognostic category may be more likely to have a specific role in the underlying immunological pathology, and as broad markers will be more useful for wider clinical care. By performing this analysis we can create a shortlist of biomarkers on which to focus. Indeed, only a few markers fall into this group, but perhaps they should receive most attention for future validation in preference to other markers. *ACAN* aggrecan core protein cartilage-specific core protein, *ACCP* anti-cyclic citrullinated peptide, *ACPA* anti-citrullinated protein antibodies, *ACT* alpha-1-antichymotrypsin, *AECA* anti-endothelial cell antibodies, *ANA* antinuclear antibodies, *Anti-BiP* anti-immunoglobulin binding protein/glucose regulated protein 78 (GRP78), *APO* apolioprotein, *APRIL* A proliferation-inducing ligand, *B2M* Beta -2-microglobulin, *BAFF* B-cell activating factor, *COMP* cartilage oligomeric matrix protein, *CRP* C-reactive protein, *FSTL-1* follistatin-like protein 1, *GSN* Gelsolin, *HO-1* heme oxygenase-1, *IFN* interferon, *IL-18BP* IL-18 binding protein, *LGAL* galectin, *MMP* matrix metalloproteinase, *ONP* osteopontin, *SAA* serum amyloid A, *SAP* serum amyloid P, *sICAM-1* soluble intracellular adhesion molecule-1, *sST2* soluble ST2/IL-1 receptor-like 1, *TIMP* tissue inhibitors of metalloproteinase, *TTr* transthyretin

prioritisation of identified markers for further evaluation is much more variable, and might be reported as being based on reproducibility, availability of antibodies or levels of protein expression [44]. However, too often these data are omitted, leading to bias in the selection procedure. Ling et al. detected 26 proteins in plasma from patients with SJIA, which differentiated flare from quiescence plasma, of which 18 proteins were significant, and from these the top 15 were selected for unsupervised analysis and shown to remain significant [45]. However, only a limited panel of 9/15 were further tested, chosen according to the availability of antibodies and ELISA. As there is no quantitative and unbiased approach for prioritising candidate markers, we created the novel but unvalidated BMS (Table 2) for this study.

We evaluated each identified biomarker (Table 3) using the BMS (Table 2). No biomarker had the maximum score (5/5). The highest-scoring markers (score 4/5) were HO-1, IL-6, IL-12, IL-18, osteoprotogerin (OPG), S100A12 and S100A8/A9 ($n = 7$). There were 10 and 51 biomarkers with scores of 3/5 and 2/5, respectively. A score of 3/5 or greater, therefore, identified 17 (25 %) of the total biomarkers. The highest-scoring markers grouped according to diagnostic or prognostic subgroup are indicated in Fig. 1.

Next, the 36 identified D1 biomarkers, the largest group of identified biomarkers for any of the clinical questions asked, were scored and ranked as an example to show how the BMS could prioritise candidates for further evaluation (shown in Fig. 2, scores in Table 3). Seven biomarkers scored 4/5 (as listed above) and seven others scored 3/5, while the remaining 22 markers scored 2/5. This resulted in a panel of 14 markers when the cutoff was applied at a score of 3/5 or above (or $n = 15$ when S100A8 and S100A9 were analysed as separate proteins). Further ranking of markers within these broad groups was not performed. The online Search Tool for the Retrieval of Interacting Genes/ Proteins (STRING) platform was used to identify if any of these 15 proteins had known functions in common [46]. To differing extents STRING identified direct or indirect functional link or interactions between all proteins except S100A12, FSTL-1 and COMP (when tested at the "medium" confidence level). All proteins were identified to be extracellular, consistent with their measurement in peripheral blood, and had an identified immune function role. A summary of the functions of this protein set is shown in Additional file 2: Table S2.

The biomarker panel approach

Multiplex cytokine analysis can (1) differentiate SJIA from differential diagnoses and (2) identify distinct profiles in individual patients. Identification of cytokine patterns in individual patients could lead to the identification of subphenotypes within SJIA and also provide insight into the underlying biological basis for the clinical heterogeneity seen in SJIA [47, 48]. This clinical variation and the variety in identified biomarkers supports a prevailing view that a biomarker panel is required [8]. A "multimarker approach" is already used to predict risk of cardiovascular events and the multibiomarker assessment of disease activity (MBDA) is validated for rheumatoid arthritis (RA) [49–55]. The MBDA outperforms clinical assessment alone, imaging and single biomarker measurement, and is also cost-effective, measuring 12 biomarkers in just 0.2 ml of serum. A potential panel of biomarkers has recently been identified for paediatric systemic lupus erythematosus, which had good predictive value for detecting the complication lupus nephritis [56]. Jager et al. identified cytokine profiles in paired plasma and synovial fluid samples in 20 patients with SJIA using a bead array based multiplex immunoassay which measured 30 soluble inflammatory mediators in only 50 μl of sample and showed the blind measurement of IL-18 predicted patients with active SJIA with 93 % accuracy [57, 58]. While the identified studies in our analysis often evaluated more than one candidate marker, combinations of markers were not tested and did not feature in study hypotheses/design and/or sample numbers.

Prerequisites for clinical biomarkers

Sample-specific and method-specific factors should be considered before performing either discovery or validation studies [59]. Sample requirements differ according to the planned methodology and platform to be used [60, 61]. Some cytokines, such as IL-1β, are extremely sensitive to degradation by freeze-thawing, whereas IL-18 is comparatively more stable [61]. A clinical biomarker should also fulfil an unmet need and improve existing tests, while also being cost-effective, criteria which will also help define candidates for validation [10, 59, 62]. We did not investigate the cost-effectiveness of markers. However, the validation and clinical use of many of the biomarkers, as described, is limited by the cost and/or local availability of diagnostic tests.

Validation of biomarkers

Most candidate markers (86 %) were identified in a single study and/or by a single group, respectively. While this indicates that multiple groups are working on SJIA biomarkers, each with different strategies, it also reflects a lack of current understanding of the pathology of SJIA. Methods of biomarker verification, as intermediary steps towards validation, become increasingly important as new and improved biomarker discovery techniques result in large numbers of candidates [35, 63]. Identification of the same biomarker by multiple research groups could be seen as a verification step, suggesting a false positive finding to be less likely. Other verification factors might include confirmation that a candidate biomarker can be robustly measurable in peripheral blood, or the use of specific verification methods such as proteomic mass-spectrometry-based selected reaction monitoring (SRM) analysis [18]. SRM measures multiple target proteins, identified from discovery studies or existing literature simultaneously, without requiring specific antibodies as with antibody-based validation techniques, but it does not replace validation.

Biomarker validation, most frequently performed using antibody-based assays, is a difficult, costly and time-consuming process [35]. An example of validation is the included study by Rothmund et al. which compared different assays for measuring S100-proteins in JIA [21, 64]. Biomarker validation, also termed "qualification", can be separated from clinical validation as a process referring more specifically to the process of linking biomarkers to a clinical endpoint based on evidence and statistical analysis [65]. Validation is widely acknowledged to be a more difficult process than identification, due to the requirement of large numbers of samples of well-defined patients from populations not used in the discovery step. An example use of a validated diagnostic biomarker or panel could allow earlier diagnosis of SJIA, allowing treatment to be started during the "window of opportunity", the time point early enough in disease that intensive targeted treatment could be used to achieve early disease remission [8, 29, 66]. We therefore focused on identifying potentially clinically relevant diagnostic or prognostic biomarkers for SJIA from studies addressing specific clinical questions.

Conclusions

There remains a need for the simultaneous evaluation of multiple biomarkers and an unbiased method of selecting candidate biomarkers for further evaluation. The parallel use of different methodological platforms such as microbead arrays (e.g. Luminex xMAP), aptamer-based assay or label-free liquid mass spectrometry (LC-MS/MS) could improve the spectrum of detected proteins [67], while the BMS used here is an example of how candidate markers could be prioritised. Markers that exclude SJIA would also be useful in the clinical setting. In particular, markers diagnostic for the main differential diagnoses of SJIA, such as the causes of fever of unknown origin, which might include infection or malignancy, would help exclude SJIA as a diagnosis. While this review was not designed to explore markers of differential diagnoses of SJIA, including them in a potential multi-marker panel would likely improve such a diagnostic assay.

Sixty-eight unique candidate markers evaluated for the management of SJIA were identified by this literature review. Only one identified study was a validation study and very few identified biomarkers were evaluated by more than one study group. Therefore, there is a clear and urgent need to confirm and consolidate findings from discovery studies and validate findings. The use of emerging technologies, with collaborative efforts, may ultimately help achieve the goal of validating new diagnostic or prognostic biomarkers, or panels of biomarkers, for improving the management of SJIA.

Abbreviations

ACPA, anti-citrullinated protein antibodies; ANA, antinuclear antibodies; APRIL, A proliferation-inducing ligand; BAFF, B-cell activating factor; BMS, biomarker scoring system; COMP, cartilage oligomeric matrix protein; CRP, C-reactive protein; ELISA, enzyme-linked immunosorbent assay; FMF, familial Mediterranean fever; FSTL-1, follistatin-like protein 1; HC, healthy controls; HO-1, heme oxygenase-1; IFN, interferon; IL, interleukin; IL-18BP, IL-18 binding protein; JIA, juvenile idiopathic arthritis (non-systemic); LC-MS/MS, label-free liquid mass spectrometry; MAS, macrophage activation syndrome; MBDA, multibiomarker assessment of disease activity; PBMC, peripheral blood mononuclear cells; RF, rheumatoid factor; SAA, serum amyloid A; SJIA, systemic juvenile idiopathic arthritis; SRM, selected reaction monitoring; sST2, soluble ST2/IL-1 receptor-like 1; STRING, search tool for the retrieval of interacting genes/proteins platform; TNF, tumour necrosis factor; TTr, transthyretin

Acknowledgements

For assistance in accessing the literature, we thank Aisha Gohar (University Hospital Centre, Utrecht), Patrick Maschmeyer (German Rheumatism Centre, Berlin) and Bechara Mfarrej (San Rafaelle Hospital, Milan).

Funding

FG was supported by the EU FP7 EUTRAIN (European Translational Training for Autoimmunity & Immune manipulation Network) project grant (ref.289903). FG, ML and DF received funding from the EU FP7 MIAMI project grant, ref- 305266 (Monitoring innate Immunity in Arthritis and Mucosal Inflammation).

Authors' contributions

FG conceived the study and performed the literature review and analysis. DF, CK, ML and DH participated in the study design and analyses. All authors were involved in writing the manuscript and all made substantial contributions to the content and approved the final manuscript.

Authors' information

FG is a paediatric trainee and a PhD candidate and Marie Curie Fellow in the European Union FP7-funded EUTRAIN Programme (European Translational Training for Autoimmunity & Immune Manipulation Network) at the Department of Paediatric Rheumatology and Immunology, University Children's Hospital Münster, Germany. Previously she worked as an academic clinical fellow at the University of Liverpool, Alder Hey Children's National Health Service Foundation Trust, Liverpool, UK. Currently, she is investigating serum biomarkers for autoinflammatory disorders. CK graduated in Biosciences and obtained a PhD on antibody-peptide interaction studies from

Goethe-University Frankfurt, Germany. In 2009, he joined Rikard Holmdahl at Medical Inflammation Research, Karolinska Institute, Stockholm, Sweden for postdoctoral training in developing peptide-based tools for the diagnosis and treatment of rheumatoid arthritis. Following his interest in innate immune functions in inflammation, he joined DF's team at the Department of Paediatric Rheumatology and Immunology in 2012. There he leads a clinical-translational junior research group focusing on mechanistic aspects of alarmin signalling and innate and adaptive immune functions in arthritis. ML graduated in Microbiology and later, by studying the response of the avian innate immunity against bacterial and viral respiratory pathogens, gained his PhD in Biological and Biotechnical Sciences - Genetics at the University of Ljubljana, Slovenia. As a Marie Curie TRACKS (Transglutaminases: role in pathogenesis, diagnosis and therapy) postdoctoral fellow in the group of Roberto Marzari at Life Science Department, University of Trieste, Italy, he studied the transglutaminase 2 (TG2) interactome and the interaction between TG2 and celiac disease auto-antibodies. Joining DF's team in 2012, his current research interests as a senior postdoctoral researcher in the EU FP7-funded MIAMI (Monitoring innate immunity in arthritis and mucosal inflammation) project are serum biomarkers in autoinflammatory diseases, like JIA and IBD, and the mechanisms of pathogenesis and the immune response in Kawasaki and celiac disease. DH graduated in Medicine and started his residency in Paediatrics at the University of Münster, Germany in 2007. In 2008, he joined Johannes Roth as Research Associate at the Institute of Immunology, Münster, where he studied S100 proteins as biomarkers and damage-associated molecular patterns in autoinflammatory diseases, and the role of the innate immune response during *S. aureus* infection. In 2013, he joined DF at the Department of Paediatric Rheumatology and Immunology, University Children's Hospital Münster, Germany where he continues his research on autoinflammatory diseases, and is training as a paediatric rheumatologist. DF is a full professor and head of paediatric rheumatology and immunology at the University of Münster, Germany. His research focus is on clinical–translational science with an overall objective to translate the knowledge from basic science on innate immunity into tools to improve the stratification of patients, with regard to their disease characteristics and prognostic factors. He coordinates major national and international research consortia and has an active role not only in the German Society of Paediatric Rheumatology but also in international networks such as the Paediatric Rheumatology International Trials Organisation (PRINTO) and the Paediatric Rheumatology European Society (PReS). He was awarded several prizes and co-organizes major international symposia.

Competing interests
The authors declare that they have no competing interests.

Consent for publication
Each author has consented to the publication of this work.

References

1. Petty RE, Southwood TR, Manners P, Baum J, Glass DN, He X, Maldonado-Cocco J, Orozco-Alcala J, Prieur A, Suarez-Almazor ME, Woo P; International League of Associations for Rheumatology. International League of Associations for Rheumatology classification of juvenile idiopathic arthritis: second revision, Edmonton, 2001. J Rheumatol. 2004;31;390–92. http://www.jrheum.org/content/31/2/390.citation.
2. Martini A. It is time to rethink juvenile idiopathic arthritis classification and nomenclature. Ann Rheum Dis. 2012;71(9):1437–9.
3. Gattorno M, Piccini A, Lasigliè D, Tassi S, Brisca G, Carta S, et al. The pattern of response to anti-interleukin-1 treatment distinguishes two subsets of patients with systemic-onset juvenile idiopathic arthritis. Arthritis Rheum. 2008;58(5):1505–15.
4. Fall N, Barnes M, Thornton S, Luyrink L, Olson J, Ilowite NT, et al. Gene expression profiling of peripheral blood from patients with untreated new-onset systemic juvenile idiopathic arthritis reveals molecular heterogeneity that may predict macrophage activation syndrome. Arthritis Rheum. 2007;56(11):3793–804.
5. Macaubas C, Nguyen KD, Peck A, Buckingham J, Deshpande C, Wong E, et al. Alternative activation in systemic juvenile idiopathic arthritis monocytes. Clin Immunol. 2012;142(3):362–72.
6. Pascual V, Allantaz F, Arce E, Punaro M, Banchereau J. Role of interleukin-1 (IL-1) in the pathogenesis of systemic onset juvenile idiopathic arthritis and clinical response to IL-1 blockade. J Exp Med. 2005;201(9):1479–86.
7. Mellins ED, Macaubas C, Grom AA. Pathogenesis of systemic juvenile idiopathic arthritis: some answers, more questions. Nat Rev Rheumatol. 2011;7(7):416–26.
8. Hinze C, Gohar F, Foell D. Management of juvenile idiopathic arthritis: hitting the target. Nat Rev Rheumatol. 2015;11(5):290–300.
9. Smolen JS, Aletaha D, Grisar J, Redlich K, Steiner G, Wagner O. The need for prognosticators in rheumatoid arthritis. Biological and clinical markers: where are we now? Arthritis Res Ther. 2008;10(3):208.
10. Tektonidou MG, Ward MM. Validation of new biomarkers in systemic autoimmune diseases. Nat Rev Rheumatol. 2011;12:708–17.
11. Kessel C, Holzinger D, Foell D. Phagocyte-derived S100 proteins in autoinflammation: putative role in pathogenesis and usefulness as biomarkers. Clin Immunol. 2013;147(3):229–41.
12. Duurland CL, Wedderburn LR. Current developments in the use of biomarkers for juvenile idiopathic arthritis. Curr Rheumatol Rep. 2014;16(3):406.
13. Consolaro A, Varnier GC, Martini A, Ravelli A. Advances in biomarkers for paediatric rheumatic diseases. Nat Rev Rheumatol. 2015;11(5):265–75.
14. Robinson WH, Lindstrom TM, Cheung RK, Sokolove J. Mechanistic biomarkers for clinical decision making in rheumatic diseases. Nat Rev Rheumatol. 2013;9(5):267–76.
15. Oldenhuis CNAM, Oosting SF, Gietema JA, de Vries EGE. Prognostic versus predictive value of biomarkers in oncology. Eur J Cancer. 2008;44(7):946–53.
16. Søreide K. Receiver-operating characteristic curve analysis in diagnostic, prognostic and predictive biomarker research. J Clin Pathol. 2009;62(1):1–5.
17. Holzinger D, Frosch M, Kastrup A, Prince FHM, Otten MH, Van Suijlekom-Smit LWA, et al. The Toll-like receptor 4 agonist MRP8/14 protein complex is a sensitive indicator for disease activity and predicts relapses in systemic-onset juvenile idiopathic arthritis. Ann Rheum Dis. 2012;71(6):974–80.
18. Lau TYK, Power KA, Dijon S, Gardelle I De, Mcdonnell S, Duffy MJ, et al. Prioritization of candidate protein biomarkers from an in vitro model system of breast tumor progression toward clinical verification research articles. J Proteome Res. 2010;9(3):1450–9.
19. Bae CB, Suh CH, An JM, Jung JY, Jeon JY, Nam JY, et al. Serum S100A12 may be a useful biomarker of disease activity in adult-onset still's disease. J Rheumatol. 2014;41(12):2403–8.
20. Nirmala N, Grom A, Gram H. Biomarkers in systemic juvenile idiopathic arthritis: a comparison with biomarkers in cryopyrin-associated periodic syndromes. Curr Opin Rheumatol. 2014;26(5):543–52.
21. Rothmund F, Gerss J, Ruperto N, Däbritz J, Wittkowski H, Frosch M, et al. Validation of relapse risk biomarkers for routine use in patients with juvenile idiopathic arthritis. Arthritis Care Res (Hoboken). 2013;66(6):949–55.
22. Cangemi G, Pistorio A, Miano M, Gattorno M, Acquila M, Bicocchi MP, et al. Diagnostic potential of hepcidin testing in pediatrics. Eur J Haematol. 2013;90(4):323–30.
23. Foell D, Wulffraat N, Wedderburn LR, Wittkowski H, Frosch M, Gerss J, et al. Methotrexate withdrawal at 6 vs 12 months in juvenile idiopathic arthritis in remission: a randomized clinical trial. JAMA Am Med Assoc. 2010;303(13):1266–73.
24. Lotito APN, Campa A, Silva CAA, Kiss MHB, Mello SBV. Interleukin 18 as a marker of disease activity and severity in patients with juvenile idiopathic arthritis. J Rheumatol. 2007;34(4):823–30.
25. Jelusić M, Lukić IK, Tambić-Bukovac L, Dubravcić K, Malcić I, Rudan I, et al. Interleukin-18 as a mediator of systemic juvenile idiopathic arthritis. Clin Rheumatol. 2007;26(8):1332–4.
26. Shimizu M, Nakagishi Y, Yachie A. Distinct subsets of patients with systemic juvenile idiopathic arthritis based on their cytokine profiles. Cytokine. 2013;61(2):345–8.
27. De Benedetti F, Brunner HI, Ruperto N, Kenwright A, Wright S, Calvo I, et al. Randomized trial of tocilizumab in systemic juvenile idiopathic arthritis. N Engl J Med. 2012;367(25):2385–95.
28. Pascual V, Allantaz F, Patel P, Palucka AK, Chaussabel D, Banchereau J. How the study of children with rheumatic diseases identified interferon-alpha and interleukin-1 as novel therapeutic targets. Immunol Rev. 2008;223:39–59.
29. Vastert SJ, de Jager W, Noordman BJ, Holzinger D, Kuis W, Prakken BJ, et al. Effectiveness of first-line treatment with recombinant interleukin-1 receptor antagonist in steroid-naive patients with new-onset systemic juvenile idiopathic arthritis: results of a prospective cohort study. Arthritis Rheumatol (Hoboken, NJ). 2014;66(4):1034–43.

30. Ruperto N, Brunner HI, Quartier P, Constantin T, Wulffraat N, Horneff G, et al. Two randomized trials of canakinumab in systemic juvenile idiopathic arthritis. N Engl J Med. 2012;367(25):2396–406.
31. Butterfield L, Whiteside T. Cytokine Assays. Chichester: John Wiley & Sons, Ltd; 2016. p. 1–11. eLS.
32. Gaines Das RE, Poole S. The international standard for interleukin-6. J Immunol Methods. 1993;160(2):147–53.
33. Ledur A, Fitting C, David B, Hamberger C, Cavaillon J-M. Variable estimates of cytokine levels produced by commercial ELISA kits: results using international cytokine standards. J Immunol Methods. 1995;186(2):171–9.
34. Taylor P, Gartemann J, Hsieh J, Creeden J. A systematic review of serum biomarkers anti-cyclic citrullinated Peptide and rheumatoid factor as tests for rheumatoid arthritis. Autoimmune Dis. 2011;2011:815038.
35. Gibson DS, Rooney ME, Finnegan S, Qiu J, Thompson DC, Labaer J, et al. Biomarkers in rheumatology, now and in the future. Rheumatology (Oxford). 2012;51(3):423–33.
36. Hügle B, Hinze C, Lainka E, Fischer N, Haas J-P. Development of positive antinuclear antibodies and rheumatoid factor in systemic juvenile idiopathic arthritis points toward an autoimmune phenotype later in the disease course. Pediatr Rheumatol Online J. 2014;12(1):28.
37. Shin JI, Kim KH, Chun JK, Lee TJ, Kim KJ, Kim HS, et al. Prevalence and patterns of anti-nuclear antibodies in Korean children with juvenile idiopathic arthritis according to ILAR criteria. Scand J Rheumatol. Informa UK Ltd UK. 2008;37(5):348–51.
38. Aletaha D, Neogi T, Silman AJ, Funovits J, Felson DT, Bingham CO, et al. 2010 Rheumatoid arthritis classification criteria: an American College of Rheumatology/European League Against Rheumatism collaborative initiative. Arthritis Rheum. 2010;62(9):2569–81.
39. Gilliam BE, Chauhan AK, Low JM, Moore TL. Pediatric rheumatology. Measurement of biomarkers in juvenile idiopathic arthritis patients and their significant association with disease severity: a comparative study. Clin Exp Rheumatol. 2008;26(3):492–7.
40. Berntson L, Nordal E, Fasth A, Aalto K, Herlin T, Nielsen S, et al. Anti-type II collagen antibodies, anti-CCP, IgA RF and IgM RF are associated with joint damage, assessed eight years after onset of juvenile idiopathic arthritis (JIA). Pediatr Rheumatol Online J. 2014;12:22.
41. Cummings J, Raynaud F, Jones L, Sugar R, Dive C. Fit-for-purpose biomarker method validation for application in clinical trials of anticancer drugs. Br J Cancer. 2010;103(9):1313–7.
42. Swan AL, Stekel DJ, Hodgman C, Allaway D, Alqahtani MH, Mobasheri A, et al. A machine learning heuristic to identify biologically relevant and minimal biomarker panels from omics data. BMC Genomics. 2015;16 Suppl 1:S2.
43. Anderson NGL, Anderson NGL. The human plasma proteome: history, character, and diagnostic prospects. Mol Cell Proteomics. 2002;1(11):845–67.
44. Solé X, Crous-Bou M, Cordero D, Olivares D, Guinó E, Sanz-Pamplona R, et al. Discovery and validation of new potential biomarkers for early detection of colon cancer. PLoS One. 2014;9(9):e106748.
45. Ling XB, Park JL, Carroll T, Nguyen KD, Lau K, Macaubas C, et al. Plasma profiles in active systemic juvenile idiopathic arthritis: Biomarkers and biological implications. Proteomics. 2010;10(24):4415–30.
46. STRING: functional protein association networks [Internet]. [cited 2016 Jan 7]. Available from: http://string-db.org/. Accessed 27 July 2016.
47. van den Ham H-J, de Jager W, Bijlsma JWJ, Prakken BJ, de Boer RJ, Van Den Ham H, et al. Differential cytokine profiles in juvenile idiopathic arthritis subtypes revealed by cluster analysis. Rheumatology (Oxford). 2009;48(8):899–905.
48. Eng SWM, Duong TT, Rosenberg AM, Morris Q, Yeung RSM. The biologic basis of clinical heterogeneity in juvenile idiopathic arthritis. Arthritis Rheumatol (Hoboken, NJ). 2014;66(12):3463–75.
49. Wang TJ, Gona P, Larson MG, Tofler GH, Levy D, Newton-Cheh Ch, et al. Multiple biomarkers for the prediction of first major cardiovascular events and death. N Eng J Med. 2006;355(25):2631–9.
50. Eastman PS, Manning WC, Qureshi F, Haney D, Cavet G, Alexander C, et al. Characterization of a multiplex, 12-biomarker test for rheumatoid arthritis. J Pharm Biomed Anal. 2012;70:415–24.
51. Curtis JR, van der Helm-van Mil AH, Knevel R, Huizinga TW, Haney DJ, Shen Y, et al. Validation of a novel multibiomarker test to assess rheumatoid arthritis disease activity. Arthritis Care Res (Hoboken). 2012;64(12):1794–803.
52. Centola M, Cavet G, Shen Y, Ramanujan S, Knowlton N, Swan KA, et al. Development of a multi-biomarker disease activity test for rheumatoid arthritis. PLoS One. 2013;8(4):e60635.
53. Bakker MF, Cavet G, Jacobs JW, Bijlsma JWJ, Haney DJ, Shen Y, et al. Performance of a multi-biomarker score measuring rheumatoid arthritis disease activity in the CAMERA tight control study. Ann Rheum Dis. 2012;71(10):1692–7.
54. Michaud K, Strand V, Shadick NA, Degtiar I, Ford K, Michalopoulos SN, et al. Outcomes and costs of incorporating a multibiomarker disease activity test in the management of patients with rheumatoid arthritis. Rheumatology (Oxford). 2015;54(9):1640–9.
55. Segurado OG, Sasso EH. Vectra DA for the objective measurement of disease activity in patients with rheumatoid arthritis. Clin Exp Rheumatol. 2014;32(Suppl. 85):S29–S34.
56. Smith E, Oni L, Midgley A, Ekdawy D, Corkhill R, Jones C, et al. Demonstration of an "excellent" biomarker panel for identifying active lupus nephritis in children. Ann Rheum Dis. 2015;331.
57. de Jager W, Hoppenreijs EPAH, Wulffraat NM, Wedderburn LR, Kuis W, Prakken BJ. Blood and synovial fluid cytokine signatures in patients with juvenile idiopathic arthritis: a cross-sectional study. Ann Rheum Dis. 2007;66(5):589–98.
58. De Jager W, Velthuis H, Prakken BJ, Rijkers GT, Kuis W. Simultaneous detection of 15 human cytokines in a single sample of stimulated peripheral blood mononuclear cells simultaneous detection of 15 human cytokines in a single sample of stimulated peripheral blood mononuclear cells. Clin Diagn Lab Immunol. 2003;10(1):133–9.
59. Sturgeon C, Hill R, Hortin GL, Thompson D. Taking a new biomarker into routine use–a perspective from the routine clinical biochemistry laboratory. Proteomics Clin Appl. 2010;4(12):892–903.
60. Gillio-Meina C, Cepinskas G, Cecchini EL, Fraser DD. Translational research in pediatrics II: blood collection, processing, shipping, and storage. Pediatrics. 2013;131(4):754–66.
61. de Jager W, Bourcier K, Rijkers GT, Prakken BJ, Seyfert-Margolis V. Prerequisites for cytokine measurements in clinical trials with multiplex immunoassays. BMC Immunol. 2009;10(1):52.
62. Van den Bruel A, Cleemput I, Aertgeerts B, Ramaekers D, Buntinx F. The evaluation of diagnostic tests: evidence on technical and diagnostic accuracy, impact on patient outcome and cost-effectiveness is needed. J Clin Epidemiol. 2007;60(11):1116–22.
63. Gibson DS, Finnegan S, Pennington S, Qiu J, LaBaer J, Rooney ME, Duncan MW. Chapter 8: Validation of Protein Biomarkers to Advance the Management of Autoimmune Disorders. In: Huang F-P, editor. Autoimmune Disorders - Current Concepts and Advances from Bedside to Mechanistic Insights. InTech; 2011. p. 614. ISBN 978-953-307-653-9. doi:10.5772/1851.
64. Hunter DJ, Losina E, Guermazi A, Burstein D, Lassere MN, Kraus V. A pathway and approach to biomarker validation and qualification for osteoarthritis clinical trials. Curr Drug Targets. 2010;11(5):536–45.
65. Lee JW, Devanarayan V, Barrett YC, Weiner R, Allinson J, Fountain S, et al. Fit-for-purpose method development and validation for successful biomarker measurement. Pharm Res. 2006;23(2):312–28.
66. Nigrovic PA. Review: is there a window of opportunity for treatment of systemic juvenile idiopathic arthritis? Arthritis Rheumatol (Hoboken, NJ). 2014;66(6):1405–13.
67. McArdle A, Butt AQ, Szentpetery A, Jager W De, Roock S de, FitzGerald O, et al. Technical brief. Developing clinically relevant biomarkers in inflammatory arthritis: a multi-platform approach for serum candidate protein discovery. Proteomics Clin Appl. 2015;1–20.
68. Simonini G, Matucci Cerinic M, Cimaz R, Anichini M, Cesaretti S, Zoppi M, et al. Evidence for immune activation against oxidized lipoproteins in inactive phases of juvenile chronic arthritis. J Rheumatol. 2001;28(1):198–203.
69. El-Sayed ZA, Saleh MT, Al-Wakkad AS, Sherief LS, AM N e-D. Cartilage proteoglycan aggrecan as a predictor of joint damage in juvenile rheumatoid arthritis. East Mediterr Health J. 2001;7(6):992–1003.
70. Bloom BJ, Toyoda M, Petrosian A, Jordan S. Anti-endothelial cell antibodies are prevalent in juvenile idiopathic arthritis: implications for clinical disease course and pathogenesis. Rheumatol Int. 2007;27(7):655–60.
71. Bodman-Smith MD, Fife MF, Wythe H, Corrigal VM, Panayi GS, Wedderburn LR, et al. Anti-BiP antibody levels in juvenile idiopathic arthritis (JIA). Rheumatology (Oxford). 2004;43(10):1305–6.
72. Ozawa R, Inaba Y, Mori M, Hara R, Kikuchi M, Higuchi R, et al. Definitive differences in laboratory and radiological characteristics between two subtypes of juvenile idiopathic arthritis: systemic arthritis and polyarthritis. Mod Rheumatol. 2012;22(4):558–64.
73. Gheita TA, Bassyouni IH, Emad Y, el-Din AMN, Abdel-Rasheed E, Hussein H. Elevated BAFF (BLyS) and APRIL in juvenile idiopathic arthritis patients: relation to clinical manifestations and disease activity. Joint Bone Spine. 2012;79(3):285–90.

74. Kounami S, Yoshiyama M, Nakayama K, Okuda M, Okuda S, Aoyagi N, et al. Macrophage activation syndrome in children with systemic-onset juvenile chronic arthritis. Acta Haematol. 2005;113(2):124–9.
75. Simonini G, Azzari C, Gelli AMG, Giani T, Calabri GB, Leoncini G, et al. Neprilysin levels in plasma and synovial fluid of juvenile idiopathic arthritis patients. Rheumatol Int. 2005;25(5):336–40.
76. Galeotti L, Adrian K, Berg S, Tarkowski A, Bokarewa M, Silvia Q. Pediatric rheumatology. Circulating survivin indicates severe course of juvenile idiopathic arthritis. Clin Exp Rheumatol. 2008;26(2):373–8.
77. Nakajima S, Naruto T, Miyamae T, Imagawa T, Mori M, Nishimaki S, et al. Improvement of reduced serum cartilage oligomeric matrix protein levels in systemic juvenile idiopathic arthritis patients treated with the anti-interleukin-6 receptor monoclonal antibody tocilizumab. Mod Rheumatol. 2009;19(1):42–6.
78. Urakami T, Manki A, Inoue T, Oda M, Tanaka H, Morishima T. Clinical significance of decreased serum concentration of cartilage oligomeric matrix protein in systemic juvenile idiopathic arthritis. J Rheumatol. 2006;33(5):996–1000.
79. Bloom BJ, Alario AJ, Miller LC. Persistent elevation of fibrin D-dimer predicts long term outcome in systemic juvenile idiopathic arthritis. J Rheumatol. 2009;36(2):422–6.
80. Wilson DC, Marinov AD, Blair HC, Bushnell DS, Thompson SD, Chaly Y, et al. Follistatin-like protein 1 is a mesenchyme-derived inflammatory protein and may represent a biomarker for systemic-onset juvenile rheumatoid arthritis. Arthritis Rheum. 2010;62(8):2510–6.
81. Gorelik M, Fall N, Altaye M, Barnes MG, Thompson SD, Grom AA, et al. Follistatin-like protein 1 and the ferritin/erythrocyte sedimentation rate ratio are potential biomarkers for dysregulated gene expression and macrophage activation syndrome in systemic juvenile idiopathic arthritis. J Rheumatol. 2013;40(7):1191–9.
82. Karagiozoglou-Lampoudi T, Trachana M, Agakidis C, Pratsidou-Gertsi P, Taparkou A, Lampoudi S, et al. Ghrelin levels in patients with juvenile idiopathic arthritis: relation to anti-tumor necrosis factor treatment and disease activity. Metabolism. 2011;60(10):1359–62.
83. Bobek D, Grčević D, Kovačić N, Lukić IK, Jelušić M. The presence of high mobility group box-1 and soluble receptor for advanced glycation end-products in juvenile idiopathic arthritis and juvenile systemic lupus erythematosus. Pediatr Rheumatol Online J. 2014;12(1):50.
84. Takahashi A, Mori M, Naruto T, Nakajima S, Miyamae T, Imagawa T, et al. The role of heme oxygenase-1 in systemic-onset juvenile idiopathic arthritis. Mod Rheumatol. 2009;19(3):302–8.
85. Shimizu M, Yachie A. Compensated inflammation in systemic juvenile idiopathic arthritis: role of alternatively activated macrophages. Cytokine. 2012;60(1):226–32.
86. Put K, Avau A, Brisse E, Mitera T, Put S, Proost P, et al. Cytokines in systemic juvenile idiopathic arthritis and haemophagocytic lymphohistiocytosis: tipping the balance between interleukin-18 and interferon-γ. Rheumatology. 2015;54(8):1507–17.
87. Ferreira RA, Silva CHM, Silva DAO, Sopelete MC, Kiss MHB, Mineo JR, et al. Is measurement of IgM and IgA rheumatoid factors (RF) in juvenile rheumatoid arthritis clinically useful? Rheumatol Int. 2007;27(4):345–9.
88. Shahin AA, Shaker OG, Kamal N, Hafez HA, Gaber W, Shahin HA. Circulating interleukin-6, soluble interleukin-2 receptors, tumor necrosis factor alpha, and interleukin-10 levels in juvenile chronic arthritis: correlations with soft tissue vascularity assessed by power Doppler sonography. Rheumatol Int. 2002;22(2):84–8.
89. Yilmaz M, Kendirli SG, Altintas D, Bingöl G, Antmen B. Cytokine levels in serum of patients with juvenile rheumatoid arthritis. Clin Rheumatol. 2001;20(1):30–5.
90. Chen O, Shan N, Zhu X, Wang Y, Ren P, Wei D, et al. The imbalance of IL-18/IL-18BP in patients with systemic juvenile idiopathic arthritis. Acta Biochim Biophys Sin Shanghai. 2013;45(4):339–41.
91. Shimizu M, Yokoyama T, Yamada K, Kaneda H, Wada H, Wada T, et al. Distinct cytokine profiles of systemic-onset juvenile idiopathic arthritis-associated macrophage activation syndrome with particular emphasis on the role of interleukin-18 in its pathogenesis. Rheumatology (Oxford). 2010;49(9):1645–53.
92. Maeno N, Takei S, Nomura Y, Imanaka H, Hokonohara M, Miyata K. Highly elevated serum levels of interleukin-18 in systemic juvenile idiopathic arthritis but not in other juvenile idiopathic arthritis subtypes or in Kawasaki disease: comment on the article by Kawashima et al. Arthritis Rheum. 2002;46(9):2539–41. author reply 2541–2.
93. Aggarwal A, Agarwal S, Misra R. Chemokine and chemokine receptor analysis reveals elevated interferon-inducible protein-10 (IP)-10/CXCL10 levels and increased number of CCR5+ and CXCR3+ CD4 T cells in synovial fluid of patients with enthesitis-related arthritis (ERA). Clin Exp Immunol. 2007;148(3):515–9.
94. Ezzat MHM, El-Gammasy TMA, Shaheen KYA, Osman AOY. Elevated production of galectin-3 is correlated with juvenile idiopathic arthritis disease activity, severity, and progression. Int J Rheum Dis. 2011;14(4):345–52.
95. Bica BERG, Gomes NM, Fernandes PD, Luiz RR, Koatz VLG. Nitric oxide levels and the severity of juvenile idiopathic arthritis. Rheumatol Int. 2007;27(9):819–25.
96. Sarma PK, Misra R, Aggarwal A. Elevated serum receptor activator of NFkappaB ligand (RANKL), osteoprotegerin (OPG), matrix metalloproteinase (MMP)3, and ProMMP1 in patients with juvenile idiopathic arthritis. Clin Rheumatol. 2008;27(3):289–94.
97. Masi L, Ricci L, Zulian F, Del Monte F, Simonini G, Capannini S, et al. Serum osteopontin as a predictive marker of responsiveness to methotrexate in juvenile idiopathic arthritis. J Rheumatol. 2009;36(10):2308–13.
98. Tomoum HY, Mostafa GA, El-Shahat EMF. Autoantibody to heterogeneous nuclear ribonucleoprotein-A2 (RA33) in juvenile idiopathic arthritis: clinical significance. Pediatr Int. 2009;51(2):188–92.
99. Gheita TA, El-Gazzar II, El Shazly RI, El-Din AMN, Abdel-Rasheed E, Bassyouni RH. Elevated serum resistin in juvenile idiopathic arthritis: relation to categories and disease activity. J Clin Immunol. 2013;33(1):297–301.
100. Foell D, Wittkowski H, Hammerschmidt I, Wulffraat N, Schmeling H, Frosch M, et al. Monitoring neutrophil activation in juvenile rheumatoid arthritis by S100A12 serum concentrations. Arthritis Rheum. 2004;50(4):1286–95.
101. Shenoi S, Ou J-N, Ni C, Macaubas C, Gersuk VH, Wallace CA, et al. Comparison of biomarkers for systemic juvenile idiopathic arthritis. Pediatr Res International Pediatric Research Foundation, Inc. 2015;78(5):554–9.
102. Wittkowski H, Frosch M, Wulffraat N, Goldbach-Mansky R, Kallinich T, Kuemmerle-Deschner J, et al. S100A12 is a novel molecular marker differentiating systemic-onset juvenile idiopathic arthritis from other causes of fever of unknown origin. Arthritis Rheum. 2008;58(12):3924–31.
103. Frosch M, Ahlmann M, Vogl T, Wittkowski H, Wulffraat N, Foell D, et al. The myeloid-related proteins 8 and 14 complex, a novel ligand of toll-like receptor 4, and interleukin-1beta form a positive feedback mechanism in systemic-onset juvenile idiopathic arthritis. Arthritis Rheum. 2009;60(3):883–91.
104. Bleesing J, Prada A, Siegel DM, Villanueva J, Olson J, Ilowite NT, et al. The diagnostic significance of soluble CD163 and soluble interleukin-2 receptor alpha-chain in macrophage activation syndrome and untreated new-onset systemic juvenile idiopathic arthritis. Arthritis Rheum. 2007;56(3):965–71.
105. Singh A, Vastert SJ, Prakken BJ, Illges H. Decreased levels of sCD21 and sCD23 in blood of patients with systemic-juvenile arthritis, polyarticular-juvenile arthritis, and pauciarticular-juvenile arthritis. Rheumatol Int. 2012;32(6):1581–7.
106. Lehmberg K, Pink I, Eulenburg C, Beutel K, Maul-Pavicic A, Janka G. Differentiating macrophage activation syndrome in systemic juvenile idiopathic arthritis from other forms of hemophagocytic lymphohistiocytosis. J Pediatr. 2013;162(6):1245–51.
107. Reddy W, Myles A, Cheekatla SS, Singh S, Aggarwal A. Soluble CD25 in serum: a potential marker for subclinical macrophage activation syndrome in patients with active systemic onset juvenile idiopathic arthritis. Int J Rheum Dis. 2014;17(3):261–7.
108. Chen C, Tsao C, Ou L, Yang M, Kuo M, Huang J. Comparison of soluble adhesion molecules in juvenile idopathic arthritis between the active and remission stages. Ann Rheum Dis. 2002;61:167–70.
109. De Benedetti F, Vivarelli M, Pignatti P, Oliveri M, Massa M, Pistorio A, et al. Circulating levels of soluble E-selectin, P-selectin and intercellular adhesion molecule-1 in patients with juvenile idiopathic arthritis. J Rheumatol. 2000;27(9):2246–50.
110. Bloom BJ, Nelson SM, Eisenberg D, Alario AJ. Soluble intercellular adhesion molecule-1 and E-selectin as markers of disease activity and endothelial activation in juvenile idiopathic arthritis. J Rheumatol. 2005;32(2):366–72.
111. Ishikawa S, Shimizu M, Ueno K, Sugimoto N, Yachie A. Soluble ST2 as a marker of disease activity in systemic juvenile idiopathic arthritis. Cytokine. 2013;62(2):272–7.
112. El-Gamal YM, Heshmat NM, El-Kerdany TH, Fawzy AF. Serum thrombomodulin in systemic lupus erythematosus and juvenile idiopathic arthritis. Pediatr Allergy Immunol. 2004;15(3):270–7.
113. Muzaffer MA, Dayer J-M, Feldman BM, Pruzanski W, Roux-Lombard P, Schneider R, et al. Differences in the profiles of circulating levels of soluble tumor necrosis factor receptors and interleukin 1 receptor antagonist reflect the heterogeneity of the subgroups of juvenile rheumatoid arthritis. J Rheumatol. 2002;29(5):1071–8.

14

Whole blood expression profiling from the TREAT trial: insights for the pathogenesis of polyarticular juvenile idiopathic arthritis

Kaiyu Jiang[1], Laiping Wong[1], Ashley D. Sawle[2], M. Barton Frank[3], Yanmin Chen[1], Carol A. Wallace[4,5] and James N. Jarvis[1,5*]

Abstract

Background: The Trial of Early Aggressive Therapy in Juvenile Idiopathic Arthritis (TREAT trial) was accompanied by a once-in-a-generation sample collection for translational research. In this paper, we report the results of whole blood gene expression analyses and genomic data-mining designed to cast light on the immunopathogenesis of polyarticular juvenile idiopathic arthritis (JIA).

Methods: TREAT samples and samples from an independent cohort were analyzed on Affymetrix microarrays and compared to healthy controls. Data from the independent cohort were used to validate the TREAT data. Pathways analysis was used to characterize gene expression profiles. Furthermore, we correlated differential gene expression with new information about functional regulatory elements within the genome to develop models of aberrant gene expression in JIA.

Results: There was a strong concordance in gene expression between TREAT samples and the independent cohort. In addition, rheumatoid factor (RF)-positive and RF-negative patients showed only small differences on whole blood expression profiles. Analysis of the combined samples showed 158 genes represented by 176 probes that showed differential expression between TREAT subjects at baseline and healthy controls. None of the differentially expressed genes were encoded within linkage disequilibrium blocks containing single nucleotide polymorphisms known to be associated with risk for JIA. Functional analysis of these genes showed functional associations with multiple processes associated with innate and adaptive immunity, and appeared to reflect overall suppression of STAT1–3/interferon response factor-mediated pathways.

Conclusions: Despite their limitations, whole blood expression profiles clearly distinguish children with polyarticular JIA from healthy controls. Whole blood expression profiles identify several immunologic pathways of biologic relevance that will need to be pursued in homogeneous cell populations in order to clarify mechanisms of pathogenesis.

Keywords: Juvenile idiopathic arthritis, Microarray, Whole blood, Gene expression, Pathogenesis

* Correspondence: jamesjar@buffalo.edu
[1]Department of Pediatrics, University at Buffalo Jacobs School of Medicine and Biomedical Sciences, Clinical & Translational Research Center, 875 Ellicott St., Buffalo, NY, USA
[5]Genetics, Genomics, and Bioinformatics Program, University at Buffalo Jacobs School of Medicine and Biomedical Sciences, Buffalo, NY, USA
Full list of author information is available at the end of the article

Background

The Trial of Early Aggressive Therapy in Juvenile Idiopathic Arthritis (TREAT; ClinicalTrials.gov registry #NCT00443430) was an National Institute of Health (NIH) funded clinical trial [1] that compared two therapeutic regimens for treatment of newly-diagnosed polyarticular juvenile idiopathic arthritis (JIA). One treatment arm used methotrexate (MTX) as an initial therapy, while the other used a combined regimen of MTX, the tumor necrosis factor (TNF) inhibitor etanercept (ET), and oral prednisone. As part of the TREAT trial, whole blood was collected for RNA expression studies at specific time points during the course of the first year of therapy. Using whole blood expression data from the TREAT subjects, we have previously reported on the feasibility of developing expression-based prognostic biomarkers for children with the polyarticular form of JIA [2]. However, the whole blood gene expression data also provide a window through which we might also gain valuable insights into both the pathogenesis of JIA and the underlying biology of treatment response, both of which are currently poorly understood.

While whole blood (and buffy coat) expression data are inherently "noisy" (among other things, they reflect gene expressions in multiple cells and cell subsets), there are both technical [3, 4] and computational approaches [5] that can be used to improve the signal-to-noise ratio in whole blood expression data and derive meaningful mechanistic insights. Furthermore, projects like the NIH Encyclopedia of Functional DNA Elements (ENCODE) and Roadmap Epigenomics have provided investigators with a wealth of information from which to derive mechanistic insights from gene expression data. In this study, we used whole blood gene expression data derived from baseline samples from children enrolled in the TREAT study, coupled with data-mining from public resources, to identify novel pathways that contribute to JIA disease pathogenesis.

Methods

Patient samples

We have previously described the TREAT baseline samples [2]. Patients entered the TREAT trial between October 2007 and November 2009 [1]. All children fit international criteria for polyarticular-onset JIA [6]. Parents of these children gave informed written consent to provide samples for translational uses, and the protocol to use these specimens was approved by the TREAT study oversight committee and the University of Oklahoma Institutional Review Board. The patients included 19 boys and 45 girls, aged 2–14 years. ANA were detected in 30 of the girls and 10 of the boys. Approximately 2.5 ml of blood was collected at the time of enrollment (month 0) prior to treatment in a PAXgene tube (PreAnalytiX GmbH, Hilden, Germany). Samples were stored at −80 °C. A summary of patient ages and characteristics is shown in Table 1.

Healthy control samples

Controls consisted of 8 healthy girls and 11 healthy boys between the ages of 7 and 13 years recruited from the OU Children's Physicians General Pediatrics clinic. The protocol for obtaining these specimens was approved by the University of Oklahoma IRB (#13205). Anesthesia for the phlebotomy was provided using topical lidocaine/prilocaine solution. These samples are hereafter referred to as healthy children (HC).

Independent cohort

In addition to the above, whole blood PAXgene specimens were obtained from an independent cohort of children with newly diagnosed, polyarticular-onset JIA recruited from the University of Oklahoma Health Sciences Center pediatric rheumatology clinic. These children ranged in age from 3 years to 15 years and consisted of 4 boys and 6 girls. All patients in this cohort were rheumatoid factor (RF)-negative. These samples are hereafter referred to as the Oklahoma cohort (OK). Table 2 summarizes the characteristics of these patients.

All research procedures were carried out strictly following the IRB-approved protocols.

RNA processing

RNA was purified from whole blood PAXgene specimens using a PAXgene Blood RNA kit (Qiagen, Valencia, CA, USA) as recommended by the manufacturer, including a DNAse (Qiagen) step to remove genomic DNA. Globin transcripts, which reduce labeling efficiency of whole blood cell RNA and decrease signal-to-noise ratios on microarrays [7], were reduced using GLOBINclear-Human (Ambion, Austin, TX, USA). Final RNA preparations were suspended in RNase-free water, quantified spectrophotometrically, and analyzed for RNA integrity by

Table 1 Phenotypic characteristics of patients at month 0 (baseline)

	Arm 1	Arm 2
Female	19 (63.3 %)	26 (76.5 %)
Male	11 (36.7 %)	8 (23.5 %)
Aged 2–6 years	7	5
Aged 7–11 years	11	15
Aged 12–16 years	12	14
Age (years), mean ± SD	10.5 ± 4.5	11.4 ± 3.6
RF-positive	9 (30 %)	12 (35.3 %)
ANA-positive	22 (73.3 %)	18 (52.9 %)[a]

Values are given as *n* (%) unless otherwise indicated
[a]One missing value
ANA Antinuclear antibody, *RF* rheumatoid factor, *SD* standard deviation

Table 2 Characteristics of JIA patients from the Oklahoma cohort

Patient number	Age	Sex	RF status	ANA status
1	9 years	F	Negative	Negative
2	12 years	F	Negative	Negative
3	9 years	M	Negative	Negative
4	11 years	F	Negative	Positive
5	7 years	F	Negative	Negative
6	3 years	F	Negative	Positive
7	8 years	M	Negative	Negative
8	14 years	M	Negative	Negative
9	15 years	F	Negative	Positive
10	4 years	M	Negative	Negative

ANA Antinuclear antibody, *F* female, *JIA* juvenile idiopathic arthritis, *M* male, *RF* rheumatoid factor

capillary gel electrophoresis (Agilent 2100 Bioanalyzer; Agilent Technologies, Palo Alto, CA, USA).

Microarray analysis

cRNA was produced from reverse transcribed cDNA using the Illumina® TotalPrep RNA Amplification Kit (Ambion, Inc., Austin, TX, USA), hybridized to Illumina WG-6 v3 or Illumina HT-12 v4 human whole genome microarrays, and stained according to the manufacturer's directions. Array hybridizations were undertaken in three separate batches. The first batch consisted of the 19 healthy controls and 26 baseline samples hybridized on Illumina WG-6 v3 arrays. The second batch consisted of the remaining patient samples hybridized to Illumina HT-12 v4 arrays. The independent cohort of OK samples were hybridized on Illumina WG-6 v3 slides. Gene microarray data have been made available to the scientific public (GEO Accession Number GSE55319).

Statistical analysis

All statistical analyses were carried out in R (www.r-project.org). To facilitate statistical analyses relative to healthy controls, it was necessary to combine data from different array batches. Due to the difference in the arrays it was necessary to create combined datasets using only those probes that were present on both array formats. Illumina probe IDs were used to identify 39,426 common probes. Datasets were variance stabilized and normalized using robust spline normalization via the *lumi* package [8, 9]. Prior to statistical analysis non-responding probes were filtered out of the datasets using the detection p value provided by the Illumina quality control metrics to eliminate probes not responding at higher than background levels.

Differential gene expression analysis was performed using the *limma* package [10, 11]. The false discovery rate (FDR) was estimated using the method described by Benjamini and Hochberg [11]. Statistical significance of gene expression was determined at FDR ≤0.05. Gene lists of interest were exported from R and uploaded to Ingenuity IPA (Ingenuity Systems, Inc., Redwood City, USA) for further functional analysis.

Network analyses of differentially expressed genes from whole blood expression profiles

We used the Ingenuity Pathway Analysis (IPA) software (Ingenuity Systems®, Redwood City, CA, USA; IPA Summer Release, June, 2015) for network analysis, with differentially expressed (DE) genes as input following the default setting of a maximum 35 genes per network. IPA network generation transforms the query genes into a set of relevant networks based on its extensive, curated Ingenuity Pathway Knowledge Base database [12, 13]. IPA utilizes a multi-stage heuristic algorithm in constructing networks through an iterative process that optimizes both interconnectivity and number of query genes under the constraint of network size. Briefly, IPA constructs networks using gene connectivity with other genes under the assumption that the gene with the highest number of connections is the most important and, thus, has the most influence. These connections represent regulatory interactions that may be either direct (e.g., the protein product of gene "A" directly regulates the expression of gene "B") or indirect (genes "A" and "B" are regulated by the same transcription factor). The last step of IPA network construction is score calculation using the Fisher Exact test on a hypergeometric distribution. The Fisher Exact test in IPA defines the null hypothesis as being a similar proportion of query genes map to a network in the same proportion as the entire reference gene set map to the network. A network score is derived from a p value (score = −log10 p value) that indicates the probability of the query genes (defined as target molecules in IPA) in a network being randomly associated within a connecting network. It is important to note that the network score does not infer network quality; it simply indicates the fitness between a reference network and the network of query genes.

Linking genetic and expression data

The recent completion of a genome-wide fine mapping study for JIA [14] extends the list of previously known disease-associated genetic variants [15] and provided us with the opportunity to determine whether there is a genetic linkage to gene expression in JIA. Using the bedtools program [16] we intersected DE genes identified in the comparison between JIA and HC with linkage disequilibrium (LD) blocks of JIA-associated single nucleotide polymorphisms (SNPs) extracted from the JIA fine mapping study [14] as well as other known regions of risk as reviewed by Hersh and Prahalad [15]. We obtained LD block information from the SNAP database (http://www.broadinstitute.org/mpg/snap) using the 1000 genome project pilot1 and HapMap3 with a cutoff of $r^2 < 0.9$ and a distance limit of 500 bases.

Results

Correlation of TREAT samples with the Oklahoma cohort

From the TREAT study we analyzed 44 baseline samples from 28 RF-negative patients and 16 RF-positive patients, plus 19 control samples from healthy children. In addition, we analyzed independent samples from 10 RF-negative patients (the OK cohort). Oklahoma and TREAT data were first normalized without using the COMBAT algorithm that we previously applied to the TREAT data to filter out batch effects [2], as there is only one condition (baseline) in the OK subjects for comparison and, thus, the algorithm cannot differentiate between biological variation and technical variation (batch effects). Our assumption was that batch effects would weaken the statistical correlation relative to the true biological situation, and any correlation we might find using this approach would thus be significant.

We first created a scatter plot correlating the OK and TREAT expression values for all probes (Fig. 1). As shown in the figure, there are four distinct groups of probes: 1) probes that appeared to match well (roughly, x = y); 2) probes with low expression in the Oklahoma cohort but demonstrating a range of expression in TREAT subjects (seen along the bottom of the graph); 3) probes that showed low expression in the TREAT subjects but a range of expression values in the Oklahoma patients (a small number running up the left-hand side of the plot); and 4) a small scattering of probes in between.

We then asked whether those probes that are low in one set but high in the other may reflect poor quality in the arrays, especially for low-expression probes. To investigate this possibility, we used Illumina array GenomeStudio software, which calculates and reports a detection p value representing the confidence that a given transcript is expressed above the background defined by negative control probes. The cut-off we used for trimming probes from the arrays prior to differential expression analysis was to only select probes with $p \leq 0.01$. The histograms in Fig. 2 show the distribution of the probe qualities in the two datasets. For each probe we counted the number of arrays on which it had a detection p value ≤ 0.01. Using this approach, we identified multiple poor quality probes on the both array sets.

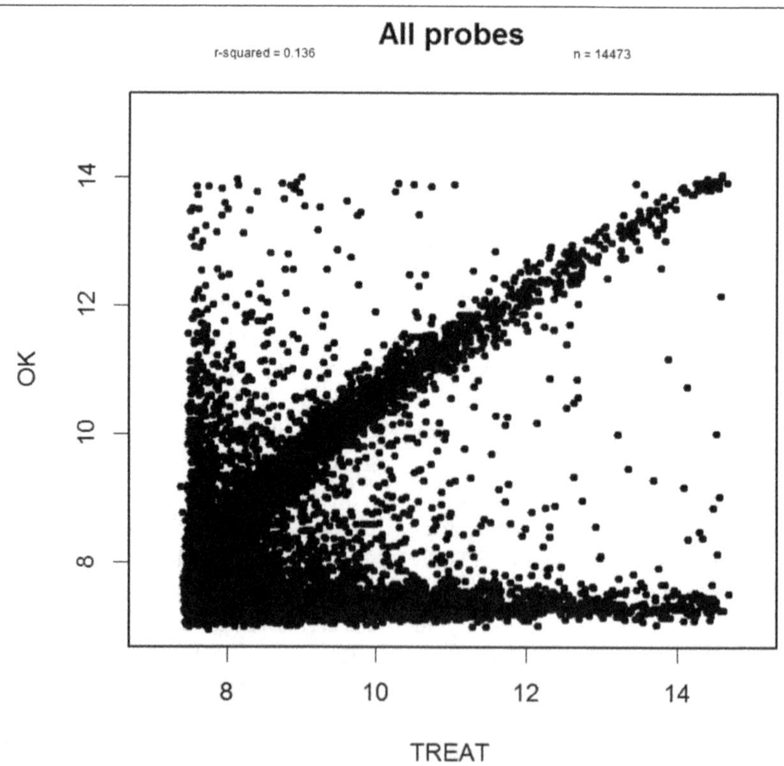

Fig. 1 Correlation between gene expression of probes between Oklahama (*OK*) and TREAT data. Four observations are shown; first, at x = y, probes correlate well; second, with y < 8, probes with low expression in the Oklahoma data but a range of expression in the TREAT data; third, when x < 8, probes with low expression in the TREAT data but a range of expression in the Oklahoma data; and, lastly, random scatters of probes in between Oklahoma and TREAT data

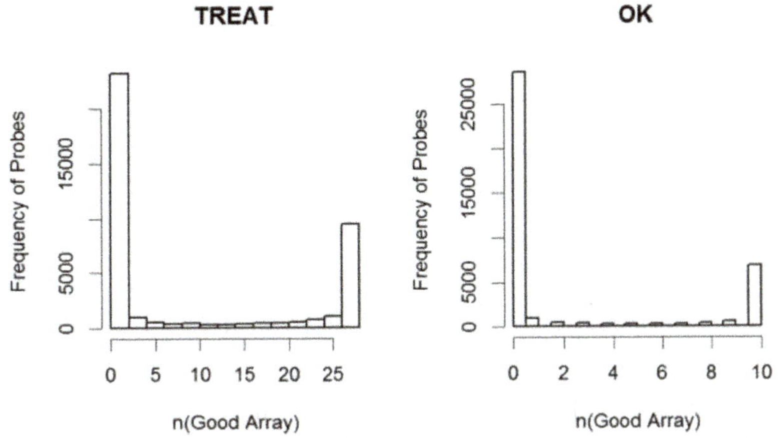

Fig. 2 Distribution of probe qualities in TREAT data (*left*) and Oklahoma data (*OK*; *right*)

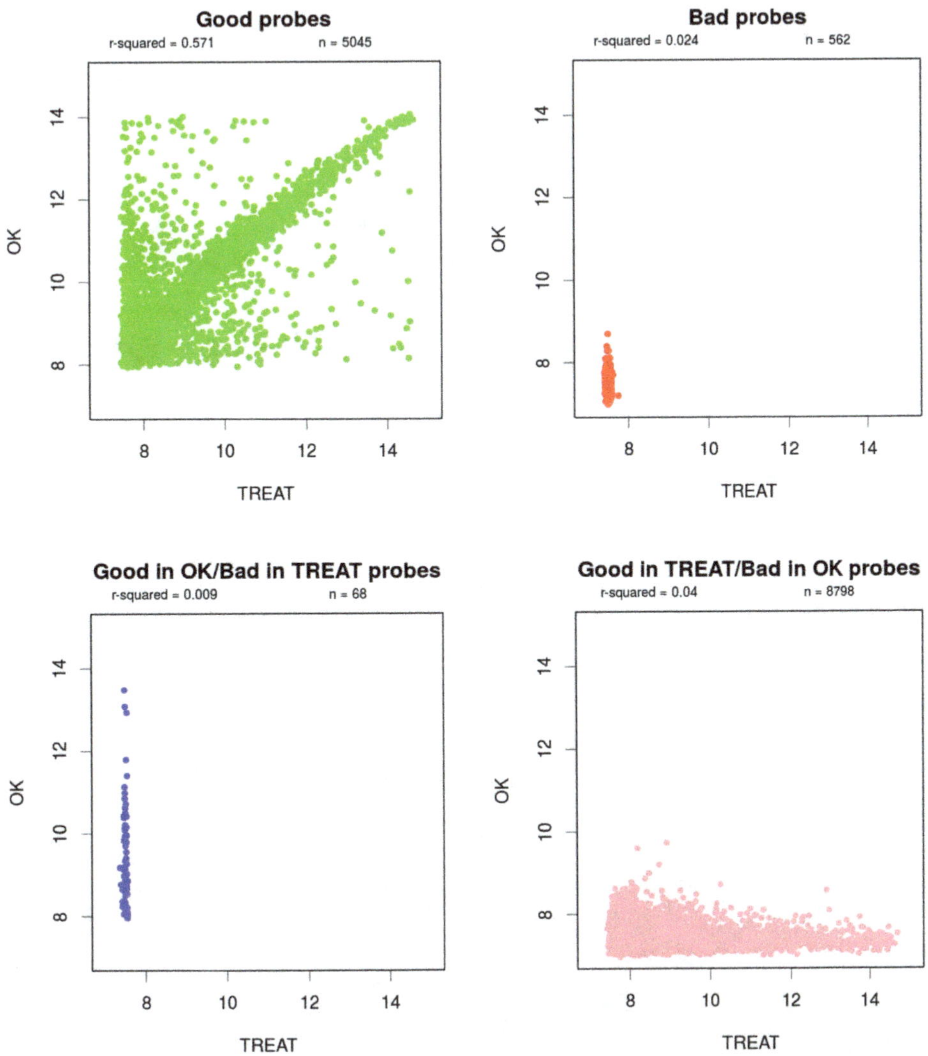

Fig. 3 Correlation of probes between TREAT and Oklahoma (*OK*) for (*top left*) good probes with good quality in both datasets and (*top right*) bad quality probes in both datasets. *Bottom left*, good probes in TREAT but bad in Oklahoma; *bottom right*, good probes in Oklahoma but bad in TREAT. Using probes that are high quality in both datasets improves correlation between the two datasets

Table 3 Differentially expressed genes in juvenile idiopathic arthritis between RF-positive and RF-negative patients

Probe_ID	Symbol	Mean expression RF⁻ (Log2)	Mean expression RF⁺ (Log2)	Fold change (Log2)	FDR
ILMN_1690443	C14orf82	8.775	9.284	−0.509	0.046
ILMN_1717594	DKFZp761E198	8.567	9.061	−0.493	0.028
ILMN_1721113	HLA-C	9.43	10.126	−0.696	0.04
ILMN_1778202	FLJ40722	11.76	12.259	−0.499	0.032
ILMN_1806165	HSPA6	10.943	11.429	−0.486	0.036
ILMN_1912662		11.38	11.896	−0.516	0.038
ILMN_2243516	C11orf63	10.335	10.939	−0.604	0.036
ILMN_2285713	TDP1	10.931	11.421	−0.49	0.015

FDR false discovery rate, *RF⁻* rheumatoid factor negative, *RF⁺* rheumatoid factor positive

Upon splitting the probes into groups based on their quality, we discerned that there were technical issues creating the two unmatched tails. In the comparison, we required that all 10 of the Oklahoma arrays be good quality (Fig. 3). Using this approach, we found that good probes (top left) displayed good quality in both datasets and bad quality probes were bad in both. Selecting only probes that are high quality in both datasets significantly improves the r^2 (0.627 for our two datasets).

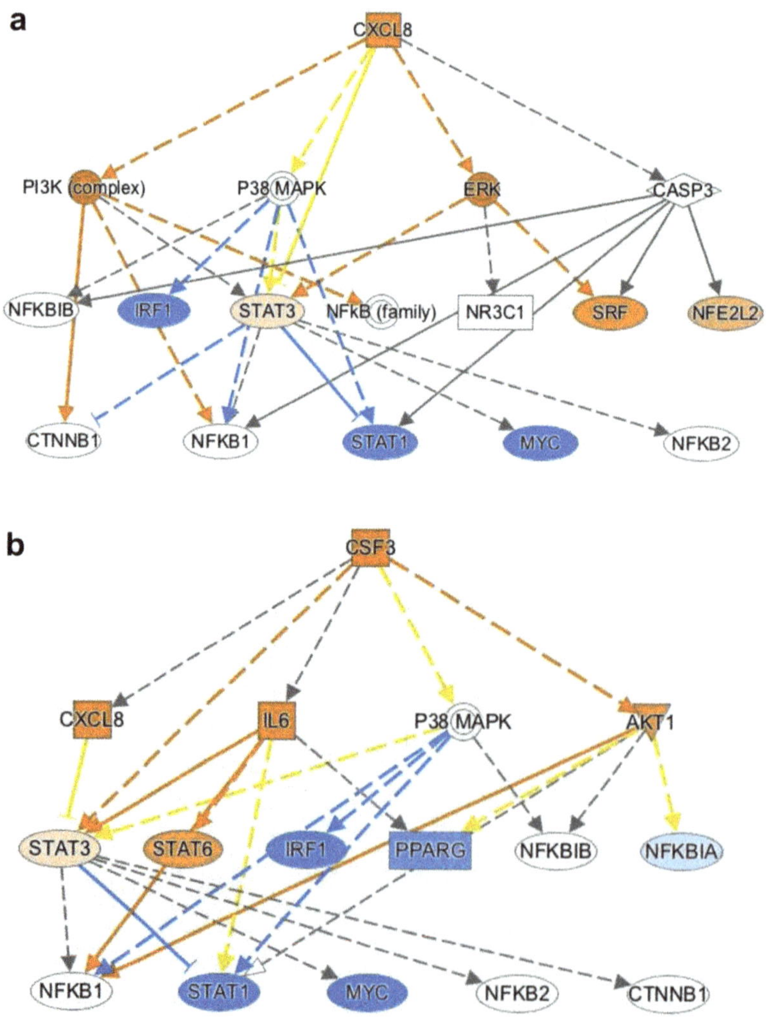

Fig. 4 Mechanistic network derived from differential gene expression analysis of upstream regulators of differentially expressed genes using IPA and comparing untreated to healthy controls. Nodes in *orange* reflect predicted activation, while those in *blue* are predicted to be inhibited based on the patterns of differential gene expression. Upstream regulators CXCL8 (**a**) and CSF3 (**b**) show an activation pattern

We also note that in our biomarker paper [2] we were able to corroborate gene expression in the TREAT and Oklahoma cohorts using quantitative polymerase chain reaction (qPCR) [11]. Having assured ourselves of the reproducibility of the array results, we proceeded to data analysis.

Differential gene expression

We first compared RF-positive ($n = 16$) and RF-negative ($n = 28$) samples. We found only 7 genes represented on 8 probes that showed differential expression between these groups; these genes are shown in Table 3. These results are consistent with our previous observation that RF-positive and RF-negative samples group together when analyzed through hierarchical cluster analyses [2]. For this reason, we determined that it would be reasonable to analyze all 44 samples (RF-positive and RF-negative) as a group.

There were 158 genes represented by 176 probes that showed differential expression with at least a 1.4-fold difference, with an FDR of 0.05, when TREAT study subjects were compared with healthy control children. The analysis of these genes using the Ingenuity database showed particular enrichment for genes regulating leukocyte adhesion and extravasation. This pattern is reflected in the network shown in Fig. 4a, demonstrating a pattern of interleukin (IL)-8 CXCL8 activation. IL-8 is produced by multiple leukocyte subsets, including macrophages [17, 18], as well as other cell types such as endothelial cells [19]. IL-8 acts through multiple G protein-coupled receptors and is a potent chemoattractant for neutrophils. It is interesting to note that we have recently demonstrated that G protein-coupled receptor signaling networks showed extensive re-organization when TREAT study subjects responded to therapy [5]. Patterns of gene expression reflect regulation by CSF3, which, like IL-8, is a potent activator of neutrophils (Fig. 4b). We have previously shown that neutrophils in JIA show aberrant patterns of activation that are linked to the metabolic pathways through which neutrophils produce myeloperoxidase and superoxide ion [20].

The baseline TREAT expression data also reflect activation of adaptive immune responses through CD3–T-cell receptor-mediated signaling, as shown in Fig. 5. T cells have long been accepted as mediators of JIA pathogenesis [21], and thus this finding was expected.

It is interesting to note that, at the same time, the expression data simultaneously reflect a pattern that we have previously identified from RNA sequencing data in human neutrophils [22]: an apparent suppression of interferon response factor (IRF)-mediated pathways leading to a suppression of type1 and type 2 interferons, as shown in Fig. 6. This pattern of suppression reflects a broader suppression of Toll-like receptor (TLR)9 activation, as shown in Fig. 7. The TREAT expression data suggest a previously unrecognized role for transforming growth factor (TGF)B1 in JIA, although its role in adult rheumatoid disease has been long recognized [23], and we have shown that TGFB1 is overexpressed in children with active JIA on therapy compared with children who have achieved clinical remission on medication [24]. These findings suggest aberrant patterns of activation and/or gene regulation within the adaptive immune system.

Linking genetic and expression data

The search for overlaps between the DE genes identified in the comparison between healthy controls and baseline TREAT subjects and LD blocks containing JIA-associated SNPs yielded no DE genes within any of the observed LD blocks. We next determined the closest LD blocks to

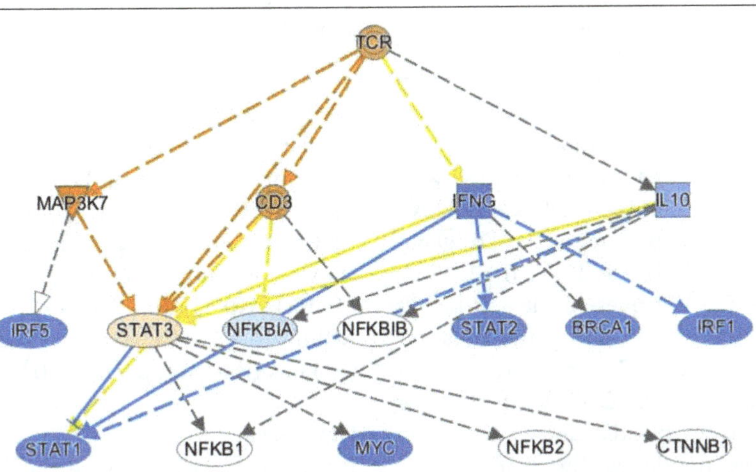

Fig. 5 Mechanistic network derived from differential gene expression analysis of upstream regulators of differentially expressed genes using IPA and comparing untreated JIA to healthy controls. Nodes in *orange* reflect predicted activation, while those in *blue* are predicted to be inhibited based on the patterns of differential gene expression. CD3–T-cell receptor (*TCR*) activation is predicted from the pattern of gene expression

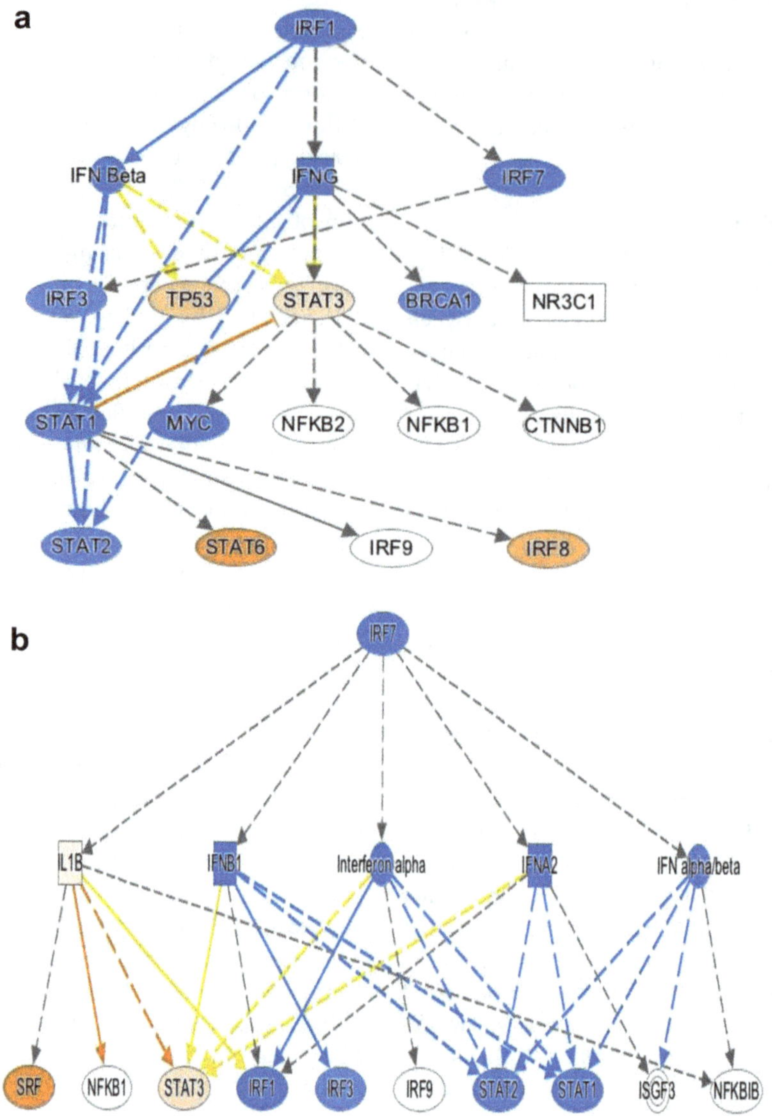

Fig. 6 Mechanistic network derived from differential gene expression analysis using IPA and comparing untreated JIA to healthy controls. Nodes in *orange* reflect predicted activation, while those in *blue* are predicted to be inhibited based on the patterns of differential gene expression. Suppression of IRF1 (**a**) and IRF7 (**b**) regulated networks is predicted from this analysis

the DE genes, and identified 75 LD blocks containing JIA-associated SNPs situated near 38 DE genes, with distances ranging between 345 and 390 kilobases. Next, we interrogated the upstream regulators of the DE genes as identified on Ingenuity analysis, i.e., IRF1, IRF3, IRF5, STAT1, STAT2, and STAT3. We queried the LD blocks containing the JIA-associated SNPs using the bedtools program. We downloaded ENCODE transcription factor binding site (TFBS) data from UCSC Genome Browser ENCODE data at http://hgdownload.cse.ucsc.edu/goldenPath/hg19/encodeDCC/wgEncodeRegTfbsClustered/and extracted TFBSs of the regulators of interest. Intersection analysis demonstrated that 53 LD blocks containing JIA-associated SNPs overlapped 232 TF binding sites for the regulators of interest. We applied Fisher's Exact test for enrichment analysis of TF binding sites overlapping with the LD blocks containing JIA-associated SNPs using all ENCODE TF binding sites as background. This analysis showed no statistically significant evidence for enrichment of IRF1, IRF3, IRF5, STAT1, STAT2, or STAT3 binding within the LD blocks containing JIA-associated SNPs (Fisher's Exact test p value 0.091).

Discussion

In this paper, we analyzed the TREAT whole blood gene microarray data in an attempt to gather insights into disease mechanisms in polyarticular JIA. We found that the whole blood expression profiles reflect complex

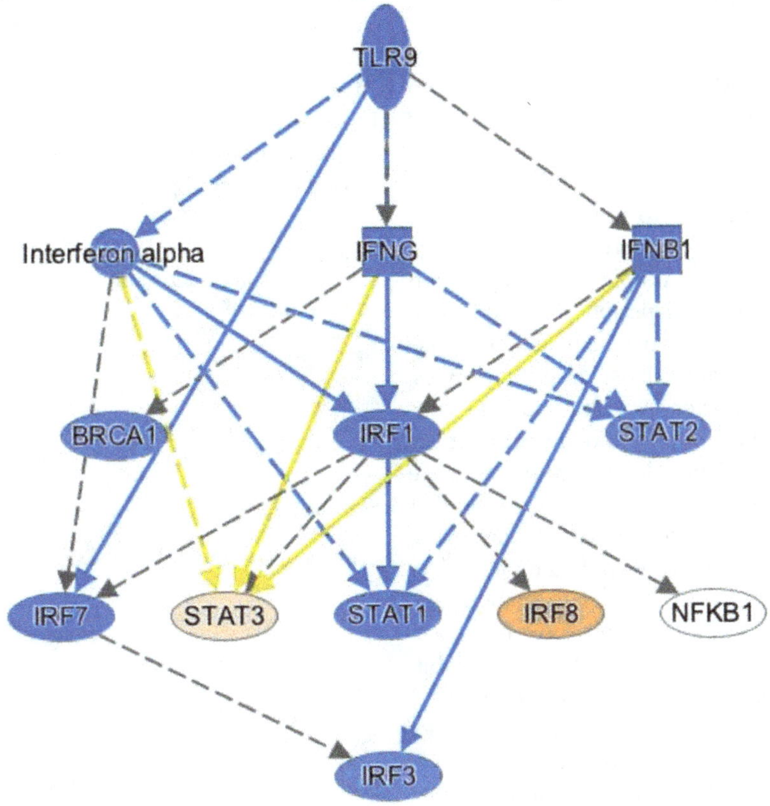

Fig. 7 Mechanistic network derived from differential gene expression analysis using IPA and comparing untreated JIA to healthy controls. Nodes in *orange* reflect predicted activation, while those in *blue* are predicted to be inhibited based on the patterns of differential gene expression. Suppression of TLR9-regulated networks is predicted from this analysis

interactions between innate and adaptive immunity, a finding that is consistent with our previous reports that both peripheral blood mononuclear cell (PBMC) [24] and neutrophil [25] gene expression profiles are abnormal in untreated children with JIA. We were not able to answer the question of whether the innate or adaptive immune aberrations are primary. While an increasing body of data shows that neutrophils are important mediators of adaptive immune responses [26–31], it is equally plausible that the transcriptional aberrations we see in neutrophils are the result of an altered cytokine milieu generated from altered T-cell function. In support of the idea that the neutrophil defect is a primary aspect of the disease is our finding that neutrophil gene expression profiles in JIA patients remain distinctly abnormal even after PBMC profiles begin to resemble those of healthy children in response to therapy [32].

These findings are also significant for what they do not tell us. Among the 158 genes that showed differential expression between baseline TREAT samples and those of healthy controls, none was located within LD blocks where there is known genetic risk for JIA [14, 15], nor are the identified LD blocks enriched for binding sites for the TFs that the whole blood expression data suggest may be important regulators of the differentially expressed genes. This finding corroborates published work demonstrating that most of the genetic risk for JIA lies within the non-coding genome [14]. We have recently demonstrated that most of the regions identified by Hinks et al. [14] are enriched (above genome background) for H3K4me1/H3K27ac-marked enhancers that can be identified in both neutrophils and CD4+ T cells [33]. Thus, if polyarticular JIA, like many complex diseases, can be characterized by the presence of so-called expression quantitative trait loci (eQTL) [34], it seems likely that the loci that most strongly influence expression will be located in non-promoter regulatory regions (e.g., enhancers, insulators, and so forth) and reflect complex layers of transcriptional control rather than perturbed function of the protein products of specific genes.

Our findings here suggest potentially useful targets for therapy in JIA. For example, the broad suppression of type 1 and type 2 interferon responses in JIA may reflect overall suppression of TLR9-mediated processes. TLR9 is an intracellular pattern recognition receptor that detects highly methylated DNA, which is common in bacterial and viral genomes (and relatively rare in mammalian genomes) [35]. In recent years, TLR9 has become an attractive therapeutic target for immune modulation in immune diseases [36, 37], as well as cancer [38–42]. Given these findings, it is hardly surprising that hydroxychloroquine, which suppresses TLR9 pathways [43, 44], has been shown to be ineffective in JIA. The TREAT whole blood expression data suggest that strategies to augment TLR9 responses might be more promising.

There are obviously limitations to these data and their interpretation. The first is the inherent "noisiness" of whole blood expression profiles. Whole blood expression profiles represent an amalgam of peripheral blood cells, including abundant leukocyte subtypes such as neutrophils and platelets, and less abundant cells such as monocytes, natural killer (NK) cells, and even circulating CD34+ cells [45]. Furthermore, while the complete blood counts of the TREAT baseline subjects did not deviate from the range typically seen in children of the same age, it is possible that the differences in expression profiles reflect expansion of small leukocyte subsets not typically identified on complete blood counts performed in a standard clinical laboratory. The noisiness and relative insensitivity of whole blood expression profiling can be reduced by removing globin genes before the RNA labeling step [3, 46], as we did here, but this step reduces only a small portion of the complexity that limits the utility of whole blood expression data. Leukocyte subset transcriptomes show a considerable degree of specificity, reflecting the specific immunologic functions of each cell type. Thus, while there are considerable commonalities in the transcriptomes and regulatory regions of peripheral blood leukocytes [47–49], it is likely that there are critical elements of leukocyte function/dysfunction in polyarticular JIA (e.g., B cells, monocytes, Th17 cells) that simply cannot be identified on whole blood expression profiling. Thus, while whole blood or blood leukocyte expression profiling has been invaluable in allowing us to develop a mechanistic understanding of significant pathologic disturbances, such as sepsis or blunt trauma [50], it seems likely that complex functional genomics approaches of specific leukocyte subsets will be required to fully elucidate the pathogenesis of more subtle phenotypes where inflammation is chronic and more indolent, as is the case in polyarticular JIA [22].

Conclusions

Whole genome expression profiling of untreated children with polyarticular JIA reveals complex transcriptional differences when compared with healthy controls. Activation of leukocyte chemotaxis/extravasation pathways and neutrophil activation by CSF3 are reflected in whole blood transcription analyses. At the same time, suppression of STAT1–3/IRF pathways, as we have previously reported in JIA neutrophils [22], is revealed in the whole blood expression profile. None of the genes that showed differential expression between children with JIA and healthy control children is encoded within LD blocks containing known JIA-associated SNPs. These findings suggest that genetic risk loci for JIA either exert their effects before the disease phenotype emerges or involves more subtle and complex layers of transcriptional regulation (e.g., by *trans*-acting enhancers [33]) than can be discerned from whole blood expression profiles.

Abbreviations

DE, differentially expressed; ET, etanercept; FDR, false discovery rate, HC, healthy children; IL, interleukin; IPA, Ingenuity Pathway Analysis; IRF, interferon response factor; JIA, juvenile idiopathic arthritis; LD, linkage disequilibrium; MTX, methotrexate; NIH, National Institute of Health; OK, independent Oklahoma cohort; PBMC, peripheral blood mononuclear cell; RF, rheumatoid factor; SNP, single nucleotide polymorphism; TFBS, transcription factor binding site; TGF, transforming growth factor; TLR, Toll-like receptor; TREAT, Trial of Early Aggressive Therapy in Juvenile Idiopathic Arthritis

Acknowledgments

This study was supported by NIH grants R01 AI-084200, R01 AR-060604 (JNJ) and R01-AR 049762 (CAW).

Authors' contributions

KJ and YC performed the wet lab experiments. This included sample processing, RNA purification, and ascertainment of RNA purity. LW, ADS, and KJ performed data analysis. This included differential gene expression analysis and corroboration of the OK and TREAT cohorts (ADS), querying of LD blocks for DE genes and TF binding (LW), and Ingenuity Pathway analysis (KJ). MBF was responsible for performing microarray procedure and assisted in data analysis and interpretation. This included RNA labeling and hybridization procedures as well as preliminary statistical procedures to monitor quality of hybridization reactions. CAW was the principal investigator on the TREAT study and assisted in data interpretation. JNJ designed and organized this study and assisted in data analysis and interpretation. All authors assisted in drafting and revising the manuscript, and read and approved the manuscript.

Competing interests

The authors declare that they have no competing interests.

Author details

[1]Department of Pediatrics, University at Buffalo Jacobs School of Medicine and Biomedical Sciences, Clinical & Translational Research Center, 875 Ellicott St., Buffalo, NY, USA. [2]Irving Cancer institute, Columbia University College of Physicians and Surgeons, 1130 Saint Nicholas Ave., New York, NY 10032, USA. [3]Oklahoma Medical Research Foundation, Arthritis & Clinical Immunology Program, 800 NE 13th St., Oklahoma City, OK 73104, USA. [4]Division of Rheumatology, Seattle Children's Hospital and Research Institute, 4800 Sand Point Way NE, MA.7.110, Seattle, WA 98105, USA. [5]Genetics, Genomics, and Bioinformatics Program, University at Buffalo Jacobs School of Medicine and Biomedical Sciences, Buffalo, NY, USA.

References

1. Wallace CA, Giannini EH, Spalding SJ, et al. Trial of early aggressive therapy in polyarticular juvenile idiopathic arthritis. Arthritis Rheum. 2012;64:2012–21.
2. Jiang K, Sawle AD, Frank MB, et al. Whole blood gene expression profiling predicts therapeutic response at six months in patients with polyarticular juvenile idiopathic arthritis. Arthritis Rheumatol. 2014;66:1363–71.
3. Liu J, Walter E, Stenger D, Thach D. Effects of globin mRNA reduction methods on gene expression profiles from whole blood. J Mol Diagn. 2006;8:551–8.
4. Chai V, Vassilakos A, Lee Y, Wright JA, Young AH. Optimization of the PAXgene blood RNA extraction system for gene expression analysis of clinical samples. J Clin Lab Anal. 2005;19:182–8.
5. Du N, Jiang K, Sawle AD, et al. Dynamic tracking of functional gene modules in treated juvenile idiopathic arthritis. Genome Med. 2015;7:109.

6. Petty RE, Southwood TR, Manners P, et al. International League of Associations for Rheumatology classification of juvenile idiopathic arthritis: second revision, Edmonton, 2001. J Rheumatol. 2004;31:390–2.
7. Cobb JP, Mindrinos MN, Miller-Graziano C, et al. Application of genome-wide expression analysis to human health and disease. Proc Natl Acad Sci U S A. 2005;102:4801–6.
8. Du P, Kibbe WA, Lin SM. lumi: a pipeline for processing Illumina microarray. Bioinformatics. 2008;24:1547–8.
9. Lin SM, Du P, Huber W, Kibbe WA. Model-based variance-stabilizing transformation for Illumina microarray data. Nucleic Acids Res. 2008;36:e11.
10. Smyth GK. Linear models and empirical Bayes methods for assessing differential expression in microarray experiments. Stat Appl Genet Mol Biol. 2004;3:Article3.
11. Benjamini Y, Hochberg Y. Controlling the false discovery rate: a practical and powerful approach to multiple testing. J R Stat Soc B. 1995;57:289–300.
12. Calvano SE, Xiao W, Richards DR, et al. A network-based analysis of systemic inflammation in humans. Nature. 2005;437:1032–7.
13. Ficenec D, Osborne M, Pradines J, et al. Computational knowledge integration in biopharmaceutical research. Brief Bioinform. 2003;4:260–78.
14. Hinks A, Cobb J, Marion MC, et al. Dense genotyping of immune-related disease regions identifies 14 new susceptibility loci for juvenile idiopathic arthritis. Nat Genet. 2013;45:664–9.
15. Hersh AO, Prahalad S. Immunogenetics of juvenile idiopathic arthritis: a comprehensive review. J Autoimmun. 2015;64:113–24.
16. Quinlan AR, Hall IM. BEDTools: a flexible suite of utilities for comparing genomic features. Bioinformatics. 2010;26:841–2.
17. Bhardwaj RS, Eblenkamp M, Berndt T, Tietze L, Klosterhalfen B. Role of HSP70i in regulation of biomaterial-induced activation of human monocytes-derived macrophages in culture. J Mater Sci Mater Med. 2001;12:97–106.
18. Xu H, Lai W, Zhang Y, et al. Tumor-associated macrophage-derived IL-6 and IL-8 enhance invasive activity of LoVo cells induced by PRL-3 in a KCNN4 channel-dependent manner. BMC Cancer. 2014;14:330.
19. Teofoli P, Lotti T. Cytokines, fibrinolysis and vasculitis. Int Angiol. 1995;14:125–9.
20. Jarvis JN, Petty HR, Tang Y, et al. Evidence for chronic, peripheral activation of neutrophils in polyarticular juvenile rheumatoid arthritis. Arthritis Res Ther. 2006;8:R154.
21. Grom AA, Hirsch R. T-cell and T-cell receptor abnormalities in the immunopathogenesis of juvenile rheumatoid arthritis. Curr Opin Rheumatol. 2000;12:420–4.
22. Jiang K, Sun X, Chen Y, Shen Y, Jarvis JN. RNA sequencing from human neutrophils reveals distinct transcriptional differences associated with chronic inflammatory states. BMC Med Genomics. 2015;8:55.
23. Pohlers D, Beyer A, Koczan D, et al. Constitutive upregulation of the transforming growth factor-beta pathway in rheumatoid arthritis synovial fibroblasts. Arthritis Res Ther. 2007;9:R59.
24. Knowlton N, Jiang K, Frank MB, et al. The meaning of clinical remission in polyarticular juvenile idiopathic arthritis: gene expression profiling in peripheral blood mononuclear cells identifies distinct disease states. Arthritis Rheum. 2009;60:892–900.
25. Jarvis JN, Jiang K, Frank MB, et al. Gene expression profiling in neutrophils from children with polyarticular juvenile idiopathic arthritis. Arthritis Rheum. 2009;60:1488–95.
26. Beauvillain C, Delneste Y, Scotet M, et al. Neutrophils efficiently cross-prime naive T cells in vivo. Blood. 2007;110:2965–73.
27. Puga I, Cols M, Barra CM, et al. B cell-helper neutrophils stimulate the diversification and production of immunoglobulin in the marginal zone of the spleen. Nat Immunol. 2012;13:170–80.
28. Sun J, Dodd H, Moser EK, Sharma R, Braciale TJ. CD4+ T cell help and innate-derived IL-27 induce Blimp-1-dependent IL-10 production by antiviral CTLs. Nat Immunol. 2011;12:327–34.
29. Hock BD, Taylor KG, Cross NB, et al. Effect of activated human polymorphonuclear leucocytes on T lymphocyte proliferation and viability. Immunology. 2012;137:249–58.
30. Harwood NE, Barral P, Batista FD. Neutrophils—the unexpected helpers of B-cell activation. EMBO Rep. 2012;13:93–4.
31. Odobasic D, Kitching AR, Yang Y, et al. Neutrophil myeloperoxidase regulates T-cell-driven tissue inflammation in mice by inhibiting dendritic cell function. Blood. 2013;121:4195–204.
32. Jiang K, Frank M, Chen Y, Osban J, Jarvis JN. Genomic characterization of remission in juvenile idiopathic arthritis. Arthritis Res Ther. 2013;15:R100.
33. Jiang K, Zhu L, Buck MJ, et al. Disease-associated single-nucleotide polymorphisms from noncoding regions in juvenile idiopathic arthritis are located within or adjacent to functional genomic elements of human neutrophils and CD4+ T cells. Arthritis Rheumatol. 2015;67:1966–77.
34. Gibson G, Powell JE, Marigorta UM. Expression quantitative trait locus analysis for translational medicine. Genome Med. 2015;7:60.
35. Yasuda K, Richez C, Uccellini MB, et al. Requirement for DNA CpG content in TLR9-dependent dendritic cell activation induced by DNA-containing immune complexes. J Immunol. 2009;183:3109–17.
36. Kline JN. Eat dirt: CpG DNA and immunomodulation of asthma. Proc Am Thorac Soc. 2007;4:283–8.
37. Klinman DM. Adjuvant activity of CpG oligodeoxynucleotides. Int Rev Immunol. 2006;25:135–54.
38. Rosa R, Melisi D, Damiano V, et al. Toll-like receptor 9 agonist IMO cooperates with cetuximab in K-ras mutant colorectal and pancreatic cancers. Clin Cancer Res. 2011;17:6531–41.
39. Berger R, Fiegl H, Goebel G, et al. Toll-like receptor 9 expression in breast and ovarian cancer is associated with poorly differentiated tumors. Cancer Sci. 2010;101:1059–66.
40. Vaisanen MR, Vaisanen T, Jukkola-Vuorinen A, et al. Expression of toll-like receptor-9 is increased in poorly differentiated prostate tumors. Prostate. 2010;70:817–24.
41. Ronkainen H, Hirvikoski P, Kauppila S, et al. Absent Toll-like receptor-9 expression predicts poor prognosis in renal cell carcinoma. J Exp Clin Cancer Res. 2011;30:84.
42. Takala H, Kauppila JH, Soini Y, et al. Toll-like receptor 9 is a novel biomarker for esophageal squamous cell dysplasia and squamous cell carcinoma progression. J Innate Immun. 2011;3:631–8.
43. Katz SJ, Russell AS. Re-evaluation of antimalarials in treating rheumatic diseases: re-appreciation and insights into new mechanisms of action. Curr Opin Rheumatol. 2011;23:278–81.
44. Brewer EJ, Giannini EH, Kuzmina N, Alekseev L. Penicillamine and hydroxychloroquine in the treatment of severe juvenile rheumatoid arthritis. Results of the USA-USSR double-blind placebo-controlled trial. N Engl J Med. 1986;314:1269–76.
45. Stroncek DF, Clay ME, Smith J, et al. Composition of peripheral blood progenitor cell components collected from healthy donors. Transfusion. 1997;37:411–7.
46. Field LA, Jordan RM, Hadix JA, et al. Functional identity of genes detectable in expression profiling assays following globin mRNA reduction of peripheral blood samples. Clin Biochem. 2007;40:499–502.
47. Weinstein JS, Lezon-Geyda K, Maksimova Y, et al. Global transcriptome analysis and enhancer landscape of human primary T follicular helper and T effector lymphocytes. Blood. 2014;124:3719–29.
48. Lin H, Joehanes R, Pilling LC, et al. Whole blood gene expression and interleukin-6 levels. Genomics. 2014;104:490–5.
49. Powell JE, Henders AK, McRae AF, et al. Genetic control of gene expression in whole blood and lymphoblastoid cell lines is largely independent. Genome Res. 2012;22:456–66.
50. Xiao W, Mindrinos MN, Seok J, et al. A genomic storm in critically injured humans. J Exp Med. 2011;208:2581–90.

15

Chromatin landscapes and genetic risk for juvenile idiopathic arthritis

Lisha Zhu[1†], Kaiyu Jiang[3†], Karstin Webber[2], Laiping Wong[3], Tao Liu[1,4], Yanmin Chen[3] and James N. Jarvis[3,4*]

Abstract

Background: The transcriptomes of peripheral blood cells in children with juvenile idiopathic arthritis (JIA) have distinct transcriptional aberrations that suggest impairment of transcriptional regulation. To gain a better understanding of this phenomenon, we studied known JIA genetic risk loci, the majority of which are located in non-coding regions, where transcription is regulated and coordinated on a genome-wide basis. We examined human neutrophils and CD4 primary T cells to identify genes and functional elements located within those risk loci.

Methods: We analyzed RNA sequencing (RNA-Seq) data, H3K27ac and H3K4me1 chromatin immunoprecipitation-sequencing (ChIP-Seq) data, and previously published chromatin interaction analysis by paired-end tag sequencing (ChIA-PET) data to characterize the chromatin landscapes within the known JIA-associated risk loci.

Results: In both neutrophils and primary CD4+ T cells, the majority of the JIA-associated linkage disequilibrium (LD) blocks contained H3K27ac and/or H3K4me1 marks. These LD blocks were also binding sites for a small group of transcription factors, particularly in neutrophils. Furthermore, these regions showed abundant intronic and intergenic transcription in neutrophils. In neutrophils, none of the genes that were differentially expressed between untreated patients with JIA and healthy children were located within the JIA-risk LD blocks. In CD4+ T cells, multiple genes, including *HLA-DQA1*, *HLA-DQB2*, *TRAF1*, and *IRF1* were associated with the long-distance interacting regions within the LD regions as determined from ChIA-PET data.

Conclusions: These findings suggest that genetic risk contributes to the aberrant transcriptional control observed in JIA. Furthermore, these findings demonstrate the challenges of identifying the actual causal variants within complex genomic/chromatin landscapes.

Keywords: JIA, Neutrophils, CD4 + T cells, SNP LD blocks, Functional elements, Epigenetic regulation

Background

One of the significant findings to emerge from translational studies of polyarticular juvenile idiopathic arthritis (JIA) has been the observation that peripheral blood cells in children with this disease have distinctly abnormal expression profiles. These abnormalities can be observed in neutrophils [1], peripheral blood mononuclear cells (PBMC) [2], and whole blood expression profiles [3], and do not correct even when children achieve remission [4]. In neutrophils, the transcriptional abnormalities are linked to perturbations in fundamental metabolic processes [5]. Furthermore, both hypervariable gene analyses [6] and contingency analyses [5] suggest that these transcriptional aberrations reflect impairment of the mechanisms through which transcription is regulated and coordinated on a genome-wide basis [7].

In addition to identifying transcriptional abnormalities, there has also been considerable progress in our ability to identify genetic risk in JIA [8, 9]. Furthermore, we are beginning to understand the contribution that genetic variance makes to the heterogeneity of clinical response to first-line agents such as methotrexate [10]. However, taking genetic risk information and integrating it into a coherent, testable hypothesis of disease pathogenesis has remained challenging. A recent genetic fine mapping study by Hinks et al. [11] illustrates that challenge.

* Correspondence: jamesjar@buffalo.edu
†Equal contributors
[3]Department of Pediatrics, Jacobs School of Medicine and Biomedical Sciences, University at Buffalo, Buffalo, NY, USA
[4]Genetics, Genomics, & Bioinformatics Program, Jacobs School of Medicine and Biomedical Sciences, University at Buffalo, Buffalo, NY, USA
Full list of author information is available at the end of the article

While these authors were able to identify multiple previously unknown regions of genetic risk for JIA using the Illumina Immunochip, the majority of the risk-associated variants were located within non-coding regions of the genome. In this regard, JIA resembles almost every other complex trait that has been studied using genome-wide association studies (GWAS) [12, 13], including immunologic/autoimmune diseases [14]. Thus, although it is common to identify genetic risk loci in terms of the closest protein-coding gene, we are learning that the genome is far more complex than previously imagined, and that the presence of a risk-conferring single nucleotide polymorphism (SNP) near a specific gene is not *prima facie* evidence that the causal variants have anything to do with that particular gene [15].

We have previously demonstrated how the field might begin to make sense of the wealth of genetic data that are being generated by GWAS and fine mapping studies [16], and how understanding genetic risk might provide additional insight into the transcriptional abnormalities seen in JIA. We recently demonstrated that the majority of the disease-associated SNPs identified in a genetic fine mapping study by Hinks et al. that are situated within the non-coding genome are located within linkage disequilibrium (LD) blocks that are enriched for H3K4me1/H3K27ac histone marks, epigenetic signatures associated with enhancer function, in both neutrophils and CD4+ T cells. Several of these same LD blocks contain non-coding RNAs that were identified on RNA sequencing (RNA-Seq) and verified by reverse transcriptase polymerase chain reaction (rtPCR) [16].

Our earlier paper focused entirely on the novel risk regions identified in the Hinks study [11]. In the current study, we examined additional regions of genetic risk as recently reviewed by Hersh et al. [8] and Herlin et al. [9]. We demonstrated how understanding the transcriptome and functional, non-coding genome allows us to better understand the nature of genetic risk in JIA and the well-described transcriptional aberrations. In the current paper, we examine the chromatin landscapes in both CD4+ T cells and neutrophils. The former are widely accepted as important mediators of the pathobiology of JIA [17], and the latter have become the subject of increasing interest from the standpoint of the role(s) in childhood-onset rheumatic diseases [18]. We used publically available genomic data and our own RNA-Seq data to gain mechanistic insights into JIA disease processes from genetic risk data.

Methods

Defining LD regions

SNPs used in this query are listed in Table 1 and were previously reviewed by Hersh et al. [8], Herlin et al. [9] and Hinks et al. [11]. We used an SNP Annotation And Proxy search (SNAP) database (http://www.broadinstitute.org/mpg/snap) [19] to define LD blocks based on the location of each SNP. In brief, we used the settings as follows: SNP dataset: 1000 Genome pilot 1 and HapMap 3 (release 2), r^2 threshhold: 0.9, Population Panel: CEU, Distance limit: 500. We selected the smallest number as our start location and the largest number as our stop location for each defined LD block.

Analysis of neutrophil RNA-Seq data

We queried neutrophil RNA-seq data from previously published RNA-seq studies [16, 20, 21] by uploading the data into the University of California Santa Cruz (UCSC) Genome Browser. The previously defined LD blocks were queried and visually inspected for signal representing intronic and intergenic transcripts as described in our previous paper [16]. We then selected two representative transcripts (one intronic and one intergenic) to confirm the presence of non-coding transcripts in these regions.

Verification of non-coding RNA transcripts identified in neutrophils within the JIA-associated LD blocks

Complementary DNA was synthesized from total RNA using an iScript cDNA Synthesis kit (Bio-Rad). rt-PCR was performed using a HotStar Master PCR kit (Qiagen) with a Veriti thermocycler (Life Technologies) and included a control with no reverse transcription to exclude the possibility of an artifactual result due to contaminating genomic DNA. The temperature profile consisted of an initial step of 95 °C for 10 minutes, followed by 35 cycles of 95 °C for 30 seconds, 60 °C for 30 seconds and 72 °C for 30 seconds, and then a final step of 72 °C for 10 minutes. PCR products were resolved in 1.5% agarose gel. The nucleotide sequences of the primers were as follows: for ncTNFa (chr6: 31,544,379-31,544,485), 5′-CCTAATTCTG GGTTTGGGTTTGGG-3′ (forward) and 5′-CCTACTT TCACCTCCATCCATCCT-3′ (reverse); for ncSTAT4 (chr2:191,915,516-191,915,617), 5′- GTCTTGTGCAACT TCTTCCTTTC-3′ (forward) and 5′- ACCCTGTGACTG TTTGAGATTAC-3′ (reverse).

ENCODE transcription factor binding site (TFBS) enrichment

ENCODE TFBS data were downloaded from UCSC Genome Browser ENCODE data (http://hgdownload.cse.ucsc.edu/goldenPath/hg19/encodeDCC/wgEncodeReg TfbsClustered/). Only the TFBS information annotated for blood cells was used. The whole genome was binned to 100 bp bins and intersected with H3K4me1 or H3K27ac peak regions, which were used as background. Fisher's exact test was applied to test the significance of the enrichment of TFBS of each transcription factor within H3K4me1 or H3K27ac peaks in LD blocks

Table 1 Histone marks in the SNP LD blocks in neutrophils and CD4 + T cells

LD region	SNP	Neutrophils		CD4 + T cells	
		H3K4me1 mark	H3K27ac mark	H3K4me1 mark	H3K27ac mark
chr1: 206940310 - 206947167	rs1800896	Y	N	Y	Y
chr1: 25197155 - 25203390	rs4648881	Y	N	Y	N
chr11: 36336263 - 36371757	rs4755450, rs7127214	N	N	N	N
chr12: 111884608 - 111932800	rs3184504	Y	Y	Y	Y
chr12: 112486818 - 112906415	rs17696736	Y	Y	Y	Y
chr13: 40299842 - 40368601	rs7993214, rs9532434	N	N	Y	N
chr13: 43056036 - 43066523	rs34132030	N	N	N	N
chr16: 11400900 - 11435990	rs66718203	Y	Y	Y	N
chr18: 12821903 - 12880206	rs7234029	Y	Y	Y	Y
chr2: 100806514 - 100837567	rs10194635, rs6740838, rs1160542	Y	N	Y	Y
chr2: 191900449 - 191935804	rs3821236	Y	Y	Y	Y
chr2: 191943742 - 191970120	rs7574865	N	N	Y	N
chr22: 24234493 - 24237862	rs755622	Y	Y	Y	Y
chr3: 119125202 - 119243934	rs4688013, rs4688011	Y	Y	Y	Y
chr3: 46253650 - 46350716	rs79893749	Y	Y	Y	Y
chr4: 123141054 - 123548068	rs17388568	Y	Y	Y	Y
chr6: 112359543 - 112448654	rs2280153	Y	Y	Y	Y
chr6: 137959235 - 138006504	rs6920220	N	N	Y	N
chr6: 31492453 - 31543031	rs1800629	N	Y	Y	Y
chr7: 22774437 - 22811384	rs6946509, rs7808122	N	N	N	N
chr7: 28152193 - 28243473	rs10280937, rs73300638	Y	Y	Y	Y
chr9: 123636121 - 123723351	rs10818488	Y	Y	Y	Y
chr9: 123640500 - 123706382	rs2900180	Y	Y	Y	Y

SNP single nucleotide polymorphism, *LD* linkage disequilibrium, *chr* chromosome, *Y* yes, *N* no

compared to other regions with H3K4me1 or H3K27ac peaks across the whole genome. We set the cutoff of the false discovery rate (FDR) to 0.05 for all the analyses.

Identification of H3K4me1/H327ac histone marks within LD regions

We used H3K4me1/H3K27ac ChIP-Seq data previously generated by our group from neutrophils of healthy adults [16] as our reference source for H3K4me1/H3K27ac genomic locations in neutrophils [GEO:GSE66896]. The H3K4me1/H3K27ac ChIP-Seq data reported on the Roadmap Epigenomics collection were used as our reference source for H3K4me1/H3K27ac genomic locations in CD4+ T cells [GEO:GSE198927]. The intersection of H3K4me1/H3K27ac peaks within LD regions was obtained using the bedtools intersect procedure [22] as described in our previous paper [16].

Identifying chromatin interactions in CD4+ T cells within JIA risk loci

Functional DNA elements such as enhancers do not always regulate the nearest gene. Indeed, in a recent study of chromatin conformation using HiC in T and B cell lines, Martin et al. [15] showed that >80% of long distance chromatin interactions occurred at distances >500 kb. We therefore queried an existing chromatin interaction analysis by paired-end tag sequencing (ChIA-PET) dataset for CD4+ T cells (GSE32677) [23] to determine chromatin interactions within the JIA-associated risk loci. This dataset used H3K4me2 as a marker for active enhancers, and thus provides a means of estimating those genes/gene networks that are regulated by specific enhancers or groups of enhancers. The chromosome coordinates for the observed 6520 long-distance chromatin interactions were converted from hg18 to hg19 using UCSC Genome browser LiftOver tool (http://www.genome.ucsc.edu/cgi-bin/hgLiftOver). For these analyses, we queried all known JIA-associated risk regions.

Identifying molecular pathways of disease-associated SNPs

One means of using genetic risk data to provide mechanistic insights is to identify specific biological pathways encompassed by SNP-associated genes [24, 25]. However, there is a considerable breadth of opinion about what constitutes an SNP-associated gene, as the actual causal variants may be a considerable distance (in genomic terms) from the risk-associated SNP. We therefore used the method of Brodie et al. [26] to identify molecular pathways encompassed by JIA-associated SNPs across broad genomic distances. We queried regions 200 kb upstream and downstream of the JIA-associated SNPs, as outlined previously [24] to define genes and pathways associated with JIA risk SNPs.

Results

Our previous work had queried new SNPs recently identified in a genetic fine mapping study published by Hinks et al. [4]. In the current study, we queried SNPs that were identified in reviews by Hersh et al. [8] and Herlin et al. [9] and those SNPs in Hinks et al. [11] that have not been analyzed in previous work and have established associations with JIA (Table 1). We used these SNPs to generate LD blocks using the SNAP database [19] and examined the functional genomic elements within these defined regions. We included SNPs located within non-coding regions of the genome (introns or intergenic areas), i.e., the majority of the JIA-associated SNPs.

Verification of non-coding transcripts within neutrophils in JIA-associated LD blocks

Review of RNA-Seq data using the UCSC Genome Browser suggested the presence of multiple non-coding RNA transcripts in neutrophils within the JIA-associated LD blocks. We used rtPCR to confirm the presence of two of these transcripts, i.e., those within the LD blocks containing the rs3821236 and rs1800629 SNPs. Figure 1 shows detectable expression of these transcripts in neutrophils from a healthy child and a patient with JIA. This finding corroborates the idea that the additional JIA-associated LD blocks queried in the current paper contain functional, non-coding RNA transcripts, and corroborates the findings from our earlier paper [16].

Location of H3K4me1/H3K27ac marks within LD blocks

For these analyses, we examined only those LD blocks not previously examined in our earlier paper [16] as noted in "Methods". We identified LD blocks for all of the 30 risk SNPs, which were located in a total of 23 LD blocks. For those 23 LD blocks, we examined whether there are functional elements located in neutrophils or CD4+ T cells within these risk-conferring regions.

Our first analyses were in neutrophils. Of the 23 risk loci, 16 LD blocks contained H3K4me1 marks, while 14

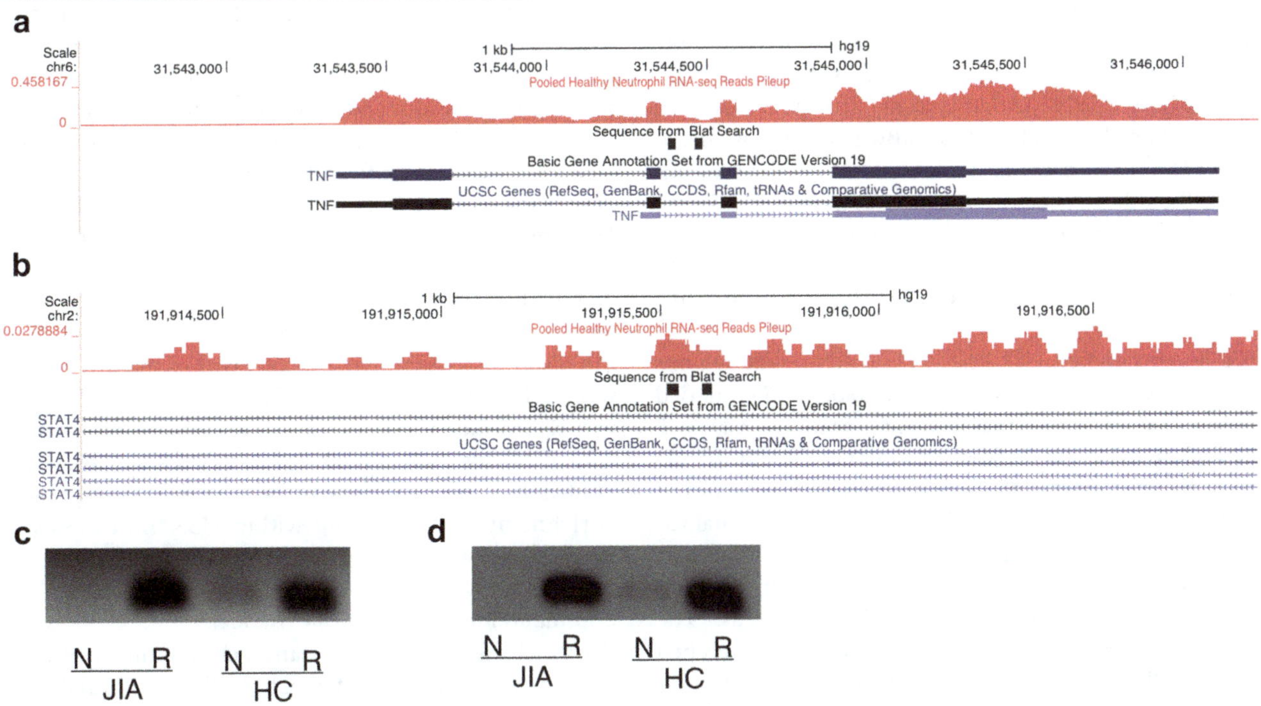

Fig. 1 University of California Santa Cruz (*UCSC*) Genome Browser screen shot showing abundant intronic transcription in the *TNF* gene (**a**) and in the *STAT4* gene (**b**) within introns. *Black bars* indicate the region amplified by PCR experiments, as described in "Methods." **c**, **d** Agarose gel images showing qualitative PCR amplification of intronic transcription (ncRNA) in the *TNF* gene (**c**) and in the *STAT4* gene (**d**) in neutrophils. *N* neutrophil RNA not subjected to reverse transcription, *R* neutrophil RNA subjected to reverse transcription prior to amplification. Neutrophils were isolated from patients with juvenile idiopathic arthritis (*JIA*) and healthy children (*HC*). Absence of signal in PCR amplifications that were performed without prior reverse transcription indicates that the signal was not being produced by contaminating DNA

LD blocks contained H3K27ac marks; 13 LD blocks contained both H3K4me1 and H3K27ac marks (Table 1). In all, 17 out of the 23 LD blocks contained either H3K4me1 or H3K27ac marks. The H3K4me1 and H3K27ac marks were significantly enriched in these LD block regions compared with non-LD block regions as determined by Fisher's exact test (p value <2.2e-16 for both H3K4me1 and H3K27ac marks).

Representative screen shots from the UCSC genome browser within two of the LD regions of interest are shown in Fig. 2. The LD block containing rs755622, for example (Fig. 2a), includes the promoter for the macrophage inhibitory factor (*MIF*) gene, but this region is also rich in transcription factor (TF) binding regions and contains H3K4me1/H3K27ac histone marks. Elevated MIF has been identified in patients with all three major JIA subtypes [27], although MIF is most elevated in children with the oligoarticular and systemic forms of the disease. Similarly, the neutrophil chromatin landscape around rs2900180 (Fig. 2b) has considerable genomic complexity. There is an expressed gene within this region, i.e., the TNF receptor-associated factor 1 (TRFA1)); there has been strong interest in the TNF signaling pathways since the efficacy of anti-TNF therapies was demonstrated in children with JIA [28]. At the same time, this region contains both H3K4me1/H3K27 marked enhancers and abundant TF binding not isolated to the TRAF promoter.

Similarly, Additional file 1: Figure S1 shows multiple functional elements adjacent to potentially disease-relevant genes such as PTPN2 (Additional file 1: Figure S1A) and NFkB inhibitor-like protein 1 (NFkBIL1, Additional file 1: Figure S1B). Thus, these findings corroborate our previous report [9] on the genetic risk regions identified in the Hinks paper [11], i.e., the genetic risk largely encompasses regions of the genome rich in functional elements that serve to regulate and coordinate transcription on a genome-wide basis.

We next examined H3K4me1/H3K27ac marked regions in CD4+ T cells in those same 23 LD blocks. We queried whether there are functional elements located in CD4+ T cells within these risk-conferring regions. Of the 23 LD blocks, 20 contained H3K4me1 marks and 15 contained H3K27ac marks. All of the 15 LD blocks that contained H3K27ac marks also contained H3K4me1 marks (Table 1). Thus, 20 out of 23 of the LD blocks contained either H3K27ac or H3K4me1 marks in CD4+ T cells. The H3K27ac and H3K4me1 marks are significantly enriched in these LD block regions compared with non-LD block regions as determined by Fisher's exact test (p value <2.2e-16 for both H3K27ac and H3K4me1 marks).

Transcription factor enrichment within the LD blocks

While H3K4me1/H3K27ac marks themselves do not unambiguously identify functional enhancers [29], the appearance of TFBS within H3K4me1/H3K27ac-marked regions is strong supportive evidence that these regions are functional [30]. Therefore, for each of the 38 LD blocks containing the 51 JIA-associated risk SNPs, we queried whether there was significant enrichment for TF binding in the H3K27ac/H3K4me1 marked regions. In these analyses, we included genetic risk information from the Hinks, Hersh, and Herlin papers. Thus, to determine whether there was additional evidence that the H3K4me1/H3K27ac marked regions within the JIA-associated LD blocks had functional significance, we queried whether there were significantly enriched TFBS within those loci compared to other genomic regions that have H3K4me1/H3K27ac marks.

For neutrophils, we observed highly enriched TF binding in promoter regions (defined as (-5 K, 1 K) of TSS) within these LD blocks. TFs that were particularly enriched included POLR2A, CHD1 and TAF1 (Fig. 3a). We noted that RUNX3 binding was also enriched within the H3K27ac-marked regions (Fig. 3a), an interesting finding in that the RUNX3 locus itself is associated with risk of JIA. This locus is characterized, in neutrophils, by dense intergenic TF binding, the presence of both H3K4me1 and H3K27ac peaks overlapping with the TF binding regions, and both intronic and intergenic RNA transcripts (not yet verified by rtPCR experiments; see Additional file 2: Figure S3). These findings suggest complex relationships between enhancers and promoters, and perhaps non-coding RNA transcripts, leading to complex levels of gene regulation in neutrophils in health and in disease states such as JIA.

For CD4+ T cells, we observed a limited number of TFBS that were significantly enriched in the LD blocks conferring risk of JIA that co-localized with H3K27ac/H3K4me1 histone marks (Fig. 3b). These regions were seen almost exclusively in promoters, defined as -5 K -1 K of the transcription start site (TSS). These transcription factors included POLR2A and GTF2F1. The majority of the distal (non-promoter) regions within these LD blocks were relatively depleted of TFBS. Thus, the LD blocks with H3K27ac/H3K4me1 marks are not highly enriched with TFs. This finding contrasts with what we observed in neutrophils, as noted above, where there is significant enrichment of TF binding within H3K4me1/H3K27ac-marked regions.

Chromatin interactions in JIA risk loci

We used the 6520 long-distance chromatin interactions from a previously-reported ChIA-PET data analysis of CD4+ T cells [23] to define chromatin interactions in all the JIA-associated LD blocks. We identified 11 LD blocks that contained 48 long-range interactions. We noted that all six of the interaction regions within the LD block containing the SNP, rs10818488, are identical to the regions within the LD block of rs2900180. Thus, 42 unique

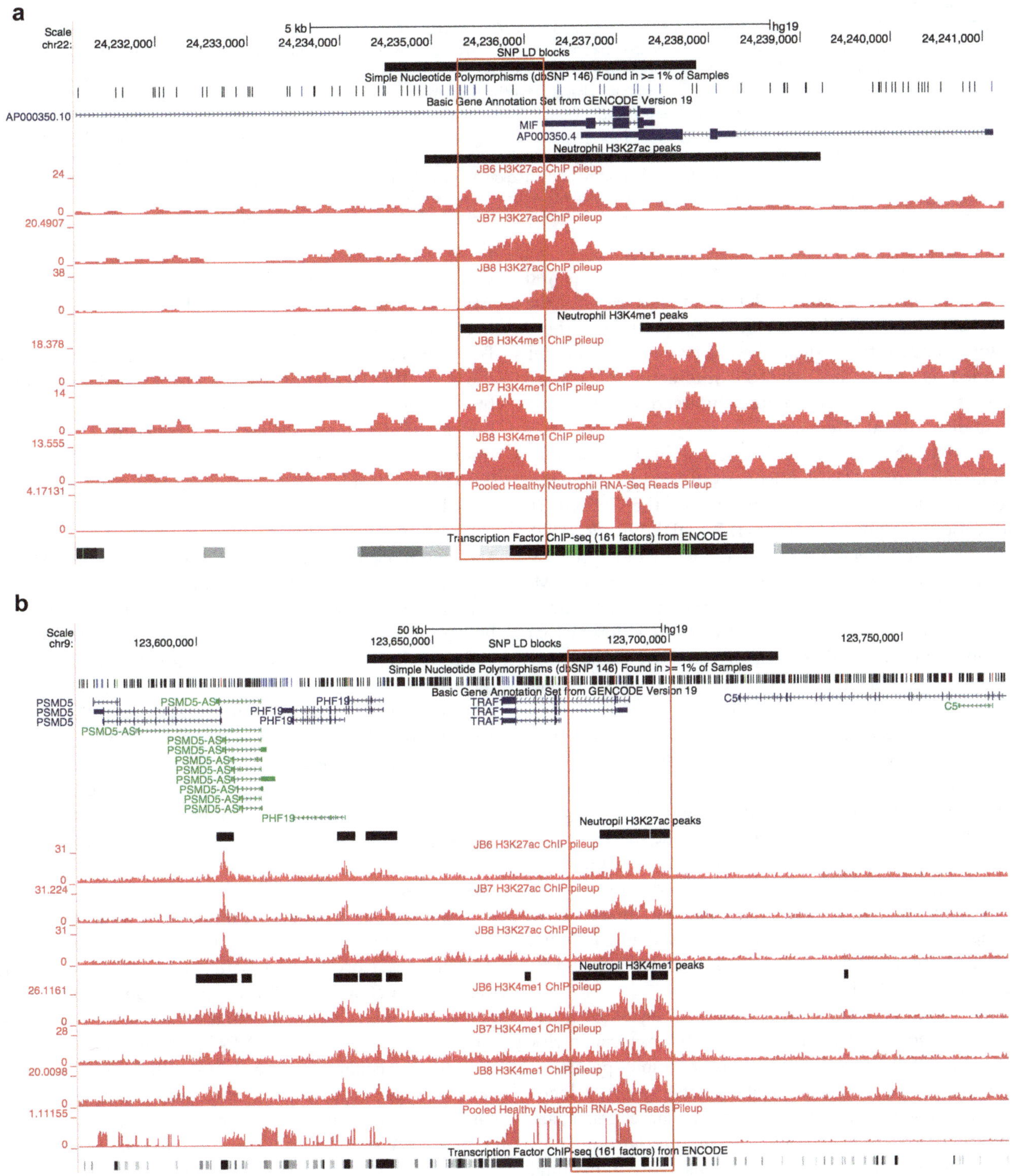

Fig. 2 (See legend on next page.)

(See figure on previous page.)

Fig. 2 Representative screen shots from the University of California Santa Cruz Genome Browser show functional elements within neutrophil genomes. *Black horizontal bar* (*top*) represents the linkage disequilibrium (*LD*) blocks of the corresponding genome-wide association study single nucleotide polymorphism (*SNP*). *Black horizontal bars* between individual tracks represent H3K27ac and H3K4me1 peak regions generated from chromatin immunoprecipitation-sequencing (*ChIP-Seq*) data. *Gray bars* at the bottom of each image represent the transcription factor ChIP-seq of 161 factors from ENCODE with factorbook motifs. **a** LD block of rs755622 in neutrophils. Note there are expressed genes within this LD block, and the LD block contains H3K27ac and H3K4me1 regions with multiple potential transcription factor binding site (TFBS) within those regions. **b** LD block of rs2900180 in neutrophils. Note that there is one gene, the tumor necrosis factor receptor-associated factor (*TRAF1*), which is expressed within this LD block. This LD block also contains both H3K27ac and H3K4me1 peak regions with multiple TFBS within those regions. Potential active enhancers (region containing both H3K27ac and H3K4me1 peak regions) are highlighted in *red*. *MIF* macrophage inhibitory factor

long-range interactions remained, 11 of which displayed more than one interaction within or intersected with the same LD blocks (Additional file 3: Table S1). For these 42 long-range interactions, 20 were promoter-promoter (defined as (-5 K, 1 K) of TSS) interactions, 21 were promoter-distal (non-promoter) interactions, and one was a distal-distal interaction.

We next analyzed the ChIA-PET data in light of transcriptomes from CD4+ T cells derived from healthy children. We identified several genes within the CHIA-PET interacting regions, including ILB, DDX39B, RASSF5 and JAK1, which demonstrated high levels of expression (average fragments per kilobase of transcript (FPKM) >100). We noted that there are multiple small RNA molecules (snoRNA, miRNA, misc_RNA, snRNA) that are encoded within these regions, but the sequencing libraries were not prepared to detect their presence because the FPKM of those molecules is zero.

Among the 42 long-range interactions, 66 regions contained both H3K4me1 and H3K27ac marks, while 2 regions contained only H3K27ac marks and 11 contained only H3K4me1 marks; only 5 of the interacting regions contained neither H3K4me1 nor H3K27ac marks. There were in all 61 genes associated with these long-range interacting regions. The genes associated with regions containing both H3K4me1 and H3K27ac marks have average higher FPKM than those genes that contained only H3K4me1 marks or those with no histone marks (Additional file 4: Figure S2).

The ChIA-PET data point to complex layers of interaction and gene regulation within the JIA-associated risk loci. Note, for example, there are multiple points of interaction between the IRF1 and Corf56 genes, a locus that also encodes a Y-RNA species. These genes are physically adjacent to one another on chromosome 5, as shown in Fig. 4a. This region is dense with functional elements, including an H3K4me1/H3K27ac-marked enhancer, dense transcription factor binding, and multiple DNase1 hypersensitivity sites. It is interesting to note that our previous work from whole blood expression profiles of untreated patients with JIA suggested an important role for IRF1 networks in the pathogenesis of JIA [3]. Equally interesting is the physical interaction detected between the HLADQB1 and HLADQB2 loci. Association between JIA risk and class II HLA alleles has been long recognized, although the alleles at the DRB1 locus are thought to have stronger effects than those at the DQB1 or DQB2 loci [31]. The genome browser shot in Fig. 4b demonstrates the complexity of this locus. Complex interactions between TRAF1 and multiple adjacent genes (C5, PHF19, and CNTRL), and TRAF1 intragenic interactions were also observed on the ChIA-PET data by Chepelev et al. [23].

Enriched molecular pathways of disease-associated SNPs

We used the method of Brodie et al. [24] and the PANTHER database [32] to identify significantly enriched biological processes and pathways for the 246 protein-coding genes and processed transcripts associated with the 51 JIA risk SNPs. Using a cutoff of a Bonferroni-adjusted p value <0.05, the enriched PANTHER pathways are related to interleukin signaling and inflammation mediated by chemokine and cytokine signaling. The enriched biological processes involve antigen processing and presentation, cellular defense response and other immunologically relevant processes (Additional file 5: Table S2).

Discussion

In this paper, we mined existing datasets in order to gain a better understanding of the nature of genetic risk in JIA and therefore gain a better understanding of the transcriptional abnormalities that we and others have previously observed in untreated patients. We found that most of the JIA-associated SNPs lie within the non-coding genome, in regions that are dense with TF binding sites, DNaseI hypersensitive sites, epigenetic signatures of enhancer function, and, in the case of neutrophils, non-coding RNA transcripts. These findings strongly support the idea that genetic risk in JIA is determined by aberrant regulation of gene expression rather than the improper function of proteins mediated by an improper amino acid substitution. This idea is now gaining broad acceptance in the field of autoimmunity [33], and may provide the basis for understanding the transcriptional abnormalities seen in a broad spectrum of peripheral blood cells in JIA. These findings also demonstrate the importance of considering

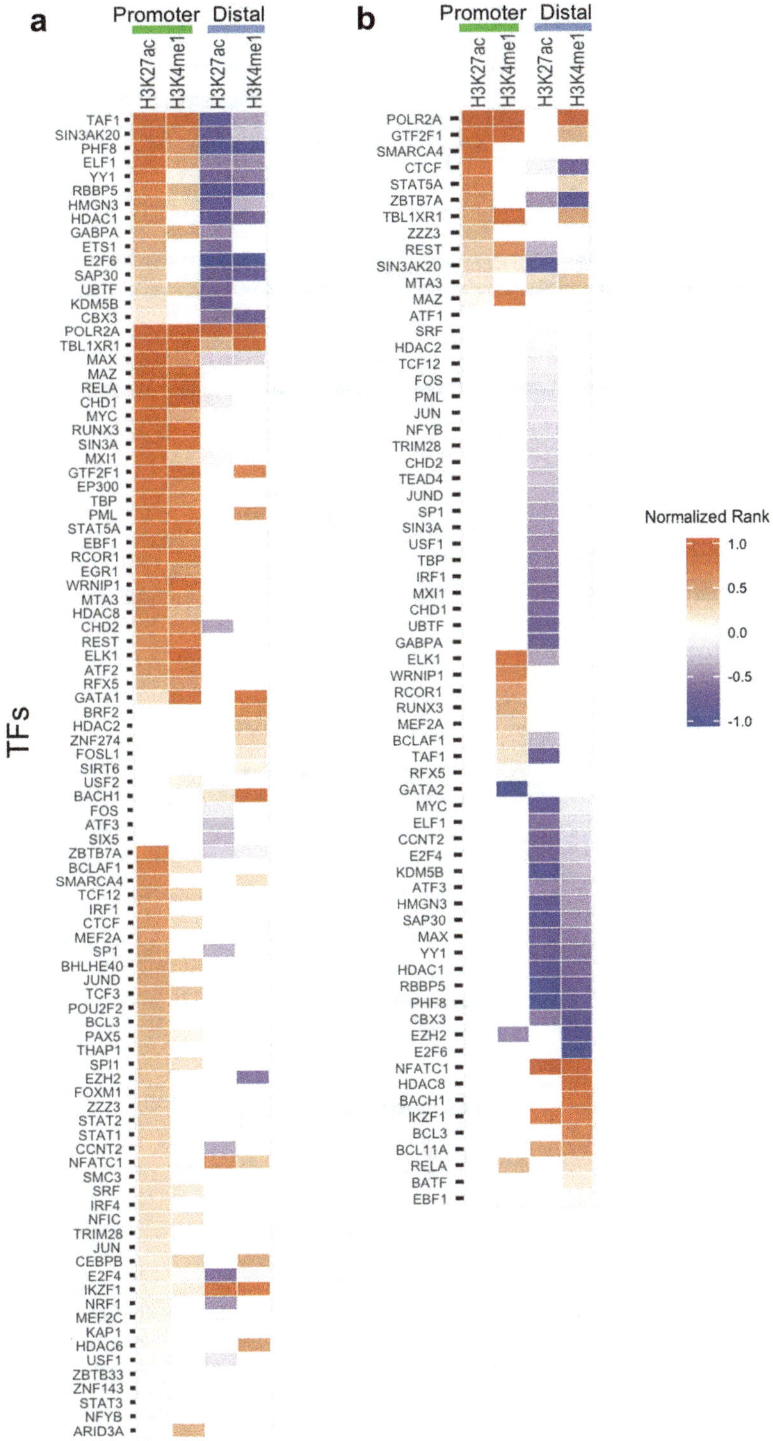

Fig. 3 Enrichment of transcription factors (*TFs*) in H3K4me1/H3K27ac mark regions. Heatmap of significantly enriched TFs with their transcription factor binding sites (TFBS) in H3K27ac or H3K4me1 peak regions in neutrophil cells (**a**) and CD4 + T cells (**b**), considering promoter and distal regions separately. TFs are ranked according to false discovery rate (FDR) (the lowest FDR with the highest rank) and normalized to (0,1) by dividing the absolute highest rank value for enrichment (*red*) and depletion (*blue*) separately. (normalized rank >0 = enrichment, <0 = depletion)

the chromatin context around disease-associated SNPs, which may have no functional association at all with the "nearest gene."

At the completion of the Human Genome Project, there was some surprise and even a little dismay at how little of the genome contains protein-encoding genes.

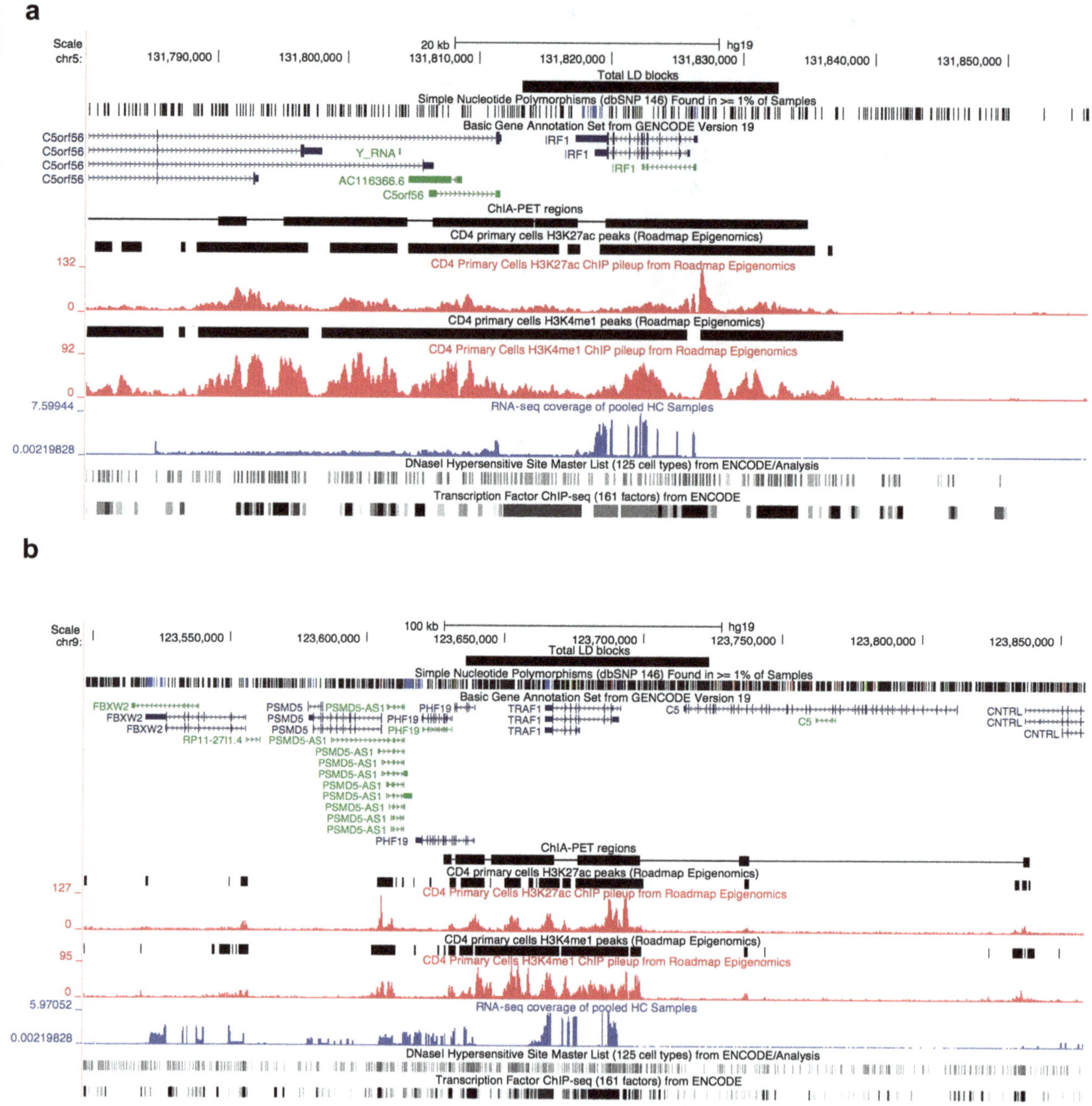

Fig. 4 a Genome browser shot of the interferon regulatory factor 1 (*IRF1*)/C5orf56 locus in CD4 primary T cells, which is an epigenetically rich region showing dense transcription factor binding, multiple DNase1 hypersensitivity sites, and active enhancers with both H3K27ac and H3K4me1 marks. **b** TNF receptor-associated factor 1 (*TRAF1*) locus with rich epigenetic architecture in this locus, including multiple transcription factor binding sites, DNase1 hypersensitive sites, and active enhancers (H3K27ac and H3K4me1 marked regions). *CNTRL* control, *HC* healthy children

When the entire project was completed, only approximately 2% of the DNA was found to encode proteins [34]. One of the transformative findings from the ENCODE and Roadmap Epigenomics projects has been the discovery of the richness of the non-coding genome. Enhancers, insulators, CCCTC binding factor (CTCF) binding sites (which regulate chromatin conformation), etc., are broadly distributed throughout the genome and demonstrate that the processes of regulating gene expression and coordinating expression on a genome-wide basis is extraordinarily complex [35]. The field of immunology is now making considerable progress in identifying these functional elements and how they regulate transcription and therefore immune responses [36].

The findings from ENCODE and Roadmap Epigenomics, and the work we describe here, demonstrate that identifying specific causal variants in JIA is going to be an ongoing challenge. A primary reason for this is the complexity of the risk loci. While many of these loci encompass genes that are of strong immunologic interest (e.g., MIF, TRAF1, PTNP2, NFkBIL1), these same loci are also rich in other functional elements that regulate transcription on a global basis. For example, Fig. 2a is a simplified genome browser screen shot that shows the neutrophil chromatin landscape around rs755622. While the actual SNP is within the promoter of the MIF gene, the entire LD block contains both H3K4me1 and H3K27ac histone marks (strong evidence for an active enhancer in this region) and rich TF binding that is not localized exclusively to the promoter. Similar genomic features can also be seen in this region in CD4+ T cells (data not shown).

We also found a large degree of complexity around rs2900180 (Fig. 2b), and rs2847293/rs7234029, which are in the same LD block. The region containing rs2847293/ rs7234029 is of broad general interest to the field of immunology, as this LD block includes the *PTPN2* gene. While PTPN2 is generally considered a regulator of T cell responses, this protein tyrosine phosphatase is broadly expressed in innate immune cells, including in neutrophils, where it serves as a negative regulator of cytokine signaling [37]. However, the PTPN2 locus is also characterized by H3K4me1/H3K27ac-marked enhancers in neutrophils and CD4+ T cells, and an apparent non-coding RNA molecule in the intron between the first and second exons in neutrophils (Additional file 1: Figure S1A). Thus, while it is tempting to focus on the protein-encoding genes within these regions as the location of the causal variants that lead to perturbed immune function, our data invite other interpretations. Enhancers, for example, may function at considerable distances (in genomic terms) from the genes they regulate, and often do not regulate the closest gene [38, 39]. This idea is shown in the recent work of Martin et al. [15]. Using Hi-C chromatin conformation capture, these authors demonstrated that >80% of long-distance chromatin interactions within T and B cell lines occurred at distances >500 Mb. Thus, until there is more solid experimental evidence to indicate otherwise, we must be open to the possibility that it is the enhancer function of these regions and/or the function of the ncRNA that are perturbed by genetic variance rather than specific functions or regulation of the nearby proteins.

This idea is corroborated by our analysis of the published CD4+ T cells ChIA-PET dataset. ChIA-PET uses crosslinked DNA to identify physical interactions between regions of DNA, which may either be in close proximity or many Mb apart on a specific chromosome (or even regions that are on different chromosomes) [23, 40]. The dataset we queried used H3K4me2 as a general mark for active enhancers. We found that the JIA-associated genetic risk loci display abundant and complex physical interactions with (usually) nearby genomic elements. The region encoding the TRAF1 gene is emblematic of this complexity. We detected interactions between an H3K4me2-marked region adjacent to the TRAF1 gene and at least three other genes. These genes included C5, the 5th component of the complement cascade, an important inflammatory mediator. The region also interacts with PHF19, which is itself a regulator of gene expression. PHF19 is a member of the polycomb repressive complex-2 (PRC-2) that is involved in gene silencing [41]. The significance of the interaction between the TRAF1 region and CNTRL (formerly for as CEP110), a centrosomic protein [42] is not immediately clear.

ENCODE also revealed that much of the genome is transcribed, and that many (if not most) of these non-coding RNA species are functional. In rheumatology, miRNA are the best-known of these non-coding RNA families, as numerous papers have shown links between specific miRNA molecules and specific immunologic features of the rheumatic diseases (e.g., [43]). Our own work has recently shown extensive re-wiring of mRNA-miRNA networks within JIA neutrophils [44]. However, the non-coding RNA world is broad, and includes RNA species that regulate chromatin accessibility [45], perform enhancer functions [46–48], and encode for small peptides [49]. Our current work also demonstrates the presence of at least two intronic, non-coding RNA molecules in the JIA-associated genetic risk loci. Such transcripts are abundant in neutrophils [50] and may regulate the decay of otherwise unstable mRNA transcripts [47]. The specific roles of these transcripts in neutrophil biology and/or the pathogenesis of JIA remain to be clarified. Their presence, however, serves to demonstrate that the localization of a disease-associated polymorphism within a specific gene does not necessarily mean that genetic risk is conferred by alterations in the protein-coding function of that gene.

The findings we report here provide an explanation for an observation that we have recently reported: differentially expressed genes in JIA are not situated within the LD blocks that confer genetic risk [3]. Using whole blood gene expression data from subjects of a National Institutes of Health-funded clinical trial, corroborated by an independent patient cohort, we reported that among >150 genes that were differentially expressed in patients and healthy controls, none were encoded within the LD blocks associated with JIA risk. Thus, the mechanisms through which genetic variance leads to perturbed gene expression are likely to be more complex than was previously considered. While it is possible that a different result might be obtained using RNA-Seq data from purified cell populations, the large number of gene-regulatory elements in the risk loci also invites us to consider that much of the genetic risk may be mediated by perturbation of long-range interactions, as suggested by the data reported by Martin et al. [15].

This paper adds to the mounting evidence that suggests that the field of pediatric rheumatology may require a fundamental re-assessment of theories on the pathogenesis of JIA. Long accepted as an "autoimmune disease" triggered by the recognition of a "self" peptide by the adaptive immune system, new evidence from the fields of genetics and genomics ought to prompt a reconsideration of this view. We propose, instead, that JIA emerges because of genetic and epigenetically mediated alterations in leukocyte genomes. These alterations, we propose, involve both innate and adaptive immune systems and lead to expression of inflammatory mediators in the absence of the external signals normally required to initiate or sustain an inflammatory response. Our work in both whole blood buffy coats [6] and neutrophils [5] is consistent with that interpretation of the available gene expression and genetic data.

Conclusions

We demonstrated that the known genetic risk loci for JIA are enriched for multiple functional elements within the non-coding genome of human neutrophils. These functional elements include rich TF binding sites, H3K4me1 and H3K27ac-marked enhancers, and non-coding RNAs. We believe that these data and newer understanding of genetic risk and genome function invite new understanding of JIA pathogenesis, and may provide the basis for radical new approaches to therapy.

Additional files

Additional file 1: Figure S1. Genome browser screen shots. Chromatin organization around PTPN2 and NFKBIL2 loci. (TIFF 20832 kb)

Additional file 2: Figure S3. Genome browser screen shots. Chromatin organization around the RUNX3 locus. (TIFF 10898 kb)

Additional file 3: Table S1. Summary of ChIA-PET peak regions intersecting with JIA-associated LD blocks. (XLSX 68 kb)

Additional file 4: Figure S2. Genes associated with these long-range interacting regions from CD4+ T cell ChIA-PET data. The genes associated with regions containing both H3K4me1 and H3K27ac marks have average higher FPKM than those genes that contained only H3K4me1 marks or those with no histone marks. (TIFF 17228 kb)

Additional file 5: Table S2. Enriched biological functions of genes within JIA-associated LD blocks. (XLS 28 kb)

Abbreviations

bp: Base pair(s); ChIA-PET: Chromatin interaction analysis by paired-end tag sequencing; ChIPseq: Chromatin immunoprecipitation-sequencing; FDR: False discovery rate; FPKM: fragments per kilobase of transcript; GWAS: Genome-wide association studies; JIA: Juvenile idiopathic arthritis; LD: Linkage disequilibrium; MIF: Macrophage inhibitory factor; ncRNA: Non-coding RNA; rtPCR: reverse transcriptase polymerase chain reaction; SNP: Single nucleotide polymorphism; SNAP: SNP Annotation And Proxy search; TF: Transcription factor; TFBS: Transcription factor binding site; TNF: tumor necrosis factor; TRAF: tumor necrosis factor receptor-associated factor; TSS: transcription start site; UCSC: University of California Santa Cruz

Acknowledgements

None applicable.

Funding

This work was supported by R01-AR060604 from the National institutes of Health (USA).

Authors' contributions

LZ and KW performed the primary bioinformatics analyses. KJ designed the primers and performed rtPCR for non-coding transcripts. LW assisted in the bioinformatics analysis. YC assisted with RNA preparation for both neutrophils for the PCR experiments. TL oversaw and directed the bioinformatics analysis performed by KW and LZ. JNJ designed the study, directed its implementation, and directed data analysis and interpretation. All authors read and approved the final manuscript.

Competing interests

The authors declare that they have no competing interests.

Ethics approval and consent to participate

Data analysis for this paper was performed on previously acquired datasets that have been published and are available in public databases (see "Availability of data and materials"). Neutrophil ChIPseq and RNA-Seq data were generated by our own research group. All research on human subjects was reviewed and approved by the University of Oklahoma and the University at Buffalo Woman & Children's Institutional Review Boards (IRB), protocol #MODCR00000010. All research was conducted in accordance with the IRB-approved protocols. Written informed consent was obtained from the parents of children (patients and controls) participating in this study. For children between the ages of 7 and 17 years, assent documents were also executed. Written informed consent was obtained from the patient/parent for publication of their individual details and accompanying images in this manuscript. The consent form is held by the authors and is available for review by the Editor-in-Chief.

Author details

[1]Department of Biochemistry, Jacobs School of Medicine and Biomedical Sciences, University at Buffalo, Buffalo, NY, USA. [2]Graduate Program in Biological Sciences, Jacobs School of Medicine and Biomedical Sciences, University at Buffalo, Buffalo, NY, USA. [3]Department of Pediatrics, Jacobs School of Medicine and Biomedical Sciences, University at Buffalo, Buffalo, NY, USA. [4]Genetics, Genomics, & Bioinformatics Program, Jacobs School of Medicine and Biomedical Sciences, University at Buffalo, Buffalo, NY, USA.

References

1. Jarvis JN, Jiang K, Frank MB, Knowlton N, Aggarwal A, Wallace CA, McKee R, Chaser B, Tung C, Smith LB, et al. Gene expression profiling in neutrophils from children with polyarticular juvenile idiopathic arthritis. Arthritis Rheum. 2009;60:1488–95.
2. Knowlton N, Jiang K, Frank MB, Aggarwal A, Wallace C, McKee R, Chaser B, Tung C, Smith L, Chen Y, et al. The meaning of clinical remission in polyarticular juvenile idiopathic arthritis: gene expression profiling in peripheral blood mononuclear cells identifies distinct disease states. Arthritis Rheum. 2009;60:892–900.
3. Jiang K, Wong L, Sawle AD, Frank MB, Chen Y, Wallace CA, Jarvis JN. Whole blood expression profiling from the TREAT trial: insights for the pathogenesis of polyarticular juvenile idiopathic arthritis. Arthritis Res Ther. 2016;18:157.
4. Jiang K, Frank M, Chen Y, Osban J, Jarvis JN. Genomic characterization of remission in juvenile idiopathic arthritis. Arthritis Res Ther. 2013;15:R100.
5. Jarvis JN, Petty HR, Tang Y, Frank MB, Tessier PA, Dozmorov I, Jiang K, Kindzelski A, Chen Y, Cadwell C, et al. Evidence for chronic, peripheral activation of neutrophils in polyarticular juvenile rheumatoid arthritis. Arthritis Res Ther. 2006;8:R154.
6. Dozmorov I, Knowlton N, Tang Y, Shields A, Pathipvanich P, Jarvis JN, Centola M. Hypervariable genes–experimental error or hidden dynamics. Nucleic Acids Res. 2004;32:e147.

7. Komili S, Silver PA. Coupling and coordination in gene expression processes: a systems biology view. Nat Rev Genet. 2008;9:38–48.
8. Hersh AO, Prahalad S. Immunogenetics of juvenile idiopathic arthritis: A comprehensive review. J Autoimmun. 2015;64:113–24.
9. Herlin MP, Petersen MB, Herlin T. Update on genetic susceptibility and pathogenesis in juvenile idiopathic arthritis.EMJ. Rheumatol. 2014;1:73–83.
10. Moncrieffe H, Hinks A, Ursu S, Kassoumeri L, Etheridge A, Hubank M, Martin P, Weiler T, Glass DN, Thompson SD, et al. Generation of novel pharmacogenomic candidates in response to methotrexate in juvenile idiopathic arthritis: correlation between gene expression and genotype. Pharmacogenet Genomics. 2010;20:665–76.
11. Hinks A, Cobb J, Marion MC, Prahalad S, Sudman M, Bowes J, Martin P, Comeau ME, Sajuthi S, Andrews R, et al. Dense genotyping of immune-related disease regions identifies 14 new susceptibility loci for juvenile idiopathic arthritis. Nat Genet. 2013;45:664–9.
12. Maurano MT, Humbert R, Rynes E, Thurman RE, Haugen E, Wang H, Reynolds AP, Sandstrom R, Qu H, Brody J, et al. Systematic localization of common disease-associated variation in regulatory DNA. Science. 2012;337:1190–5.
13. Schaub MA, Boyle AP, Kundaje A, Batzoglou S, Snyder M. Linking disease associations with regulatory information in the human genome. Genome Res. 2012;22:1748–59.
14. Farh KK, Marson A, Zhu J, Kleinewietfeld M, Housley WJ, Beik S, Shoresh N, Whitton H, Ryan RJ, Shishkin AA, et al. Genetic and epigenetic fine mapping of causal autoimmune disease variants. Nature. 2015;518:337–43.
15. Martin P, McGovern A, Orozco G, Duffus K, Yarwood A, Schoenfelder S, Cooper NJ, Barton A, Wallace C, Fraser P, et al. Capture Hi-C reveals novel candidate genes and complex long-range interactions with related autoimmune risk loci. Nat Commun. 2015;6:10069.
16. Jiang K, Zhu L, Buck MJ, Chen Y, Carrier B, Liu T, Jarvis JN. Disease-associated single-nucleotide polymorphisms from noncoding regions in juvenile idiopathic arthritis are located within or adjacent to functional genomic elements of human neutrophils and CD4+ T cells. Arthritis Rheumatol. 2015;67:1966–77.
17. Grom AA, Hirsch R. T-cell and T-cell receptor abnormalities in the immunopathogenesis of juvenile rheumatoid arthritis. Curr Opin Rheumatol. 2000;12:420–4.
18. Huttenlocher A, Smith JA. Neutrophils in pediatric autoimmune disease. Curr Opin Rheumatol. 2015;27:500–4.
19. Johnson AD, Handsaker RE, Pulit SL, Nizzari MM, O'Donnell CJ, de Bakker PI. SNAP: a web-based tool for identification and annotation of proxy SNPs using HapMap. Bioinformatics. 2008;24:2938–9.
20. Hui-Yuen JS, Zhu L, Wong LP, Jiang K, Chen Y, Liu T, Jarvis JN. Chromatin landscapes and genetic risk in systemic lupus. Arthritis Res Ther. 2016;18:281.
21. Jiang K, Sun X, Chen Y, Shen Y, Jarvis JN. RNA sequencing from human neutrophils reveals distinct transcriptional differences associated with chronic inflammatory states. BMC Med Genomics. 2015;8:55.
22. Quinlan AR, Hall IM. BEDTools: a flexible suite of utilities for comparing genomic features. Bioinformatics. 2010;26:841–2.
23. Chepelev I, Wei G, Wangsa D, Tang Q, Zhao K. Characterization of genome-wide enhancer-promoter interactions reveals co-expression of interacting genes and modes of higher order chromatin organization. Cell Res. 2012;22:490–503.
24. Wang K, Li M, Hakonarson H. Analysing biological pathways in genome-wide association studies. Nat Rev Genet. 2010;11:843–54.
25. Brodie A, Tovia-Brodie O, Ofran Y. Large scale analysis of phenotype-pathway relationships based on GWAS results. PLoS One. 2014;9:e100887.
26. Brodie A, Azaria JR, Ofran Y. How far from the SNP may the causative genes be? Nucleic Acids Res. 2016;44:6046–54.
27. Meazza C, Travaglino P, Pignatti P, Magni-Manzoni S, Ravelli A, Martini A, De Benedetti F. Macrophage migration inhibitory factor in patients with juvenile idiopathic arthritis. Arthritis Rheum. 2002;46:232–7.
28. Lovell DJ, Giannini EH, Reiff A, Cawkwell GD, Silverman ED, Nocton JJ, Stein LD, Gedalia A, Ilowite NT, Wallace CA, et al. Etanercept in children with polyarticular juvenile rheumatoid arthritis. Pediatric Rheumatology Collaborative Study Group. N Engl J Med. 2000;342:763–9.
29. Creyghton MP, Cheng AW, Welstead GG, Kooistra T, Carey BW, Steine EJ, Hanna J, Lodato MA, Frampton GM, Sharp PA, et al. Histone H3K27ac separates active from poised enhancers and predicts developmental state. Proc Natl Acad Sci U S A. 2010;107:21931–6.
30. Alexander RP, Fang G, Rozowsky J, Snyder M, Gerstein MB. Annotating non-coding regions of the genome. Nat Rev Genet. 2010;11:559–71.
31. Hollenbach JA, Thompson SD, Bugawan TL, Ryan M, Sudman M, Marion M, Langefeld CD, Thomson G, Erlich HA, Glass DN. Juvenile idiopathic arthritis and HLA class I and class II interactions and age-at-onset effects. Arthritis Rheum. 2010;62:1781–91.
32. Mi H, Muruganujan A, Casagrande JT, Thomas PD. Large-scale gene function analysis with the PANTHER classification system. Nat Protoc. 2013;8:1551–66.
33. Michailidou K, Beesley J, Lindstrom S, Canisius S, Dennis J, Lush MJ, Maranian MJ, Bolla MK, Wang Q, Shah M, et al. Genome-wide association analysis of more than 120,000 individuals identifies 15 new susceptibility loci for breast cancer. Nat Genet. 2015;47:373–80.
34. The ENCODE Project Consortium. An integrated encyclopedia of DNA elements in the human genome. Nature, 2012;489:57–74.
35. Gandin V, Sikstrom K, Alain T, Morita M, McLaughlan S, Larsson O, Topisirovic I. Polysome fractionation and analysis of mammalian translatomes on a genome-wide scale. J Vis Exp. 2014;17. doi:10.3791/51455.
36. Winter DR, Jung S, Amit I. Making the case for chromatin profiling: a new tool to investigate the immune-regulatory landscape. Nat Rev Immunol. 2015;15:585–94.
37. Spalinger MR, McCole DF, Rogler G, Scharl M. Role of protein tyrosine phosphatases in regulating the immune system: implications for chronic intestinal inflammation. Inflamm Bowel Dis. 2015;21:645–55.
38. Shlyueva D, Stampfel G, Stark A. Transcriptional enhancers: from properties to genome-wide predictions. Nat Rev Genet. 2014;15:272–86.
39. Levine M, Cattoglio C, Tjian R. Looping back to leap forward: transcription enters a new era. Cell. 2014;157:13–25.
40. Li G, Cai L, Chang H, Hong P, Zhou Q, Kulakova EV, Kolchanov NA, Ruan Y. Chromatin interaction analysis with paired-end tag (ChIA-PET) sequencing technology and application. BMC Genomics. 2014;15 Suppl 12:S11.
41. Brien GL, Gambero G, O'Connell DJ, Jerman E, Turner SA, Egan CM, Dunne EJ, Jurgens MC, Wynne K, Piao L, et al. Polycomb PHF19 binds H3K36me3 and recruits PRC2 and demethylase NO66 to embryonic stem cell genes during differentiation. Nat Struct Mol Biol. 2012;19:1273–81.
42. Ou YY, Mack GJ, Zhang M, Rattner JB. CEP110 and ninein are located in a specific domain of the centrosome associated with centrosome maturation. J Cell Sci. 2002;115:1825–35.
43. Liang D, Shen N. MicroRNA involvement in lupus: the beginning of a new tale. Curr Opin Rheumatol. 2012;24:489–98.
44. Hu Z, Jiang K, Frank MB, Chen Y, Jarvis JN. Complexity and specificity of the neutrophil transcriptomes in juvenile idiopathic arthritis. Sci Rep. 2016; 6:27453.
45. Li LC. Chromatin remodeling by the small RNA machinery in mammalian cells. Epigenetics. 2014;9:45–52.
46. Birnbaum RY, Clowney EJ, Agamy O, Kim MJ, Zhao J, Yamanaka T, Pappalardo Z, Clarke SL, Wenger AM, Nguyen L, et al. Coding exons function as tissue-specific enhancers of nearby genes. Genome Res. 2012;22: 1059–68.
47. Li W, Notani D, Rosenfeld MG. Enhancers as non-coding RNA transcription units: recent insights and future perspectives. Nat Rev Genet. 2016;17:207–23.
48. Ahituv N. Exonic enhancers: proceed with caution in exome and genome sequencing studies. Genome Med. 2016;8:14.
49. Pauli A, Rinn JL, Schier AF. Non-coding RNAs as regulators of embryogenesis. Nat Rev Genet. 2011;12:136–49.
50. Wong JJ, Ritchie W, Ebner OA, Selbach M, Wong JW, Huang Y, Gao D, Pinello N, Gonzalez M, Baidya K, et al. Orchestrated intron retention regulates normal granulocyte differentiation. Cell. 2013;154:583–95.

16

Methotrexate polyglutamates as a potential marker of adherence to long-term therapy in children with juvenile idiopathic arthritis and juvenile dermatomyositis

Ahmed F. Hawwa[1,2], AbdelQader AlBawab[1,3], Madeleine Rooney[4], Lucy R. Wedderburn[5,6,7], Michael W. Beresford[8] and James C. McElnay[1*]

Abstract

Introduction: Methotrexate (MTX) is a cornerstone of treatment in a wide variety of inflammatory conditions, including juvenile idiopathic arthritis (JIA) and juvenile dermatomyositis (JDM). However, owing to its narrow therapeutic index and the considerable interpatient variability in clinical response, monitoring of adherence to MTX is important. The present study demonstrates the feasibility of using methotrexate polyglutamates (MTXPGs) as a biomarker to measure adherence to MTX treatment in children with JIA and JDM.

Methods: Data were collected prospectively from a cohort of 48 children (median age 11.5 years) who received oral or subcutaneous (SC) MTX therapy for JIA or JDM. Dried blood spot samples were obtained from children by finger pick at the clinic or via self- or parent-led sampling at home, and they were analysed to determine the variability in MTXPG concentrations and assess adherence to MTX therapy.

Results: Wide fluctuations in MTXPG total concentrations (>2.0-fold variations) were found in 17 patients receiving stable weekly doses of MTX, which is indicative of nonadherence or partial adherence to MTX therapy. Age ($P = 0.026$) and route of administration ($P = 0.005$) were the most important predictors of nonadherence to MTX treatment. In addition, the study showed that MTX dose and route of administration were significantly associated with variations in the distribution of MTXPG subtypes. Higher doses and SC administration of MTX produced higher levels of total MTXPGs and selective accumulation of longer-chain MTXPGs ($P < 0.001$ and $P < 0.0001$, respectively).

Conclusions: Nonadherence to MTX therapy is a significant problem in children with JIA and JDM. The present study suggests that patients with inadequate adherence and/or intolerance to oral MTX may benefit from SC administration of the drug. The clinical utility of MTXPG levels to monitor and optimise adherence to MTX in children has been demonstrated.

* Correspondence: j.mcelnay@qub.ac.uk
[1]Clinical and Practice Research Group, School of Pharmacy, Queen's University Belfast, 97 Lisburn Road, BT9 7BL Belfast, UK
Full list of author information is available at the end of the article

Introduction

Methotrexate (MTX) is an effective disease-modifying antirheumatic drug (DMARD) widely used in children to treat a variety of autoimmune and inflammatory conditions, including juvenile idiopathic arthritis (JIA) and juvenile dermatomyositis (JDM) [1–6]. Owing to its efficacy and cost-effectiveness, MTX is likely to remain a cornerstone of treatment [5, 7]. However, because of the considerable interpatient variability in clinical response, absorption difficulties and a wide spectrum of side effects, monitoring of adherence to MTX is important [4, 8–11].

MTX is a prodrug activated intracellularly to form methotrexate polyglutamates (MTXPGs) through sequential addition of glutamic acid residues by the enzyme folylpolyglutamate synthase (FPGS) [12, 13]. Within the cell, MTXPGs bind to and inhibit dihydrofolate reductase and other folate pathway enzymes required for purine and pyrimidine synthesis, thereby providing anti-inflammatory effects [14, 15]. Polyglutamation of MTX promotes its retention intracellularly, resulting in enhanced inhibitory effects against its target enzymes. Compared with MTX itself, long-chain MTXPGs have been shown to confer much more potent inhibition of target enzymes within folate metabolism [13, 16, 17]. The clinical value of monitoring serum concentrations of the parent drug is therefore very limited and generally not practical, because approximately 95 % of MTX dose is metabolised within 24 h of administration [13, 18, 19]. However, monitoring MTXPGs as a surrogate biomarker for drug exposure offers a potential tool to assess adherence to long-term therapy in patients with chronic inflammatory conditions (due to their long half-life of elimination) [20, 21]. Evidence suggests that MTXPGs may be associated with the efficacy and toxicity of MTX treatment in rheumatoid arthritis, and some investigators have advocated routine monitoring of MTXPGs for that reason [22–25].

Apart from one recent study in children with JIA [26], adherence rates to MTX treatment in paediatric patients with rheumatologic diseases, including JIA and JDM, have not been previously reported. Studies investigating MTX adherence in adult rheumatology patients have been based mainly on prescription data [27–29], electronic pill counts [30] or self-reported measures [31]. Reported nonadherence to medications in adult patients with JIA ranges from 8 to 48 %, with rates fluctuating depending on the time of evaluation and method used for adherence assessment [32–37]. Risk factors for lack of adherence could include demographic variables such as the patient's being an adolescent or having low socioeconomic status [32, 34, 38], having concerns about side effects of administered drug or lack of belief about the necessity of treatment [31, 39].

In the present study, adherence to MTX treatment in a cohort of children with JIA and JDM was evaluated. A method for measuring MTXPG concentrations using the novel dried blood spot (DBS) sampling technique was developed by our group [40] and applied in the present study to evaluate adherence to prescribed MTX therapy in children. A secondary aim of the study was to characterise the pattern of variability in MTXPG concentrations and determine the clinical variables and biochemical parameters that could predict the observed variability in MTX metabolite levels.

Methods

Study population

A total of 49 paediatric patients with JIA or JDM were recruited into this study from three paediatric outpatient rheumatology clinics in three different centres: (1) Musgrave Park Hospital, Belfast, Northern Ireland; (2) Alder Hey Children's NHS Foundation Trust, Liverpool, UK; and (3) Great Ormond Street Hospital for Children NHS Foundation Trust, London. Patients between the ages of 4 and 17 years who were receiving stable MTX weekly doses [oral or subcutaneous (SC)] for at least 2 months were identified for inclusion in the study.

Participants were asked to provide one DBS sample for analysis of MTX metabolite content during a regularly scheduled clinic visit. Samples were collected by finger prick from each child by spotting drops of blood (two spots per child) directly onto a Guthrie card. For children 5 years of age or older, parents and/or older children were also asked to take two additional DBS samples at home 4 weeks apart, dry them overnight at room temperature and mail them to our laboratory in prepaid mailer kits for analysis.

Accurate information about MTX dosing and times of sampling were recorded prospectively during the clinic visit using bespoke collection forms. The following data were also collected from patient case notes and clinical chemistry records and recorded in these collection forms: age, weight, height, medical history (date of diagnosis, other medical conditions and current medications), biochemical parameters, clinical outcome and records of side effects experienced (e.g., nausea and vomiting). For samples obtained at home, the mailer kits included appropriate collection forms mailed to the patient and/or the patient's parent in advance of the sampling time, with clear instructions on how to take the sample and fill in the form.

Ethical considerations

The study was approved by the Office for Research Ethics Committees in Northern Ireland (reference number 10/NIR03/33). Patients were included in the study only after their parents or legal guardians had been fully informed and had signed the study consent form. In addition, verbal or written assent was obtained from older children (≥6 years) before enrolment into the study.

Measurement of methotrexate polyglutamate concentrations

DBS concentrations of MTX active metabolites (MTXPGs up to the fifth order of glutamation, $MTXPG_5$) were measured by using a selective and sensitive reverse-phase liquid chromatography–tandem mass spectrometry (LC-MS/MS) methodology that we previously developed and validated [40]. Intraday and interday coefficients of variation were less than 15 %, and the limits of detection for individual MTXPGs ($MTXPG_{1-5}$) and total concentration of methotrexate polyglutamate ($MTXPG_{total}$) were determined at 1.6 nmol/L and 1.5 nmol/L, respectively.

Differences in MTXPG concentrations between patients were evaluated as a function of age, sex, diagnosis and route of administration (SC or oral). To differentiate the effect of these factors from dose- or weight-related changes, MTXPG concentrations were normalised by administered dose of MTX (per kilogram of patient weight or per square metre of body surface area) and expressed as nanomoles per litre per milligram or nanomoles per litre per milligram per square metre.

Assessment of adherence

The pattern of variability in MTXPG levels as a function of time was evaluated over two consecutive 4-week intervals during which patients were receiving stable MTX doses. Nonadherence was assumed if a patient had wide variations (≥2.0-fold) in MTXPG levels on different occasions while prescribed the same dose of MTX. A ratio of 2.0-fold was chosen as the cutoff point because similar values have been suggested for identifying patients nonadherent to long-term therapy in chronic diseases [41, 42].

Statistical analysis

Statistical analysis was performed using IBM SPSS version 21 software (IBM SPSS, Armonk, NY, USA). The results were expressed as the median and range values or as frequencies. Descriptive statistics were used to characterise the variability in individual $MTXPG_{1-5}$ and $MTXPG_{total}$ concentrations between different groups of patients. Univariate associations between MTXPG concentrations and demographic or clinical characteristics were analysed using the Mann–Whitney *U* test or the Kruskal–Wallis test, as appropriate. Group differences in the proportion of patients with ≥2.0-fold variation in their MTXPG levels were explored using χ^2 tests with 1 degree of freedom or Fisher's exact test, as appropriate. Comparison of the median fold ratio of highest to lowest MTXPG concentration was performed using the Mann–Whitney *U* test. All analyses were two-sided, with *P* values <0.05 considered significant.

Results

Demographic characteristics of the study population

Of the 49 patients recruited into the study, 32 (65 %) had an underlying diagnosis of JIA and 17 had JDM. The median age (range) of the population was 11.5 years (4–17 years), and 67 % were female. All patients were being treated with weekly MTX (median 0.31 mg/kg, equivalent to 10.2 mg/m^2) for long durations (median 2.8 years, 5 months–10 years), and 41 % were receiving SC MTX. One patient did not provide a DBS sample at the clinic and therefore was not included in the analysis. Of the patients included in the analysis ($n = 48$), 40 (83 %) provided at least two DBS samples during the study period and 60 % received oral folic acid supplementation (median dose 5 mg/week). The demographic and clinical characteristics of the study participants are shown in Table 1.

Distribution of methotrexate polyglutamate concentrations and effect of administered dose

In our cohort of 48 patients with clinic DBS samples, the median $MTXPG_{total}$ was 91.5 nmol/L (range 3.5–470.4 nmol/L). Analysis of the correlation between $MTXPG_{total}$ and individual MTXPG subtypes revealed a very high correlation ($R = 0.91$, $P < 0.0001$) between total MTXPGs and MTX triglutamate ($MTXPG_3$). Considerable internal correlations of the concentrations within

Table 1 Demographic and clinical characteristics of study patients

Characteristics	Values[a] ($n = 49$)
Age (yr)	11.5 (4–17)
Sex [females, n (%)]	33 (67.3 %)
Weight (kg)	41 (13.4–119.7)
Height (cm)	146 (95–178)
MTX weekly dose (mg)	13.75 (7.5–20)
MTX weekly dose (mg/kg)	0.31 (0.08–0.67)
MTX weekly dose (mg/m^2)[b]	10.2 (4.1–15.5)
Number of medications prescribed	5 (1–8)
Number of side effects recorded	3 (1–2)
Pain scale[c]	0.9 (0–7.1)
General evaluation scale[c]	0.5 (0–8.2)
CMAS score[d]	51.5 (42–55)

[a]Values represent median (range), except where indicated otherwise
[b]Surface area was calculated using the Mosteller method [59]
[c]Pain scale and general evaluation scores were obtained from the patients' Childhood Health Assessment Questionnaire
[d]Childhood Myositis Assessment Scale (CMAS) score was recorded for children with JDM

each MTXPG subgroup were also observed; that is, short-chain MTXPGs $MTXPG_{1-2}$ were highly correlated with each other ($R = 0.73$, $P < 0.0001$), as were very long chain polyglutamates $MTXPG_{4-5}$ ($R = 0.61$, $P < 0.0001$).

The median concentration of $MTXPG_{total}$ was significantly greater when higher MTX doses were administered ($R = 0.27$, $P = 0.0007$). This appears to be attributable to selective accumulation of long-chain $MTXPG_3$ ($R = 0.28$, $P = 0.0005$) and very long chain $MTXPG_{4-5}$ ($R = 0.39$–0.42, $P < 0.0001$) at the expense of short-chain $MTXPG_{1-2}$. This was confirmed by the percentage change in individual MTXPGs (relative to $MTXPG_{total}$) as a function of MTX dose (Fig. 1a). Interestingly, concurrent administration of higher folic acid doses was associated with increased concentrations of shorter-chain $MTXPG_{1-2}$ ($R = 0.36$–0.42, $P = 0.002$). Similarly to previous reports [43], the dose of MTX was higher in patients taking folic acid supplementation.

Association of methotrexate polyglutamate levels with clinical variables

Bivariate analysis revealed significantly higher $MTXPG_{total}$ concentrations in patients who had MTX administered by the SC route than among patients who received the drug orally (median 114.1 nmol/L after SC administration vs. 75.5 nmol/L after oral administration; $P < 0.0001$). When corrected for the dose administered (i.e., relative to 1 mg/kg or 1 mg/m^2 weekly doses of MTX), the difference in $MTXPG_{total}$ concentrations stratified by route of administration remained significant (median concentration 307.8 nmol/L/mg/kg vs. 236.2 nmol/L/mg/kg dose after SC and oral administration, respectively; $P = 0.004$; such concentrations are equivalent to 11.0 nmol/L/mg/m^2 vs. 7.41 nmol/L/mg/m^2, respectively; $P = 0.002$).

Furthermore, marked differences in the distribution of individual MTXPG concentrations according to the route of administration were observed. Both normal and dose-adjusted concentrations of long-chain $MTXPG_3$ and longer-chain $MTXPG_{4-5}$ were higher in patients who received SC MTX than in patients receiving MTX. Evaluation of the proportions of individual MTXPG subtypes (relative to $MTXPG_{total}$) also supported these findings. The median proportions of long-chain $MTXPG_3$ and $MTXPG_4$ were higher in patients treated subcutaneously ($P = 0.002$ and $P < 0.0001$ for $MTXPG_3$ and $MTXPG_4$, respectively), whereas the short-chain $MTXPG_{1-2}$ made up larger proportions of MTXPGs in patients treated orally ($P = 0.001$ and $P < 0.0001$ for $MTXPG_1$ and $MTXPG_2$, respectively) (Fig. 1b).

$MTXPG_{total}$ concentrations did not change significantly with age ($P > 0.05$), despite the fact that older children received significantly lower doses (per kilogram and per square metre) of MTX ($P < 0.0001$). When corrected for dose administered, however, both $MTXPG_{total}$ and individual MTXPGs were significantly higher in older children receiving MTX ($P < 0.0001$ for $MTXPG_{total}$; $P < 0.01$ for $MTXPG_{1-2}$; and $P < 0.001$ for $MTXPG_{3-5}$) (Fig. 1c). These findings are indicative of lower clearance rates of MTXPGs in older children than in younger children.

Whether the patient had an underlying diagnosis of JIA or JDM was significantly associated with varying proportions of individual MTXPG subtypes. In particular, patients who had a diagnosis of JIA had significantly greater proportions of short-chain $MTXPG_{1-2}$ ($P < 0.005$), whereas long-chain $MTXPG_3$ and very long-chain $MTXPG_4$ made up larger proportions of total MTXPGs in patients diagnosed with JDM ($P < 0.001$ and $P = 0.009$, respectively). Such differences could reflect the fact that higher numbers of patients were treated orally in the JIA subgroup (64 % treated orally in the JIA subgroup vs. 41 % in the JDM subgroup).

Association of methotrexate polyglutamate levels with biochemical parameters

Increased dose-normalised $MTXPG_{total}$ levels were associated with greater antiarthritic effect and improved likelihood of disease control, as suggested by reduced levels of the inflammation markers C-reactive protein ($P = 0.026$) and erythrocyte sedimentation rate (ESR; $P = 0.033$), in patients who had higher accumulation of $MTXPG_{total}$ concentrations.

Assessment of adherence to methotrexate therapy

Highest and lowest MTXPG levels were recorded for each patient who had at least two measurements of their metabolite levels during the study period ($n = 40$). Nonadherence or partial adherence to MTX therapy was identified in 17 (42.5 %) of the patients, in whom greater than 2.0-fold variations in $MTXPG_{total}$ concentrations were observed. Of these 17 patients, 5 (29 %) were male and 12 (71 %) were female. They ranged in age from 7 to 17 years (median 14 years). At the time the samples were taken, these children were supposed to be taking between 10 and 20 mg weekly MTX doses without change for at least 5 months. Of note, highest to lowest MTXPG ratios, indicative of nonadherence, were significantly greater in patients receiving smaller doses (measured as milligrams per square metre) ($P < 0.031$) (Fig. 2). This suggests that patients with lower disease activity (in whom doses were not increased as they grew) could be associated with an increased risk of poor adherence to therapy. This was particularly apparent when patients were given MTX orally in the present study (Fig. 2). Overall, the results suggest that nearly half of children may fail to fully comply with MTX doses as prescribed during their long-term therapy.

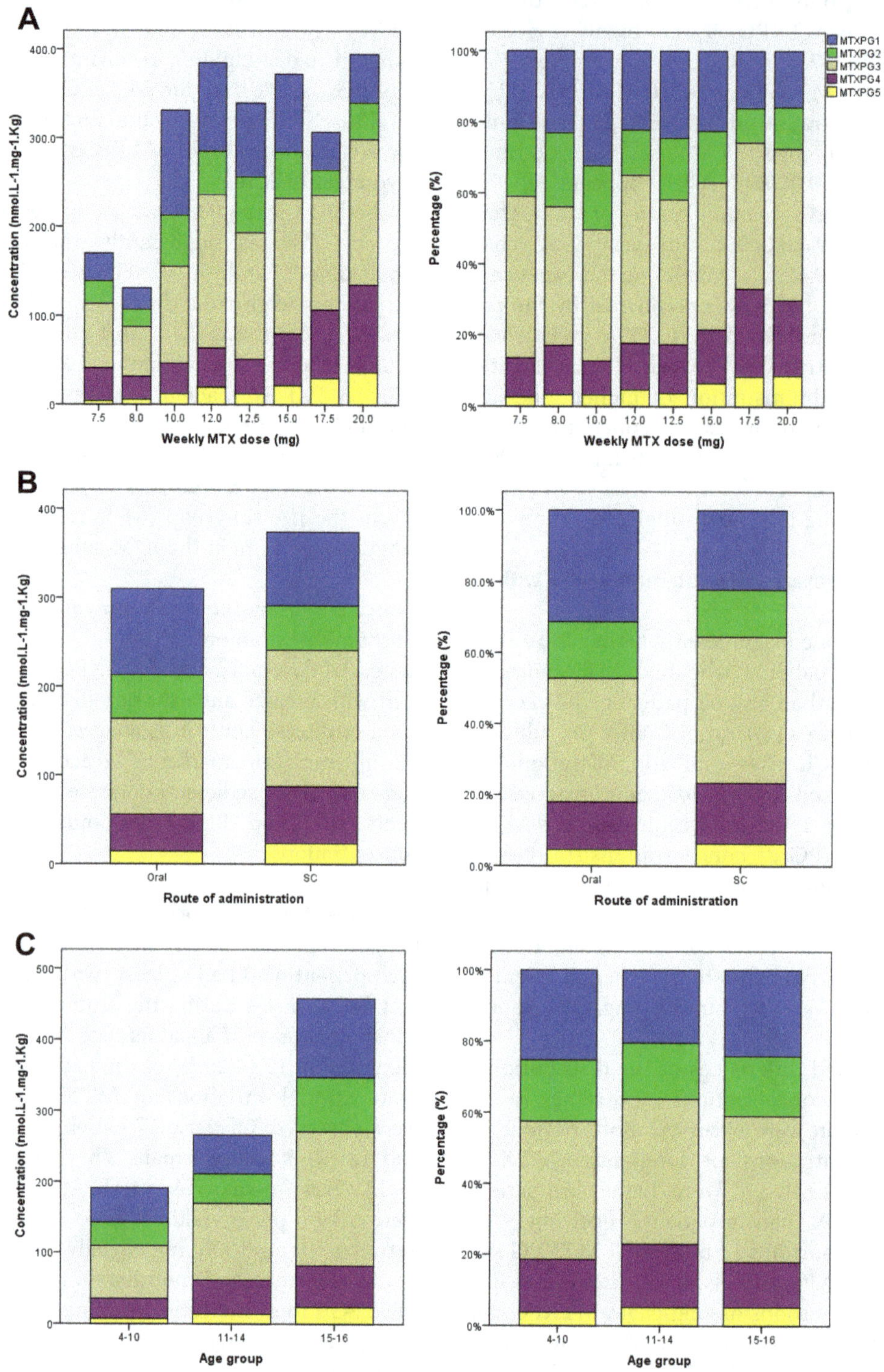

Fig. 1 Effect of administered dose (**a**), route of administration (**b**) and patient age (**c**) on the distribution of methotrexate (MTX) polyglutamates in children receiving long-term MTX therapy

Effect of route of administration and age of child on adherence to methotrexate

Univariate analyses showed that both the route of administration and patient age were significantly associated with nonadherence to MTX treatment (Fig. 2). A higher proportion of patients who received SC MTX were found to be adherent to their medication. Only 17.6 % had greater than 2.0-fold variation in their MTXPG levels after SC administration versus 60.8 % of patients who received MTX orally ($P = 0.005$).

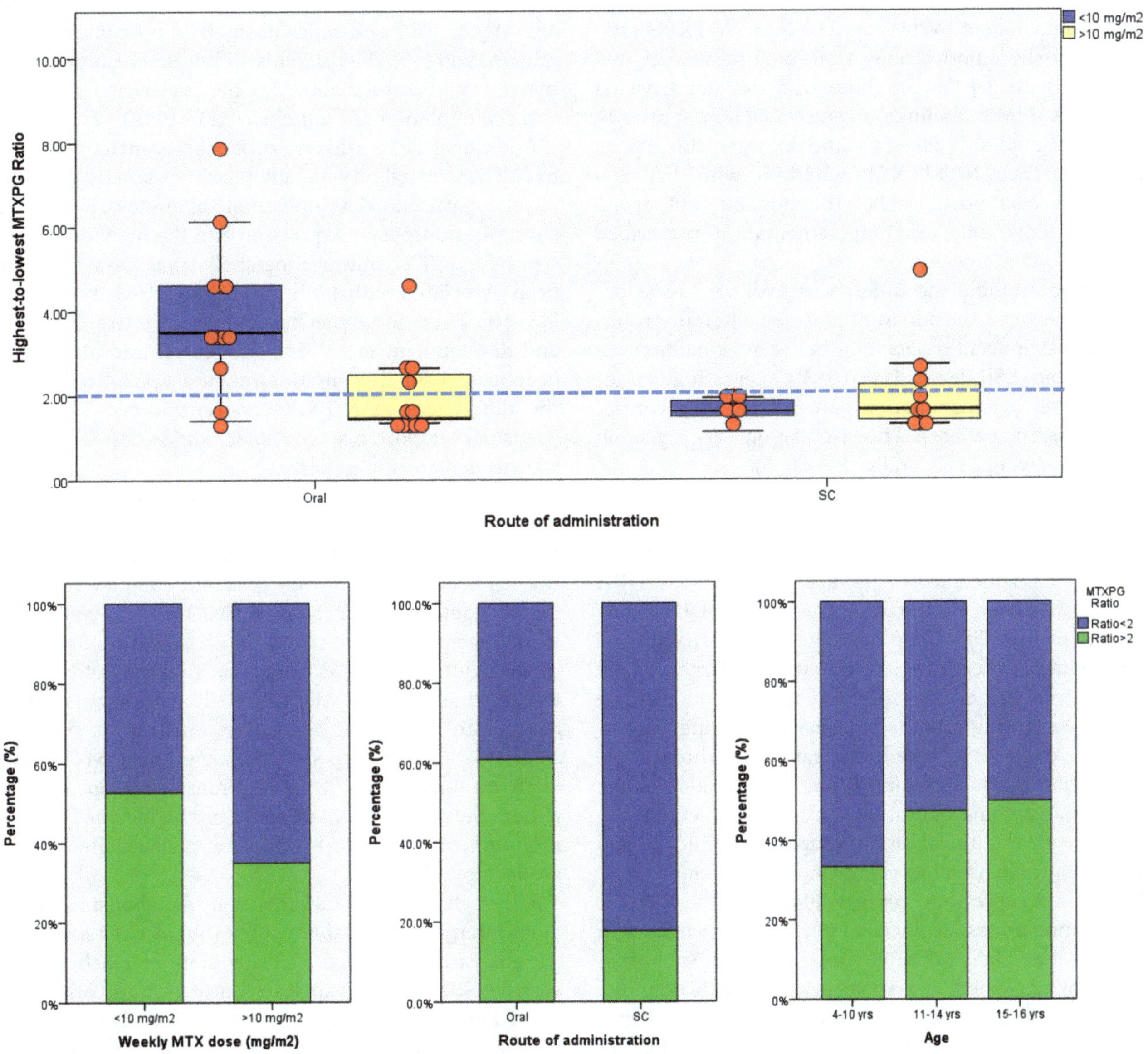

Fig. 2 Comparison of the effects of weekly methotrexate (MTX) dose, route of administration and patient age on the highest to lowest methotrexate polyglutamate (MTXPG) ratio recorded in children receiving long-term MTX therapy. *Dashed reference line* represents a ratio >2.0-fold, which is indicative of wide fluctuations in MTXPG concentration

Furthermore, adolescents and older children were more likely than younger children to be nonadherent to their prescribed medication; older age was significantly correlated with greater MTXPG ratio ($R = 0.35$, $P = 0.026$).

Sex as a variable was similarly distributed between adherent and nonadherent patients. In addition, there were no statistically significant differences in the underlying diagnosis (JIA vs. JDM) or other obvious sociodemographic characteristics between the nonadherent group and the remainder of the cohort ($P > 0.05$).

Association of nonadherence with biochemical parameters and gastrointestinal toxicity

The frequency of MTX-related gastrointestinal (GI) side effects (particularly the presence of nausea or vomiting) in nonadherent patients compared with the rest of the cohort were evaluated only in a subset of patients, because reports of nausea and vomiting were recorded only prospectively in 19 patients of those enrolled in the study. Of these 19 patients, 9 reported nausea, vomiting or other GI side effects at some stage during the study. Seven (78 %) of these patients had greater than 2.0-fold variation in their MTXPG levels and therefore were considered nonadherent to therapy. The mean MTXPG ratio in patients who reported nausea or vomiting was 3.5-fold compared with 2.4-fold in those who did not have GI complaints. These findings suggest that the presence of MTX-related side effects could increase the risk of poor adherence to MTX in children with JIA and JDM. It is also possible that the nonadherent group did not follow folic acid supplementation prescribed to reduce MTX toxicity.

Finally, examining the differences in biochemical parameters between the adherent and nonadherent groups showed a significant association between nonadherence and elevated ESR levels ($P < 0.043$), suggesting an increased level of inflammation and poor disease control in nonadherent patients. This association was higher in patients receiving MTX orally ($P = 0.035$).

Discussion

To our knowledge, this is the first study in which the extent of MTX adherence in paediatric patients with JIA and JDM has been evaluated on the basis of DBS measurement of MTXPGs. The approach using DBS proved an acceptable alternative to the use of larger whole blood or red blood cell sample quantities and had the advantage of being minimally invasive, allowing parents and older children to take blood samples at home. The combination of sparse sampling and low sample volume helped to overcome ethical and practical difficulties associated with traditional blood sampling in children and was shown to be useful in estimating adherence.

Similarly to previous reports [44, 45], the present study demonstrates significant interpatient variability in total and individual MTXPG concentrations. Such variability was explained, at least in part, by MTX administered dose, route of delivery and patient age. Higher MTX doses were associated with greater percentage of longer-chain $MTXPG_{3-5}$ at the expense of short-chain $MTXPG_{1-2}$. Such selective enrichment of longer-chain MTXPGs at higher doses is consistent with recent observations in children with JIA and children with acute lymphoblastic leukaemia [45–47]. Similarly, MTXPG distribution differed by the route of administration: Patients receiving SC MTX had higher overall levels of MTXPGs as well as selective accumulation of longer-chain MTXPGs. This route-dependent distribution of MTXPGs persisted when concentrations were corrected relative to administered dose (measured as milligrams per kilogram or milligrams per square metre). A plausible explanation for such route-specific and dose-dependent accumulation of long-chain MTXPGs could be the higher concentrations produced following SC delivery or higher-dose administration of MTX. It has been suggested that higher concentrations can result in a more pronounced folate-depleted state in cells, which activates a feedback mechanism that upregulates polyglutamation [45]. The stability of longer-chain polyglutamates would in turn allow for the preferential retention and accumulation of long-chain $MTXP_{3-5}$.

Additional factors likely to be significant contributors to MTXPG variability include pharmacokinetic variation, physiological and developmental differences in oral absorption, transporter expression and the individual genotypes for MTX multiple metabolic pathways that have been associated with both efficacy and toxicity of MTX [48–50]. Because of the importance of folate in growth and development in children, concurrent administration of folic acid supplementation might also explain some of the differences in MTXPG concentrations. This is of particular importance in older children with higher growth demands in puberty.

Folic acid supplementation is routinely given to reduce potential side effects in patients receiving MTX [51, 52]. However, because MTX and folate are transported by the same transporter within cells and compete for FPGS for polyglutamation, it is suggested that higher intracellular folate levels may trump MTX retention and affect its polyglutamation [53, 54]. The present study shows that folic acid use in MTX-treated children was associated with increased concentrations of short-chain $MTXPG_{1-2}$ at the expense of longer-chain $MTXPG_{4-5}$. Such an impact on MTX biotransformation leads to either reduced MTX efficacy or higher MTX dose requirements to achieve the same clinical effect in the absence of folic acid.

Although inherited differences in metabolism may explain interpatient variability, they should not cause intrapatient variability once a steady state is reached. Such variability is hard to explain on any grounds other than not taking the medication as prescribed. Other factors, such as diet and alcohol intake, in teenagers could aggravate this behaviour of nonadherence to prescribed medicines. An approach to detect nonadherence in the present study was therefore to study patients at different times while they were prescribed the same dose of MTX by the same route. If there were a wide variation in $MTXPG_{total}$ concentrations at steady state, this would most likely be a reflection of poor adherence.

According to this method, nearly half the patients had wide fluctuations in their MTXPG concentrations indicative of partial adherence or nonadherence. Interestingly, doses received by nonadherent children in the present study were significantly lower (measured as milligrams per square metre) than those prescribed to children who were assumed to be adherent to MTX therapy. This increased variability can be explained partly by the children dosed with the lowest oral doses, because such doses will have a greater proportion of short-chain MTXPGs that are susceptible to more significant and rapid concentration shifts. It could also indicate that children who received lower doses did not perceive a high necessity for MTX therapy, owing to their low disease activity, and therefore were less likely to take their medication consistently. Conversely, lower doses could indicate an attempt to improve adherence in patients who were more prone to MTX side effects. Further studies are required, however, to confirm these hypotheses.

Other risk factors for nonadherence to MTX therapy include GI side effects associated with the administration of MTX. Seven of the nine patients who reported nausea and vomiting at some stage during the present study had greater than 2.0-fold variation in their MTXPG levels and therefore were considered nonadherent to therapy. Such side effects can be diminished with SC administration of MTX. Patients receiving the drug subcutaneously are therefore expected to show better adherence than those treated orally [55]. Indeed, compared with patients who received the drug orally, a higher proportion of patients who received SC MTX in the present study were found to be adherent to their medication. A possible explanation for better adherence with the SC mode of administration could be the greater antiarthritic effect and better clinical outcome among patients following SC MTX administration compared with those taking oral MTX, as reported in previous studies [55–57]. However, an obvious difference impacting adherence is the fact that SC administration is more likely to be provided by a caregiver and thus is more likely to be observed.

In the present study, adherence did not relate to sex or disease type. However, a significant association between older age of children and nonadherence was established. This is concordant with previous studies that recognised adolescents as having lower adherence than younger children because of their growing autonomy [32, 34, 58]. Older children and adolescents, therefore, should be monitored carefully, particularly when they experience less severe symptoms during the stable phases of their disease. In general, adherent patients had better disease control throughout the study. This was supported by elevated ESR levels, a marker of inflammation, in nonadherent patients.

A precise, sensitive and selective LC-MS/MS assay was used for determination of MTXPGs in the present study. Although LC-MS/MS-based methods are increasingly used in clinical laboratories, the cost involved in sample preparation and access to the instrument might limit its use for routine monitoring of adherence in the clinical setting. Another limitation of the current assay is inability to measure the intracellular levels of relevant folate species. The novel DBS sampling, on the other hand, has the advantage of being both convenient for home sampling and a direct objective measure of adherence. An additional obvious benefit is the lower blood volume requirement applicable for monitoring MTXPGs in children.

Conclusions

The present study is unique in being the first detailed analysis of MTXPG levels based on DBS measurements in JIA and JDM. Our data highlight the significance of nonadherence to MTX therapy in patients with JIA and JDM and demonstrate the feasibility of measuring MTXPGs in DBS samples as a potential tool to monitor adherence. We also explored the pattern of variability in MTXPG concentrations and its association with clinical variables and additional biochemical parameters pertaining to disease activity and MTX side effects. The findings warrant further investigation into the clinical utility of MTXPG levels to guide therapy and optimise adherence to MTX treatment in children. Furthermore, the study highlights the importance of understanding the potential barriers to MTX adherence in order to help manage the disease and improve patients' quality of life.

Abbreviations

CMAS: Childhood Myositis Assessment Scale; DBS: Dried blood spot; DMARD: Disease-modifying antirheumatic drug; ESR: Erythrocyte sedimentation rate; FPGS: Folylpolyglutamate synthase; GI: Gastrointestinal; JDM: Juvenile dermatomyositis; JIA: Juvenile idiopathic arthritis; LC-MS/MS: Liquid chromatography–tandem mass spectrometry; MTX: Methotrexate; MTXPG: Methotrexate polyglutamate; $MTXPG_{1-5}$: Individual methotrexate polyglutamates up to the fifth order of polyglutamation; MTXPGtotal: Total concentration of methotrexate polyglutamate; SC: Subcutaneous.

Competing interests

The authors declare that they have no competing interests.

Authors' contributions

JCM, AFH, AA, MR, LRW and MWB contributed to the conception and design of the study and the acquisition and/or interpretation of data. AA, AFH and JCM performed the experiments and contributed to the acquisition and/or analysis of data and drafting of the manuscript. JCM, AFH, AA, MR, LRW and MWB substantially contributed to revising the manuscript critically and gave approval of the final manuscript.

Acknowledgements

The authors acknowledge funding received from Arthritis Research UK (http://www.arthritisresearchuk.org/) under grant 19421. LRW is supported by grants from Great Ormond Street Children's Charity (grant V1304), Arthritis Research UK (grant 20164) and the National Institute for Health Research–funded Biomedical Research Centre Great Ormond Street Hospital NHS Foundation Trust. The funders had no role in the study design, data collection and analysis, decision to publish, or preparation of the manuscript.

Author details

[1]Clinical and Practice Research Group, School of Pharmacy, Queen's University Belfast, 97 Lisburn Road, BT9 7BL Belfast, UK. [2]Aston Pharmacy School, Aston University, Birmingham, UK. [3]Faculty of Pharmacy, Al Zaytoonah University, Amman, Jordan. [4]Centre for Infection and Immunity, School of Medicine and Biomedical Sciences, Queen's University Belfast, Belfast, UK. [5]Institute of Child Health, University College London, London, UK. [6]Arthritis Research UK Centre for Adolescent Rheumatology, University College London, University College London Hospital, London, UK. [7]Department of Rheumatology, Great Ormond Street Hospital NHS Foundation Trust, London, UK. [8]Department of Women's and Children's Health, Institute of Translational Medicine, University of Liverpool, The Alder Hey Children's NHS Foundation Trust, Liverpool, UK.

References

1. Murray KJ, Lovell DJ. Advanced therapy for juvenile arthritis. Best Pract Res Clin Rheumatol. 2002;16:361–78.
2. Saag KG, Teng GG, Patkar NM, Anuntiyo J, Finney C, Curtis JR, et al. American College of Rheumatology 2008 recommendations for the use of nonbiologic and biologic disease-modifying antirheumatic drugs in rheumatoid arthritis. Arthritis Rheum. 2008;59:762–84.
3. Ruperto N, Murray KJ, Gerloni V, Wulffraat N, de Oliveira SK, Falcini F, et al. A randomized trial of parenteral methotrexate comparing an intermediate dose with a higher dose in children with juvenile idiopathic arthritis who failed to respond to standard doses of methotrexate. Arthritis Rheum. 2004;50:2191–201.
4. Lambert CM, Sandhu S, Lochhead A, Hurst NP, McRorie E, Dhillon V. Dose escalation of parenteral methotrexate in active rheumatoid arthritis that has been unresponsive to conventional doses of methotrexate: a randomized, controlled trial. Arthritis Rheum. 2004;50:364–71.
5. Ramanan AV, Whitworth P, Baildam EM. Use of methotrexate in juvenile idiopathic arthritis. Arch Dis Child. 2003;88:197–200.
6. Pilkington CA, Wedderburn LR. Paediatric idiopathic inflammatory muscle disease: recognition and management. Drugs. 2005;65:1355–65.
7. Weinblatt ME, Kaplan H, Germain BF, Block S, Solomon SD, Merriman RC, et al. Methotrexate in rheumatoid arthritis: a five-year prospective multicenter study. Arthritis Rheum. 1994;37:1492–8.
8. Cohen S, Cannon GW, Schiff M, Weaver A, Fox R, Olsen N, et al. Two-year, blinded, randomized, controlled trial of treatment of active rheumatoid arthritis with leflunomide compared with methotrexate. Arthritis Rheum. 2001;44:1984–92.
9. Becker ML, Rosé CD, Cron RQ, Sherry DD, Bilker WB, Lautenbach E. Effectiveness and toxicity of methotrexate in juvenile idiopathic arthritis: comparison of 2 initial dosing regimens. J Rheumatol. 2010;37:870–5.
10. Ortiz-Alvarez O, Morishita K, Avery G, Green J, Petty RE, Tucker LB, et al. Guidelines for blood test monitoring of methotrexate toxicity in juvenile idiopathic arthritis. J Rheumatol. 2004;31:2501–6.
11. Dougados M, Combe B, Cantagrel A, Goupille P, Olive P, Schattenkirchner M, et al. Combination therapy in early rheumatoid arthritis: a randomised, controlled, double blind 52 week clinical trial of sulphasalazine and methotrexate compared with the single components. Ann Rheum Dis. 1999;58:220–5.
12. Kremer JM. Toward a better understanding of methotrexate. Arthritis Rheum. 2004;50:1370–82.
13. Chabner BA, Allegra CJ, Curt GA, Clendeninn NJ, Baram J, Koizumi S, et al. Polyglutamation of methotrexate: is methotrexate a prodrug? J Clin Invest. 1985;76:907–12.
14. Cutolo M, Sulli A, Pizzorni C, Seriolo B, Straub RH. Anti-inflammatory mechanisms of methotrexate in rheumatoid arthritis. Ann Rheum Dis. 2001;60:729–35.
15. Cronstein BN, Naime D, Ostad E. The antiinflammatory mechanism of methotrexate. Increased adenosine release at inflamed sites diminishes leukocyte accumulation in an in vivo model of inflammation. J Clin Invest. 1993;92:2675–82.
16. Allegra CJ, Chabner BA, Drake JC, Lutz R, Rodbard D, Jolivet J. Enhanced inhibition of thymidylate synthase by methotrexate polyglutamates. J Biol Chem. 1985;260:9720–6.
17. Schroder H, Fogh K. Methotrexate and its polyglutamate derivatives in erythrocytes during and after weekly low-dose oral methotrexate therapy of children with acute lymphoblastic leukemia. Cancer Chemother Pharmacol. 1988;21:145–9.
18. Bannwarth B, Pehourcq F, Schaeverbeke T, Dehais J. Clinical pharmacokinetics of low-dose pulse methotrexate in rheumatoid arthritis. Clin Pharmacokinet. 1996;30:194–210.
19. Ravelli A, Di Fuccia G, Molinaro M, Ramenghi B, Zonta L, Regazzi MB, et al. Plasma levels after oral methotrexate in children with juvenile rheumatoid arthritis. J Rheumatol. 1993;20:1573–7.
20. Dervieux T, Orentas Lein D, Marcelletti J, Pischel K, Smith K, Walsh M, et al. HPLC determination of erythrocyte methotrexate polyglutamates after low-dose methotrexate therapy in patients with rheumatoid arthritis. Clin Chem. 2003;49:1632–41.
21. Dalrymple JM, Stamp LK, O'Donnell JL, Chapman PT, Zhang M, Barclay ML. Pharmacokinetics of oral methotrexate in patients with rheumatoid arthritis. Arthritis Rheum. 2008;58:3299–308.
22. Angelis-Stoforidis P, Vajda FJ, Christophidis N. Methotrexate polyglutamate levels in circulating erythrocytes and polymorphs correlate with clinical efficacy in rheumatoid arthritis. Clin Exp Rheumatol. 1999;17:313–20.
23. Cronstein B. How does methotrexate suppress inflammation? Clin Exp Rheumatol. 2010;28:S21–3.
24. Dervieux T, Furst D, Lein DO, Capps R, Smith K, Caldwell J, et al. Pharmacogenetic and metabolite measurements are associated with clinical status in patients with rheumatoid arthritis treated with methotrexate: results of a multicentred cross sectional observational study. Ann Rheum Dis. 2005;64:1180–5.
25. Dervieux T, Furst D, Lein DO, Capps R, Smith K, Walsh M, et al. Polyglutamation of methotrexate with common polymorphisms in reduced folate carrier, aminoimidazole carboxamide ribonucleotide transformylase, and thymidylate synthase are associated with methotrexate effects in rheumatoid arthritis. Arthritis Rheum. 2004;50:2766–74.
26. Pelajo CF, Sgarlat CM, Lopez-Benitez JM, Oliveira SK, Rodrigues MC, Sztajnbok FR, et al. Adherence to methotrexate in juvenile idiopathic arthritis. Rheumatol Int. 2012;32:497–500.
27. Harley CR, Frytak JR, Tandon N. Treatment compliance and dosage administration among rheumatoid arthritis patients receiving infliximab, etanercept, or methotrexate. Am J Manag Care. 2003;9:S136–43.
28. Grijalva CG, Chung CP, Arbogast PG, Stein CM, Mitchel Jr EF, Griffin MR. Assessment of adherence to and persistence on disease-modifying antirheumatic drugs (DMARDs) in patients with rheumatoid arthritis. Med Care. 2007;45:S66–76.
29. Harrold LR, Andrade SE. Medication adherence of patients with selected rheumatic conditions: a systematic review of the literature. Semin Arthritis Rheum. 2009;38:396–402.
30. Waimann CA, Marengo MF, de Achaval S, Cox VL, Garcia-Gonzalez A, Reveille JD, et al. Electronic monitoring of oral therapies in ethnically diverse and economically disadvantaged patients with rheumatoid arthritis: consequences of low adherence. Arthritis Rheum. 2013;65:1421–9.
31. de Thurah A, Norgaard M, Harder I, Stengaard-Pedersen K. Compliance with methotrexate treatment in patients with rheumatoid arthritis: influence of patients' beliefs about the medicine: a prospective cohort study. Rheumatol Int. 2010;30:1441–8.
32. April KT, Feldman DE, Platt RW, Duffy CM. Comparison between children with juvenile idiopathic arthritis and their parents concerning perceived treatment adherence. Arthritis Rheum. 2006;55:558–63.
33. Degotardi PJ, Revenson TA, Ilowite NT. Family-level coping in juvenile rheumatoid arthritis: assessing the utility of a quantitative family interview. Arthritis Care Res. 1999;12:314–24.
34. Feldman DE, de Civita M, Dobkin PL, Malleson P, Meshefedjian G, Duffy CM. Perceived adherence to prescribed treatment in juvenile idiopathic arthritis over a one-year period. Arthritis Rheum. 2007;57:226–33.
35. Litt IF, Cuskey WR. Compliance with salicylate therapy in adolescents with juvenile rheumatoid arthritis. Am J Dis Child. 1981;135:434–6.
36. Rapoff MA, Belmont JM, Lindsley CB, Olson NY. Electronically monitored adherence to medications by newly diagnosed patients with juvenile rheumatoid arthritis. Arthritis Rheum. 2005;53:905–10.
37. Sturge C, Garralda ME, Boissin M, Dore CJ, Woo P. School attendance and juvenile chronic arthritis. Br J Rheumatol. 1997;36:1218–23.
38. Skoglund KA, Söderhall S, Beck O, Peterson C, Wennberg M, Hayder S, et al. Plasma and urine levels of methotrexate and 7-hydroxymethotrexate in children with ALL during maintenance therapy with weekly oral methotrexate. Med Pediatr Oncol. 1994;22:187–93.
39. Donovan JL, Blake DR. Patient non-compliance: deviance or reasoned decision-making? Soc Sci Med. 1992;34:507–13.
40. Hawwa AF, Albawab A, Rooney M, Wedderburn LR, Beresford MW, McElnay JC. A novel dried blood spot-LCMS method for the quantification of methotrexate polyglutamates as a potential marker for methotrexate use in children. PLoS One. 2014;9:e89908.
41. Davies HA, Lennard L, Lilleyman JS. Variable mercaptopurine metabolism in children with leukaemia: a problem of non-compliance? BMJ. 1993;306:1239–40.
42. Hawwa AF, Millership JS, Collier PS, McCarthy A, Dempsey S, Cairns C, et al. The development of an objective methodology to measure medication adherence to oral thiopurines in paediatric patients with acute lymphoblastic leukaemia—an exploratory study. Eur J Clin Pharmacol. 2009;65:1105–12.

43. van Ede AE, Laan RF, Rood MJ, Huizinga TW, van de Laar MA, van Denderen CJ, et al. Effect of folic or folinic acid supplementation on the toxicity and efficacy of methotrexate in rheumatoid arthritis: a forty-eight week, multicenter, randomized, double-blind, placebo-controlled study. Arthritis Rheum. 2001;44:1515–24.
44. Stamp LK, O'Donnell JL, Chapman PT, Zhang M, Frampton C, James J, et al. Determinants of red blood cell methotrexate polyglutamate concentrations in rheumatoid arthritis patients receiving long-term methotrexate treatment. Arthritis Rheum. 2009;60:2248–56.
45. Becker ML, van Haandel L, Gaedigk R, Lasky A, Hoeltzel M, Stobaugh J, et al. Analysis of intracellular methotrexate polyglutamates in patients with juvenile idiopathic arthritis: effect of route of administration on variability in intracellular methotrexate polyglutamate concentrations. Arthritis Rheum. 2010;62:1803–12.
46. Adam de Beaumais T, Dervieux T, Fakhoury M, Medard Y, Azougagh S, Zhang D, et al. The impact of high-dose methotrexate on intracellular 6-mercaptopurine disposition during interval therapy of childhood acute lymphoblastic leukemia. Cancer Chemother Pharmacol. 2010;66:653–8.
47. Dervieux T, Zablocki R, Kremer J. Red blood cell methotrexate polyglutamates emerge as a function of dosage intensity and route of administration during pulse methotrexate therapy in rheumatoid arthritis. Rheumatology (Oxford). 2010;49:2337–45.
48. Campalani E, Arenas M, Marinaki AM, Lewis CM, Barker JN, Smith CH. Polymorphisms in folate, pyrimidine, and purine metabolism are associated with efficacy and toxicity of methotrexate in psoriasis. J Invest Dermatol. 2007;127:1860–7.
49. Warren RB, Smith RL, Campalani E, Eyre S, Smith CH, Barker JN, et al. Genetic variation in efflux transporters influences outcome to methotrexate therapy in patients with psoriasis. J Invest Dermatol. 2008;128:1925–9.
50. Warren RB, Smith RL, Campalani E, Eyre S, Smith CH, Barker JN, et al. Outcomes of methotrexate therapy for psoriasis and relationship to genetic polymorphisms. Br J Dermatol. 2009;160:438–41.
51. Ortiz Z, Shea B, Suarez Almazor M, Moher D, Wells G, Tugwell P. Folic acid and folinic acid for reducing side effects in patients receiving methotrexate for rheumatoid arthritis. Cochrane Database Syst Rev. 2000;2:CD000951.
52. Ortiz Z, Shea B, Suarez-Almazor ME, Moher D, Wells GA, Tugwell P. The efficacy of folic acid and folinic acid in reducing methotrexate gastrointestinal toxicity in rheumatoid arthritis: a metaanalysis of randomized controlled trials. J Rheumatol. 1998;25:36–43.
53. Jolivet J, Faucher F, Pinard MF. Influence of intracellular folates on methotrexate metabolism and cytotoxicity. Biochem Pharmacol. 1987;36:3310–2.
54. Kennedy DG, Van den Berg HW, Clarke R, Murphy RF. The effect of leucovorin on the synthesis of methotrexate poly-γ-glutamates in the MCF-7 human breast cancer cell line. Biochem Pharmacol. 1985;34:2897–903.
55. Braun J, Kästner P, Flaxenberg P, Währisch J, Hanke P, Demary W, et al. Comparison of the clinical efficacy and safety of subcutaneous versus oral administration of methotrexate in patients with active rheumatoid arthritis: results of a six-month, multicenter, randomized, double-blind, controlled, phase IV trial. Arthritis Rheum. 2008;58:73–81.
56. Hamilton RA, Kremer JM. Why intramuscular methotrexate may be more efficacious than oral dosing in patients with rheumatoid arthritis. Br J Rheumatol. 1997;36:86–90.
57. Todd DJ, Weinblatt ME. Oral versus parenteral administration of methotrexate for the treatment of active RA. Nat Clin Pract Rheumatol. 2008;4:342–3.
58. Staples B, Bravender T. Drug compliance in adolescents: assessing and managing modifiable risk factors. Paediatr Drugs. 2002;4:503–13.
59. Mosteller RD. Simplified calculation of body-surface area. N Engl J Med. 1987;317:1098.

17

MRP8/14 serum levels as a predictor of response to starting and stopping anti-TNF treatment in juvenile idiopathic arthritis

Janneke Anink[1*], Lisette W. A. Van Suijlekom-Smit[1], Marieke H. Otten[1], Femke H. M. Prince[1], Marion A. J. van Rossum[2], Koert M. Dolman[3], Esther P. A. H. Hoppenreijs[4], Rebecca ten Cate[5], Simona Ursu[6], Lucy R. Wedderburn[6], Gerd Horneff[7], Michael Frosch[8], Thomas Vogl[9], Faekah Gohar[10], Dirk Foell[10], Johannes Roth[9] and Dirk Holzinger[10]

Abstract

Introduction: Approximately 30 % of juvenile idiopathic arthritis (JIA) patients fail to respond to anti-TNF treatment. When clinical remission is induced, some patients relapse after treatment has been stopped. We tested the predictive value of MRP8/14 serum levels to identify responders to treatment and relapse after discontinuation of therapy.

Methods: Samples from 88 non-systemic JIA patients who started and 26 patients who discontinued TNF-blockers were analyzed. MRP8/14 serum levels were measured by in-house MRP8/14 ELISA and by Bühlmann Calprotectin ELISA at start of anti-TNF treatment, within 6 months after start and at discontinuation of etanercept in clinical remission. Patients were categorized into responders (ACRpedi ≥ 50 and/or inactive disease) and non-responders (ACRpedi < 50) within six months after start, response was evaluated by change in JADAS-10. Disease activity was assessed within six months after discontinuation.

Results: Baseline MRP8/14 levels were higher in responders (median MRP8/14 of 1466 ng/ml (IQR 1045–3170)) compared to non-responders (median MRP8/14 of 812 (IQR 570–1178), p < 0.001). Levels decreased after start of treatment only in responders (p < 0.001). Change in JADAS-10 was correlated with baseline MRP8/14 levels (Spearman's rho 0.361, p = 0.001). Patients who flared within 6 months after treatment discontinuation had higher MRP8/14 levels (p = 0.031, median 1025 ng/ml (IQR 588–1288)) compared to patients with stable remission (505 ng/ml (IQR 346–778)). Results were confirmed by Bühlmann ELISA with high reproducibility but different overall levels.

Conclusion: High levels of baseline MRP8/14 are associated with good response to anti-TNF treatment, whereas elevated MRP8/14 levels at discontinuation of etanercept are associated with higher chance to flare.

Introduction

Addition of biologic agents for treatment of juvenile idiopathic arthritis (JIA) has brought the treatment goal of inactive disease into reach even for JIA patients not responding to conventional disease-modifying anti-rheumatic drugs (DMARDs). However, 30–40 % of patients treated with biologic agents do not achieve this treatment goal for unknown reasons [1–3]. Several clinical parameters have been found to be associated with response to etanercept, a TNF-alpha inhibitor and the first biologic agent to be approved for the treatment of JIA [4, 5]. These include patient characteristics, such as age and gender, and disease characteristics, such as number of active joints, extent of disability and disease duration. However, as none of these factors are perfectly able to distinguish between responders and non-responders, these clinical characteristics in themselves are not sufficient to guide treatment decisions. A more tailored approach to drug choice, based upon use of validated biomarkers in combination with clinical parameters, could facilitate early remission induction for more children. Measurement of serum inflammatory proteins before starting treatment with a biologic agent may be valuable to separate children with a high chance of good response from poor responders or

* Correspondence: j.anink@erasmusmc.nl
[1]Department of Pediatrics/ Pediatric Rheumatology, Erasmus MC Sophia Children's Hospital Rotterdam, Rotterdam, The Netherlands
Full list of author information is available at the end of the article

non-responders. In addition, biomarkers could be of help in identifying patients in clinical remission who can successfully discontinue treatment.

The myeloid related protein (MRP) complex 8/14 (S100A8/9, also known as calprotectin) is released from activated monocytes and phagocytes. MRP8/14 is a ligand to toll-like receptor 4 (TLR-4), has a pro-inflammatory effect on phagocytes and endothelial cells [6] and is an important factor in mediating osteoclastic bone destruction in experimental arthritis [7]. MRP8/14 serum levels correlate with disease activity in JIA patients [8], can be used to identify subclinical disease activity, and are associated with flares in JIA patients in clinical remission on methotrexate (MTX) [9, 10]. In addition, this biomarker correlates closely to response to treatment in patients with systemic JIA [11] and is able to predict good response to MTX in a subset of patients with non-systemic JIA [12].

Whether MRP8/14 is also associated with response to TNF-alpha inhibitors in patients with non-systemic JIA, or can predict flares after discontinuation of etanercept after successful treatment when clinical remission is achieved, is unknown. Therefore, in the present study we prospectively evaluated the relationship between the clinical course of JIA after anti-TNF treatment and after discontinuation of etanercept and serum levels of MRP8/14.

Methods

Study population

Serum samples were included from patients with non-systemic JIA who were biologic-agent-naïve, starting either etanercept or adalimumab, and included in the Dutch Arthritis and Biologicals in Children (ABC) Register (n = 68), German Registry for Biologics in Pediatric Rheumatology (BIKER) (n = 12) or Childhood Arthritis Response to Medication Study (CHARMS) from the United Kingdom (n = 8). Additionally samples from 26 patients at discontinuation of etanercept in remission were collected ((ABC register (n = 8), BIKER register (n = 18)). The list of participating hospitals can be found in the Acknowledgements section. Patients fulfilled the International League of Associations for Rheumatology criteria for JIA [13]. Patients diagnosed with systemic JIA have been described elsewhere [11].

The ABC register is a multicenter prospective observational study that aimed to include all JIA patients in the Netherlands who initiated biologic agents. The study protocol was approved by the Medical Ethics Committee at Erasmus MC Rotterdam and by all participating hospitals [3]. The German BIKER register was founded with the same objective, after approval by the ethics committee of the University Halle [1]. The CHARMS study (approved by the Institute of Child Health/Great Ormond Street NHS Trust Ethics Committee) included JIA patients at the start of treatment with new disease-modifying medication for active arthritis [12]. For all studies, written informed consent was obtained. In all three studies patient and disease characteristics were recorded at the start of biologic treatment. Changes in disease activity, medication use and adverse events were followed prospectively. These included the JIA core set variables: physician's global assessment (PGA) of disease activity on a visual analog scale (VAS) (range 0–10 cm, 0 best score), childhood health assessment questionnaire (CHAQ) (range 0–3, 0 best score), the global assessment of well-being VAS completed by patients/parents (range 0–10 cm, 0 best score, number of joints with active arthritis and joints with limited motion and erythrocyte sedimentation rate (ESR)). Additionally pain was assessed using a VAS completed by parents/patients. Anti-TNF treatment was prescribed according to standard dosing for pediatric JIA patients.

Response to treatment, inactive disease and flare

The effect of treatment was assessed using the ACR pediatric response criteria [14]. A modified definition for inactive disease was used and defined as no active arthritis, no systemic features, no uveitis, normal ESR (≤20 mm/h), and physician's global assessment of disease activity indicating no disease activity (defined as a score ≤1.0 cm) [15]. The modified definition includes PGA with an increased threshold, because in daily practice we experience a fear of physicians to set the disease activity at zero, as while the disease is inactive, patients are not cured and still require medication. Patients were divided into responders who achieved at least an ACRpedi50 response (subdivided into ACRpedi50, ACRpedi70 or inactive disease) and non-responders (patients with no response or an ACRpedi30 response) within 6 months after start of treatment (median time of follow-up evaluation was 3.2 months (IQR 2.6 – 5.0). Additionally, response to treatment was evaluated using change on the continuous juvenile arthritis disease activity score (JADAS)-10 score, a composite score based on four of the disease activity variables (PGA, VAS wellbeing (parent/patient), active joint count and ESR). JADAS-10 was assessed at the start and within 6 months after the start of treatment [16].

Patients who discontinued treatment were all in remission on medication (defined as a period of ≥6 months of continuous inactive disease, using the modified Wallace criteria as described above) [17]. For evaluation of the association between MRP 8/14 levels at discontinuation and flaring after discontinuation, we defined flare as having at least three of the following: a physician or patient VAS ≥20 mm, ≥1 active joints, any worsening on the CHAQ and ≥30 % worsening of ESR and limited joints [18, 19]. Patients who had flares no longer fulfilled the modified Wallace criteria. Patients who did not have flares still met these criteria.

Determination of MRP8/14 serum levels

Serum levels of MRP8/14 complexes were determined by ELISA. For comparison with earlier studies, internal control sera were used as a reference in all ELISA studies. MRP8/14 serum levels in healthy pediatric controls have been repeatedly measured with our in-house ELISA with results in the range of 310 ± 40 ng/ml [11]. Additionally, MRP8/14 levels were also measured using the commercially available Bühlmann MRP8/14 Calprotectin ELISA (Bühlmann Laboratories Schönenbuch, Zwitserland) to investigate inter-assay variation. The readers of the assay were blinded to diagnosis and disease activity. Treating physicians were blinded to the MRP8/14 serum levels.

Statistical analysis

Patients starting etanercept and adalimumab were analyzed together, as the number of patients treated with adalimumab was too small to analyze separately. Although the two drugs are different in structure, both drugs are TNF-alpha blockers, and we therefore expect the effect on MRP8/14 levels in responders/non-responders to be comparable. Descriptive statistics are presented as absolute frequencies, as median values and IQR, or as mean and SD, as appropriate. The chi-square test was used to compare categorical characteristics of responders with those of non-responders. The Mann–Whitney *U* test was used for comparison of continuous variables. Correlations between serum level of MRP8/14 and clinical variables were assessed using Spearman's correlation coefficient. Correlation between the in-house ELISA and the Bühlmann ELISA was assessed using Pearson's correlation coefficient. The Wilcoxon signed rank test was used to analyze differences in MRP8/14 levels at paired time points. Receiver operator characteristic (ROC) analyses were performed to determine optimal cutoff levels separately for both assays to predict response to treatment and flare within 6 months after treatment discontinuation. Cutoff values were determined using the Youden index [20].

Univariate logistic regression models were fitted to assess the association between treatment response and baseline MRP8/14 levels. Linear regression was used to evaluate the relationship between change in JADAS-10 disease activity and baseline MRP8/14 serum levels. Change in JADAS-10 was defined as the difference between baseline and follow-up JADAS-10. Multivariable linear models were fitted for change in JADAS-10 to correct for other possible predictor variables and to assess the additional value of MRP8/14 in predicting clinical response. These variables were specified beforehand based on preexisting knowledge of their relationship with serum levels of MRP8/14 and/or the response to treatment (age at onset of JIA, baseline JADAS-10, number of previously used DMARDs, gender, baseline CHAQ score, ESR, disease duration) [4, 5, 21]. Missing data were handled using the chained equations multiple imputation command *ice* in Stata. Ten imputed datasets were created. Patients on adalimumab or etanercept were compared, and were imputed together due to having identical characteristics. Of the baseline JIA core set variable data (including VAS pain, evaluated by patient/parent) 3.6 % were missing (median of 0 missing values per patient (range 0–3). At the last available follow up within 6 months of treatment 9.3 % of the JIA core set variable data were missing (including VAS pain, median of 0 missing values per patient (range 0–7)). Analyses were performed with IBM SPSS Statistics for Windows Version 21.0, Stata/SE version 13.0 and Prism (v5, GraphPad Software, La Jolla California USA).

Results

Baseline characteristics

Baseline serum samples were available from 88 patients with non-systemic JIA to measure MRP8/14 levels with the in-house ELISA and of these 81 were available to perform both in-house and commercial ELISA. Characteristics of both the patients who started TNF inhibitors and those who discontinued etanercept are summarized in an additional table (see Additional file 1). Median MRP8/14 (ng/ml) in patients who started TNF-inhibiting treatment was 1,289 (IQR 795–2809). MRP8/14 serum levels were significantly correlated to ESR at baseline (Spearman's rho 0.440, p <0.001). Presence of rheumatoid factor, CHAQ at baseline, number of active joints and disease activity expressed as JADAS-10 were not correlated with MRP8/14 levels.

Clinical response to treatment

A total of 25 % of patients (n = 22) did not achieve an ACRpedi50 response or higher and were therefore considered non-responders to treatment. The remaining 66 patients were responders. Of these 66 patients, 46 achieved ACRpedi70, and 31 patients reached a state of inactive disease. Mean JADAS-10 score at the last available follow up within 6 months (median 3.2 months (IQR 2.6 – 5.0)) was 5.7 (±5.4).

Baseline characteristics of responders and non-responders are shown in Table 1. No significant differences were found between responders and non-responders. Data on the use of concomitant medication can be found in Additional file 1: Table S1A. There were no significant differences between responders and non-responders in concomitant medication such as systemic steroids (32 % of responders vs 18 % of non-responders, p = 0.388) or DMARDs (91 % of responders vs 73 % of non-responders, p = 0.064).

MRP8/14 serum levels and response to treatment

Baseline MRP8/14 serum levels were higher in responders (median MRP8/14 of 1466 ng/ml (IQR 1045–3170))

Table 1 Differences in baseline characteristics between responders and non-responders

Baseline characteristic	Responders (n = 66)	Non-responders (n = 22)
Female gender, n (%)	48 (73)	18 (82)
Age at onset of JIA in years, median (IQR)	10.0 (4.2–12.3)	9.4 (3.5–13.7)
Disease duration in years, median (IQR)	2.4 (1.1–4.9)	2.3 (0.8–7.7)
JADAS-10, median (IQR)	20 (14–21)	17 (11–22)
CHAQ score, median (IQR)	1.5 (0.7–2.2)	1.3 (0.6-2.0)
Number of active joints, median (IQR)	11 (5–18)	8 (2–16)
ESR in mm/h, median (IQR)	16 (9–28)	12 (7–18)
Number of previously used DMARDs, median (IQR)	1 (1–2)	1 (1–2)

JIA juvenile idiopathic arthritis, *JADAS* juvenile arthritis disease activity score, *IQR* interquartile range, *ESR* erythrocyte sedimentation rate, *CHAQ* child health assessment questionnaire, *DMARDs* disease modifying anti-rheumatic drugs

compared to non-responders (median MRP8/14 of 812 ng/ml (IQR 570–1178), p < 0.001) (Fig. 1). If we only compare patients who achieved inactive disease with those not achieving inactive disease, these differences are also present: inactive disease vs no inactive disease: median MRP 8/14 at start (ng/ml) 2287 (IQR 1053–3672) vs 1174 (IQR 704–2030), p = 0.005.

On univariate logistic regression this resulted in an odds ratio of 1.5 (95 % CI 1.1, 2.1) for achieving at least an ACRpedi 50 response per 500 units of MRP (ng/ml). Baseline MRP8/14 serum levels were significantly associated with change in JADAS-10 on linear regression analysis (β = 0.636 per 500 unit increase in ng/ml, 95 % CI 0.254, 1.018, $p = 0.001$).

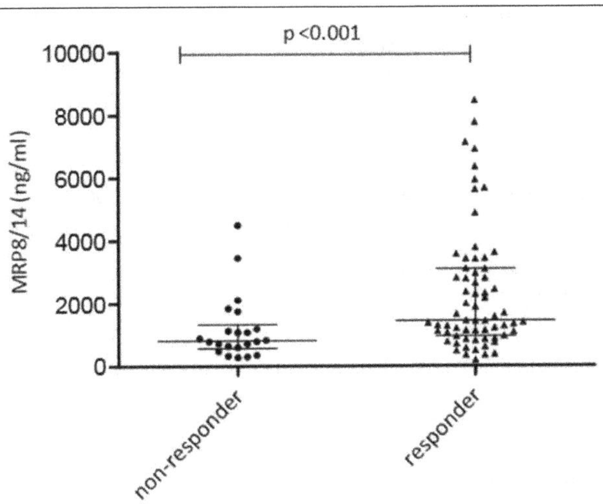

Fig. 1 Differences in myeloid related protein (*MRP*)8/14 serum levels between non-responders and responders before starting treatment

Use of MRP8/14 as a prognostic marker for response to treatment

Based on receiver operator characteristic (ROC) curve analysis, a cutoff value was identified for prediction of response to treatment (ACR pedi50 or higher). Sensitivity, specificity and likelihood ratios are given in Table 2.

Added value of MRP8/14 in prediction of response

We constructed a multivariable linear regression model including known predictors (age at onset of JIA, baseline JADAS-10, number of previously used DMARDs, gender, baseline CHAQ score, ESR, disease duration) and subsequently added MRP8/14 to the model. In this multivariable model MRP8/14 was still significantly associated with change in JADAS-10 (corrected β = 0.472 per 500 units increase in ng/ml, 95 % CI 0.161, 0.782, $p < 0.001$). The only other variable significantly associated with change in JADAS-10 was baseline JADAS-10 (corrected β = 0.678, 95 % CI 0.434, 0.921, $p < 0.001$). The variables in the model without MRP8/14 serum levels explained 50 % of the variance in change in JADAS-10 within 6 months of treatment ($R^2 = 0.50$). Adding MRP8/14 to this model resulted in a slightly better predictive model, with an R^2 value of 0.54 ($p = 0.004$).

Change in MRP8/14 levels after treatment

A follow-up measurement within 5 months after starting treatment was available for 43 patients; 14 of these were categorized as being non-responders. Treatment with TNF inhibitors significantly lowered MRP8/14 serum levels in responders ($p < 0.001$) (Fig. 2b), but not in non-responders (Fig. 2a). Patients who achieved inactive disease had a greater change in MRP than those who did not achieve inactive disease (median change in MRP 8/14 (ng/ml) -1034 (IQR -2723 to -401) vs -486 (IQR -1084 to 209)). Change in MRP was significantly correlated with change in JADAS10 (Spearman's rho: 0.421, $p = 0.006$). There were no significant differences in change in MRP levels after anti-TNF treatment between patients who were or were not treated concomitantly with systemic steroids and/or DMARDs.

Table 2 Sensitivity, specificity and likelihood ratios for the determined cutoff value of myeloid related protein (MRP)8/14 to predict response to anti-TNF treatment

Accuracy measure	
Cutoff level MRP8/14 (ng/ml)	1,193
Sensitivity	66 %
Specificity	81 %
Positive likelihood ratio	3.4
Negative likelihood ratio	0.4
Youden index	0.47
Area under the curve	0.76

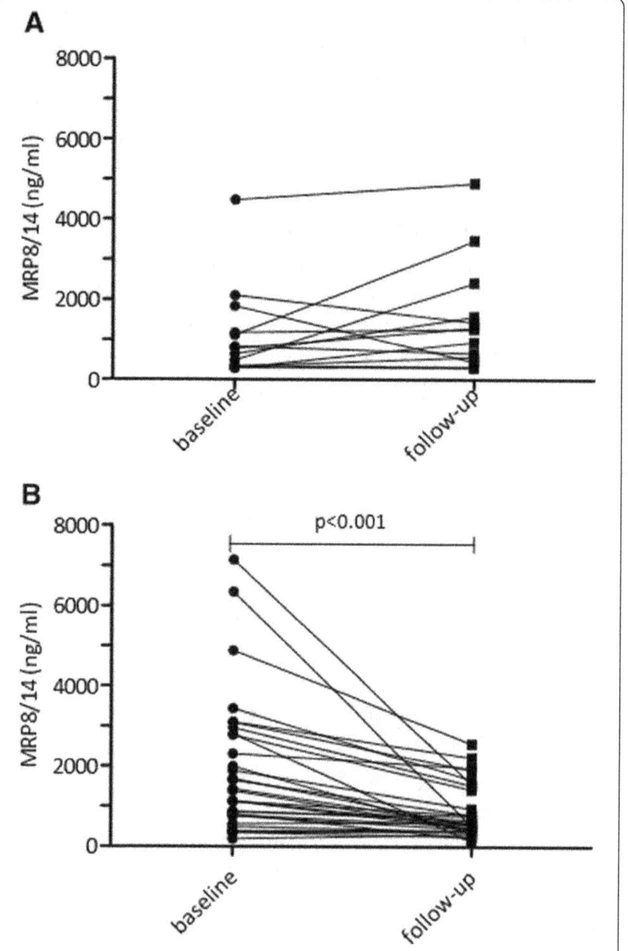

Fig. 2 a Change in myeloid related protein (*MRP*)8/14 serum levels in non-responders pre-treatment compared to levels after treatment for an average of 3.2 months. **b** Change in MRP8/14 serum levels in responders pre-treatment compared to levels after treatment for an average of 3.2 months

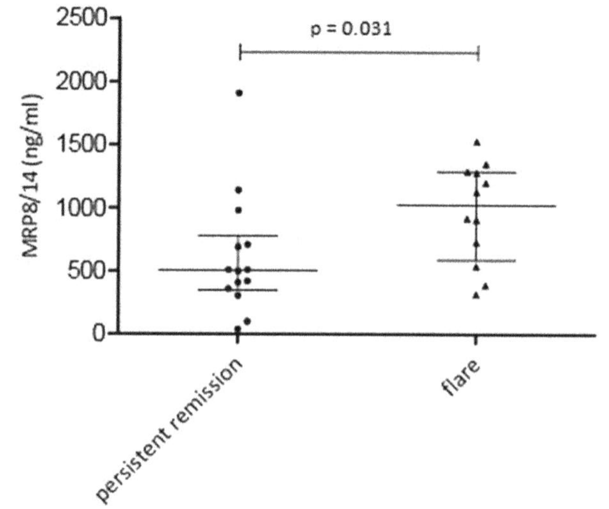

Fig. 3 Differences in myeloid related protein (*MRP*)8/14 at time of medication discontinuation between patients who then had persistent remission and patients who had flares

Association of MRP8/14 level and flare after etanercept withdrawal after successful treatment

Patients who had flares within 6 months (n = 12) after discontinuation of etanercept had higher MRP levels at discontinuation than patients who did not have flares (n = 14) ($p = 0.031$, median 1,025 ng/ml (IQR 588–1288) vs 505 ng/ml (IQR 346–778) (Fig. 3)). Patients discontinuing medication were allowed to have a PGA between 0 and 10 mm. Of the 26 patients discontinuing treatment, 14 patients had a PGA >0 (median PGA of 3). MRP levels were comparable between the patients who had a PGA of 0 and patients who had a PGA >0 at discontinuation of treatment ($p = 0.432$). Full disease activity parameters for all patients at discontinuation can be found in Additional file 1, Table S2.

The cutoff value for prediction of a flare after etanercept withdrawal and the prognostic accuracy are reported in Table 3.

Validation for routine use by commercial ELISA

Commercial MRP8/14 ELISA is available but is not validated for use as a monitoring tool for anti-TNF therapy. Therefore, we aimed to validate our findings with the commercial Bühlmann MRP8/14 Calprotectin ELISA to make MRP8/14 as a marker for anti-TNF therapy widely available. Measurements using the in-house ELISA correlated very well with those from the Bühlmann ELISA (Pearson's rho 0.902, $p < 0.001$). Although MRP8/14 levels appeared to be 3-fold to 4-fold higher when they were measured with the Bühlmann ELISA, the associations between MRP8/14 and response, on both the achievement of ACRpedi 50 or higher and on change in JADAS-10 were comparable. For predicting response to anti-TNF treatment and flares after discontinuation in clinical remission, the in-house ELISA and the Bühlmann ELISA had the same accuracy. Full results for the Bühlmann ELISA data are shown in Additional file 2.

Table 3 Sensitivity, specificity and likelihood ratios for the determined cutoff value of myeloid related protein (MRP)8/14 predicting a flare within 6 months

Accuracy measure	
Cutoff level MRP8/14 (ng/ml)	720
Sensitivity	75 %
Specificity	79 %
Positive likelihood ratio	3.5
Negative likelihood ratio	0.5
Youden index	0.54
Area under the curve (95 % CI)	0.75 (0.55, 0.95)

Discussion

In this study we show that MRP8/14 can predict response to anti-TNF treatment, although it has little additive value to other clinical factors. Patients who responded to anti-TNF treatment had higher levels of MRP8/14 at the start of that treatment than patients who did not respond. Disease activity declined more in patients with higher levels of MRP8/14. In responders, these levels decreased after initiation of treatment, and in non-responders MRP8/14 levels were constant. When the disease had become inactive and treatment with etanercept could be stopped, MRP8/14 levels appeared to be higher for patients in whom the disease flared than in patients who did not experience a flare. The prognostic accuracies of the in-house ELISA and the Bühlmann ELISA were comparable, although the cutoff levels were different.

In recent years, MRP8/14 has been widely studied as potential predictor of disease activity and response to treatment in rheumatic and other inflammatory diseases. In rheumatoid arthritis (RA), MRP8/14 has been used as a predictor for response to biologic treatment [22]. In JIA in particular, MRP8/14 levels are highly predictive of disease activity and of disease flares in systemic JIA [11]. Also in enthesitis-related arthritis there is a relationship between MRP8/14 levels and disease activity [23]. In a more heterogeneous group of JIA patients, MRP8/14 levels have been shown to predict response to MTX treatment [12]. The univariate odds ratio for achieving an ACRpedi50 response or higher following MTX treatment [12] is comparable to the odds ratio found in the present study following anti-TNF treatment. Using the same ELISA to measure MRP8/14 levels, the average serum levels of MRP8/14 in that study were higher than in our patients. Patients in the present study mostly had MRP8/14 levels comparable to patients who did not respond to MTX treatment [12]. This is not surprising as failure of MTX treatment is an eligibility criterion for treatment with biologic agents. Therefore there may be a possibility of using MRP8/14 levels to decide which patient is more likely to respond to MTX and which patient may be better off with biologic treatment right away. Unfortunately we did not have MRP8/14 serum levels for our patients at the start of MTX treatment.

There are well-established experimental ELISA protocols for MRP8/14, however, these are not available for use in routine laboratories. The commercially available Bühlmann ELISA kit has already been demonstrated to perform well in analyzing patient serum samples. To obtain reliable results in the range of MRP8/14 concentrations found at different levels of disease activity in JIA, serial dilution of individual sera to obtain reliable results is necessary [24]. In addition, the level of MRP8/14 concentrations analyzed with the two assays varied substantially. Therefore, a direct comparison of results obtained with one ELISA with a result from a different assay should not be made. Both methods were equally accurate in predicting response to treatment and flares after discontinuation in clinical remission.

For a biomarker to be used in informing therapeutic choice, it will have to fulfill certain requirements. It has to able to predict a certain outcome and the predictive value has to be validated. It has to have additional value on top of other known predictors. Additionally the prediction should have therapeutic consequences. MRP8/14 has been shown to be associated with response to treatment both in this and previous studies in JIA on both relative (ACRpedi50) and absolute measures (change in JADAS-10). Here, MRP8/14 added to the prediction of change in disease activity, though its additive value was small. Some of the responders and non-responders to treatment had comparable MRP8/14 serum levels, and sensitivity and specificity were not optimal for any cutoff value, which is in line with the study by Moncrieffe et al. [12]. Because prediction is not perfect, therapeutic decisions cannot only be based on MRP8/14 levels. However, it is unlikely that a single biomarker will ever be able to perfectly predict response in the heterogeneous pool of JIA patients. This biomarker has the advantage that it is a relatively stable protein and easily measurable in serum, in contrast to, for instance, cytokines such as TNF or IL-1beta. Therefore, MRP8/14 could play a supporting role in response prediction models for response to treatment including clinical as well as laboratory measures, which are under investigation for both JIA and RA [4, 25–29]. More importantly, MRP8/14 might be used to objectively monitor disease activity as it reflects treatment response and confirms disease activity independently from clinical parameters, and might be useful as an early marker of response in clinical trials. In the future, additional parameters are needed that could contribute to a diagnostic panel to guide treatment decisions. MRP expression could enable identification of further biomarkers by defining and dissecting treatment response groups.

For prediction of flares after discontinuation of treatment, MRP8/14 can possibly be used as a prediction tool. MRP8/14 serum levels have already been shown to be predictive of flares after the discontinuation of MTX in JIA patients [10]. We show that this is true to the same extent after stopping etanercept in patients with non-systemic JIA after inactive disease has been achieved. Additionally, we found cutoff values comparable to the earlier specified cutoff value for the in-house ELISA [10, 24]. Still, the cutoff values did not perfectly predict flare or persistent remission after discontinuation. For clinical practice this means that we have to keep searching for additional features that will provide a better prediction model.

Conclusions

In conclusion, serum levels of MRP8/14 are associated with response to treatment with etanercept in patients with non-systemic JIA. MRP8/14 serum levels decrease together with disease activity in responders to etanercept, however, it is of minor predictive value when added to a prediction model with known predictors. MRP8/14 serum levels may be useful in practice to predict flares in patients in clinical remission after cessation of etanercept. They can also be determined using a commercially available ELISA kit.

Abbreviations

ABC: Arthritis and Biologicals in Children; ACR: American College of Rheumatology; BIKER: German Registry for Biologics in Pediatric Rheumatology; CHAQ: childhood health assessment questionnaire; CHARMS: Childhood arthritis response to medication study; DMARD: disease-modifying anti-rheumatic drug; ELISA: enzyme-linked immunosorbent assay; ESR: erythrocyte sedimentation rate; IL: interleukin; IQR: interquartile range; JADAS: juvenile arthritis disease activity score; JIA: juvenile idiopathic arthritis; MRP: myeloid related protein; MTX: methotrexate; RA: rheumatoid arthritis; ROC: receiver operator characteristic; TNF: tumor necrosis factor; VAS: visual analog scale.

Competing interests

LvS has received research grants/research support from the Dutch Board of health insurances, Pfizer and Abbvie for the submitted work and outside the submitted work grants from the Dutch Arthritis Association, consultancy fees from Pfizer, Roche and Novartis, and travel grants from Pfizer and Bristol-Myers Squibb. FG is supported by EUTRAIN (ref.289903), FP7 Marie Curie Initial Training Network for Early Stage Researchers funded by the European Union. No other competing interest are reported for the submitted work; outside the submitted work, RtC has received research grants and consultancy fees from Pfizer and GH has received research grants from AbbVie, Pfizer and Roche and speaker fees from AbbVie, Novartis, Pfizer and Roche; no other relationships or activities that could appear to have influenced the submitted work are reported.

Authors' contributions

JA was involved in the conception of the study, contributed to study design, performed data analysis and interpretation and drafted the paper. MO contributed to data acquisition and study design, was involved in conception of the study and critically revised the paper. FP was involved in conception of the study, contributed to data acquisition and study design and critically revised the paper. MvR was involved in conception of the study, contributed to data acquisition and critically revised the paper. KM was involved in conception of the study, contributed to data acquisition and critically revised the paper. EH was involved in conception of the study, contributed to data acquisition, data interpretation and critically revised the paper. RtC was involved in conception of the study, contributed to data acquisition and critically revised the paper. SU was involved in conception of the study, contributed to data acquisition and critically revised the paper. LW was involved in conception of the study, study design, contributed to data acquisition and critically revised the paper. MF was involved in conception of the study, contributed to data acquisition and critically revised the paper. TV was involved in conception of the study, contributed to data acquisition and critically revised the paper. LvS contributed to study design, was responsible for study supervision and critically revised the paper. GH was involved in conception of the study, contributed to study design, data acquisition and critically revised the paper. DF was involved in conception of the study, contributed to study design, data acquisition and critically revised the paper. DH was involved in conception of the study, contributed to study design and data interpretation, drafting the paper, was responsible for study supervision, performed biomarker analysis and critically revised the paper. JR was involved in conception of the study, contributed to study design, data acquisition and critically revised the pape. FG performed biomarker analysis, was involved in data acquisition and critically revised the paper. All authors read and approved the manuscript.

Acknowledgements

Hospitals participating in this study from the ABC register are the Erasmus MC Sophia Children's Hospital Rotterdam in Rotterdam, the Academic Medical Centre Emma Children's Hospital, Reade location Jan van Breemen and the Sint Lucas Andreas Hospital in Amsterdam, the Sint Maartenskliniek and Radboud University Nijmegen Medical Centre in Nijmegen and Leiden University Medical Centre in Leiden, all in the Netherlands. Patients from the CHARMS study were all treated in Great Ormond Street Hospital for Children in London, United Kingdom. From the BIKER register, the following hospitals participated in this particular study: University Children's Hospital Muenster in Muenster, Charité-Universitaetsmedizin Berlin and the HELIOS Clinic Berlin-Buch in Berlin, Prof.-Hess-Kinderklinik, Klinikum Bremen-Mitte in Bremen, Chilrden's Hopsital St. Marien in Amberg, Asklepios Clinic Sankt Augustin in Sankt Augustin, the German Center for Pediatric and Adolescent Rheumatology in Garmisch-Partenkirchen, University Hospital Schleswig-Holstein in Kiel and the University Children's Hospital Tuebingen in Tuebingen, all in Germany. All authors thank the funding sources that made this study possible: this study was supported by a grant from Pfizer Germany and the European Union Seventh Framework Programme (EC-GA 305266 MIAMI). For maintenance and design of the ABC register it received unconditional support from the Dutch Board of Health Insurances (2003–2006), unconditional support from Pfizer (formerly Wyeth International, since 2007) and unconditional support from AbbVie (formerly Abbott, 2010–2012). The CHARMS study was funded by SPARKS UK (08ICH09), the Big Lottery Fund UK (RG/1/010135231), the NIHR-funded UK Medicines for Children Research Network and GOSH/ICH Biomedical Research Centre (BRC).

Author details

[1]Department of Pediatrics/ Pediatric Rheumatology, Erasmus MC Sophia Children's Hospital Rotterdam, Rotterdam, The Netherlands. [2]Department of Pediatrics/ Pediatric Rheumatology Academic Medical Centre Emma Children's Hospital and Reade location Jan van Breemen, Amsterdam, The Netherlands. [3]Sint Lucas Andreas Hospital and Reade location Jan van Breemen, Amsterdam, The Netherlands. [4]Sint Maartenskliniek and Radboud University Nijmegen Medical Centre, Nijmegen, The Netherlands. [5]Leiden University Medical Centre, Leiden, The Netherlands. [6]Infection, Immunity, Inflammation and Physiological Medicine Programme UCL Institute of Child Health, University College London, London, UK. [7]Centre of Pediatric Rheumatology, Department of General Pediatrics, Asklepios Clinic Sankt Augustin, Sankt Augustin, Germany. [8]German Pediatric Pain Centre, Children's and Adolescents' Hospital, Datteln, Germany. [9]Institute of Immunology, University Hospital Muenster and Interdisciplinary Centre for Clinical Research IZKF, University Hospital Muenster, Muenster, Germany. [10]Interdisciplinary Centre for Clinical Research IZKF, University Hospital Muenster, Muenster and Department of Pediatric Rheumatology and Immunology, University Children's Hospital Muenster, Muenster, Germany.

References

1. Horneff G, Schmeling H, Biedermann T, Foeldvari I, Ganser G, Girschick HJ, et al. The German etanercept registry for treatment of juvenile idiopathic arthritis. Ann Rheum Dis. 2004;63:1638–44.
2. Lovell DJ, Reiff A, Ilowite NT, Wallace CA, Chon Y, Lin SL, et al. Pediatric Rheumatology Collaborative Study G: Safety and efficacy of up to eight years of continuous etanercept therapy in patients with juvenile rheumatoid arthritis. Arthritis Rheum. 2008;58:1496–504.
3. Prince FH, Twilt M, ten Cate R, van Rossum MA, Armbrust W, Hoppenreijs EP, et al. Long-term follow-up on effectiveness and safety of etanercept in juvenile idiopathic arthritis: the Dutch national register. Ann Rheum Dis. 2009;68:635–41.

4. Otten MH, Prince FH, Armbrust W, ten Cate R, Hoppenreijs EP, Twilt M, et al. Factors associated with treatment response to etanercept in juvenile idiopathic arthritis. JAMA. 2011;306:2340–7.
5. Solari N, Palmisani E, Consolaro A, Pistorio A, Viola S, Buoncompagni A, et al. Factors associated with achievement of inactive disease in children with juvenile idiopathic arthritis treated with etanercept. J Rheumatol. 2013;40:192–200.
6. Kessel C, Holzinger D, Foell D. Phagocyte-derived S100 proteins in autoinflammation: putative role in pathogenesis and usefulness as biomarkers. Clin Immunol. 2013;147:229–41.
7. Grevers LC, de Vries TJ, Vogl T, Abdollahi-Roodsaz S, Sloetjes AW, Leenen PJ, et al. S100A8 enhances osteoclastic bone resorption in vitro through activation of Toll-like receptor 4: implications for bone destruction in murine antigen-induced arthritis. Arthritis Rheum. 2011;63:1365–75.
8. Frosch M, Strey A, Vogl T, Wulffraat NM, Kuis W, Sunderkotter C, et al. Myeloid-related proteins 8 and 14 are specifically secreted during interaction of phagocytes and activated endothelium and are useful markers for monitoring disease activity in pauciarticular-onset juvenile rheumatoid arthritis. Arthritis Rheum. 2000;43:628–37.
9. Foell D, Wulffraat N, Wedderburn LR, Wittkowski H, Frosch M, Gerss J, et al. Methotrexate withdrawal at 6 vs 12 months in juvenile idiopathic arthritis in remission: a randomized clinical trial. JAMA. 2010;303:1266–73.
10. Gerss J, Roth J, Holzinger D, Ruperto N, Wittkowski H, Frosch M, et al. Phagocyte-specific S100 proteins and high-sensitivity C reactive protein as biomarkers for a risk-adapted treatment to maintain remission in juvenile idiopathic arthritis: a comparative study. Ann Rheum Dis. 2012;71:1991–7.
11. Holzinger D, Frosch M, Kastrup A, Prince FH, Otten MH, Van Suijlekom-Smit LW, et al. The Toll-like receptor 4 agonist MRP8/14 protein complex is a sensitive indicator for disease activity and predicts relapses in systemic-onset juvenile idiopathic arthritis. Ann Rheum Dis. 2012;71:974–80.
12. Moncrieffe H, Ursu S, Holzinger D, Patrick F, Kassoumeri L, Wade A, et al. A subgroup of juvenile idiopathic arthritis patients who respond well to methotrexate are identified by the serum biomarker MRP8/14 protein. Rheumatology (Oxford). 2013;52:1467–76.
13. Petty RE, Southwood TR, Manners P, Baum J, Glass DN, Goldenberg J, et al. International League of Associations for Rheumatology classification of juvenile idiopathic arthritis: second revision, Edmonton, 2001. J Rheumatol. 2004;31:390–2.
14. Giannini EH, Ruperto N, Ravelli A, Lovell DJ, Felson DT, Martini A. Preliminary definition of improvement in juvenile arthritis. Arthritis Rheum. 1997;40:1202–9.
15. Wallace CA, Giannini EH, Huang B, Itert L, Ruperto N, Childhood Arthritis Rheumatology Research A, Pediatric Rheumatology Collaborative Study G, Paediatric Rheumatology International Trials O. American College of Rheumatology provisional criteria for defining clinical inactive disease in select categories of juvenile idiopathic arthritis. Arthritis Care Res (Hoboken). 2011;63:929–36.
16. Consolaro A, Ruperto N, Bazso A, Pistorio A, Magni-Manzoni S, Filocamo G, et al. Development and validation of a composite disease activity score for juvenile idiopathic arthritis. Arthritis Rheum. 2009;61:658–66.
17. Wallace CA, Ruperto N, Giannini E. Preliminary criteria for clinical remission for select categories of juvenile idiopathic arthritis. J Rheumatol. 2004;31:2290–4.
18. Brunner HI, Lovell DJ, Finck BK, Giannini EH. Preliminary definition of disease flare in juvenile rheumatoid arthritis. J Rheumatol. 2002;29:1058–64.
19. Ruperto N, Lovell DJ, Quartier P, Paz E, Rubio-Perez N, Silva CA, et al. Abatacept in children with juvenile idiopathic arthritis: a randomised, double-blind, placebo-controlled withdrawal trial. Lancet. 2008;372:383–91.
20. Youden WJ. Index for rating diagnostic tests. Cancer. 1950;3:32–5.
21. Albers HM, Wessels JA, van der Straaten RJ, Brinkman DM, Suijlekom-Smit LW, Kamphuis SS, et al. Time to treatment as an important factor for the response to methotrexate in juvenile idiopathic arthritis. Arthritis Rheum. 2009;61:46–51.
22. Choi IY, Gerlag DM, Herenius MJ, Thurlings RM, Wijbrandts CA, Foell D, et al. MRP8/14 serum levels as a strong predictor of response to biological treatments in patients with rheumatoid arthritis. Ann Rheum Dis. 2015;74:499–505.
23. Rahman MT, Myles A, Gaur P, Misra R, Aggarwal A. TLR4 endogenous ligand MRP8/14 level in enthesitis-related arthritis and its association with disease activity and TLR4 expression. Rheumatology (Oxford). 2014;53:270–4.
24. Rothmund F, Gerss J, Ruperto N, Dabritz J, Wittkowski H, Frosch M, et al. Validation of relapse risk biomarkers for routine use in patients with juvenile idiopathic arthritis. Arthritis Care Res (Hoboken). 2014;66:949–55.
25. Bulatovic M, Heijstek MW, Van Dijkhuizen EH, Wulffraat NM, Pluijm SM, de Jonge R. Prediction of clinical non-response to methotrexate treatment in juvenile idiopathic arthritis. Ann Rheum Dis. 2012;71:1484–9.
26. Iwamoto N, Kawakami A, Fujikawa K, Aramaki T, Kawashiri SY, Tamai M, et al. Prediction of DAS28-ESR remission at 6 months by baseline variables in patients with rheumatoid arthritis treated with etanercept in Japanese population. Mod Rheumatol. 2009;19:488–92.
27. Marotte H, Miossec P. Biomarkers for prediction of TNFalpha blockers response in rheumatoid arthritis. Joint, Bone, Spine. 2010;77:297–305.
28. Pomirleanu C, Ancuta C, Miu S, Chirieac R. A predictive model for remission and low disease activity in patients with established rheumatoid arthritis receiving TNF blockers. Clin Rheumatol. 2013;32:665–70.
29. Soderlin MK, Petersson IF, Geborek P. The effect of smoking on response and drug survival in rheumatoid arthritis patients treated with their first anti-TNF drug. Scand J Rheumatol. 2012;41:1–9.

18

Chimeric cells of maternal origin do not appear to be pathogenic in the juvenile idiopathic inflammatory myopathies or muscular dystrophy

Carol M. Artlett[1], Sihem Sassi-Gaha[1], Ronald C. Ramos[2,4], Frederick W. Miller[3] and Lisa G. Rider[3*]

Abstract

Introduction: Microchimeric cells have been studied for over a decade, with conflicting reports on their presence and role in autoimmune and other inflammatory diseases. To determine whether microchimeric cells were pathogenic or mediating tissue repair in inflammatory myopathies, we phenotyped and quantified microchimeric cells in juvenile idiopathic inflammatory myopathies (JIIM), muscular dystrophy (MD), and noninflammatory control muscle tissues.

Method: Fluorescence immunophenotyping for infiltrating cells with sequential fluorescence in situ hybridization was performed on muscle biopsies from ten patients with JIIM, nine with MD and ten controls.

Results: Microchimeric cells were significantly increased in MD muscle (0.079 ± 0.024 microchimeric cells/mm^2 tissue) compared to controls (0.019 ± 0.007 cells/mm^2 tissue, p = 0.01), but not elevated in JIIM muscle (0.043 ± 0.015 cells/mm^2). Significantly more CD4+ and CD8+ microchimeric cells were in the muscle of patients with MD compared with controls (mean 0.053 ± 0.020/mm^2 versus 0 ± 0/mm^2 p = 0.003 and 0.043 ± 0.023/mm^2 versus 0 ± 0/mm^2 p = 0.025, respectively). No differences in microchimeric cells between JIIM, MD, and noninflammatory controls were found for CD3+, Class II+, CD25+, CD45RA+, and CD123+ phenotypes, and no microchimeric cells were detected in CD20, CD83, or CD45RO populations. The locations of microchimeric cells were similar in all three conditions, with MD muscle having more microchimeric cells in perimysial regions than controls, and JIIM having fewer microchimeric muscle nuclei than MD. Microchimeric inflammatory cells were found, in most cases, at significantly lower proportions than autologous cells of the same phenotype.

Conclusions: Microchimeric cells are not specific to autoimmune disease, and may not be important in muscle inflammation or tissue repair in JIIM.

Introduction

The role of microchimeric cells in health and disease has been controversial. Microchimeric cells are acquired during pregnancy, with the transfer of cells from fetus to mother or mother to fetus. Microchimeric cells have been documented to be elevated in the peripheral blood and affected tissues of patients with autoimmune diseases, such as systemic sclerosis [1], systemic lupus erythematosus [2], neonatal lupus [3], and juvenile idiopathic inflammatory myopathies (JIIM) [4–6]. Recently, microchimeric cells were found to be elevated in specific target tissues, such as the liver in hepatitis C infection [7] and tumors, such as HER2-positive breast cancer, cervical, lung and thyroid cancer, and melanoma [8–10]. However, not all studies have documented higher levels of chimeric cells in autoimmune conditions [11] or cancer [12]. This variability suggests that they might be recruited nonspecifically to sites of inflammation and tissue injury [13, 14] or participate in tissue repair [8].

The JIIM are systemic autoimmune diseases characterized by chronic muscle inflammation and weakness. Juvenile dermatomyositis (JDM), the form of JIIM with characteristic photosensitive skin rashes, including Gottron's papules and heliotrope rash, is the most

* Correspondence: riderl@mail.nih.gov
[3]National Institute of Environmental Health Sciences, National Institutes of Health, Department of Health and Human Services, Environmental Autoimmunity Group, Program of Clinical Research, 9000 Rockville Pike, Bethesda, MD 20892, USA
Full list of author information is available at the end of the article

common of the JIIM and is thought to be mediated by CD4+ T cells, B cell and dendritic cell attack on muscle capillaries, whereas juvenile polymyositis (JPM), the form of JIIM without characteristic rashes, is thought to be mediated by CD8+ T cells on myofibers [15–17]. We previously found elevated levels of maternal microchimeric cells in muscle biopsies and peripheral blood of boys with JIIM and characterized these cells to be in the CD4+ and CD8+ peripheral T cells [4]. However, the phenotypes of the microchimeric cells in affected muscle tissues were not investigated. The current study analyzes the frequency of microchimeric cells within different inflammatory phenotypes in the muscle of JIIM and compares these findings with the nonautoimmune inflammatory muscle disorder muscular dystrophy (MD) [18] and with noninflammatory control (NIC) muscle tissue. We sought to determine whether microchimeric cells have a pathogenic or reparative role in JIIM.

Methods

Patients

All studies were performed with full Institutional Review Board approval from the National Institutes of Health and waived approval from the Institutional Review Board at Drexel University College of Medicine. All patients consented to the study. Muscle biopsies were obtained for diagnosis, and prior to initiation of therapy, from ten patients with JIIM (six JDM, four JPM), nine MD (eight Duchenne, one Becker dystrophy) and ten controls without inflammatory disease (four mitochondrial myopathies, six histologically normal) and analyzed by immunofluorescence for specific phenotypes and by fluorescence in situ hybridization (FISH) for maternal microchimeric cells. The ages of the JIIM patients ranged from 3 to 16 years [15, 16], the patients with MD from 2 to 14 years [19], and the controls from 2 to 17 years. All tissues were paraffin embedded and derived from males and were cut at 5 μM. No patient had prior blood transfusions. The size of the tissue sample ranged from 9 to 96 mm^2 in JIIM, 6 to 245 mm^2 in MD, and 20 to 62 mm^2 in the controls.

Immunofluorescence/fluorescence in situ hybridization

Before immunofluorescent staining was performed, one slide from each biopsy was stained with hematoxylin and eosin to verify the histological appearance of the tissue and the presence of inflammatory cells. Biopsies were selected based on infiltration density. The immunofluorescent assessment of the tissues was performed first, and all positive cells of each immunophenotype were documented. Tissues were stained for T cells (CD3, CD4, and CD8), T cell activation markers (CD25 and HLA Class II), memory T cells (CD45RO), naïve T cells (CD45RA), B cells (CD20) and dendritic cells (CD123 and CD83) by using antibodies from Neomarkers (Fremont, CA, USA) or Dako (Carpinteria, CA, USA). The secondary antibody carrying the Cy-2 conjugate (Jackson ImmunoResearch, West Grove, PA, USA) was used to detect the primary antibody, and sections were mounted with DAPI and viewed with a Nikon epi-fluorescent microscope with triple-band filter at 1000× magnification (Nikon Instruments, Melville, NY, USA). Positive cells were documented, and sections were processed for FISH analysis as we described previously [1]. Cells that had XX or XY nuclear probes were quantified. The sections were also assessed after FISH for other nuclei that were carrying XX probes but were negative for immunofluorescent stain. Muscle fiber nuclei were documented by morphological analyses of the muscle fiber based on the location and shape of the nucleus within the fiber. The myogenic origin was confirmed in 12 sections by actin staining. Personnel involved with muscle biopsy studies were blinded to patient diagnosis.

Characterization of microchimeric or autologous cells was determined only when both probes were evident in the nucleus (XX for microchimeric cells and XY for autologous cells). We performed immunofluorescence prior to FISH and stained the protein green. Because some immunofluorescence signal can remain after the FISH procedure, we selected red for the X chromosome. This approach left no doubt about the presence of a microchimeric cell, even if residual immunofluorescence staining was present. Biopsy sections were selected to limit the number of overlapping nuclei in the inflammatory cell infiltrates, because overlapping nuclei could result in false assignment of microchimerism due to two X chromosome probes appearing to be in the same nucleus when they are in separate nuclei. Prior to making the final assessment as to whether a cell was microchimeric or not, the entire nucleus of the cell was assessed for the presence of other probes, i.e., possible nuclei lying underneath. Only when it was confirmed that no additional probes were present, were the nuclei assigned as being microchimeric or autologous. Twelve (JIIM or MD) biopsies with many overlapping infiltrating cells without well-defined nuclei were excluded. With this careful approach to immunophenotyping and FISH we reduced the chance of over-identifying microchimeric cells due to overlapping cells and to fluorescent protein remaining after the phenotyping.

Statistical analyses

Results obtained by FISH were expressed as mean ± standard error of the mean. Differences in the frequency of positive microchimeric cells in the tissue were evaluated using Prism 5 software (GraphPad Software, San Diego, CA, USA). For nonparametric data, the Mann–Whitney rank sum t test was used to compare quantities of microchimeric cells. A p value ≤ 0.05 was considered significant; due to small sample sizes, $p = 0.051–0.06$ was considered to demonstrate a trend toward significance.

Results

Are microchimeric cells enriched in inflammatory diseases and what are their phenotypes?

Microchimeric cells were detected in nine of ten JIIM muscle biopsies, nine of nine MD biopsies, and eight of ten NIC biopsies (ten sections per biopsy). Of the total phenotyped and nonphenotyped microchimeric cells across all sections examined, the density was 0.043 ± 0.015 microchimeric cells/mm^2 of muscle tissue in JIIM, 0.079 ± 0.024/mm^2 of tissue in MD, and 0.019 ± 0.007/mm^2 of tissue in NICs (Fig. 1a). MD biopsies had significantly more microchimeric cells/mm^2 than controls ($p = 0.01$). There was a trend toward more microchimeric cells/mm^2 of muscle tissue in MD patients compared to JIIM ($p = 0.06$), but there was no difference in the density of microchimeric cells between JIIM and controls.

There were few differences in the phenotypes of the microchimeric cells and no differences in the concentration of microchimeric cells/mm^2 of muscle tissue in CD3+, Class II+, CD45RA+ or CD123+ phenotypes in patients with JIIM, MD or the controls (Fig. 1b, e, g, h). There were significantly more CD4+ and CD8+ microchimeric cells in the muscle of patients with MD compared with controls (0.053 ± 0.020/mm^2 vs. 0 ± 0/mm^2 for CD4+ microchimeric cells [Fig. 1c, $p = 0.003$] and 0.043 ± 0.023/mm^2 vs. 0 ± 0/mm^2 for CD8+ microchimeric cells [Fig. 1d,

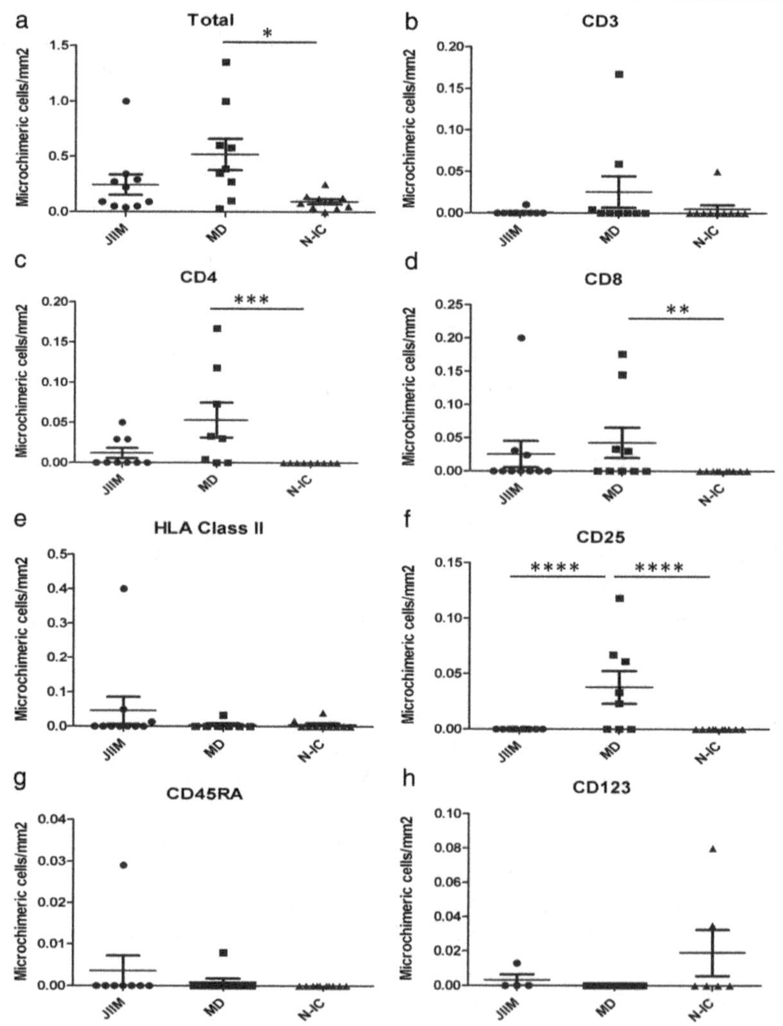

Fig. 1 Density of microchimeric cells by immunophenotype in the muscle of patients with juvenile idiopathic inflammatory myopathies (JIIM), muscular dystrophy (MD) and noninflammatory controls (N-IC). Data are presented as mean ± standard error of the mean for each immunophenotype. No microchimeric cells were identified that were positive for CD20, CD45RO or CD83 (data not shown). *JIIM* juvenile idiopathic inflammatory myopathy ($n = 10$), *MD* muscular dystrophy ($n = 9$), *N-IC* noninflammatory controls ($n = 10$). $^{*}p = 0.01$; $^{**}p = 0.025$; $^{***}p = 0.003$; $^{****}p = 0.006$. (**a**) Total microchimeric cells in tissues; (**b**) CD3 positive microchimeric cells; (**c**) CD4 positive microchimeric cells; (**d**) CD8 positive microchimeric cells; (**e**) HLA class II positive microchimeric cells; (**f**) CD25 positive microchimeric cells; (**g**) CD45RA positive microchimeric cells; (**h**) CD123 positive microchimeric cells

p = 0.025]). There was a trend toward more CD4+ microchimeric cells in MD biopsies compared with JIIM (0.053 ± 0.020/mm^2 vs. 0.012 ± 0.006/mm^2, p = 0.06); whereas the number of CD4+ microchimeric cells did not differ between JIIM and controls. The number of CD8+ microchimeric cells did not differ in the muscle tissue of patients with MD and JIIM, or JIIM and controls. MD muscle tissue had significantly more microchimeric CD25+ cells/mm^2 of tissue (0.038 ± 0.014/mm^2), whereas JIIM patients and controls did not have any detectable CD25+ microchimeric cells (Fig. 1f). None of the biopsies had microchimeric cells that were CD20+, CD45RO+ or CD83+ (not shown). Examples of phenotyped microchimeric cells are depicted in Fig. 2.

There were few differences in concentration of microchimeric cells/mm^2 in the JIIM subsets (not shown). JPM had more CD8+ microchimeric cells/mm^2 than JDM (0.064 + 0.046/mm^2 vs. 0 ± 0/mm^2; p = 0.025) and controls (0.064 + 0.046/mm^2 vs. 0 ± 0/mm^2, p = 0.004) but had similar numbers of CD8+ microchimeric cells/mm^2 as MD (p = 0.51). CD4+ microchimeric cells were detected in JDM, but not in JPM, muscle (0.022 ± 0.009/mm^2 vs. 0 ± 0/mm^2), but the concentrations did not differ significantly (p = 0.31).

Does the location of microchimeric cells differ among inflammatory muscle diseases?

Overall, 62.2 ± 5.7 % of all microchimeric cells were in the endomysial region, 26.5 ± 4.9 % in the perimysial regions and 11.3 ± 4.2 % in the perivascular regions. There were no significant differences between the percentages of microchimeric cells in the perivascular regions of JIIM or MD patients or the NIC subjects (20.8 ± 10.6 % in JIIM, 8.2 ± 4.1 % in MD, and 3.7 ± 3.5 % in controls; Fig. 3a). In the perimysial regions, microchimeric cells occurred in similar proportions between JIIM and MD patients (25.8 ± 7.4 % vs. 38.1 ± 5.6 %, p = 0.62) and between JIIM and controls (25.8 ± 7.4 % vs. 15.6 ± 10.8 %, p = 0.14). However, biopsies from MD patients had a higher percentage of microchimeric cells in the perimysial region than controls (33.9 ± 5.5 % vs. 14.0 ± 10.3 %, p = 0.014; Fig. 3b). There were no differences in the endomysial regions between JIIM or MD patients or

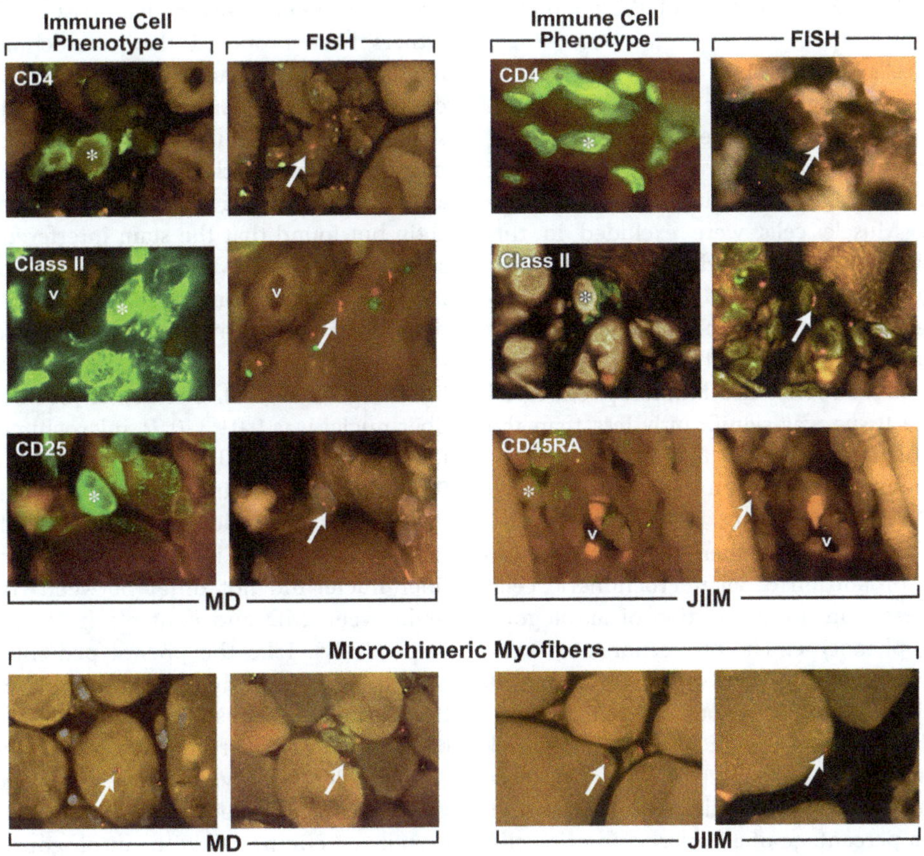

Fig. 2 Representative microchimeric cells that are expressing an immunophenotype in the muscle of patients with muscular dystrophy and juvenile idiopathic inflammatory myopathies. Examples of microchimeric cells that express a phenotype are depicted, the *left panel* in each pair is the phenotype and the *right panel* is the corresponding FISH result for that cell. *JIIM* juvenile idiopathic inflammatory myopathy, *MD* muscular dystrophy, *V* vessel. *Star* denotes the phenotype-positive cell (*green*) and the *arrows* indicate the XX probes (*red*) within that phenotyped cell

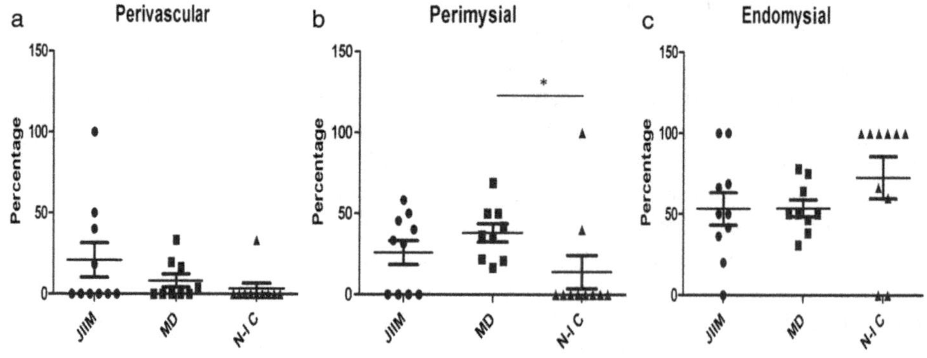

Fig. 3 Percentage of microchimeric cells at various muscle locations. Data are presented as mean of the percentage ± standard error of the mean at each location for each diagnostic group. *JIIM* juvenile idiopathic inflammatory myopathy (n = 10), *MD* muscular dystrophy (n = 9), *N-IC* noninflammatory controls (n = 10). $^{*}p = 0.014$. (**a**) Perivascular location; (**b**) Perimysial location; (**c**) Endomysial location

controls (53.3 ± 10.1 % in JIIM, 53.7 ± 5.3 % in MD, and 80.7 ± 10.8 % in controls; Fig. 3c).

The subsets of JIIM (not shown) did not differ in the percentages of microchimeric cells in the perivascular regions (14.6 ± 11.0 % in JPM vs. 25.0 ± 17.1 % in JDM, $p = 0.90$), perimysial regions (41.7 ± 4.6 % in JPM vs. 15.3 ± 10.2 % in JDM, $p = 0.15$) and endomysial regions (43.8 ± 11.9 % in JPM vs. 59.7 ± 15.6 % in JDM, $p = 0.51$).

Do microchimeric cells drive disease?

For each phenotype we determined whether microchimeric cells were enriched as a percentage of all microchimeric cells, compared to autologous cells of that phenotype as a percentage of all autologous immunophenotyped cells. Muscle cells were excluded in this analysis. An enrichment of microchimeric cells compared to autologous cells could indicate their involvement in disease pathogenesis. In most cases, the proportion of microchimeric cells of a given phenotype compared to all the microchimeric immunophenotyped cells in the muscle tissue was significantly less than the proportion of autologous cells with that phenotype as a percentage of all autologous immunophenotyped cells (Table 1). In JIIM muscle, except for CD45RA+ and CD83+ cells, the proportion of microchimeric cells for each lineage as a proportion of all microchimeric cells was significantly less than the proportion of autologous cells of that same phenotype. The proportion of microchimeric cells that were CD45RA+ compared to all microchimeric cells was similar to, but not greater than, the proportion of autologous CD45RA+ cells compared to all autologous immunophenotyped cells. In MD biopsies, the proportion of microchimeric CD3+ and Class II+ cells as a percentage of all microchimeric cells was significantly less than their autologous counterparts, with a trend toward a lower frequency of microchimeric cells in CD8+ and CD123+ lineages compared to their autologous equivalents. In the control muscle tissue, significantly fewer microchimeric cells were found in CD3+, Class II+ and the CD25+ lineages compared to these autologous lineages as a proportion of the total autologous immunophenotyped cells, with a trend toward fewer microchimeric cells of the CD8+ and CD123+ lineages.

Do microchimeric cells mediate tissue repair?

Others have proposed that microchimeric cells might mediate tissue repair. In muscle diseases, they could contribute to regenerating myofibers. Thus, we hypothesized that in JIIM and MD the proportion of microchimeric myofiber nuclei would be enriched compared to autologous myofiber nuclei. We stained 15 sections for actin but found that the stain interfered with FISH, possibly due to the overabundance of actin within these muscle sections. Consequently, we subsequently quantified maternally derived myofiber nuclei based on the morphology of the nucleus and its location within the fiber (Fig. 2, *bottom*). The density of microchimeric myofiber nuclei was 0.01 ± 0.01 microchimeric cells/mm^2 of muscle tissue in JIIM, 0.07 ± 0.03/mm^2 in MD, and 0.02 ± 0.01/mm^2 in controls. MD biopsies had significantly more microchimeric myofiber nuclei than JIIM ($p = 0.018$). The number of microchimeric myofiber nuclei did not differ between JIIM and controls or between MD and controls ($p = 0.33$ and $p = 0.18$, respectively). Like the phenotyped microchimeric cells, we found significantly fewer microchimeric muscle nuclei than autologous muscle nuclei in JIIM, MD and control biopsies. The proportion of microchimeric myofiber nuclei was significantly less than the proportion of autologous myofiber nuclei. The percentage of microchimeric myofibers compared with autologous myofibers from the same group was 0.6 ± 0.6 % in JIIM ($p = 0.002$), 3.6 ± 1.2 % in MD ($p < 0.001$) and 2.5 ± 1.4 % in controls ($p = 0.0014$) (see Fig. 2 for representative microchimeric myofibers).

Table 1 Relationship between the frequencies of microchimeric versus autologous cells of a given immunophenotype

Phenotype	JIIM	MD	NIC
% Autologous CD3+ cells of total autologous[a]	6.5 ± 2.3	9.9 ± 2.5	4.8 ± 2.7
% Microchimeric CD3+ cells of total microchimeric cells[b]	0.3 ± 0.3	2.8 ± 1.8	10 ± 10
	$p = 0.06$ (T)	$p = 0.04$	$p = 0.05$
% Autologous CD4 cells of total autologous cells	16.8 ± 6.9	12.2 ± 5.3	8.4 ± 6.6
% Microchimeric CD4 cells of total microchimeric cells	2.2 ± 1.4	7.8 ± 2.0	0 ± 0
	$p = 0.03$	$p = 0.23$	$p = 0.12$
% Autologous CD8 cells of total autologous cells	20.4 ± 5.0	12.6 ± 3.2	5.1 ± 3.2
% Microchimeric CD8 cells of total microchimeric cells	1.1 ± 0.6	6.5 ± 2.3	0 ± 0
	$p = 0.05$	$p = 0.09$	$p = 0.07$
% Autologous Class II cells of total autologous cells	21.5 ± 8.1	51.6 ± 5.9	38.0 ± 11.0
% Microchimeric Class II cells of total microchimeric cells	1.7 ± 1.1	0.8 ± 0.7	20.0 ± 13.3
	$p = 0.04$	$p < 0.001$	$p = 0.02$
% Autologous CD20 cells of total autologous cells	8.5 ± 4.4	2.7 ± 2.5	0 ± 0
% Microchimeric CD20 cells of total microchimeric cells	0 ± 0	0 ± 0	0 ± 0
	$p = 0.08$	$p = 0.3$	$p =$ NA
% Autologous CD83 cells of total autologous cells	0.1 ± 0.1	0.1 ± 0.1	0.2 ± 0.2
% Microchimeric CD83cells of total microchimeric cells	0 ± 0	0 ± 0	0 ± 0
	$p = 0.18$	$p = 0.17$	$p = 0.17$
% Autologous CD25 cells of total autologous cells	16.2 ± 5.1	9.5 ± 3.4	6.4 ± 2.8
% Microchimeric CD25 cells of total microchimeric cells	0 ± 0	7.7 ± 2.9	0 ± 0
	$p = 0.01$	$p = 0.33$	$p = 0.02$
% Autologous CD45RA cells of total autologous cells	2.3 ± 0.9	1.5 ± 0.4	3.2 ± 2.3
% Microchimeric CD45RA cells of total microchimeric cells	1.2 ± 1.1	0.9 ± 0.9	0 ± 0
	$p = 0.24$	$p = 0.26$	$p = 0.10$
% Autologous CD45RO cells of total autologous cells	6.3 ± 2.4	4.1 ± 1.1	9.0 ± 4.4
% Microchimeric CD45RO cells of total microchimeric cells	0 ± 0	0 ± 0	0 ± 0
	$p = 0.03$	$p = 0.003$	$p = 0.06$ (T)
% Autologous CD123 cells of total autologous cells	3.6 ± 1.1	1.9 ± 0.7	26.2 ± 12.2
% Microchimeric CD123 cells of total microchimeric cells	0.04 ± 0.02	0 ± 0	4.4 ± 2.3
	$p = 0.04$	$p = 0.06$ (T)	$p = 0.06$ (T)

Data are presented as mean ± standard error of the mean for each group

JIIM juvenile idiopathic inflammatory myopathy, *MD* muscular dystrophy, *NIC* noninflammatory controls; *NA* not available, *T* trend for significance

[a]Total autologous cells consists of all phenotyped cells with XY probes

[b]Total microchimeric cells consists of all cells with XX probes

Discussion

Previously we found higher frequency and number of microchimeric cells in the peripheral blood and muscle tissue of JIIM patients compared to noninflammatory or healthy control subjects, suggesting that microchimeric cells may play a role in the pathogenesis of JIIM [4, 20]. One limitation in those studies was that we did not phenotype the microchimeric cells in the tissues; however, we did find microchimeric cells in the CD4+ and CD8+ lineages in peripheral blood [4]. The current study further investigated microchimeric cells in JIIM, compared with inflammatory but nonautoimmune muscle disease (MD) and with noninflammatory control muscle and examined the immunophenotypes of microchimeric cells in muscle tissue. Our goals were to determine whether microchimeric cells play a pathogenic role in disease and/or whether they are involved in tissue repair. Persistent microchimeric cells have been found in patients with other inflammatory diseases, suggesting that these cells might be recruited nonspecifically to sites of inflammation [7–10, 13, 14].

Compared with our prior study, we found a similar frequency of JIIM muscle tissue samples containing microchimeric cells and a similar overall quantity of microchimeric cells in JIIM muscle tissue [4]. Here, we also saw a similar concentration of microchimeric cells in MD tissues, suggesting that this finding is not specific to autoimmune diseases but may be generally associated with overt inflammatory muscle disease. This suggests that the number of inflammatory microchimeric cells recruited to the site of inflammation does not depend on the total number of inflammatory cells present. MD is a genetic disease caused by mutations in dystrophin inducing muscle fiber damage, with resultant muscle necrosis and tissue inflammation [21], whereas the cause of JIIM is unknown but presumed to result primarily from an autoimmune-mediated destruction of myofibers and muscle capillaries [17]. In both diseases, tissue destruction is mediated by T and B cells, and in JDM by dendritic cells [22–24]. We were surprised to find microchimeric cells also in a high proportion of control muscle tissues, in contrast to our prior study [4]; however, in the prior study, only one muscle section was examined, whereas in the present study, ten sections from each patient's muscle tissue were examined. Microchimeric cells were not observed in every tissue section from a given patient and thus overall were considered to be a rare event.

To characterize the phenotype of microchimeric cells in JIIM and MD, we stained muscle tissue for various immunophenotypes. Overall, we detected few microchimeric cells within inflammatory phenotypes, and we did not find microchimeric cells in B cell or dendritic cell lineages, which are thought to be important in JIIM pathogenesis. Of the T cell immunophenotypes, generally the concentration of microchimeric cells was greater in MD tissues than in noninflammatory controls, and typically T cells or activated T cells were not elevated in JIIM muscle tissue. Microchimeric cells of a given phenotype did not occur more frequently than their autologous counterparts in JIIM or MD muscle tissue, compared to all microchimeric or immunophenotyped autologous cells. In terms of location, the endomysial and perivascular regions of the muscle showed similar numbers of microchimeric cells among the three groups. However, MD and JPM tissues were more likely to have microchimeric cells in the perimysium compared with controls. It is this sole finding that weakly suggests that microchimeric cells might play a pathogenic or reparative role.

We also found microchimeric cells in noninflammatory tissues and in myofibers, not only in infiltrating inflammatory cells, suggesting that these cells are resident in tissues regardless of inflammation. Tissues with maternal microchimeric cells include autoimmune and nonautoimmune thyroid [25], pancreas in type I diabetes [26], neonatal lupus heart muscle [27], tonsils and adenoids [28], cutaneous inflammatory diseases [29] and inflammatory bowel disease [30]. Normal tissues with maternal microchimeric cells include heart [27], tonsils/adenoids [28], skin diseases [29] and inflammatory bowel disease [30]; albeit at lower levels than diseased tissue of the same type, suggesting that a threshold number of microchimeric cells might be necessary to drive disease. However, in some instances microchimeric cells were found at comparable numbers in healthy tissues [6].

One hypothesis proposed by other investigators is that microchimeric cells might mediate tissue repair via microchimeric stem cells. Initially we stained for muscle fibers, but this staining procedure interfered with subsequent FISH. Therefore, we counted the numbers of microchimeric nuclei that were apparently myofibers, based on their morphological position and shape within the muscle fiber, and compared them to the numbers of autologous myofiber nuclei. We found significantly more microchimeric muscle nuclei in MD than JIIM muscle, but there were no significant differences between JIIM and controls. However, each disease class had significantly fewer microchimeric myonuclei than autologous muscle nuclei. One caveat is that we do not know how many myofibers were regenerated from autologous progenitors during the disease process [27], and this study was not designed to determine that. Overall, these results suggest that microchimeric myofibers are no more frequent than microchimeric inflammatory cells in diseased tissues, and that noninflammatory tissue resident in microchimeric myofiber nuclei are present at higher levels than observed in JIIM. This result suggests that microchimeric cells are not enriched in muscle tissue in any of these disease conditions, and that they do not mediate tissue repair at an augmented rate compared to autologous myofibers.

We stained one phenotype per FISH analysis for microchimeric cells in the tissue, but we did not stain for all cell phenotypes in the tissues. Consequently, we may have missed a microchimeric cell phenotype(s) that was noninflammatory, including muscle stem cells. We did not analyze all inflammatory phenotypes, such as macrophages, that are frequent in the inflammatory infiltrates of JIIM and MD muscle [22, 23], and some microchimeric cells did not match any of the phenotypes analyzed. The number of inflammatory cells in the JIIM samples was comparable to previously published data [22], and this suggests that the immunophenotyping was not underrepresenting inflammatory cell phenotypes. Furthermore, although we did not observe many differences in the phenotypic numbers of microchimeric cells between disease groups, only one or a small number of pathogenic microchimeric cells might be sufficient to cause disease; however, we believe this is unlikely as microchimeric cells were also present in the muscle tissue of noninflammatory controls. In addition, we did not examine the functionality of the microchimeric cells phenotyped and although microchimeric cells were found in inflammatory cells of the controls, they may have been quiescent, whereas in the inflammatory muscle diseases they may be activated, indicated by different cytokine profiles [31]. We did, however, investigate T cell activation markers, such as Class II, CD25, and memory T cell subsets, and did not detect more microchimeric cells in JIIM muscle compared to noninflammatory controls, and only MD had significantly more CD25 microchimeric cells. Finally, our sample sizes were relatively small and the study may have been underpowered to detect differences between groups.

Murine studies suggest that maternal microchimeric cells are able to manipulate the fetal immune system and promote the development of various Regulatory T cells (Tregs) that are tolerant toward the noninherited maternal antigens [32]. Additional studies using inbred mice have also reported the trafficking of alloreactive T cells in offspring and that the maternal cells can influence the fetal response to targeting specific tissues [33]. These studies were elegantly performed in mice, and whether this same phenomenon occurs to the same extent during human gestation leading to increased risk for autoimmune diseases is yet to be proved. Currently, no studies have been performed to determine whether maternal microchimerism of cells that carry noninherited shared epitopes place the JIIM cohort at a greater risk for disease, like they apparently do for rheumatoid arthritis [34]. HLA-DRB1*0301 in linkage with HLA-DQA1*0501 confers the highest susceptibility for JIIM; however, in contrast to previous studies [31], we found that HLA-DQA*0501 was not significantly associated with microchimerism [35]. Maternal microchimeric cell transfer is a frequent occurrence during fetal development [36], and these cells most likely distribute throughout all the tissues and become embedded in the bone marrow with the ability to differentiate into inflammatory cells or stromal cells upon cell damage. Thus, the presence of maternal microchimeric cells in tissues is not surprising in light of the high number of normal samples that were positive in our study and in other studies [6, 37]. Our data support the findings of Ye et al., who also reported their controls being positive for maternal microchimerism [6]. The presence of microchimeric cells in the control tissues without inflammation suggests that they are present either from fetal development if stromal in nature, or are inflammatory cells trafficking through the tissue. In contrast with Ye et al., we found the presence of some microchimeric T cells, albeit at very low percentages in our JDM samples. However, the direct role of maternal microchimeric cells in human disease is still not clear and against the complex genetic background of humans may mean that the direct role of these cells in autoimmunity may never be conclusively demonstrated.

Conclusions

Overall, our results indicate that microchimeric cells likely do not play important pathogenic roles in autoimmune or inflammatory muscle disease, nor are they seemingly involved in mediating repair of muscle tissue. Once differentiated, where there is inflammation, the autologous cells, along with their microchimeric counterparts, appear to be recruited to those sites in like manner. This study suggests that microchimeric cells are not part of the autoimmune pathogenesis in JIIM or the primary inflammatory process in MD.

Abbreviations

CD: cluster designation; FISH: fluorescence in situ hybridization; JDM: juvenile dermatomyositis; JIIM: juvenile idiopathic inflammatory myopathies; JPM: juvenile polymyositis; MD: muscular dystrophy; NIC: noninflammatory control.

Competing interests

The authors declare that they have no competing interests.

Authors' contributions

All authors contributed substantially to the manuscript. CMA was responsible for the design, data collection, experiments, and interpretation of the research. SSG and RCR were responsible for histology of the tissues and data acquisition, and critical editing of the manuscript. LGR and FWM contributed tissue samples and aided in the design of the research and data interpretation. LGR aided CMA in manuscript writing and statistical analyses. All authors have read, edited and approved the final version of the manuscript.

Acknowledgements

We thank Dr. Kathleen Patterson of Children's Hospital Medical Center, Seattle, WA, USA for the muscular dystrophy and control muscle biopsies and Dr. Ann Reed for JIIM biopsies and for staining for CD123. We also thank Drs. Christine Castro and Ira Berkower for their critical evaluation and assessment of the manuscript. This research was supported in part by the Intramural Research Program of the NIH, National Institute of Environmental Health Sciences and by a grant from The Myositis Association.

Author details

[1]Department of Microbiology and Immunology, Drexel University College of Medicine, 2900 Queen Lane, Philadelphia, PA 19129, USA. [2]Department of Medicine, Thomas Jefferson University, 1020 Walnut Street, Philadelphia, PA 19107, USA. [3]National Institute of Environmental Health Sciences, National Institutes of Health, Department of Health and Human Services, Environmental Autoimmunity Group, Program of Clinical Research, 9000 Rockville Pike, Bethesda, MD 20892, USA. [4]Present address: Agis Global, Business Development Executive, 1266 East Main Street, Stamford, CT 06902, USA.

References

1. Artlett CM, Smith JB, Jimenez SA. Identification of fetal DNA and cells in skin lesions from women with systemic sclerosis. NEJM. 1998;338:1186–91.
2. Johnson KL, McAlindon TE, Mulcahy E, Bianchi DW. Microchimerism in a female patient with systemic lupus erythematosus. Arthritis Rheum. 2001;44:2107–11.
3. Stevens AM, Hermes HM, Kiefer MM, Rutledge JC, Nelson JL. Chimeric maternal cells with tissue-specific antigen expression and morphology are common in infant tissues. Pediatr Dev Pathol. 2009;12:337–46.
4. Artlett CM, Ramos R, Jimenez SA, Patterson K, Miller FW, Rider LG. Chimeric cells of maternal origin in juvenile idiopathic inflammatory myopathies. Lancet. 2000;356:2155–6.
5. Reed AM, Picornell YJ, Harwood A, Kredich D. Chimerism in children with juvenile dermatomyositis. Lancet. 2000;356:2156–7.

6. Ye Y, van Zyl B, Varsani H, Wedderburn LR, Ramanan A, Gillespie KM. Maternal microchimerism in muscle biopsies from children with juvenile dermatomyositis. Rheumatology. 2012;51:987–91.
7. Johnson KL, Samura O, Nelson JL, McDonnell M, Bianchi DW. Significant fetal cell microchimerism in a nontransfused woman with hepatitis C: evidence for long-term survival and expansion. Hepatology. 2002;36:1295–7.
8. Fugazzola L, Cirello V, Beck-Peccoz P. Fetal microchimerism as an explanation of disease. Nat Rev Endocrinol. 2011;7:89–97.
9. Dhimolea E, Denes V, Lakk M, Al-Bazzaz S, Aziz-Zaman S, Pilichowska M, et al. High male chimerism in the female breast shows quantitative links with cancer. Int J Cancer. 2013;133:835–42.
10. Cha D, Khosrotehrani K, Kim Y, Stroh H, Bianchi DW, Johnson KL. Cervical cancer and microchimerism. Obstet Gynecol. 2003;102:774–81.
11. Khosrotehrani K, Mery L, Aractingi S, Bianchi DW, Johnson KL. Absence of fetal cell microchimerism in cutaneous lesions of lupus erythematosus. Ann Rheum Dis. 2005;64:159–60.
12. Cirello V, Perrino M, Colombo C, Muzza M, Filopanti M, Vicentini L, et al. Fetal cell microchimerism in papillary thyroid cancer: studies in peripheral blood and tissues. Int J Cancer. 2010;126:2874–8.
13. O'Donoghue K, Sultan HA, Al-Allaf FA, Anderson JR, Wyatt-Ashmead J, Fisk NM. Microchimeric fetal cells cluster at sites of tissue injury in lung decades after pregnancy. Reprod Biomed Online. 2008;16:382–90.
14. Kremer HI, Koopmans M, Baelde HJ, de Heer E, Bruijn JA, Bajema IM. Tissue chimerism in systemic lupus erythematosus is related to injury. Ann Rheum Dis. 2007;66:1568–73.
15. Shah M, Mamyrova G, Targoff IN, Huber AM, Malley JD, Rice MM, et al. The clinical phenotypes of the juvenile idiopathic inflammatory myopathies. Medicine. 2013;92:25–41.
16. Feldman BM, Rider LG, Reed AM, Pachman LM. Juvenile dermatomyositis and other idiopathic inflammatory myopathies of childhood. Lancet. 2008;371:2201–12.
17. Khanna S, Reed AM. Immunopathogenesis of juvenile dermatomyositis. Muscle Nerve. 2010;41:581–92.
18. Mercuri E, Muntoni F. Muscular dystrophies. Lancet. 2013;381:845–60.
19. Flanigan KM. The muscular dystrophies. Semin Neurol. 2012;32:255–63.
20. Artlett CM, Miller FW, Rider LG. Persistent maternally derived peripheral microchimerism is associated with the juvenile idiopathic inflammatory myopathies. Rheumatology. 2001;40:1–6.
21. Wallace GQ, McNally EM. Mechanisms of muscle degeneration, regeneration, and repair in the muscular dystrophies. Annu Rev Plant Physiol Plant Mol Biol. 2009;71:37–57.
22. Engel AG, Arahata K. Mononuclear cells in myopathies: quantitation of functionally distinct subsets, recognition of antigen-specific cell-mediated cytotoxicity in some diseases, and implications for the pathogenesis of the different inflammatory myopathies. Hum Pathol. 1986;17:704–21.
23. Tidball JG, Wehling-Henricks M. Damage and inflammation in muscular dystrophy: potential implications and relationships with autoimmune myositis. Curr Opin Rheumatol. 2005;17:707–13.
24. Lopez De Padilla CM, Vallejo AN, Lacomis D, McNallan K, Reed AM. Extranodal lymphoid microstructures in inflamed muscle and disease severity of new-onset juvenile dermatomyositis. Arthritis Rheum. 2009;60:1160–72.
25. Srivasta B, Srivasta S, Johnson KL, Samura O, Lee SL, Bianchi DW. Microchimerism of presumed fetal origin in thyroid specimens from women: a case-control study. Lancet. 2001;358:2034–8.
26. Vanzyl B, Planas R, Ye Y, Foulis A, de Krijger RR, Vives-Pi M, et al. Why are levels of maternal microchimerism higher in type 1 diabetes pancreas? Chimerism. 2010;1:45–50.
27. Stevens AM, Hermes HM, Rutledge JC, Buyon JP, Nelson JL. Myocardial-tissue-specific phenotype of maternal microchimerism in neonatal lupus congenital heart block. Lancet. 2003;362:1617–23.
28. Jonsson AM, Papadogiannakis N, Granath A, Haggstrom J, Schaffer M, Uzunel M, et al. Maternal microchimerism in juvenile tonsils and adenoids. Pediatric Res. 2010;68:199–204.
29. Khosrotehrani K, Guegan S, Fraitag S, Oster M, de Prost Y, Bodemer C, et al. Presence of chimeric maternally derived keratinocytes in cutaneous inflammatory diseases of children: the example of pityriasis lichenoides. J Invest Dermatol. 2006;126:345–8.
30. Suskind DL, Kong D, Stevens A, Wahbeh G, Christie D, Baxter-Lowe LA, et al. Maternal microchimerism in pediatric inflammatory bowel disease. Chimerism. 2011;2:50–4.
31. Reed AM, McNallan K, Wettstein P, Vehe R, Ober C. Does HLA-dependent chimerism underlie the pathogenesis of juvenile dermatomyositis? J Immunol. 2004;172:5041–6.
32. Mold JE, Michaelsson J, Burt TD, Muench MO, Beckerman KP, Busch MP, et al. Maternal alloantigens promote the development of tolerogenic fetal regulatory T cells in utero. Science. 2008;322:1562–5.
33. Roy E, Leduc M, Guegan S, Rachdi L, Kluger N, Scharfmann R, et al. Specific maternal microchimeric T cells targeting fetal antigens in beta cells predispose to auto-immune diabetes in the child. J Autoimmun. 2011;36:253–62.
34. Rak JM, Maestroni L, Balandraud N, Guis S, Boudinet H, Guzian MC, et al. Transfer of the shared epitope through microchimerism in women with rheumatoid arthritis. Arthritis Rheum. 2009;60:73–80.
35. Artlett CM, O'Hanlon TP, Lopez AM, Song YW, Miller FW, Rider LG. HLA-DQA1 is not an apparent risk factor for microchimerism in patients with various autoimmune diseases and in healthy individuals. Arthritis Rheum. 2003;48:2567–72.
36. Leveque L, Hodgson S, Peyton S, Koyama M, MacDonald KP, Khosrotehrani K. Selective organ specific inflammation in offspring harbouring microchimerism from strongly alloreactive mothers. J Autoimmun. 2014;50:51–8.
37. Jonsson AM, Uzunel M, Gotherstrom C, Papadogiannakis N, Westgren M. Maternal microchimerism in human fetal tissues. Am J Obstet Gynecol. 2008;198:325.e321–326.

19

Increased carotid artery intima-media thickness and myeloperoxidase level in children with newly diagnosed juvenile idiopathic arthritis

Jaanika Ilisson[1,2*], Maksim Zagura[3,4], Kersti Zilmer[3], Erik Salum[4], Kaire Heilman[1,5], Anneli Piir[3], Vallo Tillmann[1,2], Jaak Kals[3,6], Mihkel Zilmer[3] and Chris Pruunsild[1,2]

Abstract

Introduction: Juvenile idiopathic arthritis (JIA) is a frequent childhood rheumatic disease characterized by chronic inflammation. The latter has been related to impairment of arterial functional-structural properties, atherogenesis and later cardiovascular events. The objective of this study was to examine intima-media thickness (IMT) and the parameters of arterial stiffness in children with JIA at diagnosis and their correlation with JIA subtype and markers of inflammation and atherosclerosis.

Methods: Thirty-nine newly diagnosed patients with JIA (26 girls; mean age, 13.2 ± 2.6 years) and 27 healthy controls (9 girls; mean age, 13.6 ± 3.4 years) were included in the study. Twelve patients had oligoarthritis, fifteen had extended oligoarthritis and twelve had rheumatoid factor–negative polyarthritis. IMT of the common carotid artery was determined by ultrasonography, carotid-femoral pulse wave velocity (cfPWV) and augmentation index adjusted to a heart rate of 75 beats/min (AIx@75) were determined by applanation tonometry. The serum levels of atherosclerosis-related biomarkers, such as asymmetric dimethylarginine (ADMA), myeloperoxidase (MPO) and adiponectin, were measured by enzyme-linked immunosorbent assay.

Results: Mean IMT (0.46 ± 0.04 vs. 0.42 ± 0.04 mm; $p = 0.0003$) and MPO concentration (115.2 [95 % confidence interval {95 % CI}, 97.4–136.3] vs. 57.6 [95 % CI, 47.1–70.3] ng/ml; $p < 0.0001$) were higher in the patients with JIA than in the control subjects. The cfPWV, AIx@75 and serum ADMA and adiponectin levels did not significantly differ between the groups and JIA subtypes. Serum adiponectin level correlated negatively with AIx@75 in patients with JIA ($r = -0.38$; $p < 0.05$).

Conclusions: Patients with JIA have increased mean IMT and elevated MPO levels at early stages of the disease. AIx@75 was inversely independently associated with adiponectin level in the patients, suggesting that lower adiponectin levels might influence arterial subclinical stiffening in patients with newly diagnosed JIA.

Introduction

Juvenile idiopathic arthritis (JIA) is the most common chronic rheumatic disease in childhood, with an onset before the age of 16 years and a potential to persist into adulthood. JIA is a heterogeneous group of disorders with different disease progression and prognosis. Of the JIA subtypes, persistent oligoarthritis and monocyclic systemic arthritis have the best prognosis and polyarthritis the worst [1, 2]. Approximately 50 % of patients with JIA still have active disease and need for disease-modifying antirheumatic medications in adulthood [3–5].

Many patients with active JIA may not present with high levels of classical inflammatory markers such as C-reactive protein or erythrocyte sedimentation rate. Therefore, studies on the role of new markers (e.g., myeloperoxidase [MPO], asymmetric dimethylarginine [ADMA], adiponectin) may open some new aspects to describe inflammation in patients with JIA. MPO, ADMA and adiponectin have been linked to inflammation and/or oxidative stress [6–8]. Previous studies have shown that MPO levels are higher in patients with JIA compared with control groups [9].

* Correspondence: jaanika.ilisson@kliinikum.ee
[1]Department of Paediatrics, Faculty of Medicine, University of Tartu, Lunini 6, Tartu 51014, Estonia
[2]Children's Clinic, Tartu University Hospital, Tartu, Estonia
Full list of author information is available at the end of the article

ADMA and adiponectin have not been investigated in patients with JIA.

Atherosclerosis is considered an inflammatory disorder starting in childhood. Chronic inflammation has been suggested to play an important role in the developing of early atherosclerosis, which contributes to the development of cardiovascular disease (CVD) [10, 11].

CVD is more frequent in patients with rheumatoid arthritis (RA), and they are diagnosed at an earlier age than other patients with CVD. Mortality among RA patients is also higher than general population and is mostly due to cardiovascular diseases [12–14]. In addition to traditional risk factors for CVD, patients with a chronic inflammatory disease also have many disease-specific and drug-related risk factors [13]. Recent studies have shown that patients with RA have increased aortic stiffness, and this is correlated with markers of inflammation and aortic inflammation without any clinical signs of CVD [15, 16].

As JIA is a chronic inflammatory disease, it has long-term effects on many organ systems, including the cardiovascular system. Accordingly, it has been shown that patients with JIA have a moderate risk for premature cardiovascular events [17].

To date, only a few studies of vascular function, structural and atherosclerosis-related biomarkers in patients with JIA have been done. They have shown impaired endothelial dysfunction and alterations in vascular function compared with controls during the course of the disease [18, 19]. Satija et al. reported altered arterial wall indices in newly diagnosed patients with JIA, indicating increased arterial stiffness [20].

The aim of the present study was to evaluate intima-media thickness (IMT) and the parameters of arterial stiffness in patients with JIA at the time of diagnosis and to assess their correlation with JIA subtype and serum markers of inflammation and atherosclerosis.

Methods

Patients and controls

This cross-sectional study included 39 children with JIA (26 girls; mean age, 13.2 ± 2.6 years) who were patients of the paediatric rheumatologist at the outpatient children's clinic of Tartu University Hospital, Estonia, and 27 healthy control subjects (9 girls; mean age, 13.6 ± 3.4 years) recruited from a previous diabetes study [21]. The study group included children aged 7–18 years with newly diagnosed JIA (onset of symptoms before the 16th birthday). JIA was diagnosed according to the International League of Associations for Rheumatology criteria [22]. Twenty-seven patients had oligoarthritis (fifteen of them had extended oligoarthritis), and twelve had rheumatoid factor (RF)-negative polyarthritis. All patients were RF-negative, three were antinuclear antibody–positive and five were human leukocyte antigen B27–positive.

Healthy control subjects were defined as without known chronical illness at the time of enrolment, without acute infection and no history of using antihypertensive or lipid-lowering medications. They were matched with the patients by age (±2 years). Three of the subjects from the original control group were excluded because of greater age difference. Written informed consent was obtained from each participant and the parent or legal representative. The study was approved by the ethics committee of Tartu University.

Clinical and laboratory investigations

A full joint examination was performed by the same paediatric rheumatologist during the outpatient visit. Blood samples were obtained for nine different biochemical markers: glucose, creatinine, total cholesterol, high-density lipoprotein (HDL) cholesterol, low-density lipoprotein (LDL) cholesterol, triglycerides, ADMA, adiponectin and MPO. The first six markers are regularly used in clinical practice and were analysed in the local clinical laboratory using certified standard assays. For the last three markers, serum and plasma were stored at −80 °C until analysis. Serum ADMA concentration was determined by using a validated enzyme-linked immunosorbent assay (ELISA) kit (DLD Gesellschaft für Diagnostika und medizinische Geräte mbH, Hamburg, Germany). Serum adiponectin concentration was determined using the Human Adiponectin/Acrp30 Quantikine ELISA kit (R&D Systems Europe, Abingdon, UK). The adiponectin intraassay coefficient of variation (CV) is 4.6 %, and the interassay CV is 7.9 %. MPO was determined in serum of patients with JIA using an enzyme immunoassay test kit (catalogue number BC-1129; BioCheck, Foster City, CA, USA) and in plasma of controls using an ELISA kit (BIOXYTECH enzyme immunoassay for MPO, catalogue number 21013; OXIS Health Products, Portland, OR, USA), according to the manufacturer's instructions. MPO intraassay CV is 5.7 % and inter-assay CV 8.5 %.

Haemodynamic measurements

Brachial blood pressure (BP) and heart rate were recorded from the left arm with the subject in the supine position. BP was measured with an automated digital oscillometric BP monitor (OMRON M4-I; Omron Healthcare Europe, Hoofddorp, the Netherlands). Radial arterial pressure waveforms were obtained with a high-fidelity applanation tonometer (SPT-301B; Millar, Houston, TX, USA) applied to the wrist of the left hand. Pulse wave analysis (SCOR-Px 7.0; AtCor Medical, West Ryde, Australia) was then performed to generate a corresponding central (ascending aortic) waveform using a generalized transfer function, which has been prospectively validated for assessment of ascending aortic BP [23]. Augmentation index (AIx), mean arterial pressure (MAP), central systolic blood pressure, central diastolic blood pressure and central pulse pressure were determined by pulse wave analysis. The AIx was calculated as the difference between the second and the first systolic peaks, divided by pulse pressure and expressed in percentages [24]. The AIx values were adjusted to a heart rate of 75 beats/min (AIx@75) using a built-in algorithm in the SphygmoCor Px system (AtCor Medical). The within- and between-observer CVs for AIx@75 were 3.4 % and 7.1 %, respectively. Pulse wave velocity was measured by the foot-to-foot method using the same device. The aortic pulse wave velocity (aPWV) was determined by sequentially recording electrocardiogram-gated carotid and femoral artery waveforms, as described in detail previously [24]. The within- and between-observer CVs for aPWV were 2.3 % and 6.2 %, respectively. All measurements were made in duplicate by two trained investigators, and the mean values were used in subsequent analysis.

Assessment of carotid intima-media thickness

Carotid ultrasound for evaluation of IMT was performed using the SonoSite M-Turbo portable ultrasound device (SonoSite, Bothell, WA, USA) coupled to a 5- to 10-MHz multifrequency high-resolution linear transducer. SonoCalc software (SonoSite) was used for calculation of mean IMT values. The measurements were obtained with the subject lying down, with the head extended and slightly turned opposite to the examined carotid. Measurements were made of the common carotid artery after the examination of a longitudinal section of 10 mm at a distance of 1 cm from the bifurcation. The measurements were performed in the far wall in the lateral, anterior and posterior projections. The within- and between-observer CVs for mean IMT were 2.2 % and 5.9 %, respectively.

A standard deviation score (SDS) of IMT for each subject was calculated using height-specific IMT normative values published by Jourdan et al. [25].

Statistical analysis

Differences between the JIA and control groups were studied with analysis of variance, adjusted by sex. Because the distributions of some variables were not normally distributed, they were log-transformed for analysis as required to improve normality. The normally distributed data are presented as mean ± standard deviation; the non-normally distributed data are presented as the geometric mean with the 95 % confidence interval (CI). Multiple regression analysis was performed to investigate the independent determinants of AIx@75. To examine the associations between the variables, Pearson's correlation test was used.

We used AIx@75 as a base for power calculations for *t* tests. A total of 66 persons were targeted to enter this two-group study. The probability is 80 % that the study will detect an effect size (the smallest difference between the means) at a two-sided 0.05 significance level if the true difference between groups is 4.953 U. This is based on the assumption that the standard deviation of the response variable is 10 [26]. Differences were considered statistically different if the p value was less than 0.05. Statistical analysis was performed using the SAS version 9.2 statistical software package (SAS Institute, Cary, NC, USA).

Results

The subjects' clinical and laboratory characteristics, as well as the arterial functional-structural properties of the study groups, are presented in Table 1.

The total cholesterol, LDL cholesterol, HDL cholesterol and triglyceride levels did not differ between groups. The same was found for serum ADMA and adiponectin levels (Table 1).

The serum level of MPO was significantly higher in patients with JIA compared with the plasma MPO concentrations in control subjects (115.2 [95 % CI, 97.4–136.3] vs. 57.6 [95 % CI, 47.1–70.3] ng/ml; $p < 0.0001$).

Mean IMT values and IMT height specific SDS were higher in the patients with JIA than in the control subjects (0.46 ± 0.04 vs. 0.42 ± 0.04 mm, $p < 0.0003$; 1.694 ± 0.858 vs. 0.744 ± 0.852, $p = 0.0002$). We did not find statistically significant differences between the groups with regard to carotid-femoral pulse wave velocity (cfPWV) or AIx@75 (Table 1).

Serum ADMA and adiponectin levels, as well as the mean IMT, cfPWV and AIx@75, did not differ significantly between the JIA subtypes (data not shown).

There was a significant negative correlation between serum adiponectin level and AIx@75 in patients with JIA ($r = -0.38$; $p < 0.05$) (Fig. 1). No other statistically significant correlations were found.

In multiple regression analysis, AIx@75 was independently determined by age, MAP and adiponectin levels in patients with JIA, accounting for 29 % of its variability (R^2(adj) = 0.29; $p < 0.01$) (Table 2).

Discussion

We have demonstrated that, already at the time of JIA diagnosis, there are atherosclerosis-related changes in the arterial wall, supporting the detrimental effect of systemic inflammation on the cardiovascular system. The present study is the first clinical analysis of the relationship between adiponectin and arterial stiffness in patients with JIA. We have shown

Table 1 Clinical and laboratory data and arterial functional-structural properties in children with juvenile idiopathic arthritis and controls, adjusted by sex

Parameters	JIA group ($n = 39$)	Control group ($n = 27$)	p value
Age (yr)	13.0 ± 3.11	13.5 ± 3.08	0.5687
Body mass index (kg/m^2)	21.2 ± 4.09	20.2 ± 4.04	0.3364
Peripheral systolic blood pressure (mmHg)	112.2 ± 8.7	108.9 ± 8.6	0.1375
Peripheral diastolic blood pressure (mmHg)	57.6 ± 5.01	57.1 ± 4.96	0.7360
Mean arterial blood pressure (mmHg)	74.0 ± 5.82	73.3 ± 5.77	0.6549
Central systolic blood pressure (mmHg)	92.0 ± 7.5	90.17 ± 7.4	0.3748
Central diastolic blood pressure (mmHg)	58.5 ± 5.07	58.4 ± 5.04	0.9249
Cholesterol (mmol/L)[a]	4.1 (3.8–4.3)	4.1 (3.8–4.4)	0.8150
LDL cholesterol (mmol/L)[a]	2.24 (2.06–2.43)	2.36 (2.13–2.60)	0.4324
HDL cholesterol (mmol/L)	1.50 ± 0.40	1.71 ± 0.40	0.0415
Triglycerides (mmol/L)[a]	0.87 (0.75–1.02)	0.70 (0.59–0.84)	0.0688
ADMA (μmol/L)	0.622 ± 0.175	0.679 ± 0.173	0.2040
MPO (ng/ml)[a]	115.2 (97.4–136.3)	57.6 (47.1–70.3)	<0.0001
Adiponectin (ng/ml)[a]	8596.7 (7296.3–10,128.9)	9123.1 (7506.6–11,087.7)	0.6519
Mean IMT (mm)	0.46 ± 0.04	0.42 ± 0.04	0.0003
IMT SDS, height-specific[b]	1.694 ± 0.858	0.744 ± 0.852	0.0002
cfPWV (m/s)[a]	4.92 (4.71–5.14)	5.18 (4.90–5.47)	0.1579
Alx@75 (%)	0.642 ± 11.258	−2.042 ± 11.179	0.3811

ADMA Asymmetric dimethylarginine, *Alx@75* augmentation index values adjusted to a heart rate of 75 beats/min, *cfPWV* carotid-femoral pulse wave velocity, *HDL* high-density lipoprotein cholesterol, *JIA* juvenile idiopathic arthritis, *LDL* low-density lipoprotein cholesterol, *MPO* myeloperoxidase, *SDS* standard deviation score
Values are mean ± standard deviation unless otherwise indicated

[a]Data were log-transformed before statistical analysis and are presented as geometric mean (95 % confidence interval)

[b]Data for34 patents with JIA and 23 control were analysed as reference values and are available for the height of 140 cm and taller [25]

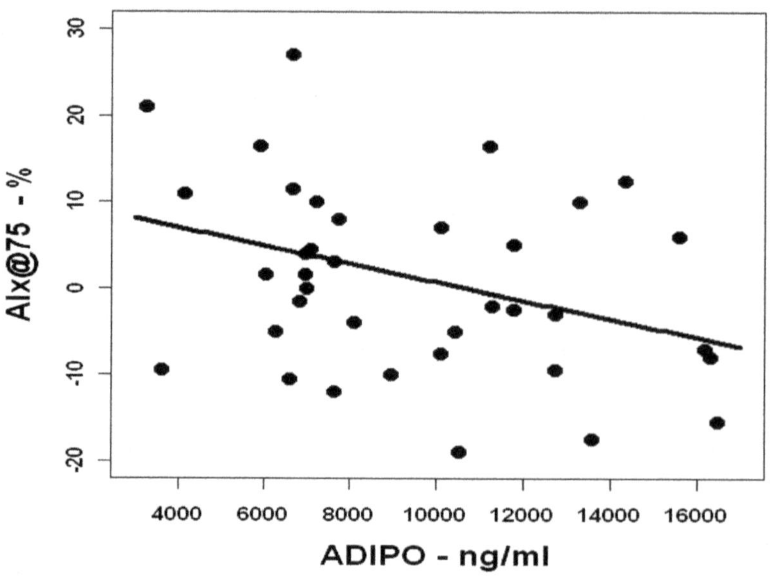

Fig. 1 Correlation between serum adiponectin (ADIPO) concentration and augmentation index values adjusted to a heart rate of 75 beats/min (Alx@75) in patients with juvenile idiopathic arthritis ($r = -0.38$; $p < 0.05$)

Table 2 Multiple regression model for patients with juvenile idiopathic arthritis with augmentation index values adjusted to a heart rate of 75 beats/min as the dependent variable

Parameter	Regression coefficient	Standard deviation	*p* value
Age	−1.71	0.62	0.009
MAP	0.73	0.27	0.01
Adiponectin	−0.001	0.0004	0.03

MAP mean arterial pressure

that AIx@75 is inversely related to adiponectin levels in a cohort of patients with JIA. This finding suggests that adiponectin might influence arterial stiffening in the early stages of the disease. In addition, we demonstrated that serum MPO is significantly higher in patients with JIA. Thus, MPO may be a sensitive marker of systemic inflammation and oxidative stress in patients with newly diagnosed JIA.

To date, IMT in patients with JIA has been reported in a few studies, with controversial results. Breda et al. reported increased mean IMT in these patients [19], whereas Vlahos et al. did not find a statistically significant difference in IMT between their JIA and control groups [18]. Comparing mean IMT between JIA subtypes, Vlahos et al. found that a systemic arthritis (high inflammatory activity) group had a thicker intima-media layer compared with the control group and the oligoarticular group [18]. Both of these studies were done in patients with previously diagnosed JIA [18, 19]. By contrast, our study was conducted with patients at the very early stage of the disease, and we demonstrated that IMT is increased in patients with JIA already in the early phase. We did not find a significant difference in IMT thickness between the oligo- and polyarticular subtypes. So far, only Breda et al. have investigated the changes in IMT longitudinally in patients with JIA. They found that after a 12-month treatment period, the mean IMT improved; that is, was less than at the start of the study [19]. This points out the importance of early, adequate, aggressive treatment of JIA to controlling the possibility of future cardiovascular events. Future investigations are needed to verify this point.

Several studies have shown that increased MPO concentration is associated with an increased risk of CVD [27, 28]. Also, studies have shown higher serum and plasma concentrations in patients with rheumatologic diseases [9, 29]. In our study, we found higher serum levels of MPO in patients with JIA already at an early stage of the disease. Thus, MPO may be a good marker of the level of inflammation, even when the classical inflammation markers are at normal levels.

ADMA acts as a natural inhibitor of nitric oxide synthase by reducing nitric oxide production. Higher levels of ADMA give rise to endothelial dysfunction and arterial stiffening [30]. The key enzyme in degradation of ADMA is dimethylarginine dimethylaminohydrolase, and its activity is downregulated by tumour necrosis factor α and has a known role in the pathogenesis of RA and JIA [31]. Higher levels of ADMA and its correlation to oxidative stress markers have been shown in patients with RA [7]. In children with other chronic diseases, such as chronic kidney disease or type 1 diabetes mellitus, elevated serum ADMA concentrations have been found [21, 32]. However, all these children already had their disease for many years. To our knowledge, the level of ADMA has not been investigated to date in patients with JIA. In our study, we did not find a significant difference in serum ADMA levels at the disease start between our patient and control groups.

Adiponectin has well-known anti-inflammatory properties. To the contrary, there are studies suggesting that hypoadiponectemia might play an important role in CVDs (e.g., hypertension) [33]. In patients with RA, adiponectin levels are higher than in patients with non-inflammatory conditions (e.g., osteoarthrosis), which is suggestive of a proinflammatory effect [8]. Alternatively, increased adiponectin might represent a compensatory response limiting further vascular injury [34]. To our knowledge, adiponectin levels have not been investigated in patients with JIA. In our study, we did not find statistically significant differences in levels of adiponectin between patients and controls, but adiponectin was inversely independently correlated with AIx@75 in patients with JIA, indicating that lower levels of adiponectin might be related to arterial stiffening already at an early stage of JIA.

In our study, there was no significant difference in cfPWV between the patients and the control subjects. These findings could be due to the fact that we studied newly diagnosed patients with JIA, whereas aortic stiffening may occur at later stages of the disease. Consistent with this hypothesis, a recent study has shown that patients with JIA with long-term active disease have increased aortic stiffness compared with control subjects [35].

The limitations of our study are the use of a historical control group, the gender difference and the absence of patients from all the JIA subtypes (although the two subgroups presented are the most frequent ones in every study group of patients with JIA), which limits extrapolation of the risk of vascular dysfunction to all patients with JIA. At the same time, we present a detailed, complex overview of different markers of inflammation, oxidative stress and arterial structural-functional properties, which describes the stage of development of subclinical atherosclerosis in these patients. Another limitation of our study is the use of generalized transfer function, which has been validated only in adults.

Conclusions

Our study shows that patients with JIA have signs of alterations in arterial structural properties already at the time of diagnosis of the disease. Independent inverse association between the atherosclerosis-related biomarker adiponectin and arterial stiffness suggests that hypoadiponectemia may influence vascular function in these patients. Further investigations are needed to clarify the risk of vascular dysfunction during the disease course and to identify children who are at increased risk of early development of atherosclerosis in adulthood.

Abbreviations

ADIPO: Adiponectin; ADMA: Asymmetric dimethylarginine; AIx: Augmentation index; AIx@75: Augmentation index values adjusted to a heart rate of 75 beats/min; aPWV: Aortic pulse wave velocity; BP: Blood pressure; cfPWV: Carotid-femoral pulse wave velocity; CI: Confidence interval; CV: Coefficient of variation; CVD: Cardiovascular disease; ELISA: Enzyme-linked immunosorbent assay; HDL: High-density lipoprotein; IMT: Intima-media thickness; JIA: Juvenile idiopathic arthritis; LDL: Low-density lipoprotein; MAP: Mean arterial pressure; MPO: Myeloperoxidase; RA: Rheumatoid arthritis; RF: Rheumatoid factor; SDS: Standard deviation score.

Competing interests

The authors declare that they have no competing interests.

Authors' contributions

JI and CP were involved in the design and conduct of the study and drafted the manuscript. MZagura conducted the haemodynamic measurements, assessment of carotid intima-media thickness and revised the manuscript. ES conducted the haemodynamic measurements, assessment of carotid intima-media thickness and helped to revise the manuscript. KH did the investigations with controls and revised the manuscript. KZ was involved in biochemical investigations and helped to revise the manuscript. AP did the biochemical analyses and revised the manuscript. JK was involved in the design of the study and revised the manuscript. MZilmer and VT were involved in the design of the study and helped to revise the manuscript. All authors read and approved the final manuscript.

Acknowledgements

This study was funded by Estonian Science Foundation Grant No. 8750, 9094, Institutional Research Funding No IUT20-42 from the Estonian Ministry of Education and Science and by the European Union through the European Regional Development Fund (RARBSTIPP). Black Sea Trade and Investment Promotion Program is not correct.

Author details

[1]Department of Paediatrics, Faculty of Medicine, University of Tartu, Lunini 6, Tartu 51014, Estonia. [2]Children's Clinic, Tartu University Hospital, Tartu, Estonia. [3]Department of Biochemistry, Institute of Biomedicine and Translational Medicine, The Centre of Excellence for Translational Medicine, Faculty of Medicine, University of Tartu, Tartu, Estonia. [4]Department of Cardiology, Faculty of Medicine, University of Tartu, Tartu, Estonia. [5]Tallinn Children's Hospital, Tallinn, Estonia. [6]Department of Vascular Surgery, Tartu University Hospital, Tartu, Estonia.

References

1. Al-Matar MJ, Petty RE, Tucker LB, Malleson PN, Schroeder ML, Cabral DA. The early pattern of joint involvement predicts disease progression in children with oligoarticular (pauciarticular) juvenile rheumatoid arthritis. Arthritis Rheum. 2002;46:2708–15.
2. Selvaag AM, Lien G, Sørskaar D, Vinje O, Førre Ø, Flatø B. Early disease course and predictors of disability in juvenile rheumatoid arthritis and juvenile spondyloarthropathy: a 3 year prospective study. J Rheumatol. 2005;32:1122–30.
3. Minden K, Niewerth M, Listing J, Biedermann T, Bollow M, Schöntube M, et al. Long-term outcome in patients with juvenile idiopathic arthritis. Arthritis Rheum. 2002;46:2392–401.
4. Flatø B, Lien G, Smerdel A, Vinje O, Dale K, Johnston V, et al. Prognostic factors in juvenile rheumatoid arthritis: a case-control study revealing early predictors and outcome after 14.9 years. J Rheumatol. 2003;30:386–93.
5. Nordal E, Zak M, Aalto K, Berntson L, Fasth A, Herlin T, et al. Ongoing disease activity and changing categories in a long-term Nordic cohort study of juvenile idiopathic arthritis. Arthritis Rheum. 2011;63:2809–18.
6. Klebanoff SJ. Myeloperoxidase: friend and foe. J Leukoc Biol. 2005;77:598–625.
7. Kwaśny-Krochin B, Głuszko P, Undas A. Plasma asymmetric dimethylarginine in active rheumatoid arthritis: links with oxidative stress and inflammation. Pol Arch Med Wewn. 2012;122:270–6.
8. Schäffler A, Ehling A, Neumann E, Herfarth H, Tarner I, Schölmerich J, et al. Adipocytokines in synovial fluid. JAMA. 2003;290:1709–10.
9. Pruunsild C, Heilman K, Zilmer K, Uibo K, Liivamägi H, Talvik T, et al. Plasma level of myeloperoxidase in children with juvenile idiopathic arthritis (a pilot study). Cent Eur J Med. 2010;5:36–40.
10. Ross R. Atherosclerosis—an inflammatory disease. N Engl J Med. 1999;340:115–26.
11. Libby P. Inflammation in atherosclerosis. Nature. 2002;420:868–74.
12. Wolfe F, Mitchell DM, Sibley JT, Fries JF, Bloch DA, Williams CA, et al. The mortality of rheumatoid arthritis. Arthritis Rheum. 1994;37:481–94.
13. del Rincón ID, Williams K, Stern MP, Freeman GL, Escalante A. High incidence of cardiovascular events in a rheumatoid arthritis cohort not explained by traditional cardiac risk factors. Arthritis Rheum. 2001;44:2737–45.
14. Aviña-Zubieta JA, Choi HK, Sadatsafavi M, Etminan M, Esdaile JM, Lacaille D. Risk of cardiovascular mortality in patients with rheumatoid arthritis: a meta-analysis of observational studies. Arthritis Rheum. 2008;59:1690–7.
15. Mäki-Petäjä KM, Hall FC, Booth AD, Wallace SM. Yasmin, Bearcroft PW, et al. Rheumatoid arthritis is associated with increased aortic pulse-wave velocity, which is reduced by anti-tumor necrosis factor-α therapy. Circulation. 2006;114:1185–92.
16. Mäki-Petäjä KM, Elkhawad M, Cheriyan J, Joshi FR, Ostör AJ, Hall FC, et al. Anti-tumor necrosis factor-α therapy reduces aortic inflammation and stiffness in patients with rheumatoid arthritis. Circulation. 2012;126:2473–80.
17. Kavey RE, Allada V, Daniels SR, Hayman LL, McCrindle BW, Newburger JW, et al. Cardiovascular risk reduction in high-risk pediatric patients: a scientific statement from the American Heart Association Expert Panel on Population and Prevention Science; the Councils on Cardiovascular Disease in the Young, Epidemiology and Prevention, Nutrition, Physical Activity and Metabolism, High Blood Pressure Research, Cardiovascular Nursing, and the Kidney in Heart Disease; and the Interdisciplinary Working Group on Quality of Care and Outcomes Research: endorsed by the American Academy of Pediatrics. Circulation. 2006;114:2710–38.
18. Vlahos AP, Theocharis P, Bechlioulis A, Naka KK, Vakalis K, Papamichael ND, et al. Changes in vascular function and structure in juvenile idiopathic arthritis. Arthritis Care Res. 2011;63:1736–44.
19. Breda L, Di Marzio D, Giannini C, Gaspari S, Nozzi M, Scarinci A, et al. Relationship between inflammatory markers, oxidant-antioxidant status and intima-media thickness in prepubertal children with juvenile idiopathic arthritis. Clin Res Cardiol. 2013;102:63–71.
20. Satija M, Yadav TP, Sachdev N, Chhabra A, Jahan A, Dewan V. Endothelial function, arterial wall mechanics and intima media thickness in juvenile idiopathic arthritis. Clin Exp Rheumatol. 2014;32:432–9.
21. Heilman K, Zilmer M, Zilmer K, Kool P, Tillmann V. Elevated plasma adiponectin and decreased plasma homocysteine and asymmetric dimethylarginine in children with type 1 diabetes. Scand J Clin Lab Invest. 2009;69:85–91.
22. Petty RE, Southwood TR, Manners P, Baum J, Glass DN, Goldenberg J, et al. International League of Associations for Rheumatology classification of juvenile idiopathic arthritis: second revision, Edmonton, 2001. J Rheumatol. 2004;31:390–2.
23. Sharman JE, Lim R, Qasem AM, Coombes JS, Burgess MI, Franco J, et al. Validation of a generalized transfer function to noninvasively derive central blood pressure during exercise. Hypertension. 2006;47:1203–8.

24. Wilkinson IB, Fuchs SA, Jansen IM, Spratt JC, Murray GD, Cockcroft JR, et al. Reproducibility of pulse wave velocity and augmentation index measured by pulse wave analysis. J Hypertens. 1998;16:2079–84.
25. Jourdan C, Wühl E, Litwin M, Fahr K, Trelewicz J, Jobs K, et al. Normative values for intima-media thickness and distensibility of large arteries in healthy adolescents. J Hypertens. 2005;23:1707–15.
26. Dupont WD, Plummer Jr WD. Power and sample size calculations: a review and computer program. Control Clin Trials. 1990;11:116–28.
27. Stamp LK, Khalilova I, Tarr JM, Senthilmohan R, Turner R, Haigh RC, et al. Myeloperoxidase and oxidative stress in rheumatoid arthritis. Rheumatology (Oxford). 2012;51:1796–803.
28. Nicholls SJ, Hazen SL. Myeloperoxidase and cardiovascular disease. Arterioscler Thromb Vasc Biol. 2005;25:1102–11.
29. Wang W, Jian Z, Guo J, Ning X. Increased levels of serum myeloperoxidase in patients with active rheumatoid arthritis. Life Sci. 2014;117:19–23.
30. Kals J, Kampus P, Kals M, Teesalu R, Zilmer K, Pulges A, et al. Arterial elasticity is associated with endothelial vasodilatory function and asymmetric dimethylarginine level in healthy subjects. Scand J Clin Lab Invest. 2007;67:536–44.
31. Ito A, Tsao PS, Adimoolam S, Kimoto M, Ogawa T, Cooke JP. Novel mechanism for endothelial dysfunction: dysregulation of dimethylarginine dimethylaminohydrolase. Circulation. 1999;99:3092–5.
32. Tain YL, Huang LT. Asymmetric dimethylarginine: clinical applications in pediatric medicine. J Formos Med Assoc. 2011;110:70–7.
33. Chow WS, Cheung BM, Tso AW, Xu A, Wat NM, Fong CH, et al. Hypoadiponectinemia as a predictor for the development of hypertension: a 5-year prospective study. Hypertension. 2007;49:1455–61.
34. Schnabel R, Messow CM, Lubos E, Espinola-Klein C, Rupprecht HJ, Bickel C, et al. Association of adiponectin with adverse outcome in coronary artery disease patients: results from the AtheroGene study. Eur Heart J. 2008;29:649–57.
35. Aulie HA, Selvaag AM, Günther A, Lilleby V, Molberg O, Hartmann A, et al. Arterial haemodynamics and coronary artery calcification in adult patients with juvenile idiopathic arthritis. Ann Rheum Dis. In press. 10.1136/annrheumdis-2013-204804.

Serum sclerostin in high-activity adult patients with juvenile idiopathic arthritis

Kristyna Brabnikova-Maresova[1,2], Katerina Jarosova[1,2], Karel Pavelka[1,2] and Jan J Stepan[1,2*]

Abstract

Introduction: Juvenile idiopathic arthritis (JIA) is a disease associated with loss of bone mass, deterioration in bone mass quality and an increased risk of fractures. The objective of this study was to evaluate factors that predict bone mineral density (BMD) alterations in young adult patients with active JIA before and during therapy with tumour necrosis factor α (TNFα) inhibitors.

Methods: Thirty-one patients (twelve males and nineteen females; mean age $=25.1 \pm 6.1$ years) with active JIA (mean Disease Activity Score in 28 joints (DAS28) $=6.36 \pm 0.64$; mean high-sensitivity C-reactive protein (hsCRP) $=18.36 \pm 16.95$ mg/L) were investigated. The control group consisted of 84 healthy individuals matched by sex and age. BMD, bone turnover markers and serum concentrations of soluble receptor activator of nuclear factor κB ligand, osteoprotegerin, dickkopf Wnt signalling pathway inhibitor 1 (Dkk1) and sclerostin were evaluated.

Results: Baseline BMD values in the lumbar spine, proximal femur, femoral neck and distal radius were significantly lower in patients with JIA compared to healthy control participants. Baseline sclerostin serum concentrations were significantly higher in patients with JIA compared to control participants. After 2 years of treatment with TNFα inhibitors, BMD was significantly increased in the lumbar spine. This increase correlated with a drop in DAS28 score. A statistically significant correlation between hsCRP and Dkk1 was found at baseline, as well as during the 2-year follow-up period. A significant reduction in serum sclerostin after 1 year of therapy was predictive of a drop in DAS28 score observed with a 1-year delay after reduction of serum sclerostin.

Conclusion: A significant correlation between the sclerostin serum concentration and the number of tender and swollen joints, but not BMD, supports the hypothesis that chondrocytes and cells of the subchondral bone may contribute to circulating sclerostin in JIA.

Introduction

Juvenile idiopathic arthritis (JIA) is a systemic autoimmune inflammatory connective tissue disease with onset occurring before age 16 years. It is associated with a decrease in bone mass, thinning of the cortical bone [1,2], sarcopenia [3,4] and an increased risk of fractures [5]. Bone loss may be systemic or localized to the periarticular bone due to arthritis of the affected joint. The pathophysiology of the bone mass loss may involve, in particular, the negative effect of proinflammatory cytokines, as well as treatment with glucocorticoids [6]. Thus, the loss of bone mass may reflect a disorder of bone modelling and remodelling. This process involves proinflammatory cytokines produced by the synovial membrane, which may increase bone resorption but also stimulate soluble antagonists of the canonical Wnt/β-catenin signalling pathway, including dickkopf Wnt signalling pathway inhibitor 1 (Dkk1) and sclerostin, and subsequently inhibit osteoblast proliferation, maturation and progenitor differentiation [7-20]. The significance of Wingless (Wnt) proteins in susceptibility to JIA was confirmed in a study of polymorphisms in the Wnt-1-inducible signalling pathway protein 3 (WISP3) [21]. To the best of our knowledge, no study related to circulating sclerostin or Dkk1 in patients with JIA has been published to date.

In the present study, we assessed bone mineral density (BMD) at standard skeletal sites, as well as biochemical markers of osteoclast, osteoblast and osteocyte function, in patients with persistent high-activity JIA. These parameters were assessed at baseline and after 12 months and 24 months of treatment with tumour necrosis factor α

* Correspondence: stepan@revma.cz
[1]Institute of Rheumatology, Na Slupi 4, 128 50 Prague 2, Czech Republic
[2]Department of Rheumatology, First Faculty of Medicine, Charles University in Prague, Kateřinská 32, 121 08 Prague 2, Czech Republic

(TNFα) inhibitors. Young adults with JIA were included in the study. The objective of the study was to evaluate factors that predict BMD alterations in young adult patients with active JIA being treated with TNFα inhibitors.

Methods

Study population

We conducted a prospective, open-label study in 2009 and 2010. We enrolled 31 patients with JIA (12 males and 19 females) with a mean age of 25.1 ± 6.1 years who had high disease activity determined on the basis of high-sensitivity C-reactive protein (hsCRP) level, erythrocyte sedimentation rate (ESR) and Disease Activity Score in 28 joints (DAS28). All of the included patients met the criteria of the Czech Rheumatology Society for treatment with TNFα inhibitors. At baseline, the patients were naive to anti-TNFα therapy. The basic condition for inclusion in the study was high disease activity expressed by DAS28 ≥ 3.9. Another precondition was inadequate response to one disease-modifying antirheumatic drug [22].

At the time of patient selection, a group of healthy control participants was recruited from amongst the friends, acquaintances and colleagues of the patients with JIA. In total, 100 healthy males and females were examined. Each patient with JIA was matched with three suitable control participants on the basis of sex and age (in most cases within a 2-year age difference and in isolated cases within a maximum age difference of 6 years). Nine female patients with JIA were matched with two control participants only. In this manner, 84 age- and sex-matched control participants were selected. All study participants were examined and treated at the Institute of Rheumatology in Prague.

The study was conducted in accordance with the World Medical Association Declaration of Helsinki regarding ethical conduct of research involving human subjects. The study was approved by the ethics committee of the Institute of Rheumatology, and all participants gave us their written informed consent before enrolment.

Clinical parameters

The baseline clinical status of the patients with JIA was established on the first day of TNFα inhibitor treatment. A physical examination, blood testing and BMD testing were performed on day 1 and again at 12 and 24 months. Detailed information about each patient's JIA disease course and treatment, as well as personal history, family history and fracture risk factor assessment, was obtained from the patient and the available medical documentation.

A physical examination of the patients with JIA was performed at each visit, and the number of swollen and tender joints was documented. Body height was measured using a stadiometer. Body weight was measured using an exact scale. The control participants were examined in a similar manner.

The patients with JIA were given daily supplements of 1,000 mg of calcium and 800 IU of vitamin D for a minimum of 6 months before the start of anti-TNFα treatment. The control participants did not receive any calcium or vitamin D supplements.

To maintain the same conditions for the collection of blood samples, patients and control participants were instructed to fast for 12 hours overnight while maintaining adequate hydration. At 8:00 the following morning, venous blood was collected into regular laboratory serum tubes by antecubital venepuncture. For the purposes of soluble receptor activator of nuclear factor κB ligand (sRANKL), osteoprotegerin (OPG), Dkk1 and sclerostin assays, aliquots of blood serum were frozen and stored at −80°C until analysis after the study was completed. Other laboratory parameters were measured on the day of blood collection.

For the purpose of determining JIA activity, the DAS28 score was calculated using objective clinical components (the number of swollen and tender joints among the total of 28 joints assessed), laboratory components (ESR in millimetres per hour) and subjective components (patient global health analogue scale, mm) (PGH).

Laboratory methods

The hsCRP concentration was measured by immunoturbidimetry. The interassay coefficient of variation was 1.9%.

The sRANKL, OPG, Dkk1 and sclerostin serum concentrations were measured using enzyme-linked immunosorbent assay (ELISA) kits in compliance with the manufacturer's instructions, always by the same person. The results were read using the Tecan Sunrise ELISA reader (Tecan, Männedorf, Switzerland). All samples were analysed in duplicates. The sRANKL ELISA (Biomedica Medizinprodukte, Vienna, Austria) was performed to detect free sRANKL without the OPG bond; intra- and interassay coefficients of variation were 9% and 3%, respectively; and the limit of detection was 0.02 pmol/L. The serum OPG ELISA (Biomedica Medizinprodukte) intra- and interassay coefficients of variation were 10% and 7%, respectively, and the limit of detection was 0.14 pmol/L. The Dkk1 ELISA (Biomedica Medizinprodukte) intra- and interassay coefficients of variation were 7% and 8%, respectively, and the limit of detection was 0.38 pmol/L. The serum sclerostin ELISA kit (Uscn Life Science, Wuhan, China/Cloud-Clone, Houston, TX, USA) has no significant cross-reactivity or interference between human sclerostin and analogues; the standard curve is read between 0.312 and 20 g/L. The limit of detection was 0.106 g/L, and the intra- and interassay coefficients of variation were <10% and <12%, respectively.

The bone metabolism markers osteocalcin (OC), procollagen type I N-terminal propeptide (PINP), C-terminal telopeptide of collagen type I (βCTX-I) and 25-hydroxyvitamin D_3 were measured using electrochemiluminescence-based immunoanalysis (cobas analyzer; Roche Diagnostics, Mannheim, Germany). The intraassay coefficient of variation for OC was <5% at concentrations between 11 and 40 μg/L. The intraassay coefficient of variation for PINP was <5%, and the interassay coefficient of variation was <7%, at concentrations between 20 and 90 μg/L. The intraassay coefficient of variation for βCTX-I was <7% for samples between 200 and 500 ng/L and <10% for very low βCTX-I concentration samples. The interassay coefficient of variation for βCTX-I was <9% for samples between 200 and 500 ng/L. The detection limit for βCTX-I was <10 ng/L.

Imaging parameters

Radiographs of the thoracic and lumbar spine (anteroposterior and lateral) were obtained. BMDs of the lumbar spine, proximal hip, femoral neck and distal forearm were measured by dual-energy X-ray absorptiometry using a bone densitometer (Prodigy; GE Healthcare, Waukesha, WI, USA). The same technician performed all measurements using the same instrument, and the same physician performed all assessments. The short-term *in vivo* coefficients of variation for lumbar spine, total femur, femoral neck and distal radius were 0.7%, 0.9%, 1.8% and 0.9%, respectively. The long-term coefficient of variation using the Hologic phantom was 0.31%. Daily scanning of a phantom showed an absence of machine drift during the study. BMD was expressed in grams per square centimetre.

Statistical analysis

Data for continuous variables were expressed as the mean ± SD or the median with a 75% confidence interval (CI). Bivariate analyses were performed by using Student's *t*-test and Pearson's correlation coefficients to analyse the relationships between the dependent variables. Following anti-TNFα treatment, changes in the monitored parameters (BMD at individual skeletal locations at 12 and 24 months, laboratory parameters at 6, 12 and 24 months) were compared using one-way repeated-measures analysis of variance (ANOVA). These changes in the JIA group were compared with those in the control group by using one-way ANOVA. A stepwise multiple linear regression analysis was performed to create a multivariate summary model of the determinants of dependent variables. All assumptions of the linear regression analysis were also examined. Results at the level of P =0.05 were considered significant. All analyses were performed using a SigmaPlot 10 software package (Systat Software, Erkrath, Germany).

Results

The basic clinical and laboratory characteristics of the participants are listed in Tables 1, 2 and 3. In female patients with JIA, the average age of menarche was 13.1 ± 1.2 years. No significant differences in anthropometric parameters were observed between the control participants and patients with JIA. In males and females with JIA, significant sex-based differences were identified in body height, DAS28 score, OC, PINP, βCTX-I and BMD in the distal radius (Table 2). In patients with JIA, the disease had been diagnosed at approximately age 10.3 ± 4.8 years, and it had lasted on average for 14.6 ± 9.1 years at the time of the study. The cervical spine was affected in seven patients. None of the patients in the study had vasculitis or lung impairment. Six patients tested positive for antinuclear antibodies. The polyarticular form of JIA was present in sixteen patients. Four patients were rheumatoid factor–positive, and twelve were rheumatoid factor–negative. The enthesitis-related form of JIA was present in nine patients; the extended oligoarticular form was present in four patients; and the psoriatic form was present in two patients. Eighteen patients were in functional class I, four were in functional class II, five were in functional class III and four were in functional class IV. The mean Health Assessment Questionnaire score (1978) was 0.97 ± 0.60, and the mean EuroQol questionnaire score 5D was 0.56 ± 0.27. Before the start of anti-TNFα treatment, all of the patients with JIA were treated with disease-modifying antirheumatic drugs. Twenty-three patients were given methotrexate at an average dose of 16.8 ± 3.4 mg/wk; four patients were treated with leflunomide, two patients were treated with sulphasalazine; one patient was treated with sulphasalazine and hydroxychloroquine sulphate; and one patient was treated with cyclosporine A. Twelve patients were receiving glucocorticoid therapy (prednisone in ten patients and methylprednisolone in two patients). The average daily dose of glucocorticoids was 6.6 ± 4.3 mg; the median dose was 5 mg/day; and the dose range was 4 to 20 mg/day. Fourteen of the patients with JIA had taken glucocorticoids in the past, but did not during the course of this study. Five of the patients with JIA did not take glucocorticoids at any time.

At baseline, the BMD values (g/cm^2) in all of the measured skeletal locations in patients with JIA were significantly lower compared to the healthy control participants (Table 3). A significant negative correlation between BMD in the femoral neck and the use of glucocorticoids (r = −0.40, P <0.05) and the disease duration (r = −0.48, P <0.005) was established for the baseline values. There was a statistically significant positive correlation between Dkk1 (r =0.36, P <0.05) and disease activity expressed by means of hsCRP. Following adjustment for sex, glucocorticoid treatment and disease duration, there was a significant correlation between DAS28 values and levels of OC (P =0.005) and OPG (P =0.32), but not βCTX-I. The baseline βCTX-I values were dependent on sex only (P <0.001). No significant association between sclerostin serum concentrations and other monitored variables was found, except for a

Table 1 Anthropometric and clinical characteristics of patients with juvenile idiopathic arthritis and control participants[a]

	Patients with JIA (n =31)	Control participants (n =84)	P-value
Males/females (n)	12/19	36/48	0.692
Age (yr)	25.1 ± 6.1	23.8 ± 4.5	0.405
Height (cm)	170.5 ± 9.8	173.3 ± 9.3	0.145
Weight (kg)	68.0 ± 12.5	69.2 ± 12.5	0.884
BMI (kg/m^2)	23.4 ± 3.9	22.9 ± 3.0	0.435
Vertebral fractures (n)	5	0	<0.001
Nonvertebral fractures (n)	6	0	<0.001
Family hip fracture history (n)	0	0	
Smoking (n)	7	13	0.372
Alcohol abuse (n)	0	0	
Glucocorticoids (n)	12	0	<0.001
Menarche (yr)	13.1 ± 1.2	12.9 ± 1.1	0.994
Contraception in females (n)	11	23	0.462
25(OH)D (nmol/L)	54.3	2.4	0.029
	(20.2 to 168.7)	(30.7 to 64.9)	
PTH (pmol/L)	4.8	5.9	0.004
	(1.3 to 8.8)	(4.7 to 7.6)	
Oestradiol (pmol/L)	98.7	103.2	0.438
	(18.4 to 541.1)	(56.4 to 260.3)	

[a]Displayed are numbers or means ± SD and/or medians and 75% CIs. Characteristics with zero value were not statistically calculated. BMI: Body mass index; JIA: Juvenile idiopathic arthritis; 25(OH)D: 25-hydroxyvitamin D_3; PTH: Parathyroid hormone.

correlation between serum sclerostin and oestradiol concentrations, following adjustment for sex (P =0.022).

In the course of the study, 18 patients were treated with infliximab, 8 patients were treated with etanercept and 5 patients were treated with adalimumab. The values of individual variables are provided in Table 3. The correlations among variables measured at baseline and in the course of treatment are given in Table 4.

The values of BMD (g/cm^2) increased in all of the measured skeletal locations compared to baseline values after the first year and after the second year of TNFα inhibitor treatment, respectively, by 2.9 ± 4.7% and by 4.6 ± 6.3% in the lumbar spine, by 0.8 ± 3.2% and by 1.0 ± 4.0% in the total proximal femur, and by 0.3 ± 3.9% and by 1.1 ± 5.0% in the femoral neck. However, the BMD increase was significant in the lumbar spine only (Table 3). An increase in spinal BMD after 2 years was significantly predicted by a reduction in DAS28 score after the first year of treatment (P =0.003), and this correlation did not change after adjustment for sex, age, body height, treatment with glucocorticoids or disease duration (Figure 1). Even after 2 years of TNFα inhibitor treatment, however, the lumbar spine BMD remained lower than that in the control group (Table 3).

Before the start of anti-TNFα treatment, serum sclerostin concentrations were significantly higher than those in the control group. Serum sclerostin dropped significantly after as little 1 year of treatment (Table 3). Serum sclerostin concentrations did not correlate with ESR or hsCRP levels (Table 4). A significant correlation was found between the number of tender joints and serum sclerostin concentration after adjustment for ESR, sex and glucocorticoid therapy (r =0.40, P <0.001). The correlation between the values of DAS28 and serum sclerostin concentration before treatment and during anti-TNFα treatment (Figure 2, Table 4) remained significant after adjustment for treatment with glucocorticoids (r =0.37, P =0.002). There was a significant positive correlation between hsCRP levels (after adjustment for treatment with glucocorticoids) and Dkk1 serum concentrations (r =0.40, P <0.001) after 2 years of anti-TNFα treatment.

A significant negative correlation was observed between serum βCTX-I concentrations and BMD at the total proximal femur (r = −0.44, P <0.001) and the femoral neck (r = −0.41, P <0.001). These correlations lost their significance after adjustment for age, sex, body height, disease duration and treatment with glucocorticoids, however.

Discussion

Testing of patients with JIA with high disease activity confirmed that they had significantly lower BMD in all of the

Table 2 Clinical characteristics of patients with juvenile idiopathic arthritis by sex[a]

	Men with JIA (n =12)	Women with JIA (n =19)	P-value
Age (yr)	21	26	0.079
	(19.75 to 26.5)	(20.5 to 32.8)	
Height (cm)	178.8 ± 7.6	165.2 ± 7.0	<0.001
Weight (kg)	73.3 ± 11.7	64.6 ± 12.1	0.059
BMI (kg/m^2)	22.9 ± 2.9	23.7 ± 4.5	0.559
Disease duration (yr)	11.0 ± 8.2	16.9 ± 9.4	0.087
Vertebral fractures (n)	3	2	
Nonvertebral fractures (n)	2	4	
Smoking (n)	3	4	
Glucocorticoids (n)	3	9	0.230
Menarche (yr)		13.1 ± 1.2	
Contraception (n)		11	
hsCRP (mg/L)	9.65	13.78	0.395
	(5.84 to 44.78)	(6.78 to 24.21)	
DAS28	6.07	6.44	0.041
	(5.63 to 6.52)	(6.15 to 7.04)	
ESR (mm/hr)	24.5	26.0	0.670
	(17.0 to 54.0)	(24.0 to 34.5)	
Swollen joints (n)	11.0	12.0	0.263
	(7.5 to 13.5)	(9.0 to 18.3)	
Tender joints (n)	13.5	17.0	0.038
	(10.0 to 15.0)	(12.3 to 21.5)	
PGH (mm)	67.5	69.0	0.947
	(60.0 to 74.5)	(53.8 to 77.5)	
Osteocalcin (μg/L)	24.3	14.3	0.016
	(20.2 to 28.0)	(11.3 to 23.0)	
PINP (μg/L)	57.6	40.1	0.003
	(46.3 to 85.6)	(19.9 to 46.4)	
βCTX-I (μg/L)	0.54	0.23	<0.001
	(0.43 to 0.87)	(0.14 to 0.36)	
PTH (pmol/L)	4.08	4.80	<0.001
	(1.73 to 6.05)	(2.50 to 6.15)	
Lumbar spine BMD (g/cm^2)	1.018	1.075	0.392
	(0.913 to 1.201)	(1.012 to 1.221)	
Total femur BMD (g/cm^2)	0.938	0.877	0.073
	(0.887 to 1.131)	(0.764 to 0.916)	
Femoral neck BMD (g/cm^2)	0.934	0.875	0.092
	(0.853 to 1.132)	(0.805 to 0.948)	
Distal radius BMD (g/cm^2)	0.751	0.667	0.030
	(0.677 to 0.792)	(0.606 to 0.704)	

[a]Displayed are numbers or means ± SD and/or medians and 75% CIs. BMD: Bone mineral density; BMI: Body mass index; βCTX-I: C-terminal telopeptide of collagen type I; DAS28: Disease Activity Score in 28 joints; ESR: Erythrocyte sedimentation rate; hsCRP: High-sensitivity C-reactive protein; JIA: Juvenile idiopathic arthritis; 25 (OH)D: 25-hydroxyvitamin D_3; PINP: Procollagen type I N-terminal propeptide; PTH: Parathyroid hormone; PGH: patient global health.

Table 3 Disease activity, bone mineral density and laboratory variables in patients with juvenile idiopathic arthritis during tumour necrosis factor α blocker treatment and in control participants[a]

	0 (n =31)	12 months (n =31)	24 months (n =31)	Control participants (n =83)
hsCRP (mg/L)	12.09[b]	5.19[b]	4.28[b]	0.73
	(6.28 to 25.17)	(1.30 to 12.89)	(0.89 to 13.44)	(0.27 to 1.78)
ESR (mm/hr)	25.50[b]	16.00[b]	12.00[b,c]	4.00
	(20.00 to 36.00)	(4.00 to 24.00)	(4.00 to 26.00)	(2.00 to 8.00)
DAS28	6.26	2.93[c]	2.51[c]	
	(5.87 to 6.82)	(1.13 to 3.69)	(1.25 to 3.64)	
Swollen joints (n)	12.0	0.0[c]	0.0[c]	
	(9.0 to 15.5)	(0.0 to 2.0)	(0.0 to 2.0)	
Tender joints (n)	15.0	1.0[c]	0.0[c]	
	(11.3 to 17.8)	(0.0 to 2.0)	(0.0 to 2.0)	
PGH (mm)	69.0	18.0[c]	10.0[c]	
	(59.0 to 75.0)	(5.0 to 27.8)	(0 to 20.0)	
Lumbar spine BMD (g/cm^2)	1.065[b]	1.089[b,c]	1.093[b,c]	1.209
	(0.972 to 1.221)	(1.044 to 1.248)	(1.053 to 1.161)	(1.175 to 1.279)
Femur total BMD (g/cm^2)	0.909[b]	0.918[b]	0.886[b]	1.134
	(0.776 to 0.984)	(0.776 to 1.015)	(0.790 to 0.996)	(1.061 to 1.202)
Femoral neck BMD (g/cm^2)	0.899[b]	0.903[b]	0.905[b]	1.118
	(0.819 to 1.017)	(0.806 to 1.033)	(0.821 to 1.019)	(1.042 to 1.201)
Distal forearm BMD (g/cm^2)	0.690	0.712	0.707	0.713
	(0.614 to 0.761)	(0.638 to 0.769)	(0.632 to 0.762)	(0.676 to 0.768)
Osteocalcin (μg/L)	17.75	17.45	15.20	21.20
	(12.40 to 24.80)	(8.80 to 26.90)	(11.95 to 20.20)	(16.68 to 26.90)
PINP (μg/L)	46.16	46.41	51.23	50.96
	(31.96 to 59.41)	(32.01 to 88.77)	(33.66 to 72.01)	(37.10 to 81.84)
βCTX-I (μg/L)	0.35	0.33	0.33[b]	0.46
	(0.18 to 0.52)	(0.23 to 0.49)	(0.20 to 0.45)	(0.34 to 0.70)
sRANKL (pmol/L)	0.08	0.05	0.07	0.06
	(0.02 to 0.25)	(0.00 to 0.25)	(0.00 to 0.21)	(0.00 to 0.16)
OPG (pmol/L)	3.84	3.26	3.02	3.14
	(2.53 to 4.84)	(2.10 to 3.64)	(2.03 to 3.55)	(2.62 to 3.85)
sRANKL/OPG ratio	0.03	0.03	0.01	0.02
	(0.01 to 0.07)	(0.00 to 0.10)	(0.00 to 0.10)	(0.00 to 0.05)
Dkk1 (pmol/L)	28.74	24.08	21.52[b,c]	28.74
	(23.8 to 36.84)	(14.54 to 29.41)	(15.72 to 31.25)	(23.80 to 36.84)
Sclerostin (μg/L)	7.42[b]	2.06[c]	1.22[c]	1.94
	(3.57 to 15.49)	(1.00 to 3.48)	(0.30 to 3.26)	(0.62 to 5.71)

[a]BMD: Bone mineral density; BMI: Body mass index; βCTX-I: C-terminal telopeptide of collagen type I; DAS28: Disease Activity Score in 28 joints; PGH: patient global health; Dkk1: Dickkopf Wnt signalling pathway inhibitor 1; ESR: Erythrocyte sedimentation rate; hsCRP: High-sensitivity C-reactive protein; JIA: Juvenile idiopathic arthritis; 25(OH)D: 25-hydroxyvitamin D_3; OPG: Osteoprotegerin; PINP: Procollagen type I N-terminal propeptide; PTH: Parathyroid hormone; sRANKL: Soluble receptor activator of nuclear factor κB ligand. [b]Median and 75% CI with probability P <0.05 by means of one-way analysis of variance, as compared to control participants. [c]Median and 75% CI with probability P <0.05 by means of repeated-measures one-way analysis of variance within JIA group, as compared to baseline.

measured skeletal locations compared to the control group. BMD in the proximal femur depended upon disease duration and treatment with glucocorticoids [23,24]. During anti-TNFα treatment, BMD increased. A significant increase in the lumbar spine BMD after 2 years of treatment correlated with the drop in DAS28 values [25,26]. However, BMD changes should be interpreted with caution, as we did not follow up BMD in control participants, and it is unclear

Table 4 Pearson correlation coefficients for the variables measured at baseline and during tumour necrosis factor α inhibitor treatment[a]

	GCs	Duration	Lumbar spine BMD	Femur neck BMD	Dkk1	Sclerostin	hsCRP	DAS28	ESR	Tender joint counts
Sex	0.226[b]	0.311[c]	0.074	0.350[c]	0.281[c]	−0.029	−0.124	0.280	0.085[c]	0.211[b]
GCs		0.130	0.274[c]	0.391[d]	0.291[c]	0.229[b]	0.229[b]	0.416[d]	0.330[c]	0.323[c]
Duration			0.176	−0.500[d]	−0.021	0.010	0.100	0.192	0.100	0.104
Lumbar spine BMD				0.512[d]	−0.106	−0.178	−0.055	−0.121	−0.075	−0.071
Femoral neck BMD					0.017	−0.154	−0.113	−0.270[b]	−0.266[b]	−0.116
Dkk1						0.026	0.402[d]	0.113	0.244	0.071
Sclerostin							−0.011	0.317[c]	0.023	0.332[c]
hsCRP								0.318[c]	0.751[d]	0.089
DAS28									0.594[d]	0.857[d]
ESR										0.255[b]

[a]BMD: Bone mineral density; DAS28: Disease Activity Score in 28 joints; Dkk1: Dickkopf Wnt signalling pathway inhibitor 1; ESR: Erythrocyte sedimentation rate; GCs: Glucocorticoids; hsCRP: High-sensitivity C-reactive protein. [b]$P<0.05$; [c]$P<0.005$; [d]$P<0.001$.

whether peak BMD was already achieved in all patients. Furthermore, hip BMD remained unchanged and lower than in control participants.

At baseline, there was a significant positive correlation between DAS28 values and the serum concentrations of sclerostin, as well as with hsCRP, but no significant association between the values of hsCRP and sclerostin was established in this study. The association between baseline values of DAS28 and serum concentrations of OC, but not βCTX-I, suggests the inhibition of new bone mass formation in active inflammatory JIA. This is consistent with the finding that etanercept is able to activate osteoblastogenesis and new bone formation by means of Dkk1 inhibition in the rheumatoid arthritis (RA) rat model [27].

Sclerostin serum concentrations depend on genetic aspects, as well as age, sex, adiposity, kidney function and presence of diabetes mellitus [28]. In the present study, the use of an age-homogeneous group of young individuals obviated effect of age on sclerostin levels [29,30]. Although the treated patients with JIA exhibited significantly higher sclerostin serum concentrations than the control participants, no significant association between sclerostin serum concentration and any other monitored variable (for example, BMD) was found at baseline. In an arthritis mouse model, sclerostin inhibition resulted

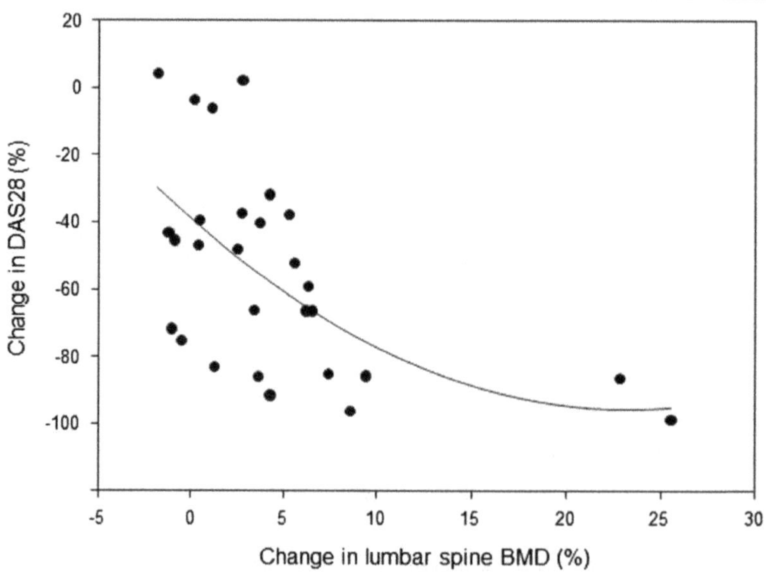

Figure 1 Correlation between percent change in Disease Activity Score in 28 joints after 1 year and change in lumbar spine bone mineral density after 2 years of tumour necrosis factor α inhibitor treatment. Change in bone mineral density (BMD) after 24 months = −1.582 − (0.112 × ΔDAS28 after 12 months) (r =0.53, P =0.003). DAS28: Disease Activity Score in 28 joints.

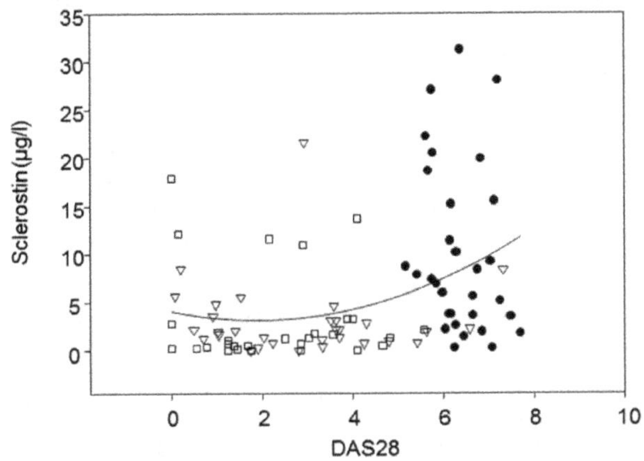

Figure 2 Correlation between the values of Disease Activity Score in 28 joints and serum sclerostin concentration before treatment and during tumour necrosis factor α inhibitor treatment. Disease Activity Score in 28 joints (DAS28) =3.332 + (0.104 × sclerostin) (r =0.32, P =0.002). Filled circles: baseline values; open triangles: 1 year of treatment; open squares: 2 years of treatment.

in a decrease in the loss of bone mass [31,32]. It is necessary, however, to point out that the values of sclerostin serum concentrations depend on the type of immunoanalysis used for measurement [33]. The literature reveals contradictory results concerning the association between sclerostin serum concentrations and BMD of the femoral neck in postmenopausal women [29,30,34,35]. The association between serum sclerostin and the risk of fractures was established in two studies in postmenopausal women [36,37], but was not evidenced in another study [34].

Significant reduction in the expression of sclerostin occurs during mechanical loading of the skeleton [38,39]. Sclerostin is not a specific product of osteocytes, however [40]. Sclerostin is also produced by chondrocytes and cementocytes [38,41], as well as in the liver, vascular wall and kidney [42,43]. Our present study in young adults with active JIA provides evidence of an association between sclerostin serum concentrations and the disease activity assessed by DAS28 values, but not by hsCRP values. Although sclerostin and Dkk1 represent relevant inhibitors of the Wnt signalling pathway and subsequently of new bone mass formation by osteoblasts [8,44-46], causal dependence between the known biological effect of sclerostin (inhibition of new bone formation) and BMD was not evidenced in our patients. Both subchondral bone cells and chondrocytes may be sources of circulating sclerostin patients with JIA. This hypothesis is supported by the finding that, in the RA model, the sclerostin inhibition by a monoclonal antibody protects the bone and cartilage from inflammatory damage [31]. This hypothesis is further supported by a significant correlation between serum sclerostin and the number of tender and swollen joints, as established in our study, whereas no significant correlation between serum sclerostin and hsCRP, ESR or Dkk1 has been identified.

Although baseline serum Dkk1 levels were not increased in patients with JIA compared to healthy control participants, there was a significant positive correlation between Dkk1 levels and disease activity expressed by hsCRP. The relationship between hsCRP and Dkk1 values was confirmed by a significant drop in both of these markers after 2 years of treatment. A similar dependence between hsCRP and Dkk1, as well as a drop in both variables, was previously described in patients with RA treated with infliximab [20]. The patients with JIA in our study did not exhibit any significant relationship between the Dkk1 serum concentrations and any of the other monitored variables at baseline or during treatment with TNFα inhibitors.

In this study, we did not find any significant increase in the serum concentrations of sRANKL, OPG or their ratio in patients with JIA compared to healthy control participants. Although studies in RA most often evidence increased sRANKL concentrations [47-49], unchanged concentrations have also been established [50]. In children with JIA, a decrease in RANKL and an increase in OPG have been demonstrated [51]. In other studies of various JIA subtypes, researchers have mentioned an increase in serum as well as synovial fluid sRANKL [15,52-54]. In the present study, sRANKL values of zero were included in the analyses, unlike in some other studies [52,54]. Also, published data about OPG serum concentrations in JIA differ to a high degree, whether they are unchanged [53], increased [51,52] or decreased [15,54]. After TNFα blocker treatment, we did not observe any deviation from baseline sRANKL levels, OPG levels or their ratio. In other studies, investigators have mentioned both sRANKL increases and decreases during treatment with TNFα blockers [55,56]. Similarly, researchers in other studies have described no changes in OPG concentrations during treatment with infliximab or etanercept [55,56].

The advantage of the present study is the prospective follow-up of an age-homogeneous group of both patients and healthy control individuals of both sexes and the testing of a range of variables that describe the quantity, remodelling and regulation of bone mass. The study is limited by the low number of patients with highly heterogeneous therapy, the use of only a single method of sclerostin serum concentration measurement and a lack of information about the source of sclerostin. Further study of local subchondral bone and cartilage expression of sclerostin could yield more valuable information on the pathogenic role of sclerostin in JIA. Incomplete assessment of potential confounding variables, including physical activity, also needs to be taken into account.

Conclusion

To our knowledge, this study is the first to establish a link between sclerostin serum concentration and the number of tender and swollen joints in patients with JIA. Furthermore, these data support the hypothesis that chondrocytes and cells of the subchondral bone may contribute to circulating sclerostin.

Abbreviations

25(OH)D: 25-Hydroxyvitamin D_3; BMD: Bone mineral density; DAS28: Disease Activity Score in 28 joints; Dkk1: Dickkopf Wnt signalling pathway inhibitor 1; ESR: Erythrocyte sedimentation rate; hsCRP: High-sensitivity C-reactive protein; JIA: Juvenile idiopathic arthritis; OC: Osteocalcin; OPG: Osteoprotegerin; PGH: Patient global health; PINP: Procollagen type I N-terminal propeptide; PTH: Parathyroid hormone; sRANKL: Soluble receptor activator of nuclear factor κB ligand; TNFα: Tumour necrosis factor α; βCTX-I: C-terminal telopeptide of collagen type I.

Competing interests

The authors declare that they have no competing interests.

Authors' contribution

KBM was responsible for study conduct, data collection and analysis, data interpretation, drafting of the manuscript and revision of the manuscript content. KJ and KP contributed to data collection and analysis and revision of the manuscript. JJS worked on the study design, study conduct, data analysis and interpretation, drafting of the manuscript and revision of the manuscript content, and takes responsibility for the integrity of the data analysis. All authors read and approved the final manuscript.

Acknowledgements

This study was supported by the Grant Agency of Charles University in Prague, Grant 84208/2008 and by Czech Republic Ministry of Health Research Grant 000 237280. The authors acknowledge Ludmila Hauptvoglova's professional cooperation and outstanding assistance with data collection.

References

1. Pepmueller PH, Cassidy JT, Allen SH, Hillman LS: **Bone mineralization and bone mineral metabolism in children with juvenile rheumatoid arthritis.** *Arthritis Rheum* 1996, **39:**746–757.
2. Lien G, Flatø B, Haugen M, Vinje O, Sørskaar D, Dale K, Johnston V, Egeland T, Førre Ø: **Frequency of osteopenia in adolescents with early-onset juvenile idiopathic arthritis: a long-term outcome study of one hundred five patients.** *Arthritis Rheum* 2003, **48:**2214–2223.
3. Felin EM, Prahalad S, Askew EW, Moyer-Mileur LJ: **Musculoskeletal abnormalities of the tibia in juvenile rheumatoid arthritis.** *Arthritis Rheum* 2007, **56:**984–994.
4. Brabnikova Maresova K, Jarosova K, Pavelka K, Stepan JJ: **The association between lean mass and bone mineral content in the high disease activity group of adult patients with juvenile idiopathic arthritis.** *BMC Musculoskelet Disord* 2014, **15:**51.
5. Burnham JM, Shults J, Weinstein R, Lewis JD, Leonard MB: **Childhood onset arthritis is associated with an increased risk of fracture: a population based study using the General Practice Research Database.** *Ann Rheum Dis* 2006, **65:**1074–1079.
6. Brabnikova Maresova K: **Secondary osteoporosis in patients with juvenile idiopathic arthritis.** *J Osteoporos* 2011, **2011:**569417. doi:10.4061/2011/569417.
7. Glass DA 2nd, Bialek P, Ahn JD, Starbuck M, Patel MS, Clevers H, Taketo MM, Long F, McMahon AP, Lang RA, Karsenty G: **Canonical Wnt signaling in differentiated osteoblasts controls osteoclast differentiation.** *Dev Cell* 2005, **8:**751–764.
8. Diarra D, Stolina M, Polzer K, Zwerina J, Ominsky MS, Dwyer D, Korb A, Smolen J, Hoffmann M, Scheinecker C, van der Heide D, Landewe R, Lacey D, Richards WG, Schett G: **Dickkopf-1 is a master regulator of joint remodeling.** *Nat Med* 2007, **13:**156–163.
9. Li Y, Li A, Strait K, Zhang H, Nanes MS, Weitzmann MN: **Endogenous TNFα lowers maximum peak bone mass and inhibits osteoblastic Smad activation through NF-κB.** *J Bone Miner Res* 2007, **22:**646–655.
10. Bodine PV, Komm BS: **Wnt signaling and osteoblastogenesis.** *Rev Endocr Metab Disord* 2006, **7:**33–39.
11. Krishnan V, Bryant HU, MacDougald OA: **Regulation of bone mass by Wnt signaling.** *J Clin Invest* 2006, **116:**1202–1209.
12. Goldring SR: **Pathogenesis of bone and cartilage destruction in rheumatoid arthritis.** *Rheumatology* 2003, **42:**ii11–ii16.
13. Hofbauer LC, Khosla S, Dunstan CR, Lacey DL, Boyle WJ, Riggs BL: **The roles of osteoprotegerin and osteoprotegerin ligand in the paracrine regulation of bone resorption.** *J Bone Miner Res* 2000, **15:**2–12.
14. Pereira RM, Falco V, Corrente JE, Chahade WH, Yoshinari NH: **Abnormalities in the biochemical markers of bone turnover in children with juvenile chronic arthritis.** *Clin Exp Rheumatol* 1999, **17:**251–255.
15. Lien G, Selvaag AM, Flatø B, Haugen M, Vinje O, Sørskaar D, Dale K, Egeland T, Førre Ø: **A two-year prospective controlled study of bone mass and bone turnover in children with early juvenile idiopathic arthritis.** *Arthritis Rheum* 2005, **52:**833–840.
16. Appel H, Ruiz-Heiland G, Listing J, Zwerina J, Herrmann M, Mueller R, Haibel H, Baraliakos X, Hempfing A, Rudwaleit M, Sieper J, Schett G: **Altered skeletal expression of sclerostin and its link to radiographic progression in ankylosing spondylitis.** *Arthritis Rheum* 2009, **60:**3257–3262.
17. Terpos E, Fragiadaki K, Konsta M, Bratengeier C, Papatheodorou A, Sfikakis PP: **Early effects of IL-6 receptor inhibition on bone homeostasis: a pilot study in women with rheumatoid arthritis.** *Clin Exp Rheumatol* 2011, **29:**921–925.
18. Garnero P, Tabassi NC, Voorzanger-Rousselot N: **Circulating Dickkopf-1 and radiological progression in patients with early rheumatoid arthritis treated with etanercept.** *J Rheumatol* 2008, **35:**2313–2315.
19. Liu YY, Long L, Wang SY, Guo JP, Ye H, Cui LF, Yuan GH, Li ZG: **Circulating Dickkopf-1 and osteoprotegerin in patients with early and longstanding rheumatoid arthritis.** *Chin Med J (Engl)* 2010, **123:**1407–1412.
20. Wang SY, Liu YY, Ye H, Guo JP, Li R, Liu X, Li ZG: **Circulating Dickkopf-1 is correlated with bone erosion and inflammation in rheumatoid arthritis.** *J Rheumatol* 2011, **38:**821–827.
21. Lamb R, Thomson W, Ogilvie E, the British Society of Paediatric and Adolescent Rheumatology, Donn R: **Wnt-1–inducible signaling pathway protein 3 and susceptibility to juvenile idiopathic arthritis.** *Arthritis Rheum* 2005, **52:**3548–3553.
22. Pavelka K, Vencovský J: **Recommendations of the Czech Society for Rheumatology for the treatment of rheumatoid arthritis.** *Czech Rheumatol* 2010, **18:**182–191.
23. Zak M, Hassager C, Lovell DJ, Nielsen S, Henderson CJ, Pedersen FK: **Assessment of bone mineral density in adults with a history of juvenile chronic arthritis: a cross-sectional long-term followup study.** *Arthritis Rheum* 1999, **42:**790–798.
24. Brik R, Keidar Z, Schapira D, Israel O: **Bone mineral density and turnover in children with systemic juvenile chronic arthritis.** *J Rheumatol* 1998, **25:**990–992.
25. Pye SR, Adams JE, Ward KA, Bunn DK, Symmons DP, O'Neill TW: **Disease activity and severity in early inflammatory arthritis predict hand cortical bone loss.** *Rheumatology* 2010, **49:**1943–1948.
26. Hoff M, Bøyesen P, Haugeberg G, Vis M, Woolf AD, Havaardsholm EA, Dijkmans BA, Kvien TK, Uhlig T, Lems WF: **High disease activity is a predictor of cortical hand bone loss in post-menopausal patients with established rheumatoid arthritis: a 5-year multicentre longitudinal study.** *Rheumatology* 2010, **49:**1676–1682.
27. Tanida A, Kishimoto Y, Okano T, Hagino H: **Etanercept promotes bone formation via suppression of Dickkopf-1 expression in rats with collagen-induced arthritis.** *Yonago Acta Med* 2013, **56:**13–19.
28. Kuipers AL, Zhang Y, Yu S, Kammerer CM, Nestlerode CS, Chu Y, Bunker CH, Patrick AL, Wheeler VW, Miljkovic I, Zmuda JM: **Relative influence of heritability, environment and genetics on serum sclerostin.** *Osteoporos Int* 2014, **25:**905–912.
29. Mödder UI, Hoey KA, Amin S, McCready LK, Achenbach SJ, Riggs BL, Melton LJ 3rd, Khosla S: **Relation of age, gender, and bone mass to circulating sclerostin levels in women and men.** *J Bone Miner Res* 2011, **26:**373–379.
30. Amrein K, Amrein S, Drexler C, Dimai HP, Dobnig H, Pfeifer K, Tomaschitz A, Pieber TR, Fahrleitner-Pammer A: **Sclerostin and its association with physical activity, age, gender, body composition, and bone mineral content in healthy adults.** *J Clin Endocrinol Metab* 2012, **97:**148–154.
31. Chen XX, Baum W, Dwyer D, Stock M, Schwabe K, Ke HZ, Stolina M, Schett G, Bozec A: **Sclerostin inhibition reverses systemic, periarticular and local bone loss in arthritis.** *Ann Rheum Dis* 2013, **72:**1732–1736.
32. Marenzana M, Vugler A, Moore A, Robinson M: **Effect of sclerostin-neutralising antibody on periarticular and systemic bone in a murine**

model of rheumatoid arthritis: a microCT study. *Arthritis Res Ther* 2013, **15**:R125.

33. Durosier C, van Lierop A, Ferrari S, Chevalley T, Papapoulos S, Rizzoli R: **Association of circulating sclerostin with bone mineral mass, microstructure, and turnover biochemical markers in healthy elderly men and women.** *J Clin Endocrinol Metab* 2013, **98**:3873–3883.
34. Garnero P, Sornay-Rendu E, Munoz F, Borel O, Chapurlat RD: **Association of serum sclerostin with bone mineral density, bone turnover, steroid and parathyroid hormones, and fracture risk in postmenopausal women: the OFELY study.** *Osteoporos Int* 2013, **24**:489–494.
35. Polyzos SA, Anastasilakis AD, Bratengeier C, Woloszczuk W, Papatheodorou A, Terpos E: **Serum sclerostin levels positively correlate with lumbar spinal bone mineral density in postmenopausal women—the six-month effect of risedronate and teriparatide.** *Osteoporos Int* 2012, **23**:1171–1176.
36. Arasu A, Cawthon PM, Lui LY, Do TP, Arora PS, Cauley JA, Ensrud KE, Cummings SR, and the Study of Osteoporotic Fractures Research Group: **Serum sclerostin and risk of hip fracture in older Caucasian women.** *J Clin Endocrinol Metab* 2012, **97**:2027–2032.
37. Ardawi MS, Rouzi AA, Al-Sibiani SA, Al-Senani NS, Qari MH, Mousa SA: **High serum sclerostin predicts the occurrence of osteoporotic fractures in postmenopausal women: the Center of Excellence for Osteoporosis Research Study.** *J Bone Miner Res* 2012, **27**:2592–2602.
38. Moester MJC, Papapoulos SE, Löwik CWGM, van Bezooijen RL: **Sclerostin: current knowledge and future perspectives.** *Calcif Tissue Int* 2010, **87**:99–107.
39. Robling AG, Niziolek PJ, Baldridge LA, Condon KW, Allen MR, Alam I, Mantila SM, Gluhak-Heinrich J, Bellido TM, Harris SE, Turner CH: **Mechanical stimulation of bone *in vivo* reduces osteocyte expression of Sost/sclerostin.** *J Biol Chem* 2008, **283**:5866–5875.
40. Winkler DG, Sutherland MK, Geoghegan JC, Yu C, Hayes T, Skonier JE, Shpektor D, Jonas M, Kovacevich BR, Staehling-Hampton K, Appleby M, Brunkow ME, Latham JA: **Osteocyte control of bone formation via sclerostin, a novel BMP antagonist.** *EMBO J* 2003, **22**:6267–6276.
41. Chan BY, Fuller ES, Russell AK, Smith SM, Smith MM, Jackson MT, Cake MA, Read RA, Bateman JF, Sambrook PN, Little CB: **Increased chondrocyte sclerostin may protect against cartilage degradation in osteoarthritis.** *Osteoarthritis Cartilage* 2011, **19**:874–885.
42. Brunkow ME, Gardner JC, Van Ness J, Paeper BW, Kovacevich BR, Proll S, Skonier JE, Zhao L, Sabo PJ, Fu Y, Alisch RS, Gillett L, Colbert T, Tacconi P, Galas D, Hamersma H, Beighton P, Mulligan J: **Bone dysplasia sclerosteosis results from loss of the *SOST* gene product, a novel cystine knot-containing protein.** *Am J Hum Genet* 2001, **68**:577–589.
43. Rhee Y, Kim WJ, Han KJ, Lim SK, Kim SH: **Effect of liver dysfunction on circulating sclerostin.** *J Bone Miner Metab* 2014, **32**:545–549.
44. Li X, Zhang Y, Kang H, Liu W, Liu P, Zhang J, Harris SE, Wu D: **Sclerostin binds to LRP5/6 and antagonizes canonical Wnt signaling.** *J Biol Chem* 2005, **280**:19883–19887.
45. Veverka V, Henry AJ, Slocombe PM, Ventom A, Mulloy B, Muskett FW, Muzylak M, Greenslade K, Moore A, Zhang L, Gong J, Qian X, Paszty C, Taylor RJ, Robinson MK, Carr MD: **Characterization of the structural features and interactions of sclerostin: molecular insight into a key regulator of Wnt-mediated bone formation.** *J Biol Chem* 2009, **284**:10890–10900.
46. Monroe DG, McGee-Lawrence ME, Oursler MJ, Westendorf JJ: **Update on Wnt signaling in bone cell biology and bone disease.** *Gene* 2012, **492**:1–18.
47. Ziolkowska M, Kurowska M, Radzikowska A, Luszczykiewicz G, Wiland P, Dziewczopolski W, Filipowicz-Sosnowska A, Pazdur J, Szechinski J, Kowalczewski J, Rell-Bakalarska M, Maslinski W: **High levels of osteoprotegerin and soluble receptor activator of nuclear factor κB ligand in serum of rheumatoid arthritis patients and their normalization after anti-tumor necrosis factor α treatment.** *Arthritis Rheum* 2002, **46**:1744–1753.
48. Hein GE, Meister M, Oelzner P, Franke S: **sRANKL and OPG in serum and synovial fluid of patients with rheumatoid arthritis in comparison to non-destructive chronic arthritis.** *Rheumatol Int* 2008, **28**:765–769.
49. Xu S, Wang Y, Lu J, Xu J: **Osteoprotegerin and RANKL in the pathogenesis of rheumatoid arthritis-induced osteoporosis.** *Rheumatol Int* 2011, **32**:3397–3403.
50. Skoumal M, Haberhauer G, Kolarz G, Hawa G, Woloszczuk W, Klingler A, Varga F, Klaushofer K: **The imbalance between osteoprotegerin and cathepsin K in the serum of patients with longstanding rheumatoid arthritis.** *Rheumatol Int* 2008, **28**:637–641.
51. Masi L, Simonini G, Piscitelli E, Del Monte F, Giani T, Cimaz R, Vierucci S, Brandi ML, Falcini F: **Osteoprotegerin (OPG)/RANK-L system in juvenile idiopathic arthritis: Is there a potential modulating role for OPG/RANK-L in bone injury?** *J Rheumatol* 2004, **31**:986–991.
52. Sarma PK, Misra R, Aggarwal A: **Elevated serum receptor activator of NFκB ligand (RANKL), osteoprotegerin (OPG), matrix metalloproteinase (MMP) 3, and ProMMP1 in patients with juvenile idiopathic arthritis.** *Clin Rheumatol* 2008, **27**:289–294.
53. Spelling P, Bonfá E, Caparbo VF, Pereira RM: **Osteoprotegerin/RANKL system imbalance in active polyarticular-onset juvenile idiopathic arthritis: a bone damage biomarker?** *Scand J Rheumatol* 2008, **37**:439–444.
54. Agarwal S, Misra R, Aggarwal A: **Synovial fluid RANKL and matrix metalloproteinase levels in enthesitis related arthritis subtype of juvenile idiopathic arthritis.** *Rheumatol Int* 2009, **29**:907–911.
55. Sennels H, Sørensen S, Ostergaard M, Knudsen L, Hansen M, Skjødt H, Peters N, Colic A, Grau K, Jacobsen S: **Circulating levels of osteopontin, osteoprotegerin, total soluble receptor activator of nuclear factor-κB ligand, and high-sensitivity C-reactive protein in patients with active rheumatoid arthritis randomized to etanercept alone or in combination with methotrexate.** *Scand J Rheumatol* 2008, **37**:241–247.
56. Vis M, Havaardsholm EA, Haugeberg G, Uhlig T, Voskuyl AE, van de Stadt RJ, Dijkmans BA, Woolf AD, Kvien TK, Lems WF: **Evaluation of bone mineral density, bone metabolism, osteoprotegerin and receptor activator of the NFκB ligand serum levels during treatment with infliximab in patients with rheumatoid arthritis.** *Ann Rheum Dis* 2006, **65**:1495–1499.

21

Genomic characterization of remission in juvenile idiopathic arthritis

Kaiyu Jiang[1,3†], Mark Barton Frank[2†], Yanmin Chen[1,3], Jeanette Osban[2] and James N Jarvis[1,3*]

Abstract

Introduction: The attainment of remission has become an important end point for clinical trials in juvenile idiopathic arthritis (JIA), although we do not yet have a full understanding of what remission is at the cell and molecular level.

Methods: Two independent cohorts of patients with JIA and healthy child controls were studied. RNA was prepared separately from peripheral blood mononuclear cells (PBMC) and granulocytes to identify differentially expressed genes using whole genome microarrays. Expression profiling results for selected genes were confirmed by quantitative, real-time polymerase chain reaction (RT-PCR).

Results: We found that remission in JIA induced by either methotrexate (MTX) or MTX plus a TNF inhibitor (etanercept, Et) (MTX + Et) is characterized by numerous differences in gene expression in peripheral blood mononuclear cells and in granulocytes compared with healthy control children; that is, remission is not a restoration of immunologic normalcy. Network analysis of the differentially expressed genes demonstrated that the steroid hormone receptor superfamily member hepatocyte nuclear factor 4 alpha (HNF4α) is a hub in several of the gene networks that distinguished children with arthritis from controls. Confocal microscopy revealed that HNF4a is present in both T lymphocytes and granulocytes, suggesting a previously unsuspected role for this transcription factor in regulating leukocyte function and therapeutic response in JIA.

Conclusions: These findings provide a framework from which to understand therapeutic response in JIA and, furthermore, may be used to develop strategies to increase the frequency with which remission is achieved in adult forms of rheumatoid arthritis.

Keywords: juvenile idiopathic arthritis, methotrexate, TNF inhibitor, gene expression, biomarker, microarray

Introduction

The advent of biological therapies for chronic forms of arthritis has been accompanied by the hopes that: (1) therapies can be increasingly tailored to specific pathogenic pathways, decreasing unwanted side effects; and (2) by use of more targeted therapies, patients will experience more sustained periods of disease quiescence and, therefore, functional and subjective well-being. In juvenile idiopathic arthritis (JIA), the most common form of chronic arthritis in children, achieving the second of these objectives appears to be very near [1].

* Correspondence: jamesjar@buffalo.edu
† Contributed equally
[1]Department of Pediatrics, Pediatric Rheumatology Research, University of Oklahoma Health Sciences Center, Basic Sciences Education Building 235A, Oklahoma City, OK 73104, USA
Full list of author information is available at the end of the article

JIA is a term used to denote a heterogeneous group of childhood illnesses characterized by chronic inflammation and hypertrophy of synovial membranes. Distinct phenotypes are recognized based on disease presentation, clinical course, and specific biomarkers, for example, IgM rheumatoid factor [2]. However, even within carefully specified disease subtypes, considerable heterogeneity exists, especially with respect to response to therapy and overall outcome [3]. The biology underlying these differences is poorly understood, and obtaining a molecular understanding of phenotypic and therapeutic response differences is an important step toward developing individualized therapies for this family of diseases and their cognate conditions in adults.

A major advance in pediatric rheumatology has been the recognition that treatment response can be staged based on consensus criteria developed by an international panel [4], and that these stages have biological validity that can be characterized at the molecular level by gene transcriptional profiling [5-7]. Wallace *et al.* [4] defined these specific states as: active disease (AD), inactive disease (ID), clinical remission on medication (CRM), and clinical remission (CR). While true remission (CR) appears to be difficult to achieve (in the Wallace study [7], only 5% of children with the multiple-joint, polyarticular form of JIA achieved remission within 5 years of diagnosis), sustained periods of disease control (CRM) have become a reality and the target end point for childhood arthritis clinical trials. However, although achieving CRM has become commonplace in pediatric rheumatology clinical care, preliminary studies have suggested that the CRM biological state is not a return to normal, but, rather, a homeostatic state where pro-inflammatory disease networks are counterbalanced by the emergence of anti-inflammatory networks [6]. Indeed, peripheral blood gene expression abnormalities persist even in children who have been disease-free and off medication for a year or more [5,6].

Now that remission (or at least CRM) has become both the gold standard for clinical care and the end point for clinical trials for children, it is critical that we understand it at the molecular/biological level. One complication in doing so is that, while approximately 35 to 50% of children with JIA will experience CRM with the use of methotrexate (MTX) (usually in combination with nonsteroidal anti-inflammatory drugs +/- corticosteroids, used systemically or via joint injection), others will attain this state only after a biological agent, most commonly a TNF inhibitor, is added to methotrexate and the other agents [8]. However, whether the state of remission induced by MTX is, at the molecular level, identical to remission induced by the addition of a TNF inhibitor remains unknown, even though the remission phenotype is identical in each case. Answering this question is critical to our understanding of both the biology of response to therapy in JIA and toward our understanding the disease process itself. Furthermore, while there may be fundamental differences in the biology of response in adults compared to children and between the different disease entities in which anti-TNF therapies are used, the frequency with which remission (as defined here) can be achieved in children provides an excellent opportunity to understand mechanisms of response in such a way that these therapies might be manipulated in adults or in other diseases to achieve the same ends. Thus, understanding remission at the molecular level in this specific disease can be expected to have a useful impact on the multiple other chronic forms of arthritis in which immunosuppressive and anti-TNF therapies are used.

In this study, we used gene expression profiling to compare two groups of children with JIA who had achieved remission (CRM) to examine the medication-specific effects on gene transcriptional profiles.

Materials and methods

Patients and controls

This study was approved by the Oklahoma University Health Sciences Center (OUHSC) Institutional Review Board, and informed consent was obtained from all patients, or their parent/guardian, prior to the initiation of the study. We studied two independent cohorts of patients. One cohort was designated the training cohort, and the second, termed the testing cohort, was used to corroborate the results from the training cohort using quantitative, real-time PCR (qRT-PCR).

Children with polyarticular onset, rheumatoid factor (RF)-negative JIA were recruited from the OU Children's Physicians' rheumatology clinics and fit criteria for this subtype as specified by the International League of Associations for Rheumatology (ILAR) [9]. All children were on treatment at the time they were studied, and all fit criteria for CRM as defined by Wallace and colleagues [7]. That is, these children had all reached the ID state (normal physical examinations, absence of morning stiffness, and normal complete blood counts and erythrocyte sedimentation rates on laboratory monitoring studies) and, to fit criteria for CRM status, had maintained the ID state for 6 continuous months. The patients were followed every 2 to 3 months following their achieving ID, and CRM state samples were taken 6 to 8 months following the achievement of ID status. In the training cohort (for microarray), 14 children (ages 8.9 ± 3.1 years; seven females and seven males) achieved CRM with the use of MTX alone, 7 to 48 months after starting therapy. The patient comparison group in this cohort consisted of 14 other children with polyarticular JIA (ages 8.9 ± 4.2 years; 13 females and one male) who achieved CRM only after the addition of the TNF inhibitor, etanercept (Et), 11 to 48 months after the initiation of therapy. Both of these groups were compared to a group of 15 healthy children (ages 11.5 ± 2.6 years; seven female and eight male) recruited from the OU Children's Physicians' General Pediatrics clinic (Table 1).

A separate testing patient cohort of children with JIA was used to validate results from the first patient cohort. Eight of these children (ages 9.4 ± 4.7 years; eight females) achieved CRM with the use of MTX alone, 10 to 27 months from the initiation of therapy, and an additional eight children with polyarticular JIA (age 9.6 ± 4.5 years; eight females) achieved CRM only after the addition of Et, 10 to 26 months after the initiation of therapy. Eight healthy children (age 11.1 ± 2.8 years; four females and four males) were used as an independent comparison group to the testing cohort. Patient groups and characteristics are summarized in Table 1. All patients were treated

Table 1 Demographic characteristics of study participants

Training group							
Response to methotrexate			Response to methotrexate + etanercept			Healthy control	
Patients	Age	Time to CRM (month)	Patients	Age (month)	Time to CRM	Control	Age
1	9	7	1	13	20	1	16
2	16	8	2	3	24	2	18
3*	11	10	3	3	48	3	9
4	7	14	4	6	8	4	11
5	11	12	5	4	18	5	10
6*	6	15	6	5	42	6	11
7	7	32	7	14	15	7	10
8*	11	13	8	9	25	8	10
9	7	36	9	10	30	9	11
10	4	46	10	15	25	10	13
11	11	8	11	11	20	11	13
12	7	15	12	12	24	12	10
13	11	48	13	12	24	13	12
14*	6	9	14	7	11	14	12
Testing group							
Response to methotrexate			Response to methotrexate + etanercept			Healthy control	
Patients	Age (month)	Time to CRM	Patients	Age	Time to CRM (month)	Control	Age
1	12	27	1	9	24	1	12
2	5	12	2	17	10	2	15
3	12	11	3	6	17	3	8
4	14	11	4	7	26	4	9
5	16	11	5	12	26	5	8
6	5	13	6	5	18	6	11
7	4	10	7	6	24	7	15
8	7	17	8	15	16	8	11

*RNA from granulocytes was insufficient for microarray analysis. CRM, clinical remission on medication.

with naproxen, 10 mg/kg/dose, as an adjunct to their primary drugs (that is, MTX +/- Et).

Cell isolation

Whole blood was drawn into 10 mL citrated Cell Preparation Tubes (Becton Dickinson, Franklin Lakes, NJ, USA). Cell separation procedures were started within one hour from the time the specimens were drawn. Peripheral blood mononuclear cells (PBMC) were separated from granulocytes and red blood cells by density-gradient centrifugation. Red cells were removed from granulocytes by hypotonic lysis, and PBMC and granulocytes were then immediately placed in TRIzol™ reagent (Invitrogen, Carlsbad, CA, USA) and stored at -80°C.

RNA isolation, labeling and gene expression profiling

Total RNA was extracted using TRIzol™ reagent according to the manufacturer's directions. RNA was further purified using a RNeasy MiniElute cleanup kit including a DNase digest according to the manufacturer's instructions (Qiagen, Valencia, CA, USA). RNA was quantified spectrophotometrically (Nanodrop, Thermo Fisher Scientific, Wilmington, DE, USA) and assessed for quality by capillary gel electrophoresis (Agilent 2100 Bioanalyzer; Agilent Technologies, Inc., Palo Alto, CA, USA). For the training cohort, sufficient amounts of high quality RNA for use in microarrays were obtained from 43 PBMC samples obtained from 14 JIA patients treated with MTX + Et, 14 JIA patients treated with MTX alone, and 15 healthy control children. From granulocytes, a sufficient amount of high quality RNA was obtained from 12 JIA patients treated with MTX + Et, 10 JIA patients treated with MTX alone, and 13 healthy control children. RNA samples were processed using GeneChip 3' IVT Express kit and hybridized to human U133 Plus 2.0 GeneChip™ microarrays according to the manufacturer's protocol (Affymetrix, Santa Clara, CA, USA). GeneChips™ were washed and stained using an Affymetrix automated GeneChip™ 450 fluidics station and scanned with an Affymetrix 3000 7G scanner. All gene expression data has been made available publically via the Gene Expression Omnibus (accession GSE41831).

Statistical analysis and network modeling

CEL files were generated from scanned images using GeneChip™ Operating Software (GCOS, Affymetrix, version 1.3.0.037). Signal intensities were generated using JustRMA software (BRB-Array Tools). A log base 2 transformation was applied before the data were quantile normalized. Signal intensities were filtered using a log intensity variation (BRB-Array Tools) to obtain probes with the 25% highest variance across the arrays (13,668 probes) for further evaluation. Samples were divided into three groups (controls, patients treated with MTX + Et, and patients treated with MTX alone) and gene expression differences were separately evaluated in each patient group relative to controls. Differences between groups were considered statistically significant using a two-sample t test with univariate random variance model if the P value was ≤0.001 (BRB Array Tools, version 3.8.0 stable release). Statistically significant differentially expressed genes were filtered to obtain those with a minimal 1.3-fold change between groups and a mean expression level above background in at least one group. Annotations for probes were obtained from Affymetrix and were further supplemented by SOURCE [10]. These gene annotations were compared with the Gene Ontology (GO) database [11] to identify overrepresented terms using the R package GO available from Bioconductor within BRB-Array Tools [12]. A minimum of five observations in a GO class and parent class plus a minimum ratio of 2 for the observed vs. expected numbers were required for further consideration.

Interactions among differentially expressed genes in PBMC and granulocytes were analyzed using Ingenuity Pathway Analysis (IPA) software (Ingenuity Systems, Inc, Redwood City, CA, USA). Differentially expressed genes were mapped onto a global molecular network developed from information contained in the Ingenuity Pathways Knowledge Base.

Gene expression validation by quantitative real-time RT-PCR

Total RNA (described above) was reverse transcribed with iScript™ cDNA synthesis kit according to the directions of the manufacturer (Bio-Rad, Hercules, CA, USA). Real-time RT-PCR was performed using SYBR Green reagents on an ABI Prism 7000 (for the training group; Applied Biosystems, Foster City, CA, USA) or a StepOne Plus (for the testing group; Applied Biosystems, Foster City, CA, USA). The temperature profile consisted of an initial 95°C step for 10 min, followed by 40 cycles of 95°C for 15 sec, 60°C for 1 min, and then a final melting curve analysis with a ramp from 60°C to 95°C over 20 min. Gene-specific amplification was confirmed by a single peak in the ABI Dissociation Curve software. Average threshold cycle (Ct) values for GAPDH (run in parallel reactions to the genes of interest) were used to normalize average Ct values of the gene of interest. These values were used to calculate averages for each group (healthy control or patient subsets), and the relative ΔCt was used to calculate fold-change values between the groups [5]. The nucleotide sequences of the primers are listed in Table 2.

Table 2 Primers used for quantitative real-time PCR validation.

Gene symbol	Primer direction[1]	Primer sequence (5′ ~ 3′)
BIRC3	F	CATGGGTTCAACATGCCAAGTGGT
BIRC3	R	TTCATCTCCTGGGCTGTCTGATGT
C3	F	GTGGAAATCCGAGCCGTTCTCT
C3	R	GATGGTTACGGTCTGCTGGTGA
CCR2	F	AGTTCAGAAGGTATCTCTCGGTG
CCR2	R	GGCGTGTTTGTTGAAGTCACT
CCR6	F	CTGAACCCTGTGCTCTACGCTT
CCR6	R	CACAGGAGAAGCCTGAGGACTT
CD22	F	GCGCAGCTTGTAATAGTTGGTGC
CD22	R	CACATTGGAGGCTGACCGAGTT
CXCR6	F	CAGTTCAGCAAGGTCTTTCTGCC
CXCR6	R	AGGTTCACCAGGAACACATCCG
EFR3A	F	ATTCAGTGCCATGTGCCATTCCTG
EFR3A	R	GCCCGAAGTTCATCGTTGACTGTT
FOXO1	F	CTACGAGTGGATGGTCAAGAGC
FOXO1	R	CCAGTTCCTTCATTCTGCACACG
FUZ	F	AGCCAGTTGTATCCACAGCTTCTG
FUZ	R	CCGAGGATGTCTGTGTGAAGGG
GM2A	F	TCGTTCCTGGAAATGTGACCCTCA
GM2A	R	CAGCTGCCAATGTAGTCTGTGCAT
GZMA	F	CCACACGCGAAGGTGACCTTAA
GZMA	R	CCTGCAACTTGGCACATGGTTC
IER5	F	ACCTCATCAGCATCTTCGGTTCCA
IER5	R	TTCATGTCTCTCAGCACCGGCTTA
IL6ST	F	CACCCTGTATCACAGACTGGCA
IL6ST	R	TTCAGGGCTTCCTGGTCCATCA
KLRD1	F	GAGCCAGCATTTACTCCAGGAC
KLRD1	R	GCACAGAGATGCCGACTTTCGT
KMO	F	ATACTCGAGTGGCTACCTTCACAC
KMO	R	TCTGATCTTCCAGGCCAACAGCTT
NBN	F	TCTGTCAGGACGGCAGGAAAGA
NBN	R	CACCTCCAAAGACAACTGCGGA
NSMAF	F	GTCTGAACACCTTCACGAGTGG
NSMAF	R	CTGTTCAAGTCTACACCTCCTTC
RNF167	F	ATGGGTCAGTCTTTATTGCGCTGC
RNF167	R	ATCCAGCCTTCTGGGCATTTAGGA
STAT1	F	ATGGCAGTCTGGCGGCTGAATT

Table 2 Primers used for quantitative real-time PCR validation. *(Continued)*

STAT1	R	CCAAACCAGGCTGGCACAATTG
TARP	F	CCCCAAGCCCACTATTTTTC
TARP	R	TGTTGCTCTTCTTTTCTTGCC
TNFAIP6	F	TCACCTACGCAGAAGCTAAGGC
TNFAIP6	R	TCCAACTCTGCCCTTAGCCATC
TRAF3	F	AGCAGAGGTTGTGCAGAGCAGTTA
TRAF3	R	TCATCGGAACCTGACTCTTGCAGT
TRGV5	F	TGACTCAGGAAGACCAGCTC
TRGV5	R	TCTTAAAACTCCGGCCCCAC
TRIM4	F	ACGCCACACAGTGGAAGGATAAGA
TRIM4	R	TCTTCAACCAGGAAGTTGTGCAGC
TST	F	TTCCAGCTGGTGGATTCAAGGTCT
TST	R	AGAGATCCACCTTCTTGGTCTGGA
UBTF	F	ATGGATTCATAAGGCCCTGGAGCA
UBTF	R	TTTGTCCGAGAGCTGAGACCACT
XIAP	F	TGGCAGATTATGAAGCACGGATC
XIAP	R	AGTTAGCCCTCCTCCACAGTGA
ZNF277	F	AATGCAGGAAGACCGTGATGGGA
ZNF277	R	AGCGGCTCCAGGATACAATCCTTA

[1]Forward primer direction (F), reverse primer direction (R).

Confocal microscopy for hepatocyte nuclear factor 4 alpha (HNF4α)

Human PBMC and granulocytes, isolated as described above, were adhered to poly-L-lysine-coated coverslips (Sigma-Aldrich, St. Louis, MO, USA) for 30 min at room temperature. Cells were fixed with 3% formaldehyde in PBS for 10 min at room temperature. After fixation, cells were treated with 0.25% Triton X-100 in PBS for 15 min. Slides were washed twice in PBS and blocked with blocking buffer (1% BSA, 1% donkey serum, 0.3M glycine in PBS containing 0.05% Tween 20) for 30 min. PBMC were incubated with rabbit anti-human HNF4α mAb (Cell Signaling Technology, Inc., Danvers, MA, USA) plus mouse anti-human CD4 mAb (Biolegend, San Diego, CA, USA), or rabbit anti-human HNF4α mAb plus mouse anti-human CD8 mAb (Biolegend, San Diego, CA, USA), and granulocytes were incubated with rabbit anti-human HNF4α mAb plus FITC-conjugated mouse anti-human CD66b mAb (BD Biosciences, San Jose, CA, USA), overnight at 4°C. After being washed with PBS, cells were incubated with Alexa Fluor 568- or 647-conjugated secondary antibody for 45 min at room temperature. After three rinses in PBS, the coverslips were mounted onto glass slides using ProLong Gold antifade reagent (Invitrogen, Carlsbad, CA, USA) with 4',6-diamidino-2-phenylindole (Invitrogen, Carlsbad, CA, USA). Fluorescent confocal laser scanning microscopy was conducted with a Leica SP2 MP laser scanning confocal microscope using the Leica confocal software LCS Lite (Leica Microsystems HD GmbH, Mannheim, Baden-Württemberg, Germany).

Results

Our primary aim in this study was to determine whether the CRM state as achieved in a typical clinical setting results in a return to normal immune homeostasis in peripheral blood leukocytes. Preliminary studies from our research group [5,6] indicated that this was not likely, and this study, performed on a larger group of patients with independent corroboration in a second group of patients, was designed to answer that question in a definitive way and elucidate differences at the molecular level. To do this, we first compared each of the CRM groups (that is, MTX or MTX + Et) to healthy control children.

In both PBMC and in granulocytes, there were differences between children who achieved remission on MTX compared with those who achieved remission on MTX + Et relative to healthy control children. That is, although remission (CRM) is a distinct biological state, and phenotypically is indistinguishable among the groups, there were still differences in patterns of gene expression between and among the groups. For both cell types, hierarchical clustering of samples from the three groups (that is, healthy controls, children who had achieved remission on MTX, and children who had achieved remission on MTX + Et) revealed two clusters, each containing a similar proportion of samples from children in remission on MTX and healthy control children, while all but one of the samples from children who achieved remission on MTX + Et were grouped in one cluster. A 3 × 2 contingency table of these distributions revealed a nonrandom distribution of samples in both cell types (Table 3; PBMC: $X^2 = 9.86$, $P < 0.007$; granulocytes: $X^2 = 11.5$, $P < 0.003$). These results suggest that combined treatment with MTX + Et produced distinct gene expression responses that are distinct and more biologically focused at the gene expression level from the more heterogeneous responses detected among the MTX-treated

Table 3 Summary of hierarchical cluster analysis in PBMC and granulocytes from healthy control and in PBMC and granulocytes from children with JIA who achieved remission with methotrexate or methotrexate and etanercept

Cells	Group	Left Cluster	Right Cluster
PBMC	MTX + Et	1	14
	MTX	8	6
	Controls	8	7
Granulocytes	MTX + Et	13	1
	MTX	3	7
	Controls	5	7

ET, etanercept; JIA, juvenile idiopathic arthritis; MTX, methotrexate; PBMC, peripheral blood mononuclear cells.

patients, consistent with the idea that Et represents a more targeted therapy.

Differences in PBMC gene expression profiles

Gene expression differences were detected in 67 genes represented by 75 probes when PBMC from JIA patients who achieved remission using MTX alone were compared to healthy controls. Twenty-two of these genes showed higher levels of expression and 45 showed lower levels in patient compared with control samples (Table S1 in Additional file 1). Thus, MTX appears to act not merely by suppressing pro-inflammatory genes, but by a re-ordering of specific transcript levels. Not surprisingly, functional associations among the differentially expressed genes included genes whose products are active in cell-mediated immunity. This included decreased expression of signal transducer and activator of transcription 1 (*STAT1*), which plays an important role mediating the effects of interferon gamma and in TH17 cell differentiation. STAT1 is activated by IL-6, an important cytokine in the pathogenesis of JIA [13] and IL-6 is known to be modulated by methotrexate [14,15]. Similarly, the expression of complement factor B, whose expression is increased by pro-inflammatory cytokines, was decreased in MTX-responsive patient samples. The decreased expression patterns of chemokine receptor 6, granzymes A and K, and the killer cell lectin like receptor subfamily D member 1 and subfamily K member 1 transcripts suggest modulation by MTX in cells of the innate (natural killer cells) and adaptive (cytotoxic T cells) immune systems in JIA. Input of the differentially expressed genes from this analysis into IPA software revealed a statistically significant downregulation of leukocyte activation in samples from the methotrexate-responsive samples based on the downregulation of five genes: *GZMA*, which activates monocytes [16], *STAT1* whose phosphorylation leads to macrophage activation [17], *CALR*, which increases activation of dendritic cells [18], *SERPINB9*, which increases leukocyte activation [19], and *KLRK1*, which increases NK cell activation [20]. Upregulation of *CALR*, *PRDM1*, *STAT1*, *TAGAP* and *TNRC6B* has been associated elsewhere with adult rheumatoid arthritis or juvenile polyarticular arthritis [21-24]. Their downregulation here is consistent with an immunosuppressive effect of MTX across a variety of different molecules. Downregulation of *GZMA* by MTX was previously reported by Belinsky *et al.* [25].

Fifty-two genes represented by 56 different probe sets were differentially expressed in PBMC samples from patients treated with MTX + Et relative to samples from healthy controls (Table S2 in Additional file 2). Transcripts for 25 of these genes were expressed in higher levels in patients and 27 were expressed in lower levels compared with controls. GO analysis indicated an overrepresentation of products of the differentially expressed genes with roles in immunity, as expected. Of the 24 GO biological process categories obtained, 11 were related to immunity with ratios of the number of observed to expected genes varying from 4.57 to 22.05. The second-most overrepresented categories were related to histone or chromatin modification, with observed/expected ratios between 3.29 and 12.53. This finding is consistent with the hypothesis that alterations in gene expression that characterize the transition from active disease to remission may be accomplished alterations in chromatin accessibility through epigenetic alterations.

Twenty-one of the transcripts which showed differential expression when the MTX + Et group was compared with controls, including *KLRD1* and *CFB*, were also differentially expressed in the MTX alone group vs. controls, suggesting either MTX-induced changes in the expression of these genes or persistence of pre-existing expression abnormalities not corrected by either drug regimen. *AGRN* and *KLRD1*, which showed decreased expression in the patient samples, are involved in T cell activation. CFB, AGRN and KLRD1 are involved in inflammatory response, while CFB and AGRN plus PPP1R14A are involved in cell-cell interactions. The remaining 31 genes were uniquely differentially expressed in the MTX + Et vs. controls comparison (including *CD22*, *CCR6* and *TREM1* which are of immunologic interest and suggest a unique effect of Et or MTX + Et interaction) and 46 that were uniquely differentially expressed in the MTX vs. controls (including *CXCR6*, *GZMA*, *TCRGC2*, *TCRGV5*, *TCR delta* and *STAT1*, which are of immunologic interest and suggest the unique effect of MTX). The increased expression of *CD22* and decreased expression of *TREM1* which occurred in patients who responded to the combined methotrexate and etanercept therapy but not those who responded to methotrexate alone suggests an Et-dependent effect on these molecules. *CD22* is known to negatively regulate B cell activation [26,27], while *TREM1* activation in monocytes induces pro-inflammatory cytokines and chemokines such as TNF, IL-1 and IL-6 [28,29]. The transcriptional modulation of these molecules in response to these therapies should reduce inflammation and modulate immune responses in responding patients.

Differential expression of genes in granulocytes

The most striking differences in gene expression profiles of patients with JIA responding to therapy were detected in granulocytes. A total of 207 differentially expressed genes were identified when samples from patients treated with MTX + Et were compared to control samples (Table S3 in Additional file 3). This contrasts with 23 genes that were differentially expressed in patients who achieved remission on MTX relative to controls (Table S4 in Additional file 4). That is, patients achieving remission on MTX alone had granulocyte gene expression profiles that more closely resembled normal than patients treated with MTX + Et.

Four genes were upregulated in samples from patients that achieved remission with either therapeutic regimen, namely chromodomain helicase DNA-binding protein 2 (*CHD2*), RNA-binding motif protein 25 (*RBM25*), tripartite motif-containing 23 (*TRIM23*) and the *KIAA0907* gene; seven genes were downregulated in both groups of patient samples relative to controls, namely forkhead box O1 (*FOXO1*), 3-phosphoinositide-dependent protein kinase-1 (*PDPK1*), PHD finger protein 20 (*PHF20*), splicing factor, arginine/serine-rich 18 (*SFRS18*), SAPS domain family, member 3 (*SAPS3*), neutral sphingomyelinase activation associated factor (*NSMAF*), and transmembrane protein 140 (*TMEM140*). FOXO proteins have been shown to regulate the expression of the TFN-related apoptosis-inducing ligand (*TRAIL*) [30], a TNF family member that can accelerate the rate of apoptosis in neutrophils [31-33]. TNF has been shown to induce granulocyte apoptosis in a dose-dependent manner, and via differential effects on expression of Mcl-1 and Bfl-1 [34-36]. Twenty-eight statistically significant ($P < 10^{-2}$) canonical pathways were identified from the MTX + Et differentially expressed genes using IPA, many of which are directly associated with inflammation, immunity, or apoptosis (Table 4). These include the RANKL signaling pathway, which regulates bone remodeling, the caspases-dependent apoptotic TWEAK signaling pathway, the CD27 apoptotic signaling pathway, the TNFR2 signaling pathway, the antigen-presenting CD40 signaling pathway, the TNF family and immunoregulatory APRIL and BAFF signaling pathways, the glucocorticoid receptor signaling pathway, and the IL-6 signaling pathway. Many of these differentially expressed genes, such as *ATM*, *BIRC3*, *MAP2K7*, *NFKBIE*, *TRAF3* and *XIAP*, occurred in more than one signaling pathway. Based on the expression patterns of the molecules in Table 4 IPA software predicted decreased cellular apoptosis (3.24×10^{-4}). Collectively, these findings demonstrate an important role of Et in the modulation of the innate immune system of responding patients, which may have implications for this and other diseases.

Between-group comparisons

Having established that CRM is not a return to normal, we next sought to determine the degree to which the homeostatic state induced by MTX alone resembled that induced by the combination of MTX + Et.

We first examined PBMC, comparing the gene expression profiles in JIA patients in remission following treatment with combined MTX + Et to samples from patients treated with MTX alone. Six genes were identified as being differentially expressed in PBMC between these groups (Table S5 in Additional file 5). Four genes were upregulated in patients treated with the combined therapy: cardiotrophin-like cytokine factor 1 *CLCF1* complement component 3 (*C3*), nonprotein-encoding XIST antisense RNA (*TSIX*), and one gene currently lacking annotation (Affymetrix probe set ID 240861_at). Two genes were downregulated in patients using combined therapy: insulin-like growth factor 1 receptor (IGF1R) and the Y-linked protein kinase gene (PRKY).

When the granulocyte expression profiles of children who achieved remission on MTX were compared directly with those who achieved remission on MTX + Et, we found 33 genes (42 probes) that showed differences in expression. This was an expected finding, given that children who had remission on MTX alone had expression profiles that more closely resembled the healthy controls than did children who achieved remission on MTX + Et.

Differential gene expression was also detected with three different probes for the eukaryotic translation initiation factor 1A, Y-linked gene (*EIF1AY*) with no evidence of expression in the MTX + Et samples relative to the MTX alone samples, with six different probes for the nonprotein-coding × (inactive)-specific transcript *(XIST)* with expression above background only in the MTX + Et-treated samples, and with three different probes for the nibrin gene (NBN) expressed above background signal intensities in both groups. Only one gene, the insulin-like growth factor 1 receptor gene (IGF1R), was differentially expressed in both PBMC and neutrophils. However, this gene was overexpressed in granulocytes from patients treated with MTX + Et, but underexpressed in MTX + Et-treated PBMC samples. Collectively, these findings indicate very different effects of Et on different subsets of peripheral blood.

The nibrin gene was overexpressed in MTX + Et relative to both MTX only and controls, as were the genes encoding for cytochrome b-245, beta polypeptide (*CYBB*), haloacid dehalogenase-like hydrolase domain-containing 1A (*HDHD1A*), baculoviral IAP repeat-containing 3 (BIRC3), TNF receptor-associated factor 3 (*TRAF3*), and × (inactive)-specific transcript (*XIST*). The histone cluster 1, H1c (HIST1H1C) gene was found to be downregulated in MTX + Et relative to both MTX only and control samples. No overlap was found among the differentially expressed genes in the MTX only vs. MTX + Et and the MTX only vs. control samples (Table S6 in Additional file 6).

Network analysis of differentially expressed genes

Functional associations between differentially expressed genes identified above were analyzed using the IPA software. It is interesting to note that many of these networks contained hub-and-node structures characteristic of scale-free systems [37] as we have previously reported [38]. While some of these structures may be artifacts that emerge from the algorithms used by IPA to query the existing literature, there is biological coherence in many of the networks, all of which were generated in an unbiased fashion. For example, in both PBMC (Figure 1A, and

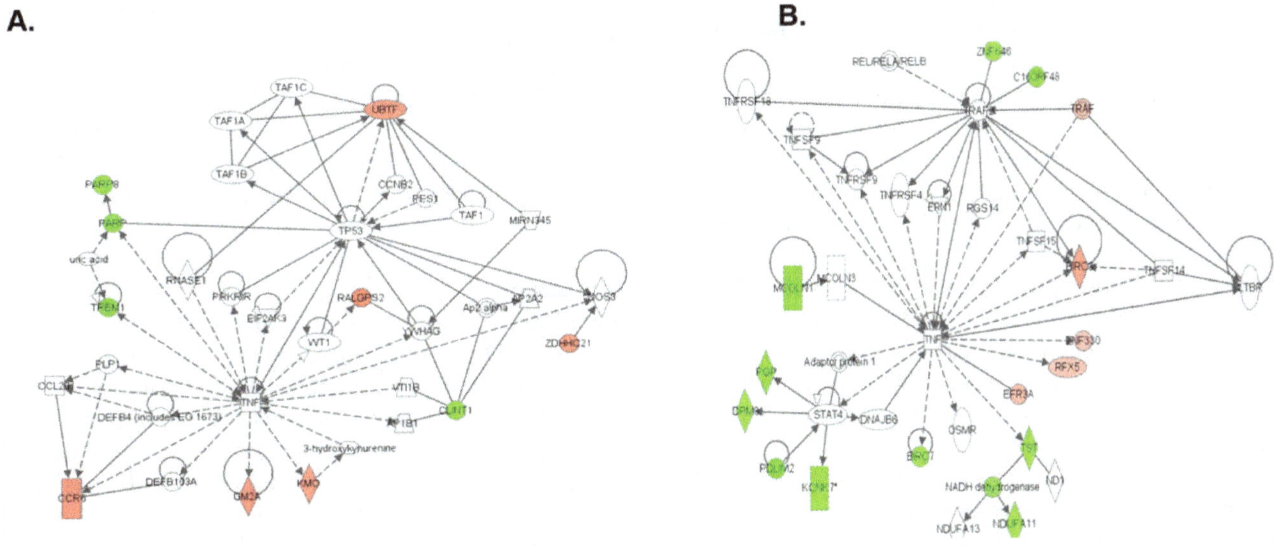

Figure 1 Networks derived from Ingenuity Pathway Analysis software of children who achieved CRM status using MTX + Et compared with healthy controls. Network analysis in PBMC is shown in **(A)** and analysis in granulocytes is shown in **(B)**. Note prominence of TNFA as a hub in these networks. Genes shown in red show higher expression in patients compared with controls, and those shown in green show lower expression..CRM, clinical remission on medication; ET, etanercept; MTX, methotrexate; PBMC, peripheral blood mononuclear cells.

Figure S1 in Additional file 7) and granulocytes (Figure 1B, and Figure S2 in Additional file 8), TNF alpha appears as a hub in at least one network, as would be predicted given Et's mechanism of action. We also noted hub-and-node structured networks derived from both types of cells that demonstrated interactions between the steroid hormone receptor/transcription factor hepatocyte nuclear factor 4 alpha (HNF4α) and differentially expressed gene products in both types of cells (Figure 2). Connections in these networks reflect HNF4α binding to DNA sequences in or adjacent to these genes that were identified by chromatin immunoprecipitation assays [39]. Because HNF4α had not been reported to be expressed in leukocytes, we undertook experiments to investigate this finding further.

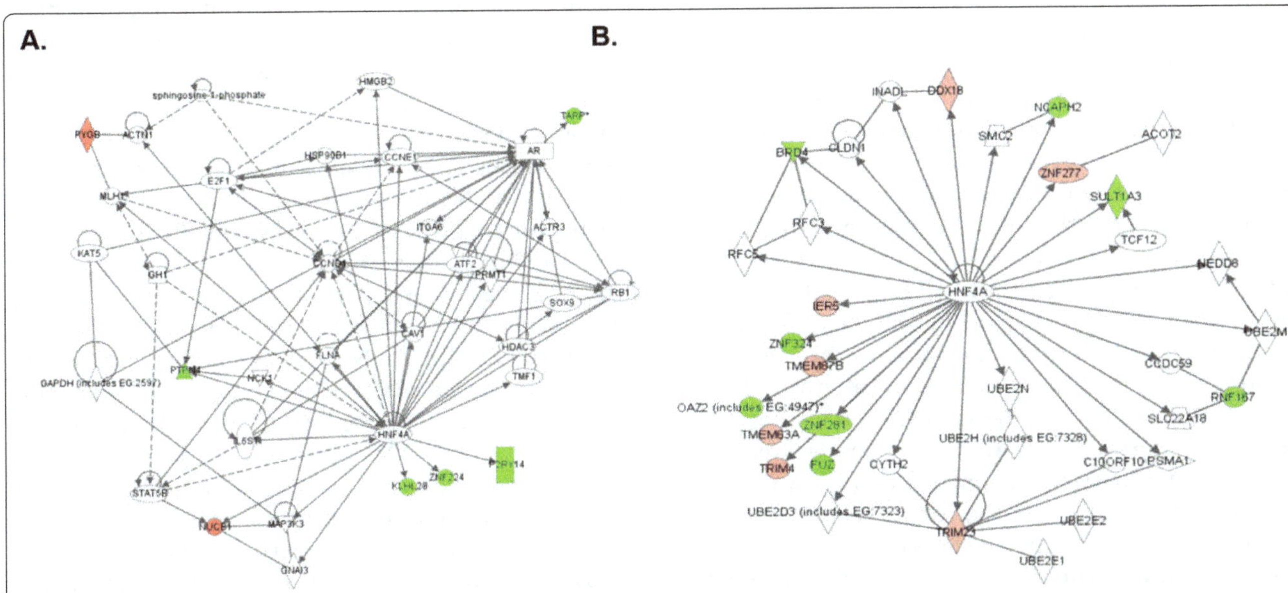

Figure 2 Network derived from Ingenuity Pathway Analysis software of children who achieved CRM status using MTX + Et (A) or MTX alone (B) compared with healthy controls. Network analysis is from PBMC (A) and granulocytes (B). Note the prominence of HNF4α as a hub in both networks. Genes shown in red show higher expression in patients compared with controls, and those shown in green show lower expression. CRM, clinical remission on medication; ET, etanercept; MTX, methotrexate; PBMC, peripheral blood mononuclear cells.

Expression of HNF4α in leukocytes

Network analyses of the microarray data suggested a role for HNF4α in regulating a number of genes associated with remission (for example, Figure 2). HNF4α is a transcription factor and a steroid hormone receptor superfamily member that is expressed mainly in liver and kidney, and at lower levels in pancreatic islets, small intestine and colon [40]. Given the relationship between HNF4α and a number of the differentially expressed genes in PBMC and granulocytes, we tested for the presence of HNF4α protein in human leukocytes using immunofluorescence microscopy. As a positive control, we observed intense nuclear and light cytoplasmic staining in human hepatocellular carcinoma HepG2 cells (Figure 3A). We next examined CD66b+ granulocytes, CD4+ T cells, and CD8+ T cells and detected HNF4α in each of these leukocyte subsets. In T cells, HNF4α immunofluorescent signals were of similar intensity in CD8+ and in CD4+ T cells and lower than intensities observed in CD66b+ granulocytes. All T cells were immunofluorescent positive for HNF4α while one-third of CD66b+ cells were positive. Staining in CD66b+ cells was primarily cytoplasmic, while nuclear and cytoplasmic staining was observed among each T cell subpopulation. All of these findings were observed in cells from healthy children, healthy adults, and children with JIA (data not shown). The findings support the hypothesis that HNF4α is expressed in each of these types of cells and indirectly corroborate the functional interaction of gene products in the networks reported above.

Validation of microarray data

We performed quantitative real-time PCR on RNA obtained from granulocytes and PBMC from the training cohort of patients and healthy controls to confirm the altered pattern of gene expression detected with microarrays. Ten differentially expressed genes identified from microarray expression patterns of PBMC were evaluated (Figure 4A). All genes were similarly over- or under-expressed using both methods. In granulocytes, nine genes that were tested by qRT-PCR exhibited agreement between microarray and quantitative real-time PCR results (Figure 4C). To further confirm the findings from the microarray results, 12 differentially expressed genes identified from microarray expression patterns in PBMC and 14 differentially expressed genes identified from microarray expression patterns in granulocytes were evaluated by quantitative real-time PCR on RNA obtained from the independent testing cohort. The PCR results confirmed the differential expression of 11 of the 12 genes in PBMC (Figure 4B, 92% validation) and 13 of the 14 genes in granulocytes (Figure 4D, 93% validation). The differentially expressed gene *CXCR6* in PBMC and *FOXO1* in neutrophils were not been validated by PCR (data not shown). Five (*IER5, FUZ, RNF167, TRIM4* and *ZNF277*) of the 13 genes we validated in granulocytes were also relevant directly to the HNF4a network mentioned above. *TARP*, which was present in the PBMC network with an *HNF4A* hub (above), was validated by PCR in both training and testing groups. Thus, PCR experiments, including those performed on an independent patient cohort, corroborated results from both the expression and network analysis data.

Discussion

Significant advances have been made in the past 10 to 15 years in the treatment of JIA. Indeed, it is now possible to achieve remission in the majority of children with even the more severe polyarticular-onset forms of this disease, although sustained periods without clinical disease can currently be achieved and maintained only by sustained use of immunosuppressive medications. While preliminary studies from our group suggested that remission (both CRM and CR) in JIA represents a distinct biological 'state' that can be recognized at the molecular level as well as clinically [6], it is critical to derive a deeper understanding of the biological meaning of these states. In particular, since children with JIA can achieve remission on different medications, it is of great interest to know whether remission achieved on MTX leads to an identical immunologic/biologic state as that achieved on a TNF inhibitor. We demonstrate here that children who have achieved the CRM state show significant differences from healthy controls, although those differences are more pronounced in the group who achieved remission on MTX + Et compared with those who achieved remission on MTX alone. The findings here corroborate our smaller, preliminary studies [22] and demonstrate that the CRM state is not a return to 'normal', but rather a re-ordering of transcriptional profiles in leukocytes (and very possibly other cells or tissues) in such a way that pro-inflammatory responses are counterbalanced by anti-inflammatory responses. Furthermore, this re-ordering occurs in cells of both the innate and adaptive immune systems. Findings in this study are thus consistent with previously published work [5,6,22,40] suggesting that, rather than being driven purely by aberrant adaptive immune processes, the pathogenesis of polyarticular JIA likely involves complex interactions between innate and adaptive immunity. For example, 21 of the differentially expressed genes in PBMC in patients (MTX + Et and MTX alone) relative to controls are known to be involved in T cell activation (*AGRN* and *KLRD1*), inflammation response (CFB, AGRN and KLRD1), and cell-cell interaction (*CFB, AGRN* and *PPP1R14A*). The differentially expressed genes in PBMC in patients (MTX alone) relative to controls are involved in T cell and NK cell proliferation (*STAT1* and *KLRK1*) and in T cell apoptosis and death (*SERPINB9, CALR, PRDM1* and *GZMA*).

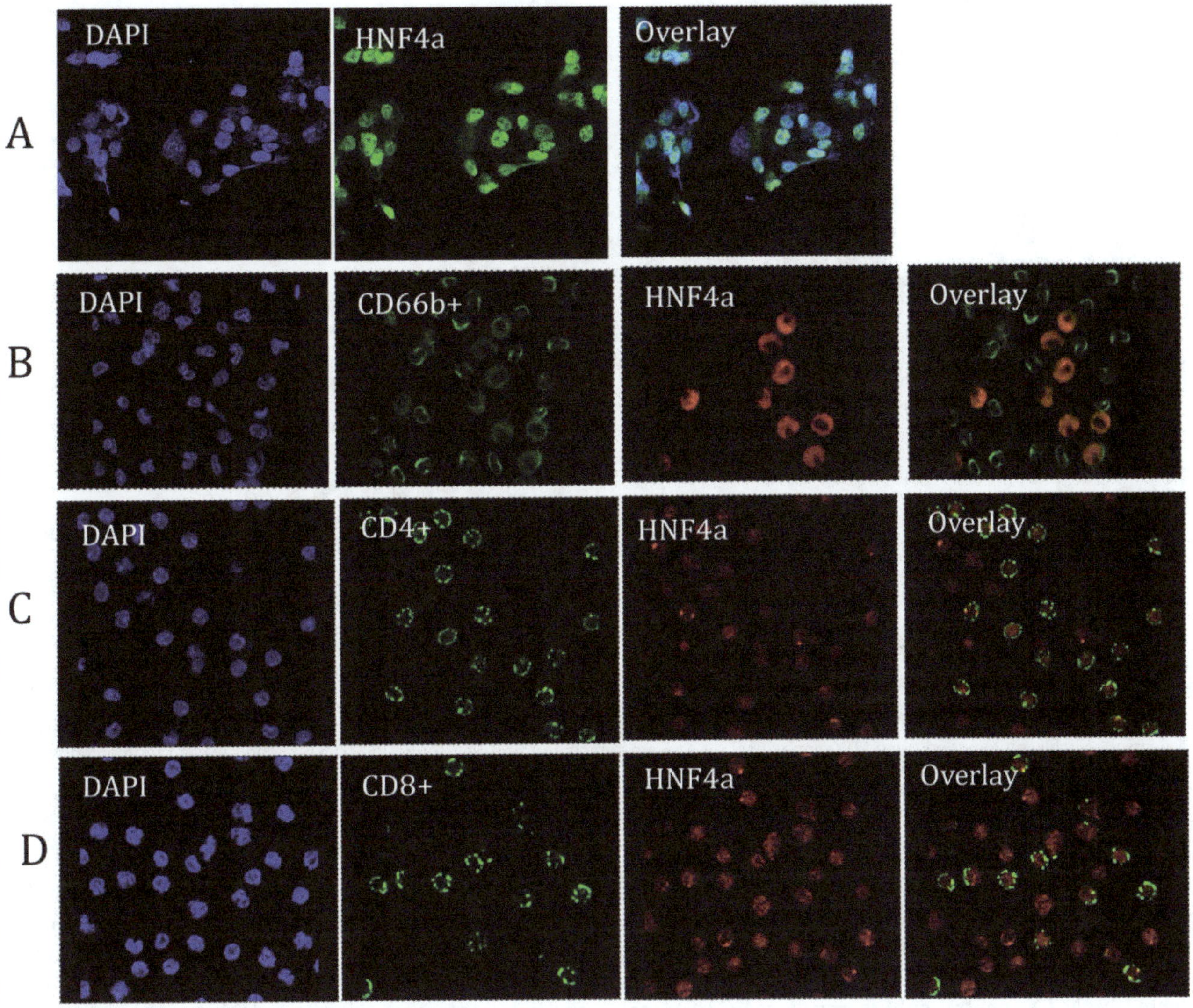

Figure 3 Expression of HNF4α in leukocytes. Indirect immunofluorescence microscopy was used to detect the expression of HNF4α. Cells were fixed in 4% paraformaldehyde and stained with antibodies against human CD4, CD8, CD66b, and HNF4α. **(A)** HepG2 cells as positive control. **(B)** Granulocytes. **(C** and **D)** Peripheral blood mononuclear cells.

The more dramatic differences between children in remission and healthy control children were observed in the expression profiles of granulocytes. This was especially true when we compared children in remission on MTX + Et with the control population. In that comparison, there were 207 genes that showed differential expression. Not surprisingly, many of the differentially expressed genes act through TNF-associated pathways. For example, *ABCF1* can be regulated by TNF-alpha and play a role in enhancement of protein synthesis and the inflammation process [41]. *TNFAIP6*, increased in JIA patient granulocytes, can be induced by pro-inflammatory cytokines such as TNF-alpha and IL-1 [42]. Enhanced levels of TNFAIP6 protein have also been found in the synovial fluid of patients with osteoarthritis and rheumatoid arthritis [43]. GCH1 protein expression and enzyme activity are strongly induced by a mixture of three pro-inflammatory cytokines, IL-1beta, TNF-alpha, and IFN-gamma [44]. XIAP belongs to a family of apoptotic suppressor proteins and acts by binding to TNF receptor-associated factors TRAF1 and TRAF2. This protein also inhibits at least two members of the caspase family of cell-death proteases, caspase-3 and caspase-7. XIAP also regulates innate immune responses by interacting with NOD1 and NOD2 through interaction with RIP2 [45,46].

Despite the large number of differentially expressed genes in granulocytes of patients who responded to MTX + Et therapy, only 23 differentially expressed genes in granulocytes were identified in patients that achieved remission on MTX relative to controls. This

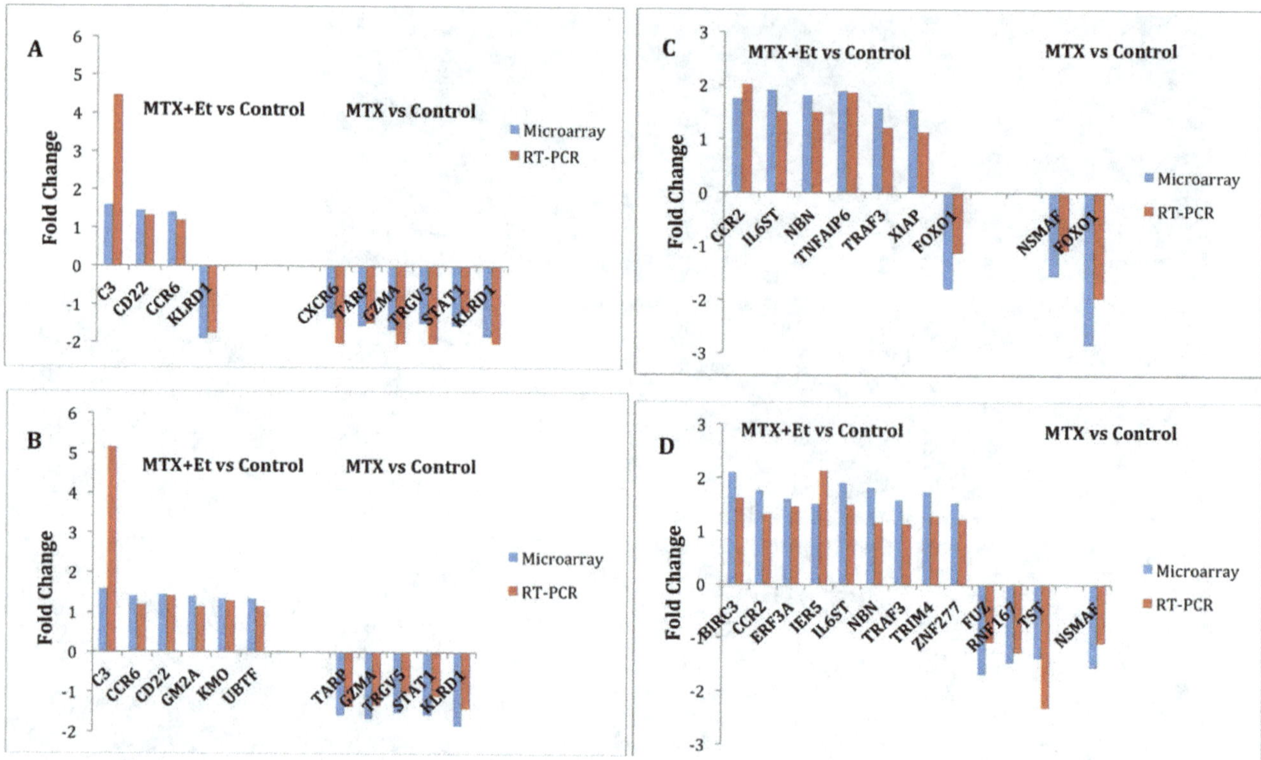

Figure 4 Validation of microarray data for selected genes by real-time PCR. (**A** and **B**) Differentially expressed genes in PBMC from JIA patients who achieved remission using MTX alone or MTX + Et were compared to healthy controls in training cohort (A) and testing cohort (B). (**C** and **D**) Differentially expressed genes in granulocytes from JIA patients who achieved remission using MTX alone or MTX + Et were compared to healthy controls in training cohort (C) and testing cohort (D). ET, etanercept; JIA, juvenile idiopathic arthritis; MTX, methotrexate; PBMC, peripheral blood mononuclear cells.

finding argues that the majority of the MTX +Et transcriptome changes were affected by Et. Nevertheless, there may be functional overlap in genes affected by these therapeutic regimens. For example, among genes affected by MTX, neutral sphingomyelinase (N-SMase) activation associated factor (*NSMAF*), downregulated in MTX-treated patient vs. control samples, is an adaptor protein that constitutively binds to TNF-R1 and is involved in TNF-induced gene expression such as IL-6 and CXCL-2, and leukocyte recruitment, contributing to the establishment of the specific immune response [47]. The effect of these drugs is not limited to TNF-related modifications. Eleven genes (*CHD2, KIAA0907, PHF20, RBM25, NSMAF, FOXO1, PDPK1, SAPS3, SFRS18, TMEM140* and *TRIM23*) were differentially expressed following treatment with MTX or MTX + Et, and participate in various cellular processes including cellular development, carbohydrate metabolism, cell morphology, cell death and gene expression.

A number of differentially expressed genes identified in this study have been shown to bind the transcription factor HNF4α [40]. HNF4α belongs to the steroid hormone receptor superfamily and is enriched in liver [48]. HNF4α contributes to regulation of a large fraction of the liver and pancreatic islet transcriptomes by binding directly to nearly half of the actively transcribed genes in those tissues and plays a role in regulating the cytokine-induced inflammatory response [41,49]. Based on the predicted interaction between HNF4α and a number of differentially expressed genes in this study, we demonstrated expression of HNF4α in leukocytes at the protein level in PBMC and granulocytes from patients with JIA and from healthy controls using immunofluorescence assays. *HNF4A* transcripts were expressed above background signal intensities on the microarrays (data not shown). Our results support the hypothesis that HNF4α controls many genes associated with remission. Although we did not see significant differences in the expression levels of *HNF4A* transcripts in leukocytes between patients and healthy controls, HNF4α may be controlled by posttranscriptional events or may act as a cofactor, interacting with other transcription factors, for example ETS-domain transcription factor ELK1, and not directly bind to DNA to regulate these genes [50]. Some ETS family proteins interact with other transcription factors (AP-1, NF-κB and Stat-5) to co-regulate the expression of cell-type-specific genes, and these interactions coordinate cellular processes in response to diverse signals from cytokines, growth factors, antigens, and cellular stresses [51]. The differences in the intracellular localization of HNF4α observed here in granulocytes and T cells remain to be explained. They may be related to the abundance of other transcriptional binding factors in such cells or to mutations or exon splice variations that are present in the *HNF4A* gene.

Together, our results demonstrate that the remission state in JIA is not the result of a normalization of immune homeostasis. Gene expression in both PBMC and granulocytes remains abnormal when patients in remission are compared with healthy control children. Furthermore, while there are some overlapping points, remission achieved on MTX differs from remission achieved on MTX + Et, especially in granulocytes, suggesting overlapping but not identical 'set points' for each of these remission states.

These findings provide insight into one of the single most important clinical features of chronic arthritis in children: the frequency of disease recurrence and the rarity of true remission (defined by the Wallace group as a full year off all medications without recurrence of disease signs or symptoms). Our studies show that the CRM state is still associated with distinct differences between children in remission (who appear to be completely normal) and perfectly healthy children. The degree to which these abnormalities reflect persistence of the underlying condition itself or a new immunologic homeostasis that emerges because of the drugs themselves is unclear, although our earlier studies [5,6] strongly suggest the latter. Longitudinal studies will be required to monitor the expression of these or other genes prior to, throughout, and after treatment to identify biomarkers that may predict which patients with JIA are likely to respond to particular therapeutic regimens to optimize therapy in the future. These findings represent the first steps in the identification of such molecules.

Conclusions

Remission (CRM) in polyarticular JIA is a distinct biological state that differs from normal. Gene expression profiles of PBMC show little differences whether the CRM state was achieved with MTX or the combination of MTX + Et. However, the CRM state in JIA neutrophils show significant differences depending on whether remission was achieved with MTX or MTX + Et. These findings therefore add evidence to the importance of neutrophils in the pathogenesis of JIA and its response to therapy.

Additional material

Additional file 1: Table S1. Differentially expressed genes in PBMC in JIA patients who achieved remission with methotrexate alone vs. controls. Genes listed more than once indicate different probes for the same gene which showed different values in expression.

Additional file 2: Table S2. Differentially expressed genes in PBMC in JIA patients who achieved remission with etanercept and methotrexate vs. controls. Genes listed more than once indicate different probes for the same gene which showed different values in expression.

Additional file 3: Table S3. Differentially expressed genes in granulocytes of JIA patients who achieved remission with methotrexate and etanercept vs. controls. Genes listed more than once indicate different probes for the same gene which showed different values in expression.

Additional file 4: Table S4. Differentially expressed genes in granulocytes of JIA patients who achieved remission with methotrexate alone vs. controls. Genes listed more than once indicate different probes for the same gene which showed different values in expression.

Additional file 5: Table S5. Differentially expressed genes in PBMC in JIA patients who achieved remission with methotrexate and etanercept vs. methotrexate alone.

Additional file 6: Table S6. Differentially expressed genes in granulocytes in JIA patients who achieved remission with methotrexate and etanercept vs. methotrexate alone. Genes listed more than once indicate different probes for the same gene which showed different values in expression.

Additional file 7: Figure S1. Interactions between products of differentially expressed genes in PBMC from patients with JIA who achieved remission using methotrexate alone (A) or Etanercept and Methotrexate (B) relative to PBMC from controls. Differentially expressed genes entered in the Ingenuity Pathway Analysis program are colored. Genes shown in red show higher expression in patients compared with controls, and those shown in green show lower expression. Genes not colored were added by the IPA program to generate these networks.

Additional file 8: Figure S2. Interactions between products of differentially expressed genes in granulocytes from patients with JIA who achieved remission using methotrexate alone (A) or Etanercept and Methotrexate (B) relative to granulocytes from controls. Differentially expressed genes entered in the Ingenuity Pathway Analysis program are colored. Genes shown in red show higher expression in patients compared with controls, and those shown in green show lower expression. Genes not colored were added by the IPA program to generate these networks.

Abbreviations

AD: active disease; BSA: bovine serum albumin; CR: clinical remission; CRM: clinical remission on medication; ET: etanercept; GO: gene ontology; ID: inactive disease; IL: interleukin; IPA: Ingenuity Pathways Analysis; JIA: juvenile idiopathic arthritis; mAB: monoclonal antibody; MTX: methotrexate; PBS: phosphate-buffered saline; qRT-PCR: quantitative real-time reverse-transcription polymerase chain reaction; PBMC: peripheral blood mononuclear cells; TNF: tumor necrosis factor.

Competing interests

The authors declare that they have no competing interests.

Authors' contribution

KJ, BF and JJ designed and executed the study, analyzed data and prepared the manuscript. YC was involved in sample acquisition and RNA preparation. JO was involved in RNA labeling and scanning. All authors read and approved the final manuscript.

Acknowledgements

Support was received from the National Institutes of Health (P20RR16478, P20RR15577, R01-AI084200 (JNJ), U19AI062629, R01-AR-060604 (JNJ)), the Oklahoma Center for the Advancement of Science and Technology (HR07-139 (JNJ)), and an Innovative Research Grant from the Arthritis Foundation (JNJ). Analyses were performed using BRB-Array Tools version 3.8.0 stable release developed by Dr. Richard Simon and BRB-Array Tools Development Team.

Authors' details
[1]Department of Pediatrics, Pediatric Rheumatology Research, University of Oklahoma Health Sciences Center, Basic Sciences Education Building 235A, Oklahoma City, OK 73104, USA. [2]Microarray Research Facility, Arthritis and Clinical Immunology Program, Oklahoma Medical Research Foundation, 840 NE 13th Street, Oklahoma City, OK 73104, USA. [3]Department of Pediatrics, Rheumatology Research, SUNY Buffalo Clinical and Translational Research Center, 875 Ellicott Street, Buffalo, NY 14203.

References

1. Ringold S, Wallace CA: **Measuring clinical response and remission in juvenile idiopathic arthritis.** *Curr Opin Rheumatol* 2007, **19**:471-476.
2. Jarvis JN: **Juvenile rheumatoid arthritis: a guide for pediatricians.** *Pediatr Ann* 2002, **31**:437-446.
3. Shenoi S, Wallace CA: **Remission in juvenile idiopathic arthritis: current facts.** *Curr Rheumatol Reports* 2010, **12**:80-86.
4. Wallace CA, Ruperto N, Giannini E, Childhood Arthritis and Rheumatology Research Alliance, Pediatric Rheumatology International Trials Organization, Pediatric Rheumatology Collaborative Study Group: **Preliminary criteria for clinical remission for select categories of juvenile idiopathic arthritis.** *J Rheumatol* 2004, **31**:2290-2294.
5. Jarvis JN, Jiang K, Frank MB, Knowlton N, Aggarwal A, Wallace CA, McKee R, Chaser B, Tung C, Smith LB, McGhee JL, Chen Y, Osban J, O'Neil KN, Centola M: **Gene expression profiling in neutrophils of children with polyarticular juvenile idiopathic arthritis.** *Arthritis Rheum* 2009, **60**:1488-1495.
6. Knowlton N, Jiang K, Frank MB, Aggarwal A, Wallace C, McKee R, Chaser B, Tung C, Smith L, Chen Y, Osban J, O'Neil K, Centola M, McGhee JL, Jarvis JN: **The meaning of clinical remission in polyarticular juvenile idiopathic arthritis: gene expression profiling in peripheral blood mononuclear cells identifies distinct disease states.** *Arthritis Rheum* 2009, **60**:892-900.
7. Wallace CA, Huang B, Bandeira M, Ravelli A, Giannini EH: **Patterns of clinical remission in select categories of juvenile idiopathic arthritis.** *Arthritis Rheum* 2005, **52**:3354-3562.
8. Shenoi S, Wallace CA: **Tumor necrosis factor inhibitors in the management of juvenile idiopathic arthritis: an evidence-based review.** *Paediatric Drugs* 2010, **12**:367-377.
9. Petty RE, Southwood TR, Manners P, Baum J, Glass DN, Goldenberg J, He X, Maldonado-Cocco J, Orozco-Alcala J, Prieur AM, Suarez-Almazor ME, Woo P: **International League of Associations for Rheumatology classification of juvenile idiopathic arthritis: second revision Edmonton, 2001.** *J Rheumatol* 2004, **31**:390-392.
10. Diehn M, Sherlock G, Binkley G, Jin H, Matese JC, Hernandez-Boussard T, Rees CA, Cherry JM, Botstein D, Brown PO, Alizadeh AA: **SOURCE: a unified genomic resource of functional annotations, ontologies, and gene expression data.** *Nucleic Acids Research* 2003, **31**:219-223.
11. Ashburner M, Ball CA, Blake JA, Botstein D, Butler H, Cherry JM, Davis AP, Dolinski K, Dwight SS, Eppig JT, Harris MA, Hill DP, Issel-Tarver L, Kasarskis A, Lewis S, Matese JC, Richardson JE, Ringwald M, Rubin GM, Sherlock G: **Gene ontology: tool for the unification of biology. The Gene Ontology Consortium.** *Nature Genet* 2000, **25**:25-29.
12. Gentleman RC, Carey VJ, Bates DM, Bolstad B, Dettling M, Dudoit S, Ellis B, Gautier L, Ge Y, Gentry J, Hornik K, Hothorn T, Huber W, Iacus S, Irizarry R, Leisch F, Li C, Maechler M, Rossini AJ, Sawitzki G, Smith C, Smyth G, Tierney L, Yang JY, Zhang J: **Bioconductor: open software development for computational biology and bioinformatics.** *Genome Biology* 2004, **5**: R80.
13. Piekorz RP, Nemetz C, Hocke GM: **Members of the family of IL-6-type cytokines activate Stat5a in various cell types.** *Biochem Biophys Res Commun* 1997, **236**:438-443.
14. Huang Q, Jin X, Gaillard ET, Knight BL, Pack FD, Stoltz JH, Jayadev S, Blanchard KT: **Gene expression profiling reveals multiple toxicity endpoints induced by hepatotoxicants.** *Mutat Res* 2004, **549**:147-167.
15. Kim YJ, Song M, Ryu JC: **Inflammation in methotrexate-induced pulmonary toxicity occurs via the p38 MAPK pathway.** *Toxicology* 2009, **256**:183-190.
16. Sower LE, Froelich CJ, Allegretto N, Rose PM, Hanna WD, Klimpel GR: **Extracellular activities of human granzyme A. Monocyte activation by granzyme A versus alpha-thrombin.** *J Immunol* 1996, **156**:2585-2590.
17. Takeda K, Akira S: **STAT family of transcription factors in cytokine-mediated biological responses.** *Cytokine Growth Factor Rev* 2000, **11**:199-207.
18. Proskuryakov SY, Konoplyannikov AG, Gabai VL: **Necrosis: a specific form of programmed cell death?** *Exp Cell Res* 2003, **283**:1-16.
19. Lovo E, Zhang M, Wang L, Ashton-Rickardt PG: **Serine protease inhibitor 6 is required to protect dendritic cells from the kiss of death.** *J Immunol* 2012, **188**:1057-1063.
20. Sutherland CL, Chalupny NJ, Schooley K, VandenBos T, Kubin M, Cosman D: **UL16-binding proteins, novel MHC class I-related proteins, bind to NKG2D and activate multiple signaling pathways in primary NK cells.** *J Immunol* 2002, **168**:671-679.
21. Andreakos E, Sacre S, Foxwell BM, Feldmann M: **The toll-like receptor-nuclear factor kappaB pathway in rheumatoid arthritis.** *Front Biosci* 2005, **10**:2478-2488.
22. Jarvis JN, Petty HR, Tang Y, Frank MB, Tessier PA, Dozmorov I, Jiang K, Kindzelski A, Chen Y, Cadwell C, Turner M, Szodoray P, McGhee JL, Centola M: **Evidence for chronic peripheral activation of neutrophils in polyarticular juvenile rheumatoid arthritis.** *Arthritis Res Ther* 2006, **8**:R154.
23. Nakamura N, Shimaoka Y, Tougan T, Onda H, Okuzaki D, Zhao H, Fujimori A, Yabuta N, Nagamori I, Tanigawa A, Sato J, Oda T, Hayashida K, Suzuki R, Yukioka M, Nojima H, Ochi T: **Isolation and expression profiling of genes upregulated in bone marrow-derived mononuclear cells of rheumatoid arthritis patients.** *DNA Res* 2006, **13**:169-183.
24. Goëb V, Thomas-L'Otellier M, Daveau R, Charlionet R, Fardellone P, Le Loët X, Tron F, Gilbert D, Vittecoq O: **Candidate autoantigens identified by mass spectrometry in early rheumatoid arthritis are chaperones and citrullinated glycolytic enzymes.** *Arthritis Res Ther* 2009, **11**:R38.
25. Belinsky GS, Parke AL, Huang Q, Blanchard K, Jayadev S, Stoll R, Rothe M, Achenie LE, Gupta RR, Wu GY, Rosenberg DW: **The contribution of methotrexate exposure and host factors on transcriptional variance in human liver.** *Toxicol Sci* 2007, **97**:582-594.
26. Cyster JG, Goodnow CC: **Tuning antigen receptor signaling by CD22: integrating cues from antigens and the microenvironment.** *Immunity* 1997, **6**:509-517.
27. Nitschke L, Carsetti R, Ocker B, Köhler G, Lamers MC: **CD22 is a negative regulator of B-cell receptor signalling.** *Curr Biol* 1997, **7**:133-143.
28. Netea MG, Azam T, Ferwerda G, Girardin SE, Kim SH, Dinarello CA: **Triggering receptor expressed on myeloid cells-1 (TREM-1) amplifies the signals induced by the NACHT-LRR (NLR) pattern recognition receptors.** *J Leukoc Biol* 2006, **80**:1454-1461.
29. Dower K, Ellis DK, Saraf K, Jelinsky SA, Lin LL: **Innate immune responses to TREM-1 activation: overlap, divergence, and positive and negative cross-talk with bacterial lipopolysaccharide.** *J Immunol* 2008, **180**:3520-3534.
30. Modur V, Nagarajan R, Evers BM, Milbrandt J: **FOXO proteins regulate tumor necrosis factor-related apoptosis inducing ligand expression. Implications for PTEN mutation in prostate cancer.** *J Biol Chem* 2002, **277**:47928-47937.
31. Renshaw SA, Parmar JS, Singleton V, Rowe SJ, Dockrell DH, Dower SK, Bingle CD, Chilvers ER, Whyte MK: **Acceleration of human neutrophil apoptosis by TRAIL.** *J Immunol* 2003, **170**:1027-1033.
32. Wright HL, Moots RJ, Bucknall RC, Edwards SW: **Neutrophil function in inflammation and inflammatory diseases.** *Rheumatology (Oxford)* 2010, **49**:1618-1631.
33. Grivennikov SI, Tumanov AV, Liepinsh DJ, Kruglov AA, Marakusha BI, Shakhov AN, Murakami T, Drutskaya LN, Förster I, Clausen BE, Tessarollo L, Ryffel B, Kuprash DV, Nedospasov SA: **Distinct and nonredundant in vivo functions of TNF produced by t cells and macrophages/neutrophils: protective and deleterious effects.** *Immunity* 2005, **22**:93-104.
34. Salamone G, Giordano M, Trevani AS, Gamberale R, Vermeulen M, Schettinni J, Geffner JR: **Promotion of neutrophil apoptosis by TNF-alpha.** *J Immunol* 2001, , **166**: 3476-3483.
35. van den Berg JM, Weyer S, Weening JJ, Roos D, Kuijpers TW: **Divergent effects of tumor necrosis factor alpha on apoptosis of human neutrophils.** *J Leukoc Biol* 2001, **69**:467-473.
36. Cross A, Moots RJ, Edwards SW: **The dual effects of TNFalpha on neutrophil apoptosis are mediated via differential effects on expression of Mcl-1 and Bfl-1.** *Blood* 2008, **111**:878-884.

37. Barbasi AL, Albert A: **Emergence of scaling in networks.** *Science* 1999, **286**:509-512.
38. Jeong H, Tombor B, Oltval ZN, Barabasi A-L: **The large-scale organization of metabolic networks.** *Nature* 2000, **407**:651-654.
39. Frank MB, Wang S, Aggarwal A, Knowlton N, Jiang K, Chen Y, McKee R, Chaser B, McGhee T, Osban J, Jarvis JN: **Disease-associated pathophysiologic structures in pediatric rheumatic diseases show characteristics of scale-free networks seen in physiologic systems: implications for pathogenesis and treatment.** *BMC Med Genomics* 2009, **2**:9-23.
40. Odom DT, Zizlsperger N, Gordon DB, Bell GW, Rinaldi NJ, Murray HL, Volkert TL, Schreiber J, Rolfe PA, Gifford DK, Fraenkel E, Bell GI, Young RA: **Control of pancreas and liver gene expression by HNF transcription factors.** *Science* 2004, **303**:1378-1381.
41. Ihara A, Yamagata K, Nammo T, Miura A, Yuan M, Tanaka T, Sladek FM, Matsuzawa Y, Miyagawa J, Shimomura I: **Functional characterization of the HNF4alpha isoform (HNF4alpha8) expressed in pancreatic beta-cells.** *Biochem Biophys Res Commun* 2005, **329**:984-990.
42. Richard M, Drouin R, Beaulieu AD: **ABC50, a novel human ATP-binding cassette protein found in tumor necrosis factor-alpha-stimulated synoviocytes.** *Genomics* 1998, **53**:137-145.
43. Wisniewski HG, Hua JC, Poppers DM, Naime D, VilEek J, Cronsteint BN: **TNF/ IL-1 -inducible protein TSG-6 potentiates plasmin inhibition by inter-alpha-inhibitor and exerts a strong anti-inflammatory effect in vivo.** *J Immunol* 1996, **156**:1609-1615.
44. Fujikado N, Saijo S, Iwakura Y: **Identification of arthritis-related gene clusters by microarray analysis of two independent mouse models for rheumatoid arthritis.** *Arthritis Res Ther* 2006, **8**:R100.
45. Chiarini A, Armato U, Pacchiana R, DalPra I: **Proteomic analysis of GTP cyclohydrolase 1 multiprotein complexes in cultured normal adult human astrocytes under both basal and cytokine-activated conditions.** *Proteomics* 2009, **9**:1850-1860.
46. Sanna MG, da Silva Correia J, Luo Y, Chuang B, Paulson LM, Nguyen B, Deveraux QL, Ulevitch RJ: **ILPIP, a novel anti-apoptotic protein that enhances XIAP-mediated activation of JNK1 and protection against apoptosis.** *J Biol Chem* 2002, **277**:30454-30462.
47. Krieg A, Correa RG, Garrison JB, Le Negrate G, Welsh K, Huang Z, Knoefel WT, Reed JC: **XIAP mediates NOD signaling via interaction with RIP2.** *Proc Natl Acad Sci USA* 2009, **106**:14524-14529.
48. Montfort A, de Badts B, Douin-Echinard V, Martin PG, Iacovoni J, Nevoit C, Therville N, Garcia V, Bertrand MA, Bessières MH, Trombe MC, Levade T, Benoist H, Ségui B: **FAN stimulates TNF(alpha)-induced gene expression, leukocyte recruitment, and humoral response.** *J Immunol* 2009, **183**:5369-5378.
49. Cheung C, Akiyama TE, Kudo G, Gonzalez FJ: **Hepatic expression of cytochrome P450s in hepatocyte nuclear factor 1-alpha (HNF1alpha)-deficient mice.** *Biochem Pharmacol* 2003, **66**:2011-2020.
50. Wang Z, Bishop EP, Burke PA: **Expression profile analysis of the inflammatory response regulated by hepatocyte nuclear factor 4 α.** *BMC Genomics* 2011, **12**:128.
51. Li R, Pei H, Watson DK: **Regulation of Ets function by protein-protein interactions.** *Oncogene* 2000, **19**:6514-6523.

Permissions

All chapters in this book were first published in AR&T, by BioMed Central; hereby published with permission under the Creative Commons Attribution License or equivalent. Every chapter published in this book has been scrutinized by our experts. Their significance has been extensively debated. The topics covered herein carry significant findings which will fuel the growth of the discipline. They may even be implemented as practical applications or may be referred to as a beginning point for another development.

The contributors of this book come from diverse backgrounds, making this book a truly international effort. This book will bring forth new frontiers with its revolutionizing research information and detailed analysis of the nascent developments around the world.

We would like to thank all the contributing authors for lending their expertise to make the book truly unique. They have played a crucial role in the development of this book. Without their invaluable contributions this book wouldn't have been possible. They have made vital efforts to compile up to date information on the varied aspects of this subject to make this book a valuable addition to the collection of many professionals and students.

This book was conceptualized with the vision of imparting up-to-date information and advanced data in this field. To ensure the same, a matchless editorial board was set up. Every individual on the board went through rigorous rounds of assessment to prove their worth. After which they invested a large part of their time researching and compiling the most relevant data for our readers.

The editorial board has been involved in producing this book since its inception. They have spent rigorous hours researching and exploring the diverse topics which have resulted in the successful publishing of this book. They have passed on their knowledge of decades through this book. To expedite this challenging task, the publisher supported the team at every step. A small team of assistant editors was also appointed to further simplify the editing procedure and attain best results for the readers.

Apart from the editorial board, the designing team has also invested a significant amount of their time in understanding the subject and creating the most relevant covers. They scrutinized every image to scout for the most suitable representation of the subject and create an appropriate cover for the book.

The publishing team has been an ardent support to the editorial, designing and production team. Their endless efforts to recruit the best for this project, has resulted in the accomplishment of this book. They are a veteran in the field of academics and their pool of knowledge is as vast as their experience in printing. Their expertise and guidance has proved useful at every step. Their uncompromising quality standards have made this book an exceptional effort. Their encouragement from time to time has been an inspiration for everyone.

The publisher and the editorial board hope that this book will prove to be a valuable piece of knowledge for researchers, students, practitioners and scholars across the globe.

List of Contributors

Sorcha Finnegan
Arthritis Research Group, Queen's University Belfast, Centre for Infection and Immunity, Health Sciences Building, 97 Lisburn Road, Belfast BT9 7BL, UK

Madeleine E Rooney
Arthritis Research Group, Queen's University Belfast, Centre for Infection and Immunity, Health Sciences Building, 97 Lisburn Road, Belfast BT9 7BL, UK
Pediatric Rheumatology, Withers Ward, Musgrave Park Hospital, 20 Stockman's Lane, Belfast BT9 7JB, UK

David S Gibson
Arthritis Research Group, Queen's University Belfast, Centre for Infection and Immunity, Health Sciences Building, 97 Lisburn Road, Belfast BT9 7BL, UK
Northern Ireland Centre for Stratified Medicine, C-TRIC Building, Altnagelvin Hospital campus, Glenshane Road, Londonderry BT47 6SB, UK

Joanne Robson
School of Biological and Biomedical Sciences, Durham University, Durham DH1 3LE, UK

Caitriona Scaife and Stephen R Pennington
Proteome Research Centre, UCD Conway Institute for Biomolecular and Biomedical Research, University College Dublin, Dublin, Ireland

Catherine McAllister
Pediatric Rheumatology, Withers Ward, Musgrave Park Hospital, 20 Stockman's Lane, Belfast BT9 7JB, UK

Kristyna Brabnikova-Maresova, Katerina Jarosova, Karel Pavelka and Jan J Stepan
Institute of Rheumatology, Na Slupi 4, 128 50 Prague 2, Czech Republic
Department of Rheumatology, First Faculty of Medicine, Charles University in Prague, Kateřinská 32, 121 08 Prague 2, Czech Republic

Koert M. Dolman
Sint Lucas Andreas Hospital and Reade location Jan van Breemen, Amsterdam, The Netherlands

Jaak Kals
Department of Biochemistry, Institute of Biomedicine and Translational Medicine, The Centre of Excellence for Translational Medicine, Faculty of Medicine, University of Tartu, Tartu, Estonia
Department of Vascular Surgery, Tartu University Hospital, Tartu, Estonia

Erik Salum
Department of Cardiology, Faculty of Medicine, University of Tartu, Tartu, Estonia

Janneke Anink, Lisette W. A. Van Suijlekom-Smit, Marieke H. Otten and Femke H. M. Prince
Department of Pediatrics/Pediatric Rheumatology, Erasmus MC Sophia Children's Hospital Rotterdam, Rotterdam, The Netherlands

Marion A. J. van Rossum
Department of Pediatrics/Pediatric Rheumatology Academic Medical Centre Emma Children's Hospital and Reade location Jan van Breemen, Amsterdam, The Netherlands

Esther P. A. H. Hoppenreijs
Sint Maartenskliniek and Radboud University Nijmegen Medical Centre, Nijmegen, The Netherlands

Rebecca ten Cate
Leiden University Medical Centre, Leiden, The Netherlands

Simona Ursu and Lucy R. Wedderburn
Infection, Immunity, Inflammation and Physiological Medicine Programme UCL Institute of Child Health, University College London, London, UK

Marion AJ van Rossum
Department of Pediatric Hematology, Immunology, Rheumatology and Infectious Disease, Emma Children's Hospital, Academic Medical Center, Meibergdreef 9, 1105 AZ Amsterdam, The Netherlands
Department of Pediatric Rheumatology, Reade location Jan van Breemen, Dr. Jan van Breeemenstraat 2, 1056 AB Amsterdam, The Netherlands

Gerd Horneff
Centre of Pediatric Rheumatology, Department of General Pediatrics, Asklepios Clinic Sankt Augustin, Sankt Augustin, Germany

Michael Frosch
German Pediatric Pain Centre, Children's and Adolescents' Hospital, Datteln, Germany

Thomas Vogl and Johannes Roth
Institute of Immunology, University Hospital Muenster and Interdisciplinary Centre for Clinical Research IZKF, University Hospital Muenster, Muenster, Germany

Faekah Gohar, Dirk Foell and Dirk Holzinger
Interdisciplinary Centre for Clinical Research IZKF, University Hospital Muenster, Muenster and Department of Pediatric Rheumatology and Immunology, University Children's Hospital Muenster, Muenster, Germany

Carol M. Artlett and Sihem Sassi-Gaha
Department of Microbiology and Immunology, Drexel University College of Medicine, 2900 Queen Lane, Philadelphia, PA 19129, USA

Ronald C. Ramos
Department of Medicine, Thomas Jefferson University, 1020 Walnut Street, Philadelphia, PA 19107, USA
Agis Global, Business Development Executive, 1266 East Main Street, Stamford, CT 06902, USA

Frederick W. Miller and Lisa G. Rider
National Institute of Environmental Health Sciences, National Institutes of Health, Department of Health and Human Services, Environmental Autoimmunity Group, Program of Clinical Research, 9000 Rockville Pike, Bethesda, MD 20892, USA

James C. McElnay
Clinical and Practice Research Group, School of Pharmacy, Queen's University Belfast, 97 Lisburn Road, BT9 7BL Belfast, UK

Ahmed F. Hawwa
Clinical and Practice Research Group, School of Pharmacy, Queen's University Belfast, 97 Lisburn Road, BT9 7BL Belfast, UK
Aston Pharmacy School, Aston University, Birmingham, UK

AbdelQader AlBawab
Clinical and Practice Research Group, School of Pharmacy, Queen's University Belfast, 97 Lisburn Road, BT9 7BL Belfast, UK
Faculty of Pharmacy, Al Zaytoonah University, Amman, Jordan

Madeleine Rooney
Centre for Infection and Immunity, School of Medicine and Biomedical Sciences, Queen's University Belfast, Belfast, UK

Lucy R. Wedderburn
Institute of Child Health, University College London, London, UK
Arthritis Research UK Centre for Adolescent Rheumatology, University College London, University College London Hospital, London, UK
Department of Rheumatology, Great Ormond Street Hospital NHS Foundation Trust, London, UK

Michael W. Beresford
Department of Women's and Children's Health, Institute of Translational Medicine, University of Liverpool, The Alder Hey Children's NHS Foundation Trust, Liverpool, UK

Lisha Zhu
Department of Biochemistry, Jacobs School of Medicine and Biomedical Sciences, University at Buffalo, Buffalo, NY, USA

Tao Liu
Department of Biochemistry, Jacobs School of Medicine and Biomedical Sciences, University at Buffalo, Buffalo, NY, USA
Genetics, Genomics, & Bioinformatics Program, Jacobs School of Medicine and Biomedical Sciences, University at Buffalo, Buffalo, NY, USA

Karstin Webber
Graduate Program in Biological Sciences, Jacobs School of Medicine and Biomedical Sciences, University at Buffalo, Buffalo, NY, USA

Kaiyu Jiang, Laiping Wong and Yanmin Chen
Department of Pediatrics, Jacobs School of Medicine and Biomedical Sciences, University at Buffalo, Buffalo, NY, USA
Department of Pediatrics, University at Buffalo Jacobs School of Medicine and Biomedical Sciences, Clinical & Translational Research Center, 875 Ellicott St., Buffalo, NY, USA

Jaanika Ilisson, Vallo Tillmann and Chris Pruunsild
Department of Paediatrics, Faculty of Medicine, University of Tartu, Lunini 6, Tartu 51014, Estonia
Children's Clinic, Tartu University Hospital, Tartu, Estonia

Kaire Heilman
Department of Paediatrics, Faculty of Medicine, University of Tartu, Lunini 6, Tartu 51014, Estonia
Tallinn Children's Hospital, Tallinn, Estonia

Kersti Zilmer, Mihkel Zilmer, Anneli Piir and Maksim Zagura
Department of Biochemistry, Institute of Biomedicine and Translational Medicine, The Centre of Excellence for Translational Medicine, Faculty of Medicine, University of Tartu, Tartu, Estonia
Department of Cardiology, Faculty of Medicine, University of Tartu, Tartu, Estonia

Ashley D. Sawle
Irving Cancer institute, Columbia University College of Physicians and Surgeons, 1130 Saint Nicholas Ave., New York, NY 10032, USA

M. Barton Frank
Oklahoma Medical Research Foundation, Arthritis & Clinical Immunology Program, 800 NE 13th St., Oklahoma City, OK 73104, USA

Carol A. Wallace
Division of Rheumatology, Seattle Children's Hospital and Research Institute, 4800 Sand Point Way NE, MA.7.110, Seattle, WA 98105, USA
Genetics, Genomics, and Bioinformatics Program, University at Buffalo Jacobs School of Medicine and Biomedical Sciences, Buffalo, NY, USA

Faekah Gohar, Christoph Kessel, Miha Lavric, Dirk Holzinger and Dirk Foell
Department of Paediatric Rheumatology and Immunology, University of Münster, Domagkstraße 3, D-48149 Münster, Germany

Timothy Beukelman, Fenglong Xie, John W. Baddley, Lang Chen, Melissa L. Mannion, Kenneth G. Saag, Jie Zhang and Jeffrey R. Curtis
The University of Alabama at Birmingham, 1720 2nd Ave S, Birmingham, AL, 35233, USA

Gerd Horneff and Ariane Klein
Department of Pediatrics, Centre of General Pediatrics and Neonatology, Asklepios Clinic Sankt Augustin, 53757 Sankt Augustin, Germany

Jens Klotsche and Kirsten Minden
German Rheumatism Research Centre Berlin, and Children's University Hospital Charité, Berlin, Germany

Hans-Iko Huppertz and Frank Weller-Heinemann
Prof Hess Children's Hospital, Bremen, Germany

Jasmin Kuemmerle-Deschner
Department of Pediatrics, University of Tuebingen, 72076 Tuebingen, Germany

Johannes-Peter Haas
German Centre for Pediatric and Adolescent Rheumatology, Garmisch-Partenkirchen, Germany

Anton Hospach
Department of Pediatrics, Section of Rheumatology, Olgahospital, Klinikum, Stuttgart, Germany

Joost Swart and Nico Wulffraat
Department of Pediatric Immunology and Rheumatology, Wilhelmina Children's Hospital, Lundlaan, 6 Utrecht, The Netherlands

Gabriella Giancane, Nicolino Ruperto, Francesca Bovis and Francesca Bagnasco
IRCCS Istituto Giannina Gaslini, Clinica Pediatrica e Reumatologia, PRINTO, Via Gaslini, 5, 16147 Genoa, Italy

Gerd Horneff
Asklepios Clinic Sankt Augustin, Arnold-Janssen strasse 29, Sankt Augustin, Germany
Department of Pediatric and Adolescents medicine, Medical faculty, University Hospital of Cologne, Kerpener Str. 62, Cologne, Germany

Bo Magnusson
Karolinska University Hospital, Pediatric Rheumatology Unit, Stockholm, Sweden

Michael Hofer
Unité Romande d'Immuno-Rhumatologie Pediatrique/Centre Hospitalier Universitaire Vaudois (CHUV), Pediatrie, University of Lausanne, Av Bugnon 46, Lausanne, Switzerland
University Hospital of Geneva, Geneva, Switzerland

Alessandro Consolaro
IRCCS Istituto Giannina Gaslini, Clinica Pediatrica e Reumatologia, via Gaslini 5, Genoa, Italy
Dipartimento di Neuroscienze, Riabilitazione, Oftalmologia, Genetica e Scienze Materno-Infantili (DiNOGMI), Università degli Studi di Genova, Genoa, Italy

Angela Pistorio
IRCCS Istituto Giannina Gaslini, Servizio di Epidemiologia e Biostatistica, via Gaslini 5, Genoa, Italy

Alberto Martini
IRCCS Istituto Giannina Gaslini, Direzione Scientifica, via Gaslini 5, Genoa, Italy
University of Genova and Istituto Giannina Gaslini, Pediatria II-PRINTO, Genoa, Italy

Arndt H. Brachat
Novartis Institutes for Biomedical Research, Basel, Switzerland

Alexei A. Grom, Hermine I. Brunner and Daniel J. Lovell
Cincinnati Children's Hospital Medical Center, PRCSG, Cincinnati, OH, USA

Nico Wulffraat
Wilhelmina Kinderziekenhuis, Department of Pediatric Immunology and Rheumatology, Utrecht, Netherlands

Pierre Quartier
Université Paris-Descartes, IMAGINE Institute, Hôpital Necker-Enfants Malades. Centre de référence national pour les Arthrites Juveniles, Unité d'Immunologie, Hématologie et Rhumatologie Pediatrique, Paris, France

Riva Brik
Rambam Medical Center, Department of Pediatrics B, Haifa, Israel

Liza McCann
Alder Hey Children's NHS Foundation Trust, Liverpool, Uk

Ken Abrams
Novartis Pharmaceuticals Corporation, East Hanover, NJ, USA

Rachelle Donn
Centre for Musculoskeletal Research, University of Manchester, Manchester M13 9PT, UK

Nanguneri R. Nirmala
Novartis Institutes for Biomedical Research, Cambridge, MA, USA

Nicolino Ruperto
Istituto Giannina Gaslini, Pediatria II-PRINTO, Genoa, Italy

Ariane Klein, Georg Werner Just and Gerd Horneff
Centre for Paediatric Rheumatology, Department of Paediatrics, Asklepios Clinic Sankt Augustin, Arnold-Janssen-Strasse 29, 53757 Sankt Augustin, Germany

Stephanie Gabriele Werner
HELIOS Klinikum Duisburg, Klinik für Rheumatologie, Duisburg, Germany

Prasad T. Oommen
Department of Pediatric Oncology, Hematology and Clinical Immunology, University Children's Hospital, Medical Faculty, Heinrich-Heine-University, Düsseldorf, Germany

Kirsten Minden
Charité University Medicine and Epidemiology Unit, German Rheumatism Research Centre, Berlin, Germany

Ingrid Becker
Institute of Medical Statistics, University of Cologne, Cologne, Nordrhein-Westfalen, Germany

Hans-Eckhard Langer
RHIO (Rheumatologie, Immunologie, Osteologie) Düsseldorf, Düsseldorf, Germany

Dirk Klee
Department of Diagnostic and Interventional Radiology, University Düsseldorf, Medical Faculty, Moorenstraße 5, 40225 Düsseldorf, Germany

Veronika Rypdal and Ellen Nordal
Department of Pediatrics, University Hospital of North Norway, Tromsø, Norway
Department of Clinical Medicine, UIT the Arctic University of Norway, Tromsø, Norway

Ellen Dalen Arnstad
Department of Clinical and Molecular Medicine, NTNU - Norwegian University of Science and Technology, Trondheim, Norway
Department of Pediatrics, Levanger Hospital, Nord-Trøndelag Hospital Trust, Levanger, Norway

Marite Rygg
Department of Clinical and Molecular Medicine, NTNU - Norwegian University of Science and Technology, Trondheim, Norway
Department of Pediatrics, St. Olavs Hospital, Trondheim, Norway

Kristiina Aalto and Suvi Peltoniemi
Hospital for Children and Adolescents, University of Helsinki, Helsinki, Finland

Lillemor Berntson
Department of Women's and Children's Health, Uppsala University, Uppsala, Sweden

Maria Ekelund
Department of Women's and Children's Health, Uppsala University, Uppsala, Sweden
Department of Pediatrics, Ryhov County Hospital, Jonkoping, Sweden

Anders Fasth
Department of Pediatrics, Institute of Clinical Sciences, Sahlgrenska Academy, University of Gothenburg, Gothenburg, Sweden

Mia Glerup and Troels Herlin
Department of Pediatrics, Aarhus University Hospital, Aarhus, Denmark

Susan Nielsen and Marek Zak
Department of Pediatrics, Rigshospitalet Copenhagen University Hospital, Copenhagen, Denmark

Martin Rypdal
Department of Mathematics and Statistics, UIT the Arctic University of Norway, Tromsø, Norway

Miriam Listing, Ina Liedmann, Martina Niewerth, Claudia Sengler and Joachim Listing
Deutsches Rheuma-Forschungszentrum Berlin, Epidemiology Unit, Charitéplatz 1, 10117 Berlin, Germany

Jens Klotsche and Kirsten Minden
Deutsches Rheuma-Forschungszentrum Berlin, Epidemiology Unit, Charitéplatz 1, 10117 Berlin, Germany
Charité - Universitätsmedizin Berlin, epartment of Rheumatology and Clinical Immunology, Berlin, Germany

Kirsten Mönkemöller
Kinderkrankenhaus Amsterdamer Straße, Kliniken der Stadt Köln gGmbH, Köln, Germany

Dirk Foell
Department of Pediatric Rheumatology and Immunology, University of Münster, Münster, Germany

Arnd Heiligenhaus
Department of Ophthalmology at St. Franziskus Hospital Münster, University of Duisburg-Essen, Duisburg, Germany

Ariane Klein and Gerd Horneff
Asklepios Klinik Sankt Augustin, Sankt Augustin, Germany

Gerd Ganser
St. Josef-Stift Sendenhorst, Sendenhorst, Germany

Johannes-Peter Haas
Deutsches Zentrum für Kinder- und Jugendrheumatologie, Garmisch-Partenkirchen, Germany

Boris Hügle, Nadine Fischer and Johannes-Peter Haas
German Center for Pediatric and Adolescent Rheumatology, Gehfeldstrasse 24, 82467 Garmisch-Partenkirchen, Germany

Anastasia Schippers, Kim Ohl, Bernd Denecke and Klaus Tenbrock
Department of Pediatrics, Universitätsklinikum Aachen, Aachen, Germany

Fabio Ticconi and Ivan G. Costa
IZKF Research Group Bioinformatics, RWTH Aachen Medical Faculty, Aachen, Germany

Bas Vastert
University Medical Center Utrecht, Utrecht, Netherlands

Janneke Anink and Lisette WA van Suijlekom-Smit
Department of Pediatrics/Pediatric Rheumatology, Sophia Children's Hospital, ErasmusMC, Wytemaweg 80, 3015 CN Rotterdam, The Netherlands

Rick R van Rijn, Mario Maas and Charlotte M Nusman
Department of Radiology, Academic Medical Center, Meibergdreef 9, 1105 AZ Amsterdam, The Netherlands

Adam Stevens, Daniel Hanson and Peter Clayton
Manchester Academic Health Sciences Centre, Royal Manchester Children's Hospital, Manchester M13 9WL, UK

Stefan Meyer
Manchester Academic Health Sciences Centre, Royal Manchester Children's Hospital, Manchester M13 9WL, UK
Stem Cell and Leukaemia Proteomics Laboratory, School of Cancer and Imaging Sciences, University of Manchester, Manchester, UK

Stefano Stagi
Health's Sciences Department, University of Florence, Florence, Italy

Loredana Cavalli, Carla Signorini and Maria Luisa Brandi
Department of Internal Medicine, Endocrinology Unit, University of Florence, Florence, Italy

Federico Bertini, Marco Matucci Cerinic and Fernanda Falcini
Department of Internal Medicine, Section of Rheumatology, Transition Clinic, University of Florence, Viale Pieraccini 18, 50139 Florence, Italy

Kaiyu Jiang and Yanmin Chen
Department of Pediatrics, Pediatric Rheumatology Research, University of Oklahoma Health Sciences Center, Basic Sciences Education Building 235A, Oklahoma City, OK 73104, USA
Department of Pediatrics, Rheumatology Research, SUNY Buffalo Clinical and Translational Research Center, 875 Ellicott Street, Buffalo, NY 14203

James N. Jarvis
Department of Pediatrics, Jacobs School of Medicine and Biomedical Sciences, University at Buffalo, Buffalo, NY, USA
Genetics, Genomics, & Bioinformatics Program, Jacobs School of Medicine and Biomedical Sciences, University at Buffalo, Buffalo, NY, USA
Clinical & Translational Research Center, 875 Ellicott St., Buffalo, NY, USA
Department of Pediatrics, Pediatric Rheumatology Research, University of Oklahoma Health Sciences Center, Basic Sciences Education Building 235A, Oklahoma City, OK 73104, USA
Department of Pediatrics, Rheumatology Research, SUNY Buffalo Clinical and Translational Research Center, 875 Ellicott Street, Buffalo, NY 14203

Mark Barton Frank and Jeanette Osban
Microarray Research Facility, Arthritis and Clinical Immunology Program, Oklahoma Medical Research Foundation, 840 NE 13th Street, Oklahoma City, OK 73104, USA

Index

www.ingramcontent.com/pod-product-compliance
Lightning Source LLC
LaVergne TN
LVHW080728210926
848485LV00003B/538
* 9 7 8 1 6 3 9 2 7 3 9 6 6 *